SECOND EDITION

# The Transformed School Counselor

**Carol A. Dahir**
*New York Institute of Technology*

**Carolyn Bishop Stone**
*University of North Florida*

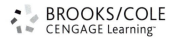

BROOKS/COLE
CENGAGE Learning™

Australia • Brazil • Japan • Korea • Mexico • Singapore • Spain • United Kingdom • United States

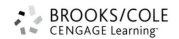
BROOKS/COLE
CENGAGE Learning

**The Transformed School Counselor,
Second Edition**
Carol A. Dahir and Carolyn Bishop Stone

Publisher/Executive Editor: Linda Schreiber-Ganster

Acquisition Editor: Seth Dobrin

Assistant Editor: Naomi Dreyer

Editorial Assistant: Suzanna Kincaid

Technology Project Manager: Elizabeth Momb

Marketing Manager: Christine Sosa

Marketing Coordinator: Gurpreet Saran

Marketing Communications Manager:
Tami Strang

Content Project Management: PreMediaGlobal

Art Director: Jennifer Wahi

Print Buyer: Linda Hsu

Rights Acquisition Specialist, Image & Text:
Don Schlotman

Production Service: PreMediaGlobal

Cover Designer: Jeff Bane, CMB design

Cover Image: Jeff Bane, CMB design

Compositor: PreMediaGlobal

For product information and technology assistance, contact us at
**Cengage Learning Customer & Sales Support, 1-800-354-9706**

For permission to use material from this text or product,
submit all requests online at **www.cengage.com/permissions**.
Further permissions questions can be emailed to
**permissionrequest@cengage.com**.

Library of Congress Control Number: 2010939167

ISBN-13: 978-1-285-19120-1

ISBN-10: 1-285-19120-X

**Brooks/Cole**
20 Davis Drive
Belmont, CA 94002-3098
USA

Cengage Learning is a leading provider of customized learning solutions with office locations around the globe, including Singapore, the United Kingdom, Australia, Mexico, Brazil, and Japan. Locate your local office at **www.cengage.com/global**.

Cengage Learning products are represented in Canada by Nelson Education, Ltd.

For your course and learning solutions, visit **www.cengage.com**.

Purchase any of our products at your local college store or at our preferred online store **www.cengagebrain.com**.

Printed in the United States of America
1 2 3 4 5 6 7 16 15 14 13

# CONTENTS

## 3  Counseling Practice in Schools  63

## 4  School Counselors as Leaders  95

## 5  School Counselors as Advocates  123

## 6  Legal and Ethical Issues for School Counselors  147

# 7  Implementing the ASCA National Model    177

## 8 Accountability and Data-Driven Decision Making   211

## 9 Diversity Matters   251

## 10 Working with Special Needs Students   284

## 11 Creating a Safe, Supportive, and Respectful School Culture and Environment  321

## 12 School Counselors as Consultants  354

## 13 School Counselors as Coordinators, Collaborators, and Managers of Resources   388

# PREFACE

The school counseling profession has undergone a transformation similar to the experiences of the academic disciplines to ensure all of our students, especially our underserved and underrepresented students, are succeeding. Since the late 1990s, the school counseling community has positioned itself as an influential partner in contemporary school improvement with the expressed purpose of eliminating barriers to educational opportunity for every student (Dahir, 2004). As school counselors address the challenge of closing the gap, they can be seen as critical players in raising student aspirations and in helping every student meet the rigors of the academic standards to achieve a quality education. Acting as agents of school and community change, school counselors can create a climate where access and support for quality and rigor is the norm (Lapan, Aoyagi, & Kayson, 2007; Stone & Dahir, 2011).

> The concept of deep restructuring is a matter of drawing up an appropriate vision of human potential and of aiming for the stars (Hillard, 1991, p. 34).

Since the Transforming School Counseling Initiative (Education Trust, 1997) was launched, the American School Counselor Association (ASCA) developed the National Standards (1997), the ASCA National Model (2003, 2005, 2012) and the School Counselor Competencies (2008), and additionally the CACREP 2009 Standards were introduced. As a result, the school counseling profession has become an integral component in this nation's educational agenda. New vision and transformed school counselors use the principles of leadership, advocacy, teaming and collaboration, and data-driven decision making to ensure a social justice mindset. The ASCA National Model reinforced this new way of thinking and working by also bringing systemic change and school counselor accountability to the attention of practitioners.

By of integrating the principles of the Transforming School Counseling Initiative at our respective universities, we realized the importance of preparing this next generation of school counselors with a solid foundation in counseling theory, techniques, and consultation skills while also grounding them in the delivery of the ASCA National Model and advocating for equitable educational opportunities for every student. The first edition of *The Transformed School*

*Counselor* has helped thousands of graduates of school counselor preparation programs across the United States to acquire the skills and knowledge necessary to become new vision practitioners who are invested in school improvement. As a result of working with this textbook both practitioners and degree candidates are grounded in contemporary and traditional theory and practice to work with a social justice mindset and implement the ASCA National Model.

The transformed school counselor acts, influences, and affects change. Throughout this textbook, you, the school counselor in training, will be challenged to take your personal vision of student success and connect it to the day-to-day realities in the place we call school. Your studies this semester will challenge you to view your sphere of influence from a systems perspective. School counselors traditionally have not seen themselves as players in systemic change. Many problems that individual students bring to the school counseling center are symptomatic of larger issues. Linking school counseling with the mission of schools connects the school counselor and the school counseling program with the achievement of *all* students.

Throughout this text you will meet dozens of practicing school counselors and read about their real experiences with delivering comprehensive, accountable, data-driven school counseling programs. Through the voices of these counseling practitioners we bring the new vision of transformed practice alive.

Transformed school counselors examine their practice and look at ways of working beyond one student at a time, focusing their attention on raising student aspirations and facilitating effective working relationships among students, faculty, parents, and community members. Transformed school counselors use data to inform their practice and use data-driven decision making to respond to the needs of today's students and schools. The key goal of this textbook is to help you understand this important way of working.

## THE BASIS FOR KNOWLEDGE AND SKILLS

Another goal of this textbook is to guide you in your acquisition of knowledge and understanding in the core content areas and the school counseling specialty of the 2009 Council for Accreditation of Counseling and Related Educational Programs (CACREP) Standards, and also with the requirements of National Council Accreditation of Teacher Education (NCATE). (See Table 1.)

## OVERVIEW OF THIS TEXTBOOK

Whether you are a first-semester graduate student acquiring an initial understanding of the scope and practice of the profession, or a professional school counselor motivated to acquire new knowledge and enhance your skills, *The Transformed School Counselor* will help you to do the following:

- Embrace a leadership mindset while acting on your beliefs and advocating for the success of every student

TABLE **1**
Matrix: CACREP and NCATE

| This Textbook | CACREP Core Content | CACREP School Counseling Specialty | NCATE |
|---|---|---|---|
| **Chapter 1:** New Vision of 21st-Century School Counseling | Social and Cultural Diversity<br>Professional Orientation and Ethical Practice | Foundations<br>Diversity and Advocacy<br>Leadership | 1. Candidate Knowledge<br>4. Diversity |
| **Chapter 2:** Counseling Theory in Schools | Social and Cultural Diversity<br>Counseling Theory<br>The Helping Relationship | Foundations<br>Counseling Prevention and Intervention | 1. Candidate Knowledge<br>4. Diversity |
| **Chapter 3:** Counseling Practice in Schools | Social and Cultural Diversity<br>Counseling Theory<br>The Helping Relationship<br>Professional Orientation and Ethical Practice<br>Group Work<br>Technology | Foundations<br>Counseling Prevention and Intervention<br>Academic Development | 1. Candidate Knowledge<br>2. Candidate Skills and Dispositions<br>3. Field Experience and Clinical Practice<br>4. Diversity |
| **Chapter 4:** School Counselors as Leaders | Professional Orientation and Ethical Practice<br>Group Work<br>Research and Program Evaluation<br>Technology | Leadership<br>Diversity and Advocacy<br>Collaboration and Consultation | 1. Candidate Knowledge<br>2. Candidate Skills and Dispositions<br>4. Diversity |
| **Chapter 5:** School Counselors as Advocates | Social and Cultural Diversity<br>Professional Orientation and Ethical Practice<br>Group Work | Leadership<br>Diversity and Advocacy<br>Collaboration and Consultation | 1. Candidate Knowledge<br>2. Candidate Skills and Dispositions<br>4. Diversity |
| **Chapter 6:** Legal and Ethical Issues for School Counselors | Professional Orientation and Ethical Practice<br>Research and Program Evaluation<br>Technology | Foundations<br>Leadership<br>Diversity and Advocacy | 1. Candidate Knowledge<br>2. Candidate Skills and Dispositions<br>4. Diversity |
| **Chapter 7:** Implementing the ASCA National Model | Social and Cultural Diversity<br>Professional Orientation and Ethical Practice<br>Career Development<br>Research and Program Evaluation<br>Technology | Counseling, Prevention, and Intervention<br>Diversity and Advocacy<br>Assessment<br>Research and Program Evaluation<br>Academic Development | 1. Candidate Knowledge<br>2. Candidate Skills and Dispositions<br>3. Field Experience and Clinical Practice<br>4. Diversity |
| **Chapter 8:** Accountability | Professional Orientation and Ethical Practice | Foundations<br>Diversity and Advocacy | 1. Candidate Knowledge<br>2. Candidate Skills and |

| | | | |
|---|---|---|---|
| and Data-Driven Decision Making | Group Work<br>Research and Program Evaluation<br>Assessment<br>Technology | Assessment<br>Research and Program Evaluation | Dispositions<br>3. Field Experience and Clinical Practice<br>4. Diversity |
| Chapter 9: Diversity Matters | Social and Cultural Diversity<br>Professional Orientation and Ethical Practice<br>Research and Program Evaluation<br>Assessment<br>Technology | Diversity and Advocacy<br>Leadership<br>Collaboration and Consultation | 1. Candidate Knowledge<br>2. Candidate Skills and Dispositions<br>4. Diversity |
| Chapter 10: Working with Special Needs Students | Appraisal and Assessment<br>Professional Orientation and Ethical Practice<br>Research and Program Evaluation | Diversity and Advocacy<br>Leadership<br>Collaboration and Consultation<br>Academic Development | 1. Candidate Knowledge<br>2. Candidate Skills and Dispositions<br>4. Diversity |
| Chapter 11: Creating a Safe, Supportive, and Respectful School Culture and Environment | Social and Cultural Diversity<br>Professional Orientation and Ethical Practice<br>Group Work<br>Research and Program Evaluation<br>Technology | Diversity and Advocacy<br>Leadership<br>Collaboration and Consultation<br>Research and Program Evaluation | 1. Candidate Knowledge<br>2. Candidate Skills and Dispositions<br>4. Diversity |
| Chapter 12: School Counselors as Consultants | Professional Orientation and Ethical Practice<br>The Helping Relationship<br>Group Work | Foundations<br>Leadership<br>Collaboration and Consultation | 1. Candidate Knowledge<br>2. Candidate Skills and Dispositions<br>3. Field Experience and Clinical Practice<br>4. Diversity |
| Chapter 13: School Counselors as Coordinators, Collaborators, and Managers of Resources | Social and Cultural Diversity<br>Professional Orientation and Ethical Practice<br>Group Work<br>Technology | Counseling, Prevention, and Intervention<br>Leadership<br>Collaboration and Consultation | 1. Candidate Knowledge<br>2. Candidate Skills and Dispositions<br>4. Diversity |
| Chapter 14: Preparing All Students to Become Career and College Ready | Social and Cultural Diversity<br>Counseling Theory<br>Career Development<br>Assessment<br>Technology | Leadership<br>Collaboration and Consultation<br>Academic Development<br>Research and Program Evaluation | 1. Candidate Knowledge<br>2. Candidate Skills and Dispositions<br>4. Diversity |

*(continued)*

TABLE **1**
Matrix: CACREP and NCATE (Continued)

| This Textbook | CACREP Core Content | CACREP School Counseling Specialty | NCATE |
|---|---|---|---|
| **Chapter 15:** Transitioning into the Field of School Counseling | Social and Cultural Diversity Professional Orientation and Ethical Practice Technology | Foundations Leadership Collaboration and Consultation | 3. Field Experience and Clinical Practice 4. Diversity |

- Use counseling, consultation, collaboration, and the coordination of services to affect the climate and culture of your school
- Advocate for a social justice agenda and promote equitable access to quality education for all students
- Implement comprehensive, standards-based accountable school counseling programs based on the ASCA National Model
- Examine data to effectively identify patterns and behaviors that impede student success
- Use technology to efficiently and effectively expand the delivery of services and communication among all stakeholders, including parents

Our focus on connecting school counseling to student achievement is not intended to be at the expense of attending to the mental health needs of students. Transformed school counseling offers new ways of working with individuals and groups that ensure balance in providing academic, career, and personal-social development.

## Content Overview

### Chapter 1: New Vision of 21st-Century School Counseling

Chapter 1 presents the challenges of the school improvement and school counseling reform agenda of the past 20 years and how schools and school counselors proactively responded to the call for providing every child with a quality education. A context is established to address what school counselors need to know and how to successfully work with every student using a social justice way of work to close the opportunity, information, and achievement gaps. Federal education agendas including No Child Left Behind and the Blueprint for Reform are discussed.

### Chapter 2: Counseling Theory in Schools

How do school counselors apply the body of knowledge of counseling theory to a school setting? Ten major counseling theories, including behavioral, cognitive behavioral approach, existentialism, gestalt, individual psychology (Adlerian), motivational interviewing, person-centered (Rogerian), rational emotive behavior therapy, reality therapy, and solution focused counseling are explored in a school context. Counseling techniques and skills are presented as they apply to the child and adolescent in a school setting.

### Chapter 3: Counseling Practice in Schools

Chapter 3 addresses the many dimensions of counseling practice including individual and group counseling and student development curriculum (classroom guidance) with students for the purpose of developmental growth, prevention, and intervention. Understanding learning styles, the use of the developmental assets, assessments, building resiliency skills, and advisory programs are some of the practices presented as components of counseling in schools.

### Chapter 4: School Counselors as Leaders

Leadership is becoming an increasingly valued and shared phenomenon at the school level. This chapter explores the unique opportunities school counselors have to develop strong leadership skills and assert their ability to influence and support success in academic achievement for all students.

### Chapter 5: School Counselors as Advocates

Involvement in social action and social intervention and a commitment to institutional improvement of schools are critical functions of the school counselor. Chapter 5 examines social justice and advocacy roles for school counselors and address the skills counselors need to examine and challenge the status quo.

### Chapter 6: Legal and Ethical Issues for School Counselors

School counselors function in an environment regulated by state and federal laws, court decisions, certification boards, and school boards. This chapter is a survey of the ethical, legal, and professional issues facing the school counselor. A case-study approach helps the student apply the American Counseling Association and American School Counselor Association's Ethical Standards for School Counselors (2010) in situations affected by federal law, court case law, state statutes, community standards, and school board rules.

### Chapter 7: Implementing the ASCA National Model

The primary focus of this chapter is to acquire the knowledge and skills to understand and implement a *comprehensive school counseling program based on the ASCA Model (2003, 2005, 2012) that provides a template for the development, implementation, and evaluation of a school counseling program. Chapter 7 includes a discussion of the *National Standards for School Counseling Programs* (ASCA, 1997) and the Partnership for 21st Century Skills, which are statements of the 21st-century knowledge and skills that students should acquire as a result of participating in a school counseling program.

### Chapter 8: School Counselor Accountability and Data-Driven Decision Making

In this age of accountability, it is essential that school counselors contribute to the school success agenda and clearly tie successful outcomes for students to their presence in the school. The accountable school counseling program utilizes student data to create vision and targeted change. MEASURE (Stone & Dahir, 2004, 2007, 2011), a six-step process for school counselor accountability, shows how to collect and analyze data to inform, improve, and evaluate the effectiveness of the school counseling programs.

### Chapter 9: Diversity Matters

Public schools are a place where children can learn to get along with others in a diverse society. Schools must become the primary institutions to create cohesion among diverse groups. Conversations about diversity in today's schools must consider the influences of culture, class, race, ethnicity, gender, socioeconomic status, sexual orientation, learning ability, and language. School counselors recognize and acknowledge personal biases and prejudices that can influence their approach to counseling, guiding, advising, and encouraging students. Personal sensitivity to diversity also helps school counselors to determine how culture influences a student's perception of the problem and the choice of intervention.

### Chapter 10: Working with Special Needs Students

School counselors believe that all children can learn and all children can achieve. All school personnel should be sensitive to the time needed to learn, especially for students who struggle to achieve a level of minimum proficiency. Using a social justice mindset, school counselors must be well-prepared to understand how to identify and work with all special populations who require special education services, exceptional education services, or 504 compliance. The school counselor's role in Response to Intervention, Positive Behavior Intervention Supports, and the Special Education process is introduced.

### Chapter 11: Creating a Safe, Supportive, and Respectful School Culture and Environment

Essential in today's rapidly changing and technologically advanced world is collaboration among school counselor and the principal, teachers, and parents to help individual students and classroom groups communicate caring and respect for one another. This chapter helps future school counselors understand the importance of climate and culture in creating positive learning communities. Topics such as helping students acquire resiliency and coping skills, bullying, cyberbullying, conflict resolution, and character education are addressed.

### Chapter 12: School Counselors as Consultants

Consultation extends the school counselor's reach by working collaboratively with the adults in a student's life who can make a major impact on the student's academic, career, and social/emotional life. Various models of consultation appropriate for the school setting are presented to help you develop the skills needed to be an effective consultant. An emphasis is placed on the benefits of the consultation role, relationship building, strategies for consultation with teachers and other school personnel, working effectively with parents, and gathering critical student information.

### Chapter 13: School Counselors as Coordinators, Collaborators, and Managers of Resources

School counselors must balance providing direct services and managing resources to offer an expanded array of opportunities for students. Coordination, collaboration, and management of resources are the mechanics or "how to" that guide your school counseling program. Particular emphasis is placed on working with student support professionals, teachers, and mental health providers in the schools and in community-based organizations.

### Chapter 14: Preparing All Students to Become College and Career Ready

Preparing students to select a career goal and guiding them to enroll in the appropriate coursework that will lead them to achieve their career goals is an important component of the work of school counselors. School counselors, in collaboration with teachers, school administrators, and parents or guardians, have a responsibility to support students to ensure that they all have options after high school and can identify the meaningful paths to the educational preparation needed to achieve in her or his chosen career. This chapter emphasizes the importance of developing a college and career readiness program as an integral component of your comprehensive school counseling program.

### Chapter 15: Transitioning into the Field of School Counseling

In addition to practical suggestions to prepare counselors-in-training for induction into the school counseling profession, Chapter 15 offers insight into the influences and trends that are driving the evolving professional orientation and the impact of the transforming school counseling initiative on school improvement. Practical "getting started" suggestions are presented that assist the new counselor in learning about the culture of the school, community, and understanding the belief system of the school where she or he will work.

## Text Organization and High-Interest Features

To enhance the usability of this textbook for counselor educators, graduate students, and practitioners, each chapter follows a consistent format.

*At the beginning of each chapter you will find:*

- *Chapter Outline*—a preview of the chapter headings.
- *Chapter Objectives*—student learner objectives aligned with the CACREP 2009 Standards, the expectations of the ASCA National Model and the Transformed School Counseling Initiative.
- *School Counselor Casebook: Getting Started*—a scenario concerning a contemporary school-based issue—such as the closing the achievement gap or creating safe school environments—followed by questions that prompt students to grapple with the issue as they read through the chapter.

*At the end of each chapter:*

- *Tech Tools*—an annotated list of chapter content–related technology resources.
- *School Counselor Casebook: Voices from the Field*—practicing school counselors respond to the scenario presented at the beginning of the chapter.
- *Chapter Summary*—a review of important chapter concepts.
- *Key Terms*—a list of important terms and the page number where each is defined in the chapter.
- *Learning Extensions*—exercises and activities designed to reinforce your comprehension and ability to put theory into practice.

*Throughout each chapter:*

- *Tables and graphs*—enhance your understanding.
- *Case studies*—bring real counselor/student stories alive.
- *Features titled* "Meet ..."—present real-life situation that every school counselor struggles with and how they apply transformed practice to everyday issues, concerns and challenges, and present real-life success stories.

## Supplemental Instructional Resources

The redesigned instructor's manual is completely web-based and organizes the tools you need to build your weekly instruction, curriculum, and activities in one place. Sample syllabi with learner objectives aligned with the 2009 CACREP and NCATE standards and week-to-week suggestions are included to help you plan your course.

This newly designed ancillary and supplements section includes presentation slides for weekly class lectures; supplemental student activities that also can serve as additional assignments to the Learning Extensions at the end of each chapter; and a complete test bank of multiple-choice and short-answer questions and essays.

# NEW TO THE 2ND EDITION

- The American School Counselor Association's National Model: A Framework for School Counseling Programs (2003, 2005, 2012) and the Transformed School Counseling Initiative that began in 1997 underpin the focus of this textbook and is evident in every chapter. This approach reinforces the essential skill set of leadership, social justice advocacy, teaming and collaboration, use of data, and technology, which are necessary to deliver an accountable comprehensive school model. The skills are emphasized in specific chapters around these topics as well as integrated throughout the text and case scenarios for reinforcement.
- The Council for Accreditation of Counseling and Related Educational Programs 2009 revised standards are aligned with each chapter. The Appendix also includes the ASCA School Counselor Competencies

(2009), which address critical skills in practice, and the recently revised ASCA Ethical Standards for School Counselors (2010).

- Each chapter starts with a new School Counselor Casebook/Scenario and concludes with a practitioner's response at the conclusion of each chapter.
- A redesigned "Diversity Matters" (Chapter 9) emphasizes influences of culture, class, race, ethnicity, gender, socioeconomic status, sexual orientation, learning ability, and language on counseling, guiding, advising, and encouraging students.
- Chapter 10, "Working with Special Needs Students," was added to the text to help school counselors identify and work with all special populations who require special education services, exceptional education services, or 504 compliance. Topics such as Response to Intervention, Positive Behavior Intervention Supports, and the Special Education process are introduced.
- The national emphasis on the topic of data-driven practice and accountability is interwoven throughout the text and expanded in Chapter 8, "School Counselor Accountability and Data Informed Practice," which emphasizes the school counselor role in using data as a tool to achieve social justice goals and align practice with building school improvement plans.
- All tables and data sets are updated to reflect the most recently available information from the National Center of Education Statistics and organizational monitoring of student achievement.
- A strong emphasis on collaboration and teaming as a critical way of work is addressed throughout the text; also highlighted is the recent research regarding principal/school counselor partnerships.
- The Tech Tools section includes the most up-to-date Web-based resources at the time of this printing.

### Wherein Lies the Future

The future of the school counseling profession resides in your hands, the next generation of school counselors. It is your words, behaviors, and actions that will transform school counseling as you contribute to school improvement and design and deliver student interventions that support, prevent, and motivate. The challenge is yours to become a school counselor who works systemically to achieve educational equity and excellence for all students. Today you begin your journey to join the ranks of the next generation. Are you up to the challenge?

## ACKNOWLEDGMENTS

We wish to extend our sincere appreciation to the thousands of counselor educators and school counselors across the country who inspired and encouraged us to create this textbook. They too believe that this next generation of school counselors will become the leaders, advocates, and systemic change agents who will continue to transform the practice of school counseling and make a significant difference in the lives of students.

We appreciate the thoughtful insight and suggestions provided by the review team, Jan Chandler, Jacksonville State University; Kimberly Desmond, Indiana University of Pennsylvania; Eleanor Farinato, Lesley College; Tim Grothaus, Old Dominion University; Aaron Hughey, Western Kentucky University; Carol A. Langelier, River College; Muriel Stockburger, Eastern Kentucky University, who helped shape the content of this second edition.

A special note of appreciation to all of our *Voices from the Field,* who generously gave their time to respond to school-based scenarios: Bridget Anderson, Tara Benevento, Michelle Brantley, Barbara Crudale, Sharon Eaves, Linda Eby, Joy Guss, Lynn Haldaman, Steven Lay, Susan McCarthy, Brenda Melton, Marjorie Miller, Kim Rodriquez, and Amy Thompson.

A special thank you is extended to the systemic change agents, leaders, and advocates, whose work is highlighted throughout the text: Leigh Bagwell, Robert Bardwell, Barbara Barry, Kathy E. Biles, Chris Bryan, Kelley Cox, Arlene Crandall, Tammy Dodson, Ada Rosario Dolch, Barbara Donnellan, Gene Eakin, Rosemary English, Victoria Felix, Harvey Harper, Melissa Hippensteel Howell, Eric Katz, Laura Lee Kinard, Karen Kolkedy, Jim MacGregor, Karen Meador, Shirin Mitsis, Mary Morseth, Christa Mussi, Carol Orso, Rose Paolino, Sejal Parikh, Philip Petrone, Lourdes Rivera, MaryBeth Schaefer, Lewis Serra, Susan Sklar, Ronald Smith, Eric Sparks, Penny Studstill, Robert Turba, Julie Van Nostrand, Ellen Bullard Whitbread, Bernadette Willette, Nan Worsowicz, and Olcay Yavuz.

We especially want to highlight the school counselors of Duval County, Florida; Rutherford County, Tennessee; Wake County, North Carolina; Lindenhurst High School, New York; and West Haven High School, Connecticut, who shared their struggles and commitment to ensure that every one of their students benefited from the work of school counselors.

A special acknowledgment and thank you goes to our editor Seth Dobrin of Brooks/Cole Cengage Learning for believing in our vision of preparing the next generation of school counselors and bringing this text to life. Also, to the Cengage Team: Naomi Dryer, Dewanshu Ranjan, Abigail Perrine, and Matt Ballantyne, who worked closely with us on editing and production of the instructional supplementals. A special thank you to Jill Cook, ASCA's assistant director for her vision and thoughtful feedback. Thank you to our wonderful team of graduate student assistants, Ofe Clarke, Zara Hunt, Sarah Lowra, Jenna Senkowsky, Tiffany Singleton, and Kristina Zemaityte, for their meticulous attention and assistance with citations, references, permissions, and editing details.

We wish to acknowledge pioneers in the school counseling field: Norman Gysbers, Curly Johnson, Patricia Martin, and Robert Myrick, whose contributions provided solid pathways to a brighter future for all students. To our families and friends who patiently supported and encouraged us every step of the way, we cannot thank you enough!

# New Vision of 21st-Century School Counseling

## CHAPTER OBJECTIVES

*By the time you have completed this chapter, you should be able to*

- examine the school improvement agenda since *A Nation at Risk* (1983) to the Blueprint for Reform (U.S. Department of Education, 2010a) and how they have affected students, teachers, parents, administrators, and school counselors;

- describe the role of counseling in today's schools;

- describe how school counseling programs can support student achievement;

- identify the many roles that the school counselor plays in a school environment, which includes counselor, leader, social justice advocate, team player and collaborator, consultant, and data-driven practitioner;

- identify examples of a school counselor in an advocacy role, as a leader and consultant, and as a collaborator and team member with students, faculty, parents, and community.

---

## School Counselor Casebook: Getting Started

### The Scenario

Jason is in 11th grade and is convinced that the next week's high school exit exam is the most important test that he will ever take. His parents, teachers, and you, his counselor, have reminded him that he still has several opportunities to pass—just in case. Jason is an average student and usually gets Cs and Bs in most of his subjects. He failed the test the first time he took it in 10th grade, saying he was overly anxious and could not think straight. Jason told you that if he cannot pass the test this time, he will just have to quit high school. He does not know what he wants to do after high school—sometimes he thinks he wants to go to college, other times he thinks that he wants a technical career. Now he thinks he should just go to work and not deal with any of this.

### Thinking about Solutions

As you read this chapter, think about how you, as a school counselor in this situation, might work with your colleagues to devise solutions and promote the necessary changes. When you come to the end of the chapter, you will have the opportunity to see how your ideas compare with a practicing school counselor's approach.

---

Every child in America deserves a world-class education. A world-class education is also a moral imperative—the key to securing a more equal, fair, and just society. We will not remain true to our highest ideals unless we do a far better job of educating each one of our sons and daughters. We will not be able to keep the American promise of equal opportunity if we fail to provide a world-class education to every child. (President Barack Obama in ESEA Blueprint for Reform, U.S. Department of Education, Office of Planning, Evaluation and Policy Development, 2010, p. 1)

## THE NEW DIRECTION FOR 21st-CENTURY SCHOOLS

Now, more than ever before, a world-class education is essential for success. The law that is known as the **No Child Left Behind Act** has been the primary statute governing the federal government's role in education since 2000.

The Blueprint for Reform is the proposed reauthorization of the Elementary and Secondary Education Act (ESEA), which has as its primary linguistic goal to ensure that every student should graduate from high school ready for college and a career, regardless of their income, race, ethnicity or background, or disability status. This educational agenda can be considered the civil rights movement of the 21st century.

America's schools may look like they are frozen: in time; students still spend much of their day as their great grandparents did sitting in desks, in rows, and listening to teachers lecture (Wallis & Steptoe, 2006). Considering the pace of change in every other aspect of life, public education is reinventing itself to make sure this next generation of learners will make the grade in the global economy. Although school buildings and classrooms may look the same as they did years ago, a multitude of influences driving the contemporary school reform agenda continue to significantly affect the teaching and learning process in today's schools. In addition to promoting academic achievement, schools today are expected to promote good citizenship by addressing the affective and personal-social developmental needs of children and youth. Violent acts in our schools are increasingly receiving attention as incidents of trauma, tragedy, and terrorism have moved from the community into the schoolhouse.

The daily vernacular of educators today includes such phrases as *accountability*, *standards-based curriculum*, *high-stakes testing*, and *closing the achievement gap*. In every state, school building, and community, **educational reform** initiatives have become the standard. Ongoing reform efforts since the mid-1990s continue to raise the expected level of achievement for students. **Accountability** is a driving force and this pressure weighs heavily on each school's staff to produce the desired results and improve in unprecedented ways. Teachers, principals, school support staff, and school counselors are actively engaged in developing and implementing annual school improvement plans to make their school a better place for children to strive and thrive.

Educational reform and school improvement are not new. Federal legislation has historically pressured school systems to examine practices and seek improvement. Thirty years ago, policymakers began drawing public attention to the mediocrity threatening American education. Monographs such as *A Nation at Risk: The Imperative for Educational Reform* (National Commission on Excellence in Education, 1983), *What Works: Research about Teaching and Learning* (U.S. Department of Education, 1987), and *The Forgotten Half: Pathways to Success for America's Youth and Young Families* (William T. Grant Commission on Work, Family and Citizenship, 1988) challenged the quality of academic preparation and levels of student achievement. In 1989, the National Governor's Association (NGA) called for an unprecedented education summit to undertake a nationwide effort at educational renewal. The NGA generated broad-based objectives, which ultimately became the foundation for six national goals for education. These efforts resulted in America 2000 (U.S. Department of Education, 1990), which was considered at that time to be the most significant statement of the federal role and responsibility in the conduct of public education since the

Johnson administration passed the first Elementary and Secondary Education Act (ESEA) of 1965 (Clinchy, 1991).

As high school graduation requirements for students of all backgrounds and levels of performance became more rigorous (Sewall, 1991), public attention shifted to the back-to-basics components of education: curriculum, teaching, and administration. Also incorporated into America 2000 was the concept of developing world-class **standards** that intended to describe what students should know and be able to do across the content areas. "In the absence of well defined and demanding standards, education in the United States has gravitated toward de facto minimum expectations. Standards would provide the basic understandings that all students need to acquire, but not everything a student should learn" (National Council on Education Standards and Testing, 1991, p. D-56).

Goals 2000: The Educate America Act (1994), which was the next iteration of ESEA, promoted "raising the bar" to improve educational achievement for all students. Goals 2000 (U.S. Department of Education, 1994) established expectations for student performance and school account-ability that led to sweeping educational changes, including the development of national voluntary academic standards across all disciplines. New curriculum standards and new measures of **high-stakes testing** spun out of reform following Goals 2000, resulting in every state establishing standards and increased graduation requirements (Marzano, 2000). The National Gover-nor's Association and the Council of Chief State Officers led an effort in which 46 states representing 80 percent of the nation's K–12 student population have formally agreed to join forces to create common academic standards in math and English language arts (U.S. Department of Education, 2010). These standards are aligned with college and work expectations, including rigorous content and skills, and are internationally benchmarked.

Changes in presidential administrations often result in reauthorization of ESEA. For instance, congressional bipartisan support for continuous comprehensive school improvement resulted in the No Child Left Behind Act (NCLB), which had as its expressed purpose closing the achievement gap between minority students and their peers. No Child Left Behind (2001) acknowledged the importance of equitable access to educational opportu-nities and sought to create settings in which all children are held to high expectations and are given the conditions necessary to achieve this goal. School counselors aligned their work with NCLB's five primary goals by contributing to a school climate that is safe and respectable (goal 4); ensuring that all students graduate (goal 5); contributing to instructional success (goals 1 and 2); and having the appropriate credentials for certification and/or licensure (goal 3).

Despite the intentions of NCLB to speak to high expectations for all students regardless of race, ethnicity, and SES, merely legislating requirements to promote change in expectations for students has not yet produced the desired outcomes. NCLB's emphasis on high-stakes testing placed unprece-dented pressure on teachers, students, and parents. Legislators, school board members, teachers, school site and district-level administrators, parents, employers, and other school and community members feel the pressure of raising academic standards and improving student academic success.

With a renewed emphasis on high school completion and the importance of postsecondary education, the U.S. Department of Education (USDOE) has called for universal literacy, acquiring 21st-century skills (Partnership for 21st Century Skills, 2006), improving high school graduation rates, and increasing access to and the completion of some postsecondary education (Duncan, 2010) as the primary agenda in the reauthorization of the Elementary and Secondary Education Act (ESEA). As this bill moves through Congress, the new ESEA will replace the No Child Left Behind Act.

The **Blueprint for Reform** (2010) builds on the significant changes embedded in the American Recovery and Reinvestment Act of 2009 around four areas: (1) improving teacher and principal effectiveness to ensure that every classroom has a great teacher and every school has a great leader; (2) providing information to families to help them evaluate and improve their children's schools, and to educators to help them improve their students' learning; (3) implementing college- and career-ready standards and developing improved assessments aligned with those standards; and (4) improving student learning and achievement in America's lowest-performing schools by providing intensive support and effective interventions (U.S. Department of Education, 2010).

State education departments were charged to examine policies to ensure that resources are available for students and schools to meet the challenges in the Blueprint for Reform, especially when the futures of individual children are at stake. Additionally, at the local level, school administrators are required to constantly rethink the allocation of existing resources and maximizing the potential of school staff to help all students achieve at these higher levels of academic success.

> The clock is ticking. Every minute of every school day, as we continue to ignore the crisis in our high schools, another 15 students will drop out of school—never to return. (Alliance for Excellent Education, 2007a)

As the economic patterns become more global and the United States produces more service and technology jobs, youth and young adults need to understand that a higher level of educational attainment is critical to their ability to compete and thrive. The prediction is that 90 percent of the fastest-growing jobs of the future will require more than a high school diploma and some postsecondary education (Alliance for Excellent Education, 2007b).

> We're losing more than a quarter of all students before graduation day—and in many urban communities, half or more of students of color are dropping out of school. 12 percent of our high schools, or 2,000 high schools, produce half of the dropouts in the country, and three-fourths of dropouts among African-American and Latino students. This is economically unsustainable and morally unacceptable. (Duncan, 2010)

Far more needs to be accomplished to guarantee each student an equitable opportunity to a quality educational experience regardless of ethnicity, race, or income.

| | |
|---|---|
| National Graduation Rate 2009 | 70.6% |
| New Jersey | 83.3% |
| Utah | 78.6% |
| Tennessee | 65.4% |
| Massachusetts | 75% |
| New York State | 62.5% |
| Florida | 60.8% |
| South Carolina | 58.8% |

FIGURE **1.1** Selected State Graduation Rates
Source: Education Week, 2010

However, as revealed in Figure 1.1, too many of our youth who begin ninth grade in U.S. schools do not complete their high school education in four years.

> We must recognize that America's achievement gap hurts not just the children who are cheated of a quality education but the nation itself. The nation's achievement gaps have imposed "the economic equivalent of a permanent national recession" on America. (Duncan, 2010)

The challenges that lie ahead are great and the data tell the story. The Condition of Education (USDOE, 2010) reported the following:

- In 2007–08, about 20 percent of all public elementary schools and 9 percent of public secondary schools were considered high-poverty schools, compared with 15 percent and 5 percent, respectively, in 1999–2000.
- Between 1988 and 2008, the percentage of Hispanic public school students increased from 11 to 22 percent. Largely as a result of this increase, the percentage of White students decreased from 68 to 55 percent over those two decades.
- In 2007–08, according to school administrators, about 28 percent of high school graduates from high-poverty schools attended four-year colleges after graduation, compared with 52 percent of high school graduates from low-poverty schools.
- The percentage of 25- to 29-year-olds who completed a bachelor's degree increased from 17 percent in 1971 to 29 percent in 2009. During this same period, bachelor's degree attainment more than doubled for Blacks (from 7 to 19 percent) and Hispanics (from 5 to 12 percent) and nearly doubled for Whites (from 19 to 37 percent).

Student diversity, including ethnicity, language, and economic means, continues to challenge educators and community-based professionals as demographics shift (Sapon-Shevon, 2001). Student opportunities are frequently stratified by race, ethnicity, and socioeconomic status (Education Trust, 2009). The projected change in demographics demands a greater focus on underrepresented populations (Figure 1.2).

As educators across the United States struggle with the growing demands of federal legislation, many will concur that raising student achievement for every student is the primary focus of **school improvement** (Martin, 2004). Closing the opportunity and information gaps for all students, including the underrepresented and underserved is a responsibility shared by all of the critical stakeholders, including school counselors. School counselors have an important role to play. As potential key players in furthering the primary goals of 21st-century schools, school counselors can become partners in systemic change and identify those students who need more to achieve. Many students are caught in the dichotomy of weak educational foundations and the expectations of rigorous academic standards; often, except for the school counselor's intervention, they may remain anonymous in their struggle to survive and succeed.

The 21st-century approach for working in schools and standards-based reform has dramatically changed the way every educator works in schools to improve student performance. When school counselors operate with the premise that they are key players in the academic success story for students, then school counseling programs are viewed as integral to student achievement (Stone & Dahir, 2004). Affecting the instructional program, motivating and raising student aspirations to achieve at high levels, and collaborating to create safe school environments are some of the ways in which school counselors can fully participate in all aspects of the implementation of the Blueprint for Reform and document efforts to help all children succeed.

Changing demographics demand greater focus on underrepresented populations.

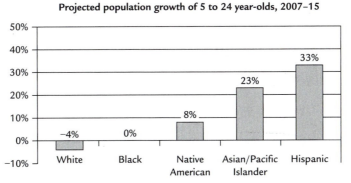

**Projected population growth of 5 to 24 year-olds, 2007–15**

Closing racial gaps in degree attainment will create more than half of the degrees necessary to raise America to first in the world in degree attainment.

FIGURE **1.2** Changing Demographics

Source: U.S. Census Bureau. Statistical Abstract of the United States: 2009 (128th edition) Washington, DC. 2008:NCHEMS

# SCHOOL COUNSELING: CHANGING WITH THE TIMES

Throughout this most recent wave of educational reform and legislative changes, relatively few areas of public education escaped the scrutiny of national attention. Yet, school counseling programs and school counselors were absent from many of the early conversations that spoke to changes in curriculum, instruction, and pedagogy. Thankfully this is no longer the situation. Since the mid-1990s the school counseling profession has undergone a transformation that parallels the call for change in schools (Education Trust, 1997). A brief retrospective examination of the history of school counseling offers insight into past perspectives and current initiatives that ultimately will influence the future.

The counseling profession first took a seat in the American schoolhouse in the late 19th century (Schmidt, 2007). Jesse Davis introduced a guidance program into a Detroit high school curriculum in 1898 to help students develop character, avoid problems, and relate vocational interests to coursework (Brewer, 1932). These efforts established the beginnings of what was to evolve from vocational guidance to school counseling. Frank Parsons, often cited as the "father of guidance," is credited as the person who began this movement. Parsons's attention to vocational guidance was coupled with his concern about society's failure to provide resources for human growth and development, especially for young people (Schmidt, 2007). In working with youth, Parsons and his followers emphasized the following:

- The individual must have a clear understanding of her or his abilities, interests, ambitions, and limitation. Thus, the counselor assists individuals in learning about their personal characteristics.
- The individual must have knowledge of the world, the opportunities and options available, and an understanding of what requirements were needed for the chosen field. The counselor here assumed an information dissemination role.
- The individual must bring together knowledge of self and the awareness of the world of work. The counselor served as a guide to help the individual develop a clear and logical path to reach her or his goal.

Parsons's influence was long-reaching and became the impetus and direction for expanding the concept of vocational guidance. World War I and its aftermath of the Great Depression resulted in a greater need for assisting students with vocational selection and placement. The term *vocational counselor,* rarely heard before the Depression, entered the educational vocabulary (Wittmer, 2000; Wittmer & Clark, 2007). Attempts to organize and expand guidance in the school setting in the 1930s led to the addition of educational and personal/social services (Gysbers, 2001). The traditional way of describing guidance as a vocational service was no longer in vogue; these newer views broadened the goals of the program and added to it the elements of counseling.

Between the Great Depression and the outbreak of World War II, new assessment instruments such as intelligence tests and vocational aptitude tests appeared on the market for employment purposes and then for use in the military. High schools began to administer intelligence measurements for children and welcomed group testing for purposes of pupil evaluation. The use of these new instruments led to the development of counseling approaches that related student traits with interest and ability. The progressive education movement, although short-lived, encouraged the school to play a greater role in the personal and social development of students (Nugent, 1994). In the 1940s major events such as the influence of Carl Rogers's client-centered theory, the impact of World War II, and the government's involvement in education strongly affected the future direction of guidance and counseling (Gladding, 2004). Mental measurement and vocational guidance further shaped the delivery and orientation of guidance services. The George-Barden Act of 1946 provided funds to support guidance and counseling in the schools and other settings.

By the middle of the 20th century, psychological assessment, mental health approaches, counseling theorists, and the beginnings of educational reform began to influence school guidance and counseling. In the 1950s, the public became fascinated with the term *IQ* (intelligence quotient) and parents thought these data would better help them understand their children's school performance. Rogerian theory focused attention almost exclusively on individual counseling with an emphasis on the counselor-client relationship. Societal pressures resulting from the stresses of the Korean War also added to the need for mental health and vocational support for adults and students alike.

In the mid-century era, professional associations emerged as strong influences and the American School Counselor Association (ASCA) became a division of the American Personnel and Guidance Association in the 1950s. Guidance work in school continued to grow and the numbers of counselors increased significantly due to a major stimulus, the National Defense Education Act of 1958 (Herr, 1979). The primary purpose of the National Defense Education Act (NDEA) was to increase funding to education to help the United States regain a competitive edge in mathematics and the sciences. Part of this funding was earmarked to augment the number of secondary school counselors. This generation of counselors was expected to have skill in therapeutic interventions that would support the student in resolving personal problems that might be a barrier to academic success; they also were required to have expertise in providing college admissions information (Perry & Schwallie-Giddis, 1993). The ultimate goal was to increase the numbers of students going on to college and pursuing careers related to math and science. This emphasis on postsecondary opportunities and individual personal support now placed an emphasis on guidance and counseling as available only to the college-bound or for those with personal problems. Also during the mid-1950s access to guidance and counseling in the junior and senior high schools became limited (Perry & Schwallie-Giddis, 1993; Rosenbaum, 1976). Increased funding for the guidance provision in NDEA in the early 1960s added elementary guidance and counseling programs as the missing link in the continuum of services from kindergarten through high school (Gysbers, 2004). The expansion of services to elementary schools ultimately led to a broader professional focus on programs and services (Schmidt, 2007).

Gilbert Wrenn's (1962) book, *The Counselor in a Changing World*, may have influenced school guidance and counseling more than any other publication (Wittmer, 2000). Wrenn asserted that the primary emphasis in counseling students should be on individual developmental needs and not only on the remedial and crisis situations in their lives. Wrenn also suggested that counselors needed to expand their knowledge of human behavior to better serve the complex needs of students. As guidance services expanded across the country, Mathewson (1962) promoted school guidance as a process that moved with the individual student and in a developmental sequence through the age of maturity (Wittmer, 2000; Wittmer & Clark, 2007). Although the strong influences of Rogerian theory on school counselor training continued (Wittmer, 2000; Wittmer & Clark, 2007) no longer was mental health practice considered the primary responsibility of the counselor in a school setting. Social pressures and the emphasis on educational student support refocused the emphasis of school counseling from individual student response and crisis intervention to a proactive series of strategies that engage every student. This resulted in the development of new models for program design and delivery systems.

The 1970s saw the advent of guidance as a comprehensive program (Dinkmeyer & Caldwell, 1970; Gysbers & Henderson, 2000; Myrick, 1997, 2000). The comprehensive program approach deemphasized clerical and administrative tasks and promoted guidance as a structured program with specific student outcomes (Gysbers & Henderson, 1994, 2000; Sink & Mc Donald, 1998). Consequently, the vast majority of state departments of education have adopted or endorsed a comprehensive approach to school counseling. Coupled with the expansion of the comprehensive model was the American School Counselor Association's proactive response to Goals 2000, the development of the **National Standards for School Counseling Programs** (American School Counselor Association [ASCA], 1997a), which positioned school counseling to play an increasingly important role in contemporary school improvement (Dahir, 2004). The widespread use of the National Standards for School Counseling Programs (ASCA, 1997a), the Education Trust's Transforming School Counseling Initiative (1997), and the ASCA National Model (2003, 2005) defined the vision and goals for the 21st-century school counseling programs and placed the school counseling program in a critical position to effectively complement academic rigor with affective development.

## DEFINING THE ROLE OF SCHOOL COUNSELING IN 21ST-CENTURY SCHOOLS

Despite the presence of more than 100,000 school counselors in every school district across the 50 states, the school counseling profession was omitted from most of the educational reform agendas of the past. Although school counselors have always focused their efforts on assisting students to improve their attitude and/or behavior to achieve greater school success and to champion for student personal/social needs, the omission was confusing and troublesome. Perhaps, as a relatively young profession, in comparison to its educational counterparts, a natural confusion existed as to the nature, function, purpose, and role of school counseling. Mathewson (1962) once referred to guidance and counseling as a search for a system characterized by statements of objectives and goals. Ryan and Zeran (1972) suggested that guidance and counseling suffered from the lack of a systematic theory to guide the practical applications of services, which significantly differ from the curriculum delivery of the academic disciplines. This could be attributed to the relatively small size of the counseling community or the poor public and professional understanding of the roles performed by school counselors (Burtnett, 1993).

Boyer (1988), in his description of the school counselor, stated:

> Today, in most high schools, counselors are not only expected to advise students about college, they are also asked to police for drugs, keep records of dropouts, reduce teenage pregnancy, check traffic in the halls, smooth out the tempers of irate parents, and give aid and comfort to battered and neglected children. School counselors are expected to do what our communities, our homes, and our churches have not been able to accomplish, and if they cannot, we condemn them for failing to fulfill our high minded expectations. (p. 3)

School district administrators, educational organizations, and foundations and state departments of education clearly dictated the functions, activities, and programs that professional school counselors should deliver to students. The assignment of non-counseling activities suggested that the role of the school counselor and the school counseling program were poorly defined and not valued by the school administration (Hart & Jacobi, 1992). This resulted in many new duties added to a counselor's already existing responsibilities (Gysbers, 2001), including tasks that were administrative or clerical in nature. "When schools fail to clearly define the counselor's role, school administrators, parents with special interests, teachers or others may feel their agenda ought to be the school counseling program's priority. The results often lead to confusion and criticisms when they are disappointed" (Cunanan & Maddy-Bernstein, 1994, p. 1). Counselors focusing their attention on the delivery of a constellation of responsive and reactive activities, and performing "random acts of guidance" (Bilzing, 1996), will serve only a small percentage of the student population.

School counselors felt compelled to accept the responsibility to address societal issues that continued to affect school-aged children (Boyer, 1988). The school counselor and the school counseling program regularly reacted, responded, and expanded to meet these needs and challenges. Thus the scope of school counseling practice continued to encompass a wide variety of diverse services offered to students from kindergarten through high school (Gysbers & Henderson, 2000). Services and activities varied from school to school and from state to state and resulted in ambiguity in the organization of school counseling (guidance) services. School counseling often was viewed as an ancillary service to support the academic goals of schooling (Gerler, 1992). From the multitude of external and internal forces influencing the profession, it is natural that school counselors have grappled with issues regarding professional title, scope of practice, and role and responsibilities as the profession defines and refines itself in 21st-century schools.

In the post–*A Nation at Risk* (1983) era, the American Counseling Association (ACA), concerned about the future of counseling in schools, put forth a series of recommendations in a report titled *School Counseling: A Profession at Risk* (ACA, 1987) and, six years later, convened a "think tank" that proposed a series of activities and functions that more clearly establish the role and relationship of the school counselor in reference to the educational system. Organizations such as the College Board produced and widely distributed monographs such as *Keeping the Options Open: Recommendations* (1986) that spoke to the ability of guidance and counseling to support and encourage student success. The ASCA continued to define the role and function of school counselors through position statements and monographs. The association (ASCA, 1994) advocated for school counselors to become agents of change and assume a leadership role in education reform. School counselors were urged to assist students to improve their attitude and/ or behavior to achieve greater academic and school success, and to champion for student needs. However, there was no external call from the educational or legislative arenas to take action, and responses to these recommendations remained solely within the confines of the school counseling community.

With a minimal amount of empirical evidence that addressed and demonstrated the effect of school counseling on student achievement, confusion about the contributions of school counseling programs to student achievement persisted. Borders and Drury (1992) suggested that school counselors played an important role in shaping the design and implementation of counseling programs to best meet individual student needs, while Whiston and Sexton (1998) noted that more research had been conducted in the areas of remediation and intervention rather than in preventing problems.

School counseling practice underwent a transformation similar to the school improvement expectations of the academic disciplines. Since the late 1990s, the school counseling community has positioned itself as an influential partner in contemporary school improvement with the expressed purpose to eliminate the barriers to educational opportunity for every student (Dahir, 2004). "The concept of deep restructuring is a matter of drawing up an appropriate vision of human potential and of aiming for the stars" (Hillard, 1991, p. 34). As school counselors addressed the challenge of "closing the gap" (No Child Left Behind, 2001) they were finally seen as critical players in raising student aspirations and focusing on helping every student meet the rigors of the academic standards to achieve a quality education.

> Research suggests that high-quality counseling services can have long-term effects on a child's well-being and can prevent a student from turning to violence and drug or alcohol abuse. High-quality school counseling services also can improve a student's academic achievement. Studies on the effects of school counseling have shown positive effects on students' grades, reducing classroom disruptions, and enhancing teachers' abilities to manage classroom behavior effectively. High-quality school counseling services also can help address students' mental health needs. (U.S. Department of Education, 2002b, p. 117)

Additionally, federally funded initiatives, including Gaining Early Awareness and Readiness for Undergraduate Programs (GEAR UP) and the Elementary and Secondary School Counseling Demonstration Act (ESCDA), offered financial support and recognized the contributions of school counseling to student educational attainment and achievement. However, much more needs to be done on the part of school counselors to highlight the effect of school counseling programs as an effective solution to closing the opportunity and information gaps.

## SCHOOL COUNSELORS ACTING AS AGENTS OF CHANGE

When school counselors embrace the ethical and moral obligation to reduce and eliminate the institutional and/or social barriers that may stand in the way of every student's academic, career, or personal-social development (Lee, 2007a; Lee & Walz, 1998; Stone, 2010a), they advance the moral dimensions of school to include a strong social justice agenda to "close the gap" especially for diverse populations of students who have been traditionally underserved or underrepresented. School counselors can no longer passively react to the challenges facing schools and youth; it is a critical time to take action and accept the challenge of contributing to the epidemic of nonschool completion (Gysbers & Henderson, 2002). Acting as agents of school and community change, school counselors can create a climate where access and support for quality and rigor is the norm (Lapan, Aoyagi, & Kayson, 2007; Stone & Dahir, 2011). By doing so, underserved and underrepresented students now have a chance of acquiring the educational skills necessary to fully participate in the 21st-century economy, i.e., graduate from high school with the preparation to engage in quality postsecondary opportunities (Johnson & Johnson, 2002; Johnson, Johnson, & Downs, 2006; Partnership for 21st Century Skills, 2006; Stone & Dahir, 2011). When school counselors place their efforts on motivating students to realize their dreams and complete high school, they are seen as powerful partners and collaborators in school improvement and champions of social justice who are bent on narrowing the opportunity and achievement gap (Johnson, Johnson, & Downs, 2006; Stone & Dahir, 2006). School counselors ensure that human relationships are nurtured, diversity is valued, and every student has the opportunity for a bright future (Figure 1.3).

## ISSUES AFFECTING TODAY'S SCHOOLS

### Pressures from the Global Economy

Many years have passed since *A Nation at Risk* (1983) and as a nation we continue the concerted effort to raise the standards in K–12 education. This push is driven by the educational needs of a 21st-century economy, rather than by the educational failures or deficiencies of the past or present (Carnevale & Desrochers, 2003a). Without efforts to better prepare today's students for postsecondary education and increase their access to college, America's economic position and global competitiveness could be in jeopardy. The restructuring of the American economy initiated in the early

| Traditional Role Focus | Transformed Role Focus |
| --- | --- |
| Individual student's concerns/issues | Proactive prevention and intervention for every student |
| Primary focus on personal/social development | Academic/career and personal social development |
| Clinical model focused on student deficits | Whole school and system concerns/issues model |
| Mental health provider for individual and small-group counseling | Academic, career, and personal-social counseling to support student learning and achievement, supporting student success |
| Postsecondary planning for interested students | All students career and college ready |
| Ancillary support personnel | Key contributor to effect change as a leader, social justice advocate, program developer |
| Works in isolation; little collaboration with teachers | Shift from "I" to the "We" mindset as a team player and collaborator with all educators and staff in the school |
| Student scheduler | Develop a program of study with students based on education and career goals |

FIGURE **1.3** The Changing Focus of the School Counselor

1980s has made postsecondary education or technical training the threshold requirement for employment, resulting in academic readiness for postsecondary education becoming the standard for adequacy in K–12 education (Education Trust, 2001). Continuing prosperity will require greater worker investment in postsecondary education and training (United States Council on Competitiveness, 2007). New technologies, new business practices, and demand for higher productivity require today's workers to learn more and learn faster than previous generations. Nearly half of all jobs created between 2006 and 2016 will require postsecondary credentials (U.S. Department of Labor, 2010). This means that less-educated workers face even greater difficulties finding a job; they suffer higher-than-average earnings volatility and are more likely to be unemployed (Postsecondary Education Opportunity, 2010). Economic data revealed 15.3 percent of workers with less than a high school diploma were unemployed compared to 10.5 percent with a high school diploma, 9 percent with an associate's degree, and 5 percent with a bachelor's degree (U.S. Department of Labor, 2010). The demand for highly skilled and educated workers has risen faster than the supply, and the U.S. Council on Competitiveness claims that continuing U.S. prosperity will require greater worker investment in postsecondary education and training

(2007). Since 1979 the economic premium paid to workers with at least some college education has increased from 42 percent to 62 percent even as the supply of workers with at least some college has doubled as a share of all workers (Bureau of Labor Statistics, 2009).

> Educators recognize that the purpose of schooling goes well beyond the means to the end of preparing students for the workforce and the implications are broad for all educators, including school counselors. Educators have cultural and political missions to ensure there is an educated citizenry to continue to defend and promote America's democratic ideals. Nevertheless, the inescapable reality is that ours is a society based on individual economic autonomy. Those who are not equipped with the knowledge and skills necessary to get, and keep, a good job are denied full social inclusion and tend to drop out of the mainstream culture, polity, and economy. Hence, if the standards-based reform movement cannot fulfill its economic mission to help youth and adults become successful workers, it also will fail in its cultural and political missions to create good neighbors and good citizens. (Carnevale & Deroscher, 2003b, p. vii)

High school graduation is now the minimum ticket to exit the cycle of poverty and provides the opportunity to earn a salary to escape the circumstances that are associated with earning a minimal income. Despite the attention in U.S. schools on improving the graduation rate, almost daily 7,000 students become dropouts, which translates to approximately 1.2 million students who will not graduate from high school with their peers annually. Lacking a high school diploma can doom a young adult to a life of periodic unemployment, government assistance, or trips in and out of the prison system (Alliance for Excellent Education, 2007a).

Twenty-first-century schools must ensure that all students acquire the attitudes, knowledge, and skills necessary to make successful transitions from grade level to grade level, to postsecondary education, and to the world after high school. By working closely with students and their families/caretakers, school counselors can help ensure that students understand the options they have after high school and maximize their postsecondary opportunities.

## The Power of Technology

Technology has changed the way students and adults access information and, more importantly, communicate with each other. Multitasking is a way of life for teenagers who use cell phones—not a computer—to access the Internet and use text messages, instant messaging, blogs, wikis, and social networking in simultaneous, synchronous real time. The Internet has created a language all its own embraced by the youth culture. Peer-to-peer communication is about instantaneous response. Conversation can at best be impersonal. Many youth seek "net speak," social network sites, and texting as safe havens or anonymous hangouts to test their sexual identity, speak their mind, escape from loneliness, and find a peer group with which to identify. Others throw their thoughts into cyberspace without considering the consequences. For today's youth it is complex, exciting, and a cutting-edge new age of exchanging information and conversation that evolves in ways that are unpredictable.

However, not all youth have access to technology for the socialization aspects described above. Many have limited access to technology and Internet in their schools and in their homes. Colin Powell referred to the problem as digital apartheid, not the digital divide, and further suggests "there is a huge gap between those who have access to the wonders of digital technology and the Internet and those who do not . . . if we don't bridge the gap between the two, the 'have nots' will be poorer and more resentful and the 'haves' will find themselves lacking the skilled workers and potential customers they need" (qtd. in Sanford, 2001, p. 32). Educational technology for many students from poor communities is a tool for liberation (Sistek-Chandler, 2001).

YouTube, computer and video games, movies, DVDs, and TV continue to influence the lives of students. The media affecting their world can often become a primary source for identifying role models and developing career awareness. Students' future goals revolve around snapshots of superheroes, sports figures, rock stars, and sitcom characters. This millennial generation has grown up with video games the way that baby boomers grew up with board games (Howe & Strauss, 2000). The media have also exposed youth to violent acts in video games, on television, and in the movies (U.S. Department of Education, 2002a).

## Swings and Shifts in Societal Issues and Values

Children and youth have a wider exposure to lifestyles and career choices than ever before in our society, and the economic boom of the last 10 years has created a previously unexperienced affluence for middle and upper income families. Purchases made by children ages 4 to 12 have tripled; and although not every child benefited from this age of affluence, the influence of media branding has resulted in tremendous peer pressure (Howe & Strauss, 2000). Teenagers are a primary target of market engineering.

American youth were made aware of the fragile nature of human life by the tragic events of September 11, 2001. The attitudes of our youth toward terrorism and respect for human life have been influenced in ways that at this time cannot be predicted. Terrorism threats are also affecting youths' connectivity to the community and eradicated some of the apathy that had previously stigmatized this generation. School violence, which was once reserved for large, inner-city systems, has erupted in our rural and suburban schools (Sandhu, 2000). Concerns for safety in school continue as a national priority were one of five goals of No Child Left Behind (2001) and were included in the Blueprint for Reform.

With youth behavior and attitudes a primary source of concern, character education was promoted as a key component of the NCLB and resulted in a new wave of character education program mandates in a majority of our 50 states (NCLB, 2001). Addressing sexual harassment and bully-proofing strategies has become part of the daily concern of school counselors in every elementary, middle/junior high, and high school across the nation. Schools now implement drug and alcohol education in elementary school. Many parents have left sex education to school personnel. Students questioning their sexual identity frequently find school an unsafe place. According to the

National Center for Missing and Exploited Children (2009), approximately one in five children received a sexual solicitation or were approached over the Internet during the past year. As demographics change and waves of immigration reach beyond urban centers, schools have turned to teaching tolerance, respect, equity, and acceptance.

A complex and ever-changing global economy, technological innovation, and complex societal influences and values have significantly affected the way all educators work with the millennial generation and those who follow in today's schools. As the defining behaviors of this generation of students gradually influence teaching, learning, and career guidance at the high school and collegiate levels, school counselors will need to assess their efforts to build and sustain relationships with this generation of students and their parents (Elam, Stratton, & Gigson, 2007). Essential to the goals of improving schools and the teaching and learning process is the school counselor, a specialist in student growth, and academic, career, and personal-social development.

## SCHOOL COUNSELING PROGRAMS: ESSENTIAL TO EVERY STUDENT'S EDUCATION

Counseling in schools in the United States has shifted its focus from a responsive services approach to one that is proactively and integrally tied to student achievement and student success (Dollarhide & Lemberger, 2006). The new paradigm for school counseling is based on a comprehensive, national standards-based defined program that emphasizes student growth, learning, and results, and also recognizes that all children growing up in America face the normal challenges of coping with everyday problems. On a daily basis school personnel encounter students who are abused, neglected, frustrated by the cycle of personal and academic failure, disabled, drug addicted, homeless, or suffering from feelings of worthlessness. Many students face emotional, physical, social, and economic barriers that inhibit successful learning.

### THE STATE OF AMERICA'S CHILDREN, 2010

### Key Facts about American Children

- Every second a public school student is suspended.
- Every 11 seconds a high school student drops out.
- Every 19 seconds a child is arrested.
- Every 32 seconds a baby is born into poverty.
- Every 41 seconds a child is confirmed as abused or neglected.
- Every minute a baby is born to a teen mother.
- Every 4 minutes a child is arrested for a drug offense.
- Every 7 minutes a child is arrested for a violent crime.
- Every 18 minutes a baby dies before her or his first birthday.
- Every 45 minutes a child or teen dies from an accident.

*(continues)*

- Every 3 hours a child or teen is killed by a firearm.
- Every 5 hours a child or teen commits suicide.
- Every 6 hours a child is killed by abuse or neglect.

*Each Day in America . . .*

- 1 in three Black and 1 in six Latino boys born in 2001 are at risk of imprisonment during their lifetime.
- 4 children are killed by abuse or neglect.
- 5 children or teens commit suicide.
- 9 children or teens are killed by firearms.
- 32 children or teens die from accidents.
- 202 children are arrested for violent crimes.
- 377 children are arrested for drug crimes.
- 1,210 babies are born to teen mothers.
- 2,109 children are confirmed as abused or neglected.
- 2,222 high school students drop out.
- 2,962 babies are born into poverty.
- 4,435 children are arrested.
- 18,493 public school students are suspended.

Source: Children's Defense Fund, 2010

Students presenting these significant needs challenge educators. These challenges raise a series of questions such as: How do we provide a quality and equitable education for students who face emotional and academic barriers? What is the responsibility of the school counselor for addressing the emotional and social barriers that inhibit student learning?

## Advancing the Academic Agenda

The purpose of the counseling program in a school setting is to impart specific skills, facilitate learning opportunities in a proactive and preventive manner, and to provide the knowledge and skills to help all students achieve school success through academic, career, and personal/social development experiences. The school counseling program promotes and enhances the learning process (Campbell & Dahir, 1997) as an integral part of the total school program (Clark & Stone, 2000a). The comprehensive school counseling program empowers school counselors to place themselves front and center in the restructuring process of their school systems, advance the academic agenda, and establish a foundation for blending affective education with educational expectations. Competency-based learning in academic, career, and personal-social development sets high expectations of achievement for every student. By addressing barriers to learning and social-emotional health, school counseling programs can successfully bridge the gap between student needs and expectations for learning (AEL, Inc., 2000).

Concerns about equitable access to educational programs are a major issue that warrant investigation as the Blueprint for Reform raises the bar of

TABLE **1.1**
Who Takes AP Tests?

| | Public K–12 Enrollment | Calculus AB | English Language and Composition | Biology |
|---|---|---|---|---|
| African American | 15% | 5% | 7% | 6% |
| Asian | 5% | 16% | 11% | 18% |
| Latino | 15% | 8% | 13% | 9% |
| Native American | 1% | <1% | 1% | <1% |
| White | 63% | 65% | 62% | 61% |
| Other | NA | 5% | 7% | 7% |
| Total | 6,604,849 | 204,546 | 277,966 | 141,321 |

Source: Education Trust, 2009.

educational expectations. School counselors are leaders and advocates who can profoundly influence students' academic achievement, aspirations, decisions, and future plans (National Office for School Counselor Advocacy, 2010). New mechanisms need to be established to help all students reach the expectations of the new Common Core Standards. What are the effective teaching and counseling practices that will help all children achieve at a higher level? Not all students come to the school environment prepared, properly nourished, and ready to learn. Table 1.1 provides a source of discussion about who will ensure that equal opportunity exists for all students despite disparity in school wealth.

At the conclusion of the 20th century the School Counselor's Role in Educational Reform (ASCA, 1994) encouraged school counselors to become catalysts for educational change and to assume and to accept a leadership role in education reform. School counselors, as partners in student achievement, also faced the test of preparing students to meet the expectations of higher academic standards and to become productive and contributing members of society. Recognizing the importance of this message, the following revised definition of school counseling was adopted by the ASCA Governing Board (1997b):

> Counseling is a process of helping people by assisting them in making decisions and changing behavior. School counselors work with all students, school staff, families, and members of the community as an integral part of the education program. School counseling programs promote school success through a focus on academic achievement, prevention and intervention activities, advocacy and social-emotional and career development. (ASCA, 1997b)

## Leaders and Advocates for School Improvement

School counselors through a leadership and social advocacy role ensure that all students have equal access to quality academic programs and the needed support to meet the demands of these challenges. School counselors call attention to situations in schools that are defeating or frustrating students, thereby hindering their success. These situations, supported by data, present an opportunity for school counselors to lead a schoolwide effort to promote equity and provide opportunity. Measurable success resulting from this effort can be documented by an increased number of students completing school with the academic preparation, career awareness, and personal/social growth essential in choosing from a wide range of substantial postsecondary options, including college (Education Trust, 1997). This is not a new message but certainly one that continues to be at the forefront of the ongoing school counselor conversation about student engagement and achievement.

> If school counselors truly believe in the worth of all children and see themselves as advocates for all students, they must step away from being "maintainers of the status quo" and become "dream-makers and pathfinders" for all students navigating their way through K–12 schools today. They must have the courage to stand up for students who may be unable to stand up for themselves in systems that have produced disparate academic results and thus, few to no postsecondary options for many students in the past. (National Office for School Counselor Advocacy, 2010)

### Partners in Educational Excellence

In collaboration with principals, teachers, other school professionals, and parents/caretakers, school counselors share the challenge of preparing students to meet the expectations of higher academic standards and become productive and contributing members of society. School counselors work toward the same goal, i.e., successful schools can provide an equitable, excellent, and challenging education for every child. As key partners in educational excellence, school counselors share the responsibility of educating all children. The school counselor is in a unique position to interact with students, faculty, administration, parents, and the community to help students build resiliency and overcome barriers to academic achievement.

## 21st-CENTURY SCHOOL COUNSELING PROGRAMS: BENEFITTING ALL STAKEHOLDERS

When school counselors implement comprehensive school counseling programs, they demonstrate a commitment to ensure every student fully participates and benefits from the program. Additionally, the program is aligned with the school's improvement goals that support improved student achievement. In this manner everyone benefits!

The benefits for school counselors are the following:

- Clarify responsibilities within the context of a school counseling program.
- Eliminate non-school counseling program activities.
- Ensure that every student has access to developmental and comprehensive school counseling programs.
- Design, deliver, and manage an accountable school counseling program.
- Demonstrate the school counselor's role as a leader, advocate, team player, data informed practitioner, and collaborator in the school setting.

- Align the school counseling program's contribution with the academic mission of the school.
- Connect the work of the school counselor to school improvement and positive school climate.
- Document students' achievement and growth in academic, career, and personal-social development.

The benefits for students are the following:

- Participate in relevant curriculum, individual student planning, and responsive services.
- Understand that they are participating in programs for both career and college readiness.
- Participate in proactive strategies and responsive interventions to minimize and eliminate educational barriers.
- Engage in targeted interventions aimed at closing the gap.
- Encourage high aspirations for every student.
- Focus their goals on future success.
- Understand the importance of rigor and results.
- Acquire attitudes, knowledge, and skills in the three counseling domains: academic, personal/social, and career as a result of participating in a school counseling program.
- Participate in a rigorous academic curriculum.
- Have equitable access to all educational opportunities.

The benefits for parents/guardians are the following:

- Acquire knowledge about their children's academic, career, and personal-social development.
- Partnership with school counselors regarding their children's learning and career goals.
- Participate in educational and informational sessions.
- Participate in ongoing communication between parent, teacher, administrators, and school counselor.
- Increase access to school and community resources.
- Gain the necessary support to help their children successfully transition from grade level to grade level.
- Receive information and assistance with the postsecondary planning process.
- Gain access to school and community resources.
- Receive opportunities for informational and support workshops.

The benefits for teachers are the following:

- Participate in an interdisciplinary team approach to address student needs and educational goals.
- Improved collaboration among school counselors and teachers to improve student achievement.
- Ongoing consultation on student needs and interventions.
- Receive direct support in the classroom to improve student achievement.

- Support improving motivation and student management in the classroom and hallways.
- Collaborate in the development of student development (guidance) lessons.
- Work together on data analysis to improve school climate and school improvement.

The benefits for student services personnel are the following:

- Utilizing the school counseling program as a means of promoting affective development.
- Using school data to develop prevention and intervention strategies.
- Collaborating for utilizing and coordinating school and community resources.
- Coordinating and sharing strategies and coordinate services.
- Building a team to design and implement prevention and intervention services.

The benefits for administrators are the following:

- Demonstrate the alignment of the school counseling program with the school's academic mission.
- Receive support from school counselor as a critical stakeholder and leader in the educational process.
- Consult to inform the School Improvement Plan and strengthen school climate and student performance/achievement.
- Receive input regarding opportunities for professional development.
- Document the link between the school counseling program and student success.
- Collaborate to improve school climate and culture.
- Promote collaboration and support for the use of data in school improvement.
- Provide for an accountability process to measure success of the school counseling program.
- Improve student growth and achievement in academic, career, and personal-social development.
- Integration of the National Standards for School Counseling Programs with the academic standards.
- Demonstrate school counselor support and involvement in the goals of the Blueprint for Reform and Race to the Top.

The benefits for the boards and departments of education are the following:

- Show the connection of school counseling to school improvement.
- Demonstrate the involvement of school counselors in data driven decision making.
- Understand the involvement and commitment of school counselors to student achievement.
- Gain insight as to the perspective of parent/guardians and students regarding their development and aspirations.

- Promote the equitable access to a quality school counseling program for every student.
- Support the rational for appropriate levels of funding and resources for school counseling.
- Rationale for supporting appropriate credential and staffing ratios.
- Provide the community with an awareness of a comprehensive and developmental school counseling.
- Understand the alignment of the comprehensive school counseling program with the district's goals.
- Document measurable results and accountability for shared responsibility for student success.

The benefits for postsecondary educational institutions are the following:

- Articulation and transition of students to postsecondary institutions.
- Expanded opportunities to collaborate with all educators to prepare every student for postsecondary opportunities.
- Encourage every student to seek a wide range of substantial, postsecondary options, including college.
- Endorse and support high aspirations and rigorous academic preparation.
- Promote equitable access to postsecondary education for every student.

The benefits for community members (community organizations, business, labor and industry) are the following:

- Offer opportunities for all community stakeholders to actively participate in the development and implementation of the school counseling program.
- Assist with the school's access to community resources.
- Connect with school stakeholders and students who affect community well-being and workforce.
- Promote collaboration and teaming to encourage citizenship, high achievement, and community pride.
- Encourage students to take pride in their community.
- Demonstrate the role the community plays in a student's education.
- Show community support, commitment to, and involvement in school improvement.

From the moment I stepped onto a school campus, I identified not with other therapists but with other educators, and like them, felt I was at the heart and soul of the educational process; not a visitor whose job it was to be a clinician, but an educator who brought unique counseling skills and specialized knowledge. As an educator, I need my counseling skills but I impact my students' through a repertoire of other powerful roles: leader, advocate, collaborator, team builder, consultant, data analyzer/consumer, systemic change agent, steward of equity and access, manager of resources, career and academic advisor, and didactic counselor. We are in a setting called schools and as a school counselor I owe a duty to my clients, students, to help them become successful learners through the application of a wide range of exciting skills. (Stone, ACA, 2003, p. 15)

School counselors, working in today's schools, share the commitment, the responsibility, and the accountability for student educational success. As key players in the school improvement arena, 21st-century school counselors can contribute in powerful ways to creating schools that nurture respect, have high aspirations, and are committed to closing the gap.

## TECH TOOLS

Effective school counselors use the power of technology to maximize their efficiency. Here are six "tech tools" you can use to maximize your own effectiveness:

- Use the World Wide Web to keep abreast of U.S. Department of Education initiatives and find out more about the new Blueprint for Reform.
- Contact the office of your school district that manages student information and discuss how you can get data in a form that will be useful to you such as attendance data disaggregated by grade level, day of the week, etc.
- Examine your local school district's website. How can you use the website to improve communication to parents and other stakeholders?
- Access your district's school report card, which describes critical student data in your school system. Use this to develop a presentation on "Student Progress in My School District."
- Discover more about achievement in the United States by exploring the Education Trust website (www.Edtrust.org), the Alliance for Excellent Education (www.all4ed.org), and other educational watchdog groups.
- Explore Postsecondary.org (www.postsecondary.org) and other websites that provide you with data that inform you about patterns in higher education enrollment. Use this information to compare these trends and patterns to those in your local high school and to inspire others to help your school improve.

---

## *School Counselor Casebook: Voices from the Field*

### The Scenario Reviewed

Jason is in 11th grade and is convinced that the next week's high school exit exam is the most important test that he will ever take. His parents, teachers, and you, his counselor, have reminded him that he still has several opportunities to pass—just in case. Jason is an average student and usually gets Cs and Bs in most of his subjects. He failed the test the first time he took it in 10th grade, saying he was overly anxious and could not think straight. Jason told you that if he cannot pass the test this time, he will just have to quit high school. He does not know what he wants to do after high school—sometimes he thinks he wants to go to college, other times he thinks that he wants a technical career. Now he thinks he should just go to work and not deal with any of this.

## A Practitioner's Approach

Here's how a practicing school counselor approached this challenge.

Jason and I have worked together since 9th grade; as his school counselor, we have talked extensively about building his confidence to achieve his educational and career goals. After chatting with Jason for a few moments, I concurred that this high school exit exam is the most important exam he has ever taken. However, I pointed out that he has prepared extensively since last year, his grades show that he certainly knows the material, and he has experience with the type of questions that will be asked on this year's test.

I thought it would help Jason if we first discussed his anxiety and then brainstormed solutions to help him feel more relaxed. By first asking him to scale his anxiety (with 1 being the most stress, 10 being very relaxed), Jason responded that he was feeling about a "3." I then asked him to think about which number he would like to be on test day. He jokingly answered, "10—and I wouldn't be taking the test!" I agreed that not taking the test would be a perfect scenario but not possible because he wants to receive his diploma. I asked him what a diploma means to him, and after a few moments of reflection, Jason shared that "graduating would mean everything to me.... I would be the first in my family to graduate, and maybe take some classes after high school." I then asked him to describe specifically how the test proctor would see Jason. Jason said he would have his pencils sharpened, calculator ready, and be wide awake. We brainstormed specific test-taking strategies that Jason would use during the test, as well as his favorite method of falling asleep and the breakfast he would eat on the test day morning.

Before Jason returned to class, I reassured him that I know planning for his future is also a concern, and that after the exam, I would work with him to find a shadowing experience in sports marketing, as he had expressed interest in this field after taking a career interest inventory as a sophomore. I also reminded Jason we would plan next year's program of study to reflect his other interest in a potential career in business. However, between now and test day, I wanted to review test-taking strategies with him daily. I asked permission to call his parents, explain the heightened anxiety Jason was experiencing about this test, and ask their support by reminding him to see me after school. Finally, I told Jason I wanted to request from his teachers practice exit exam questions. Jason shook his head, saying, "I'll have to pass this test now, if everyone is helping me. I can come by after school tomorrow for a few minutes; will you be here?"

Jason and I worked on test preparation almost every day after school. On the morning of the test, I stood outside the classroom, and as Jason came around the corner I told him, "I know you are ready to pass the high school exit exam. Go in there, focus on what we have reviewed, and just *do your best*." I looked forward to seeing him when he finished!

*Barbara Crudale is a high school counselor at South Kingstown High School in Rhode Island. She is a past president of the Rhode Island School Counselor Association and an adjunct professor at Providence College.*

# LOOKING BACK: SALIENT POINTS

## The Changing Direction of 21st-Century Schools

The most recent educational reform agenda which took a strong hold in the mid-1990s focused its attention on developing national standards across all curricula areas. This emphasis on what students should know and be able to do has also resulted in high-stakes testing in every state across the nation. Coupled with this is a growing concern over the achievement gap, which appears to be rooted in socioeconomic, racial, and ethnic differences.

## School Counseling: Changing with the Times

Throughout the earlier years of educational reform and debate, school counseling was largely ignored as part of the solution to improve student achievement and success in school. Recently counseling in schools is acknowledged for the greater role it plays in contributing to student aspirations and educational achievement. The shared purpose of creating schools in which all children are held to high expectations must be addressed if school counselors are going to help prepare all students to meet the challenges of the 21st century.

## Defining the Role of School Counseling in 21st-Century Schools

Despite the presence of more than 100,000 school counselors in every school district across the 50 states, the school counseling profession was omitted from most of the educational reform agendas of the past. Since the late 1990s, the school counseling community has positioned itself as an influential partner in contemporary school improvement with the expressed purpose to eliminate the barriers to educational opportunity for every student. However, much more needs to be done on the part of school counselors to highlight the effect of school counseling programs as a viable solution to closing the opportunity and information gaps.

## School Counselors Acting as Agents of Change

School counselors advance the moral dimensions of school to include a strong social justice agenda to "close the gap" especially for diverse populations of students who have been traditionally underserved or underrepresented. Acting as agents of school and community change, school counselors can create a climate where access and support for quality and rigor is the norm.

## Issues Affecting Today's Schools

All stakeholders have expectations of higher levels of academic achievement as **standards-based education** is the norm. The pressure is on from an ever-changing global economy. Business and industry continue to expect more from education. There is a demonstrated need for academic and effective competence in all aspects of K–12 education and a direct link between knowledge, skills, and income. Changing technology affects all aspects of our lives. The millennial generation spends its entertainment and leisure time in ways adults cannot always identify with. Shifting societal issues and values affect the way we work with youth.

### School Counseling Programs: Essential to Every Student's Education

The purpose of the counseling program in schools is to impart specific skills and facilitate learning opportunities in a proactive and preventive manner to help all students achieve school success through academic, career, and personal/social development experiences.

### Advancing the Academic Agenda

School counselors must establish a foundation for effective education, competency-based learning in academic, career, and personal-social development, and commit to high expectations of achievement for every student. Twenty-first-century school counselors support student success; help all children achieve at a higher level; change attitudes and beliefs about student achievement; and are partners in educational excellence.

### Leaders and Advocates for School Improvement

School counselors through a leadership and social advocacy role ensure that all students have equal access to quality academic programs and the needed support to meet the demands of these challenges. School counselors call attention to situations in schools that are defeating or frustrating students, thereby hindering their success.

### 21st-Century School Counseling Programs: Benefitting All Stakeholders

Everyone benefits from school counseling programs and implementing a comprehensive national standard-based school counseling program empowers school counselors to place themselves front and center of the restructuring process in their school systems.

## KEY TERMS

No Child Left Behind Act p. 2

Educational reform p. 3

Accountability p. 3

Standards p. 4

High-stakes testing p. 4

Blueprint for Reform p. 5

School improvement p. 7

National Standards for School Counseling Programs p. 10

Standards-based education p. 26

## LEARNING EXTENSIONS/MAKING CONNECTIONS

1. Education professionals are talking (and writing) about the No Child Left Behind Act (2001). This latest reauthorization of the Elementary and Secondary Education Act is driving the educational agenda in our states, districts, and schools. Use a search engine such as Google or Yahoo to find out what principals, school board members, superintendents, and parents are thinking about No Child Left Behind.

2. Read *A Nation at Risk*, which can be found online at www.ed.gov/pubs/NatAtRsk. How does this paper, written two decades ago, apply to the state of education in America today?

3. Locate your state department of education's website to review the Educational Requirements for Students. Create a table to summarize what is required at each level in elementary, middle/junior high, and high school. Carefully examine the new curriculum, assessment, promotion, and graduation requirements.

4. Think back to your high school days. Were you placed in a particular academic track? What type of academic program did you follow? What academic program did your friends follow? Did you notice differences in the various plans of study among students in your school? How did tracking affect your expectations of yourself and of your friends?

5. Talk to someone you know who works for a large organization and also to someone who works in a small business or company. Show them the Partnership for 21st Century Skills (2007). Ask them how these skills are used in their organization.

6. To explore the current state of student achievement, go to the website Edtrust.org and find the section called Education Watch National and State Reports. Why is this information important to your preparation as a school counselor?

7. The National Center for Education Statistics (NCES) maintains comprehensive data on the state of education across our nation. Find three positive improvements in the data and identify three areas that require additional improvement.

8. Examine your local school district/system's report card. What does this tell you about levels of students' performance in your community? What else might you want to know?

# Counseling Theory in Schools

## CHAPTER OBJECTIVES

*By the time you have completed this chapter, you should be able to*

- understand the purpose of counseling in schools;

- demonstrate an understanding of the major theoretical approaches to counseling that are relevant in a school setting;

- apply counseling theory to case studies;

- identify counseling techniques that are appropriate to your style and a school setting;

- explain how to utilize counseling theories and techniques to help each student achieve academic, career, and personal-social success;

- understand how to address the diverse counseling needs of students including race, ethnicity, culture, religion, sexual orientation, learning differences, and/or physical or emotional disabilities;

- explain the importance of utilizing community-based mental health resources;

- demonstrate the knowledge to identify counseling interventions appropriate to the specific needs of the student and the issue, problem, or challenge she or he faces.

---

## *School Counselor Casebook: Getting Started*

### The Scenario

Katie's dad abruptly left their home over the weekend. She has not heard from him for three days. Her second-grade teacher came to you to talk about the dramatic change in her behavior—Katie is withdrawn and cannot concentrate. How will you address her needs through individual counseling?

### Thinking about Solutions

As you read this chapter, think about how you as a school counselor would handle this situation. What plan of action might you follow? How might you use your knowledge of counseling theory and techniques to help Katie? When you come to the end of the chapter, you will have the opportunity to see how your ideas compare with a practicing school counselor's approach.

---

## COUNSELING IN THE COMPLEX WORLD OF SCHOOLS

On a daily basis, students face a fast-paced world challenged by multiple personal, social, and emotional concerns. Coping with day-to-day pressures such as trauma, grief, and loss, economic stressors, temptations of substance abuse, peer influence, and aggression in school hallways are part of the challenges of growing up in the 21st century.

Schools are microcosms of our communities and some children, streetwise and sophisticated in their knowledge about sex, drugs, and alcohol, learn to adjust and develop coping mechanisms, and acquire resiliency skills to find balance in their school, family, and community life.

For many children, their academic success is depressed by the stressors of the world in which they live. Students move through the developmental stages of physical and emotional growth faced with multiple dilemmas and complex choices. Abuse, dysfunctional home environments, blended families, hunger, poverty, violence, harassment, bullying, peer pressure, and homelessness are just some of the pressures they encounter and struggle with on a daily basis (Children's Defense Fund, 2010). For many students, the school building is a safe haven.

Schools are complex institutions and daily routines are at times confusing and frustrating for many children. Students may walk through the front door each day ready and willing to learn but, when met by external and internal pressures, their motivation, drive, and concentration are tempered or crushed. Although many children have developed the coping and resiliency skills needed to survive and even thrive, a growing number develop emotional, social, and behavioral problems that necessitate intervention. Children struggle with behavioral reconciliation whether challenged by peers, parents, teachers, or other figures of authority. Escapism has become an alternative via the world of alcohol and drugs or immersion in video games and media (Howe & Strauss, 2000). Social networking sites such as Facebook, MySpace, and Twitter offer young people the chance to interact in a completely new way while potentially fostering poor interpersonal communication skills (Rollins, 2008).

In 2010, delegates to the American Counseling Association (ACA) 20/20: A Vision for the Future of Counseling defined **counseling** as "a professional relationship that empowers diverse individuals, families, and groups to accomplish mental health, wellness, education, and career goals" (American Counseling Association, 2010; Rollins, 2010). Counseling is a complex helping process in which the counselor establishes a trusting and confidential working relationship with a student or groups of students (ACA, 1997; ASCA, 1998) to help them set goals and make changes in behavior. Students bring acting-out behaviors, lack of motivation, poor achievement, learning problems, sadness and depression, social isolation, and pressure and stress to the **counseling process**. Counseling goals address, analyze, and explore behaviors and attitudes that affect a student's ability to perform successfully in the learning community. The focus of counseling in the educational setting is on problem solving, decision making, social-emotional development, and the personal issues and concerns that affect learning and development.

The foundation and basis for the school counseling program reside in **counseling theory** and those processes and techniques relevant to the school setting. Not to be confused with advising or guidance or therapy, counseling is the most significant component of the school counseling program, and the one by which the counselor's professional identity is often established.

When trying to address the needs of overwhelming numbers of students, teachers and administrators sometimes send students to the school counselor to be "cured." When counseling is equated as a quick fix, disappointment and confusion follow when a student continues to pose problems. (Cunanan &

Maddy-Bernstein, 1994). It is difficult to eliminate or even remediate students' presenting problems when you work with the student in isolation. School counselors are needed, not to be the panacea, but rather to provide counseling toward change and delivering support to teachers, administrators, and parents in the form of facilitative collaborative interventions. Oftentimes, the person who is the most highly trained to prevent, intervene, and remediate student behavior is the school counselor.

## COUNSELING STUDENTS: PURPOSE AND LIMITATIONS

> Counseling is a confidential relationship which the counselor conducts with students individually and in small groups to help them resolve their problems and developmental concerns. (ASCA, 1999b, p. 1)

Counseling is a professional skill. Unlike conversations between friends or working with students in a guidance or advisory role, counseling is a complex process and is far more involved than simply establishing a relationship with a student and setting goals for behavioral changes. Counseling children requires the use of the helping relationship to focus on concerns that can be developmental or problem-based, help a student make decisions to correct a situation, or learn or acquire new behavioral skills to improve one's image of self (Henderson & Thompson, 2011; Schmidt, 2007; Thompson & Henderson, 2007).

Clear goals are needed when counseling students (Schmidt, 2007). George and Cristiani (1995) identified five major goals that are at the heart of most counseling theories and models:

1. Facilitate a change in behavior.
2. Improve social and personal relationships.
3. Increase one's ability to cope.
4. Learn and apply the decision making process.
5. Enrich personal growth and self-development.

These same goals can serve as a good guide for you when you become a school counselor as they are applicable to helping students, our "clients," learn to help themselves, make good decisions, and bring about positive changes in behavior.

Counseling in schools differs from therapeutic treatment in purpose and process. It usually involves short-term goals, while psychotherapeutic intervention relies on a positive therapeutic alliance influenced by the commitment of the client and the skill and talents of the clinician (Henderson & Thompson, 2011; Seligman, 2001). The focus of counseling with students is to address prevention, intervention, and developmental concerns, assist with mild disorders in educational or developmental settings, and engage students in dealing with personal, social, emotional, career, and educational decisions and behaviors (Henderson & Thompson, 2011; Thompson and Rudolph, 2000). School counselors will refer students to a mental health professional in a agency, clinic, or private practice setting when the goals of counseling are complex and require therapeutic intervention. The Education Trust defined school counseling as "a profession that focuses on the relations and interactions between students and their school environment to reduce the effects of environmental and institutional barriers that impede student academic success. School counselors foster educational equity, access, and academic success in a rigorous curriculum to ensure that all students graduate from high school ready to succeed in college and careers" (Education Trust, 2009, para. 3).

# THEORETICAL UNDERPINNINGS OF COUNSELING

To professionally and skillfully move a student through the counseling process, the school counselor needs a broad-based awareness, knowledge, and understanding of theory. Counseling is first and foremost guided by theory (Gladding, 2009). According to Gladding, theoretical understanding is an essential part of effective counseling practice. Theories help counselors organize critical data, make complex processes coherent and provide conceptual guidance for interventions. Counseling theories provide a point of reference from which the counselor develops a personal perspective of human growth, development, and behavior. The counselor selects different theories and approaches according to the models used and the assistance that a student needs. Counseling requires the acquisition of requisite skills and knowledge so that counselors can facilitate, process, and construct appropriate intervention plans. Counselors use techniques and strategies that best match their theoretical approach, philosophical orientation, the needs of their clientele, and the setting in which they work.

There are over 250 documented counseling and psychotherapy systems (Corsini & Wedding, 1995) to study, analyze, and incorporate into practice. Given that you will be working in a school setting and your clients are students, 10 theories were carefully chosen as having the greatest potential for counseling work with minors in a school setting. The theories are presented in a brief and concise manner and this chapter cannot replace comprehensive reading, study, and analysis. As you read each theory, consider referencing a counseling textbook that is specifically devoted to the study of theory. This will provide you with a much deeper intellectual awareness and understanding of theories, interventions, treatment systems, and skills associated with each. In-depth study and supervised practice in applying student growth and developmental theories will grow your confidence and effectiveness.

## The Gestalt Approach

The Gestalt approach was developed by Fritz Perls and promotes the importance of wholeness and completeness in day-to-day living. Perls (1969) purported that people strive to accomplish all that they can in their lifetime. **Gestalt theory** emphasizes the present and supports the equation now = experience = awareness = reality. Only the now exists since the past is no more, and the future has not yet revealed itself.

The phrase "the whole is greater than the sum of its parts" emphasizes the importance of wholeness or completeness. Through Gestalt therapy, the client learns to identify and analyze the smaller issues in relationship to the larger problem or situation. The client works with the present to resolve past issues and seeks her or his self-actualization that emerges through personal interaction with their environment. Problems can arise in five different ways: (1) loss of contact with the environment; (2) loss of touch with self by becoming too involved with the environment; (3) failure to put aside unfinished business; (4) finding oneself moving in several different directions; and (5) caught in conflict between doing what one thinks she or he should do vs. what one wants to do.

### Techniques

The Gestalt approach uses a repertoire of exercises and experiments. When exercises are used, the counselor guides the student through experiences that include enactment of fantasies, role-play, and psychodrama. Exercises such as "Empty Chair," "Confrontation," "I Take Responsibility," and "May I Feed You a Sentence" are intended to help the student acquire and apply newly honed skills. Other examples of different Gestalt approaches include the following:

*Dream Work*—The student fantasizes what it would be like in different parts of the dream to better understand the multiple ways of interacting with the environment.

*Empty Chair*—The student talks to an empty chair to better understand rational and irrational ways of communicating.

*Confrontation*—The student is challenged by the counselor for her or his actions or words. For example, the student is constantly smiling while masking anger or frustration.

*Making the Rounds*—This technique, often used in group counseling, involves expressing an emotion or feeling to each person in the group. The student becomes more aware of internal emotions and feelings through verbal expression.

*I Take Responsibility*—The student makes a statement about an issue or perception and completes the sentence with "... and I take responsibility for it."

*May I Feed You a Sentence*—The counselor supplies the student with a sentence to help her or him clarify thoughts and responses.

Although Gestalt techniques include free association, the counselor does not interpret or analyze. Rather the purpose is to help the student get in touch with her or his emotions through self-exploration.

### Theory into Practice

Gestalt therapy is complex and sophisticated and requires a high level of cognitive and behavioral development in students. Because life does not unfold in a controlled environment, young students may not be able to apply what they have learned in a counseling situation to a real life challenge.

Techniques such as "I Take Responsibility" can help a student sort through blaming and enabling by becoming aware that the solution lies within her or him and does not lie with parents, peers, or teachers.

The Gestalt approach helps to address situations that are current in a student's life. There is an emphasis on immediacy to make choices in the present that will affect the future, and there is no room for procrastination or putting off until tomorrow or indefinitely. However, this is a difficult concept for most young people and many adults to grasp.

### Practical Application

*During a parent-student conference, you are well aware that your seventh-grade student is sending out mixed messages. Jennifer verbally states her desire to succeed but is not doing anything concrete to get assignments in on time either during class or homework. Her mom talks about her procrastination, laziness, and even indifference to her schoolwork. When the three of you reviewed Jennifer's school records, there was nothing apparent that indicated a learning problem. Up until this year, Jennifer was a solid B to B+ student.*

Using a Gestalt approach, what techniques might work in this situation?

## The Person-Centered Approach

This theory evolving from the work of Carl Rogers (1961) focuses on the "core conditions" of genuineness, empathy, positive regard, and concreteness that are essential to all helping relationships and the counseling process. Humans are characteristically positive, forward moving, constructive, realistic, and trustworthy. Rogers also believes that people are aware, inner directed, and moving toward self-actualization from the time they are born. Rogerians believe that self-actualization is the most prevalent and motivating drive of existence and it encompasses actions that influence the total person.

**Person-centered theory** stresses that each person is capable of finding personal meaning and purpose in life and that the self is an outgrowth of what a person experiences. Self-awareness helps a person differentiate herself or himself from others, but a person needs positive regard in her or his life for a healthy self to emerge. Positive regard is love, warmth, care, respect, and acceptance.

Through the counseling process, the client learns how to deal and cope with situations. As the client begins to free herself or himself of defense mechanisms and past experiences, she or he approaches counseling with openness to self-exploration and self-awareness. Person-centered counseling assists the client to develop into a more mature, confident, and well-adapted decision maker. The client embraces a more realistic sense of self, can adapt and recover quickly from situations, and is less stressed in her or his everyday events.

### Techniques

There are three different stages of application of the theory. The nondirective stage emphasizes the development of the relationship with the student by creating a permissive and noninterventive atmosphere that creates a climate of acceptance and clarification. The second stage is known as the reflective period. During this time the student with the counselor's help tries to create nonthreatening relationships in her or his life. The counselor concentrates on responding to the student's feelings and reflects the underlying effect back to the student. During the third application, called the experimental stage, positive regard (acceptance) and congruence (genuineness) are emphasized. Other overall techniques that are used are active and passive listening, accurate reflection of thoughts and feelings, clarification, summarization, confrontation, and general and open-ended leads.

### Theory into Practice

The person-centered approach works well when treating students who exhibit mild to moderate anxiety and adjustment and interpersonal disorders. This therapy requires the student to have a complete understanding of herself or himself and her or his experiences. Therefore, it may not work well with young children or students with learning or emotional disabilities. This approach can be effective in a relatively short time; however, behavioral change may also be short term. The person-centered approach may address only surface issues and not challenge the student to explore deeper when the ultimate goal is to develop a long-lasting impact on the student.

Students with minor behavioral adjustments or mild anxiety, and older students who are just generally confused about their future direction, benefit from this approach; however, one criticism is that person-centered counseling may be too optimistic or perceived as a short-term solution for today's complex societal issues.

### Practical Application

*Michael's parents are going through a separation. Although Michael cannot remember a time in his 10 years when his parents were not arguing and fighting, he feels he is to blame and somehow he has contributed to the problem. Michael's teacher asked you to talk with Michael. At least three times this week, Michael started to cry in class when corrected for small errors on homework or class work. He also noticed that he does not seem to be hanging out with his friends as much in the lunchroom and on the playground.*

How could you use person-centered techniques to help Michael?

## The Individual Psychology Approach

**Individual psychology** was developed by Alfred Adler. However, one cannot discuss Adler's work without reference to the influence of Sigmund Freud. Adler, initially one of Freud's disciples, eventually became one of his strongest dissidents. Freud invited Adler to participate in discussion circles until such time that Adler rejected Freud's emphasis on sex, the unconscious, and the influence of the past. Although Freud's theory of psychoanalysis suggested new ways of understanding love, hate, emotions, family relations, fantasy, and sexuality, Adler purported that personality difficulties are rooted in feelings of inferiority and are derived from an individual's need for self-assertion. Adler termed his theory *individual psychology* to distinguish his work from Freud. Central to Adler's theory is the concept that social interest drives behavior. Terms such as *inferiority complex*, *social interest*, *empathy*, and *lifestyle* were coined by Adler and quickly adopted by other theorists and scholars (Gladding, 2009).

Human beings desire success; thus, all behavior is purposeful and goal-oriented. The Adlerian approach encourages the client to be well aware of her or his surroundings and environment, and the theory supports healthy development to overcome any feelings of inferiority. This theoretical orientation stresses the influence of subjective feelings as a primary motivator. The client learns to grapple with her or his conscious levels of thought and assumes responsibility for taking charge of changing behaviors.

Behavior and misbehavior are the externals and are symptomatic of the feelings that the student has internalized. Especially with misbehavior, school counselors can pay particular attention to the reasons for the behavior whether looking for attention, seeking power, revenge, or compensating for feelings of inadequacy (Dreikurs & Soltz, 1990). Schools present myriad opportunities for students to experiment with different types of behaviors and gain a sense of belonging and connectedness (Sciarra, 2004).

### Techniques

Counselors who consider themselves "Adlerian" demonstrate empathy, support, and genuine warmth toward the client. However, the counselor uses a variety of techniques to assist and encourage change in behavior such as confrontation. Confrontation challenges the client to examine her or his logic and behavior and to look at the situation she or he is in. Asking questions and attending are used to explore possibilities. For example, when a student is asked "What would be different if you _____?" she or he can respond with an answer based on what she or he wants ideally. The counselor listens and encourages the client to embrace good, positive, and realistic behaviors. Encouragement motivates the client to believe that change is possible. "Catching oneself" is a technique to teach the client to become aware of self-destructive behaviors and thoughts.

Other specialized strategies such as "pushing buttons" help the client to develop an awareness of what prompts her or his reaction and when she or he is acting in an inappropriate manner. Clients are also encouraged to set tasks and establish short-term goals to ultimately establish and attain long-term but realistic change in behavior.

### Theory into Practice

Adlerians approach behavior as goal directed and the focus for children is on immediate behavior targets rather than long-term objectives. Play therapy helps young children learn how to better express themselves, socialize, and interact with others. It also provides a vehicle for differentiating between good and bad behaviors. Drawings are also helpful to discern a child's pattern of behavior.

The Adlerian method helps the student identify more successful ways of resolving problems than what the student is currently doing in school, play, and social interactions. The counselor works with the assumption that the student can assume responsibility and acquire better ways to meet personal goals. The counselor uses questioning to frame the structured interview and explore the perspective that the student has of her or his life. Students explore their orientation in their families, confront negative behavior, establish goals, and examine social interactions. Encouragement is a critical part of the counseling process and the Adlerian method subscribes to the belief that students misbehave when they are frustrated and discouraged and have no other means to succeed. School counselors use these techniques to facilitate, change, and encourage appropriate behaviors while disregarding unwanted and unhealthy ways of responding.

### *Practical Application*

*Kara feels she is unable to do anything well. She is only comfortable in class when the teacher expects nothing from her. You ask Kara, "What do you want your teacher and classmates to know about you? Are there some things in class that you are really good at and would like everyone to know? How can we make that happen?"*

How would you approach this counseling situation if your professional orientation is Adlerian?

## The Behavioral Approach

The behavioral approach to counseling is strongly influenced by the work of B. F. Skinner and is based on the processes closely associated with overt behavior. Behavioral theory promotes the premise that all behavior is learned and that learning is effective in changing maladaptive behavior. The three main approaches in contemporary behavior therapy are the stimulus-response model, applied behavior analysis, and social-cognitive theory.

The stimulus-response model approaches behavioral change through the association of stimuli-conditioning of involuntary responses. It is sometimes called respondent learning or stimulus-response (S-R) model. The classic example that immediately comes to mind is Pavlov's dog. Salivation occurs when a bell is rung because the bell is associated with food. Behavior can also be "unlearned" through counter-conditioning in which new associations take the place of old ones.

When behavioral analysis is applied, a person is rewarded or punished for her or his actions. This is an extension of operant conditioning. A person learns to repeat what was rewarded (reinforced) and not repeat the actions that were punished.

Social-cognitive theory purports that people acquire new knowledge and behavior by observing others. It emphasizes observational learning, imitation, social modeling, and vicarious learning. Social-cognitive theory is efficient in that it saves time, energy, and effort in acquiring new skills and is most effective if the observer can relate to the model. The counselor plays multiple roles as consultant, teacher, advisor, reinforcer, and facilitator and responds in a concrete, objective, and collaborative manner. Additionally, the client is involved in every phase of counseling.

Behavioral counseling goals help clients make good adjustments to life circumstances and achieve personal and professional objectives by replacing unproductive actions (maladaptive behavior) with productive actions. The counselor and client mutually agree on goals in these four basic steps:

1. Define the problem.
2. Explore how past circumstances were handled through a developmental history.
3. Establish specific goals in small, achievable units and design learning experiences to acquire needed skills.
4. Determine the best methods for change.

### Techniques

School counselors who subscribe to a behavioral approach will apply different techniques for various situations. Many of these techniques are adapted for classroom and group experiences. For example, teachers often use positive reinforcers to yield a desired result or action. This can be translated into intrinsic or extrinsic rewards. It is important to differentiate between negative reinforcers and punishment. For example, is there a difference between a teacher "yelling" at the class vs. withholding a privilege? Would either technique result in the desired change in student behavior?

School counselors also work with students on "shaping" behavior, which is learning new ways of responding through successive approximation. In "Generalization" the counselor helps the student understand how she or he has applied the behavior outside of where it was initially learned. "Maintenance" means the student now continues the behavior without anyone else's support. "Extinction" occurs when the student eliminates behavior(s) due to the withdrawal of reinforcement.

These techniques can be applied with a student as the need arises or if the student needs more clarification of what particular situations mean:

- Behavioral rehearsal is practicing a desired behavior until it is performed the way the student wishes.
- Environmental planning is establishing an environment to promote or limit certain behaviors and help the student avoid places that she or he associates with painful memories.
- Systematic desensitization helps the client overcome anxiety in particular situations.
- Assertiveness training helps the student to express thoughts and feelings appropriately without feeling undue anxiety.
- Contingency contracts spell out the behavior to be performed, changed, or discontinued and the rewards and/or stipulations involved in the agreement.

### Theory into Practice

School counselors using behavioral techniques are actively engaged in the teaching and learning process to help the student learn, unlearn, or modify behaviors. The teaching aspect of counseling is a part of behavioral theory. It can be empowering to students, even young ones, when they see and feel tangible results for modifying or changing behavior. As a student learns to eliminate negative or distracting behavior simultaneously, she or he is encouraged to display positive behavior and the student is seen as capable of learning new ways of addressing situations. Students are empowered to know that they are capable of taking charge and learning control. Behavioral theory relies on a good working relationship between the student and counselor. Although the student extends the effort to make the desired changes, the student is encouraged, supported, and empowered to stay focused by the counselor.

### Practical Application

*Ms. Bishop has her hands full with 25 high-energy second graders. Although she feels she has created a stimulating and challenging learning environment, there are at least four students who have significant difficulty completing their assignments on time. Ms. Bishop thinks the students' problems stem from difficulties with organization and attending and not a learning disability. You offer to help the teacher set up a positive reinforcement system that will benefit the entire class and, most specifically, targeted to help these four students.*

How will you use behavioral techniques to bring about the desired results?

## The Reality Therapy Approach

Reality therapy helps clients understand the need to be psychologically strong and make healthy productive choices in their interpersonal and intrapersonal relationships. Attaining psychological strength and using productive decision making lead to autonomy and taking responsibility for the behaviors that affect oneself and others. Reality therapy encourages the client to learn how to make more effective choices and develop the skills to cope with daily stresses and problems. Individuals take ownership of realistic goals, thus accepting responsibility for their present and future. Most importantly, the counselor helps clients realize that that they cannot blame others for inappropriate decisions; reality therapy attempts to eliminate these excuses.

William Glasser (1986, 1998, 2000a), the father of reality therapy, believes that human beings operate on a conscious level and are not driven by unconscious forces or instinct. Human learning is a lifelong process based on choice. Glasser suggests that there are six criteria for healthy behavior that a person must seek. Behavior is easily completed, individually driven, has value, improves lifestyle, and is not self-critical or competitive. Choice theory is the foundation of reality therapy. Individuals self-determine the way in which they meet their needs for survival, power, fun, freedom, and belonging and choose their thoughts, actions, and emotions accordingly (Corey, 2001, 2009; Glasser, 1998, 2000a). This approach concentrates so much on the present that it tends to ignore the past and the unconscious, unlike psychoanalytic theory, which is heavily immersed in both. Reality therapy is difficult to apply to youth or adults who have problems expressing themselves or their feelings.

### Techniques

The school counselor uses active techniques such as humor, role-play, confrontation, feedback, goal setting, attending and teaching, designing plans, and composing contracts to help the student explore her or his options. The primary technique of reality therapy is teaching a student how to become responsible for personal actions. The counselor's role is to reinforce positive planning and action steps. A student begins to see how her or his behavior is unrealistic and sometimes negative. Guided by the school counselor, the student begins to understand that she or he is in control of the desired change(s).

Confrontation and role-play help the student to accept responsibility for behavior and bring past events into the here and now. Reviewing past behaviors helps the student take charge in the present and plan for the future, while establishing realistic goals to change her or his behaviors. Humor is one of the techniques used; however, it must be used respectfully. Students have fragile egos and cannot think they are being made fun of. Incorporating humor may help the student to look at the situation differently and see how unrealistic it was.

Reality therapy uses the Wants, Direction, Evaluate, Plan (WDEP) system (Wubbolding, 2000) to help the counselor and the student focus on the desired change and assess progress. The counselor identifies what the student *wants* early on in the session. The counselor shares what she or he *wants* for the student. The student takes *direction* over her or his life. *Evaluation* is the basis for reality therapy. Students learn to *evaluate* their behaviors and begin to recognize which behaviors are unproductive. Students take action to create a *plan* for changing behaviors. Reality therapy places the responsibility on the student to accomplish the goals set forth in the plan of action. The counselor never gives up on the student and the student assumes responsibility to break the cycle of failure.

### Theory into Practice

Reality therapy requires a student to accept the responsibility to determine the course of action the student will follow. Reality therapy does not dwell on the past but rather projects the students forward toward a change in action and behavior. Students may view reality therapy as empowering, believing that they have choices and there are alternatives ways to the methods used to approach a situation or problem in the past. It keeps a student focused on dealing with the "here and now" to gain self-confidence and assurance. Using role-play helps bring the future or past into the present. Reality therapy seems to work best with older children who are capable of understanding choice and demonstrating the desire to change their behavior.

### Practical Application

*At the eighth-grade team meeting last week, Mrs. Riemer, a social studies teacher, presented some concerns she has about Robbie and discovered that in all of Robbie's classes he was seeking constant attention mainly in the form of joking and clowning. Academically he is inconsistent, performing well for some teachers and not for others. Robbie is in danger of failing four out of his eight classes. You agree to meet with Robbie and explore the reasons that he is successful in some classes and not in others.*

How will you use reality therapy to help Robbie change his approach to his schoolwork and behavior?

## The REBT (Rational Emotive Behavior Therapy) Approach

First introduced by Albert Ellis in 1962 as Rational Emotive Therapy (RET), the B for "behavior" was added later as Ellis found that the use of pleasurable behaviors helped to motivate the client to be vigilant in new thinking patterns. **Rational emotive behavior therapy** (REBT) is intended to help people live balanced, productive, and more rational lives by limiting the demands that one makes of oneself. This theory concentrates on the relationship between thoughts and their effect on emotions and behaviors.

Ellis believes that if people gain insight into their thinking processes, they can change because thinking influences feelings and behavior. Ellis also suggests that people have within themselves the ability to control their thoughts, feelings, and actions. However, clients must first be aware of what they are telling themselves (self-talk) to gain control. It is the difference between saying "I act badly" and "I am bad." Demands and wishes, and words such as *should have, must, have to,* and *need to* lead to irrational thoughts and unfulfilled emotions. As the client gains a more rational thought process and positive way of thinking, she or he gains the ability to focus on altering specific behaviors instead of a total personality change. Clients begin to understand that they have the choice of what to say and do, and this becomes empowering.

### Techniques

School counselors who subscribe to REBT believe that experiences directly affect one's feelings whether they are positive, negative, neutral, or mixed. Techniques such as teaching and disputing help school counselors educate students on the anatomy of emotion. Feelings are viewed as a result of thoughts and not events. The counselor helps the student dispute irrational thoughts and students are encouraged to facilitate change in their thought patterns. Often the irrational thought is not the thought presented and the technique of inference chaining is valuable in revealing the true thought(s) that need to be confronted. School counselors guide students to come to an understanding of their behaviors through cognitive processing, guided imagery, and behavioral disputing. Each of these techniques invokes direct questions, logical reasoning, imagining real situations, and attempting behavior that is not within their norm. Students may experience role-play, homework assignments, journal writing, and bibliotherapy as part of the counseling process.

The counselor also uses the cognitive theory of disturbance to help the student understand how irrational beliefs lead to negative consequences. The ABC equation is central to REBT practice. A is the fact, an *activating* event, or the behavior or attitude on the part of a student. B is the student's *belief* that

A that causes C, the emotional and/or behavioral *consequence*. However, the student must come to understand that the reaction can be healthy or not; appropriate or not, A does not cause C. The student learns to acknowledge that she or he is largely responsible for creating her or his problems and accepts that she or he has the ability to change the outcome. Ultimately, the student understands that the problem stems from an irrational belief, works hard to counteract the irrationality, and engages in rational, emotive behavior as a way of life.

### Theory into Practice

REBT helps to restore emotional balance. This approach helps the student learn new ways of thinking, behaving, and feeling and ultimately take control of the direction the student's life is going. REBT can be used with other behavioral techniques to affectively assist students who have anxiety and adjustment disorders. The intent of REBT is to complete the process in a short-term period; therefore, it is also considered a viable theory in a school setting where time is limited. REBT is best applied with older children and adolescents who are mature enough and intellectually capable to discern reality from fictional thought processing. REBT is considered ineffective with mentally or severely emotionally disabled students or with very young children.

Changing thought patterns may not be the simplest or most compelling way to reframe emotions or behaviors. Accountability for behavior requires that students must become responsible for their own actions. Although an event can create a thought, which can lead to a consequence of action, students must assume responsibility for their own actions. REBT encourages students to be more tolerant of themselves and to strive to achieve their personal goals.

### Practical Application

*It is senior year and the college selection process is underway. Amanda is feeling pressured as to what schools she should apply. In her community, there is a lot of pressure on getting into the "right" college. It seems to be more of an issue with the parents than with the students. Although she ranks third in her class, and has an exceptional high school resume, Amanda has asked for your help in explaining to her parents that she is not interested in applying to an "ivy league school" but very much wants to study in an environment that will not put as much pressure on her and allow her to participate in co-op experiences and internships as part of her studies. With early decision deadline dates looming ahead, Amanda is very stressed out over the conversation she needs to have with her parents so she can submit her applications.*

How can using the REBT approach help Amanda communicate her personal goals to her parents?

## The Cognitive Behavior Approach

Bandura influenced **behavioral therapy** by applying the concept of conditioning to social development (1986). Social cognitive theory builds on social

## MEET ERIC KATZ: USING REBT TECHNIQUES IN A SCHOOL SETTING

Eric Katz is a high school counselor who uses REBT techniques in a school setting at the Newburgh Free Academy. Eric studied part-time at The Albert Ellis Institute for Rational Emotive Behavioral Therapy in New York City.

REBT theory provided me with a theoretical orientation and strategies that helped me to address some of the prevalent challenges when working with students such as developing a locus of control (i.e., the teacher failed me vs. what did I do that contributed to my failing) and the all or nothing thinking which is so much a part of the adolescent mindset.

Here's an example of how two of my students seemed to be very responsive to an REBT approach. The first student, Paul, suffered from chronic generalized anxiety. He would get physically ill obsessing about taking his tests. He would start with a dozen "what if I fail" type questions days before and continuing up to the day of the exam. In attacking the irrational thoughts here were, "I am going to fail this test and it will be TERRIBLE, CATASTROPHIC and I will be a TOTAL nothing." I got Paul to start to challenge his thoughts (much like weighing the evidence in a court trial) and ask himself one question: Where is the proof that I will fail this test? If I do why will this specific exam be the one that will make me a "nothing"? We looked at the facts that would dispute his thoughts: first, Paul was getting the top grades in this class, and second, he had taken many tests in the past and always tested well. We went over his assets other than exam scores that made him an attractive candidate for college admissions and likely to be a success in later life.

Kelly's situation was a much more common scenario. Kelly had been an honor student up through junior high and then began to slip academically and her attendance deteriorated. When I spoke with Kelly, she revealed to me how her father had told her "college is not for you." Like many teens, she bought into this belief and told me that no college would "want her." Here we went right to attacking her belief. In 20 minutes, I helped her find a list of 15 colleges that would admit her when she graduated. I continued meeting with her and providing a counter voice to that of her father. This year for the first time in three years, Kelly passed all her classes and is back on track to graduate on time with her class.

In using REBT, I often utilize a lot of humor to diffuse the catastrophic feelings that the students believe are overwhelming them. At times the humor is used to eliminate the thoughts that can help the student start to see that the belief is not fact. I must advise anyone who wishes to use these techniques that great care is needed. The humor taken outside of context can border on sarcasm. I want to make clear that I am only able to work this way when the quality of the relationship between the student and me is firmly established as safe and mutually respectful.

Today in the midst of my frustration trying to accommodate dozens of schedule changes and corrections, Paul stops by my office, looks at me, and says, "remember to breathe Mr. Katz, in through the nose and then let it out slowly through the mouth." Apparently, our relaxation breathing training sessions have borne fruit and the student is now the teacher.

learning theory (Mitchell & Krumboltz, 1996) and self-efficacy; it assists clients to deal with life's events and accomplish personal and professional goals. Bandura purported that faulty thinking leads to emotional and behavioral disturbances. Cognitions are a major determinant of how we feel and act. This therapeutic approach is directed toward creating cognitive and behavioral change. While the cognitive aspect focuses on thinking and understanding why a person behaves a certain way, the behavioral component focuses on doing and how to change. The client confronts faulty beliefs with the evidence that she or he gathers and evaluates.

Cognitive behavior theory is direct in style, structured, goal oriented, time limited, and focuses on problem solving. It is a process in which clients are taught to identify, evaluate, and change self-defeating or irrational thoughts that negatively affect behavior. It is a psycho-educational model that emphasizes the learning process to acquire and practice new skills, learning new ways of thinking, and acquiring new ways of coping with problems.

The psycho-educational model includes four steps. The first step is defining the problem to resolve the issue. This step involves identifying or observing what the behavior or the presenting problem is. The second step requires taking a developmental history in which both the client and the counselor are aware of past events and how behaviors and issues were addressed or resolved. The third step is to establish specific goals, beginning with smaller incremental steps that lead to achievement of the primary goal. The fourth step is to analyze the best method for change. Thus, the counselor and client can explore various behavior modifications and identify which strategies will best support an individual dealing with change.

### Techniques

Counselors who practice the cognitive behavior approach must maintain objectivity and become well-versed in a variety of strategies. Cognitive restructuring teaches students how to identify, evaluate, and change self-defeating, irrational thoughts that can negatively influence behavior. Reinforcers, both positive and negative, facilitate behavior change. Behavior modification is coupled with positive reinforcement, primarily based on behavioral conditioning. A good deed, a correct response is rewarded. Shaping is another technique that counselors use to help achieve behavior adjustments. Once a new behavior is learned the counselor can "gradually" help the student manage the new skill and build on it to improve or change behavior. Generalization helps the student transfer the learned behavior to the presenting situation at home or in school. Maintenance helps the student focus on self-control and self-manage the new or modified behaviors. Extinction occurs when the undesired behavior has been eliminated from the individual's daily routine and is no longer part of the repertoire of response. The counselor may use confrontation, time out, confirmation, and attending to facilitate the client's progress. Homework assignments and recording activities and responses aid in the purpose of understanding and changing behavior.

The cognitive aspect of this theory is more focused on "thinking," and the behavioral component supports the "doing" necessary to change behavior.

However, both aspects are essential to work effectively. The presenting problem is framed in the present and it is assumed that the student's belief system about her or his behavior is the primary cause of the disorder. The premise is simply to modify unwanted behavior. The cognitive behavioral approach is perceived as a therapeutic timesaver because it does not need to delve into the past to deal with the present; it is a learning theory that is constantly evolving. Today's society is dynamic and people and their surroundings are always in a state of flux. Students must always be conscious of falling back into bad patterns.

### Theory into Practice

Token reinforcement and behavior modification programs are familiar classroom interventions. Cognitive behavior theory adds the dimension of understanding, applying logic and using reasoning to modify and change behavioral response well beyond conditioning and rewards. Cognitive behavior theory focuses on problem-solving abilities; it helps the student identify, evaluate, and change self-defeating or irrational thoughts that negatively influence her or his behavior through cognitive restructuring. Students who are feeling defeated in learning, who have fallen prey to the cycle of failure or inappropriate behavior, or who easily succumb to peer pressure can learn and apply a new set of skills to modify or change how they respond to or cope with the situation. By selecting a "choice goal" (Bandura, 1986) the student becomes determined to carry out a specific task or achieve a particular accomplishment.

Stress inoculation helps the student acquire coping skills to help her or him handle stressful events. For example, a student with a chronic illness or disability is constantly dealing with stress events. This is partially because the student simply does not comprehend the nature of the illness or why the emotional, physical, or learning disability exists in the first place. Teaching a student about her or his illness or disability and the treatment involved is empowering. When a young person acquires skills to gain some control over a difficult situation, it is easier to cope with any negativity and challenges. Whether addressing maladaptive behaviors, stress, pressure, or debilitating conditions, cognitive behavioral theory can help students change how they respond to situations by learning and applying new and appropriate behaviors. Consideration must always be given to the developmental and maturity level of the student to ensure that the conceptual framework is within the realm of their cognitive thinking and understanding.

### Practical Application

*Jason is convinced that the high school exit exam is the most important test that he will ever take. His parents, teachers, and you, his counselor, have reminded him that he still has several opportunities to pass—just in case. Jason is an average student and usually gets Cs and Bs in most of his subjects. He failed the test the first time he took it, saying he was overly anxious and could not think straight. Jason told you that if he cannot pass the test the next time he takes it, he will just have to quit high school. He does not know what he wants to do after high school—sometimes he thinks he wants to go to college, other times he thinks that he wants a technical career. Now he thinks he should just go to work and not deal with any of this.*

How can cognitive behavioral techniques help Jason reduce his test anxiety and pass the exit exam?

## The Existential Approach

People live by the choices they make. Self-determination is freedom of choice. The founders of **existential theory** (May, 1950; Frankl, 1963; May & Yalom, 1995; Yalom, 1980) developed this theory to bring an awareness of being, responsibility, freedom, and potential to individuals. One goal of this theory is to encourage clients to take a more active role in shaping their personal reality and putting themselves first. The client is taught to shift the process of thinking from an outward to an inward approach. This results in a better understanding of the relationship between decisions and present and future actions.

Existentialists emphasize the importance of anxiety, values, freedom, and responsibility as one searches to find meaning. Because people author their lives by the choices they make, no longer can life's choices depend on the judgment of others. The client uncovers life's meaning by doing a deed, experiencing a value, or by suffering.

### *Techniques*

There are no specific techniques for the existential approach other than an assurance of the student's readiness to work in an open and inquiring manner. The counselor encourages the student to accept the truth and learn how to work through ambiguity. The counselor must remain open and self-revealing to help the student become more in touch with personal feelings and experiences. The emphasis in the relationship is on spontaneity, authenticity, and honesty. The use of confrontation, goal setting, and imagery helps the student see that everyone is responsible for her or his life and should not allow outside influences to affect choice or behavior. Issues are presented not as problems but rather as learning experiences that can motivate one to strive to succeed.

Existentialism respects diversity and places importance on an individual's ethnic and social background. Existentialism may be used in conjunction with other theories such as behavior modification and cognitive theory to assist in cases such as alcoholism and severe depression. This style of counseling is so individualized that each counselor practices in a different way and tends to be more philosophical than theoretical. Existentialism ascribes to the belief system that connects individuals to the universal problems faced by humankind such as searching for peace and confronting life's challenges through honest expression. Feelings are not classified as negative or positive; they are simply accepted. Since no two individuals are alike, this theory focuses on uniqueness.

Existentialist philosophies also can be combined with other theoretical models such as person-centered and Adlerian because both of these are sensitive to individual uniqueness and focus on the student's personal well-being and effective adjustment in society. The ultimate goal is for the student to work and live productively and peacefully in the student's current environment.

### Theory into Practice

The debate continues as to whether existentialism is a philosophy or a counseling approach—not an easy discussion to resolve. However, let's consider that the existential approach helps students realize the importance of meaning, responsibility, awareness, freedom, and potential. The student cannot be merely an observer of life but also must be a participant in meaningful personal activity. What matters most in the existential approach is the student's perception, not someone else's.

In a school setting, the counselor must be both open and inquiring; however, the student must offer the same. Students assume responsibility for their own life. Students participate in guided imagery and awareness exercises and goal setting activities similar to other models.

### Practical Application

*You have been invited by the team of eighth-grade teachers to collaborate on developing a program that will help the students make a smooth transition from middle school to high school.*

What existential approaches would you propose for classroom activities and group counseling?

## Motivational Interviewing

The **motivational interviewing** (MI) approach was originally conceptualized by William Miller and later more fully developed by Stephen Rollnick and Miller in the 1980s. It was first used in the addiction's counseling field and is now used in many different settings. Empirical research supports the effectiveness of MI for treating diverse populations for a variety of problems, including substance abuse, dietary issues, family planning, HIV prevention, etc. (Mason, 2009).

MI is defined as directive, client-centered, and eliciting change by helping clients explore and resolve ambivalence (Miller & Rollnick, 2002). Motivational interviewing places the counselor in the role of collaborator with the client and seeks to avoid power struggles that could lead to resistance. Confrontation and trying to force out feelings are discouraged (Brooks & McHenry, 2009; Rollnick & Miller, 1995; Rollnick, Miller, & Butler, 2008). In a school setting, motivational interviewing is intended to help counselors work with students who fluctuate between incongruent thoughts and behaviors (Biles & Eakin, 2010).

A school counselor using MI works to evoke the student's motivation based on the student's confidence and desire to make changes (Biles & Eakin, 2010). Although the desire may be there to make a change, there is also ambivalence in changing one's behavior or making a decision. MI normalizes ambivalence about changing and works through it as a natural part of the process of change (Rosengran, 2009).

### Techniques

There are four basic principles in the motivational interviewing approach: expressing empathy, developing a discrepancy, rolling with resistance, and support self-efficacy.

> *Expressing Empathy*—using the concept of genuineness first described by Rogers (Gladding, 2009), students who feel completely understood are less likely to experience resistance and may be more open to the counseling process.
>
> *Developing a Discrepancy*—By helping students to see the disconnect between their goals and their behaviors, change and growth may occur.
>
> *Rolling with Resistance*—Avoiding power struggles and arguments with students decreases resistance. Counselors working respectfully with students keep the door open for new possibilities while honoring their feelings and giving them the assurance that they are being heard.
>
> *Support Self-Efficacy*—Accentuating the positive and remaining hopeful when working with students during the change process can let students know that you believe in them and respect their choices.

More recently, Rollnick et al. (2008) described the principles using the acronym RULE: R—resist the righting reflex; U—understand your student's motivation; L—listen to your student; and E—empower your student. As school counselors, using RULE in your work with your students means resisting our tendency to want to fix the problems in students' lives; tapping into students' strengths and being fascinated with where their strengths and motivation come from; listening to students (with no hidden agendas or personal worldview); and empowering students to recognize their own self-efficacy and ability to be self-changers.

### Theory into Practice

Motivational interviewing has practical applications for school counselors. Often students are in the school counselor's office at the request of a teacher, an administrator, or a parent, not voluntarily. This instantly sets up a natural resistance on the part of the student. By joining effectively with the student, counselors can break down the resistance and help to initiate the change process. Students may also feel the intrinsic power differential that exists between them and a member of the school staff. Creating a climate of collaboration with the student can be a refreshing change and help them to see that the change they are potentially making is based on their own wants and needs and not on something that someone else is making them do. Therefore, their personal investment in the change process and its benefits is increased.

### Practical Application

*Kiley is a 16-year-old junior who was referred by her parents after having been caught experimenting with marijuana. She insists that she can stop any time she wants and doesn't understand what the problem is. During a career exploration exercise in sophomore year, Kiley expressed an interest in a*

## MEET KATHY BILES AND GENE EAKIN: USING MOTIVATION TO CHANGE AND ACHIEVE

Kathy Biles and Gene Eakin are counselor educators who first began using motivational interviewing (MI) and the Transtheoretical Stages of Change with middle school and high school students while working as school counselors. Kathy and Gene observed students making changes and becoming successful as a result of their working within the spirit of MI and using the principles of MI.

As school counselors, Kathy and Gene partnered with their students. While Kathy and Gene had their expertise in the school counseling arena, they believed in their students' expertise in their own lives, their circumstances, and their own strengths. Approaching your work with your students from a place of curiosity, rather than fixing, helps to identify the strengths your students already possess.

Kathy worked with middle school students individually and in pairs, using the principles and elements of MI. One memorable moment came when working with two eighth-grade boys who were participating in risky behavior and had a poor attendance record. These youth came in on a Monday morning, which had become a regular day to miss school, and requested to meet with Kathy. They wanted to talk about their confidence rulers and how they had done some things differently over the weekend. Listening, reflecting, and affirming their desire and change assisted to keep their momentum moving toward increased motivation and continued change.

During Gene's work at his high school, he conducted an MI-based group for 10 ninth graders who had earned two to six credits of a possible eight credits during first semester. These students had a 60 percent increase in credits earned during second semester and then also had a 40 percent increase in credits earned during the first semester of tenth grade, as compared with the first semester of ninth grade.

Inspired by the ninth graders' success, he then focused on 40 sophomores who were behind in credits and would not graduate if they did not start earning credits at a faster pace. Gene utilized a variety of MI strategies in his work with these students and his belief and hope was that the students had gained momentum to continue making behavior changes to succeed.

Their advice is to just begin to use MI by simply being present and listening to your students. Identify what is important to them, what they value, and the discrepancy between where they are currently and where they want to be. Our students have the ability to be self-changers.

*Kathy Biles, PhD, is a former middle school and high school counselor who is presently a counselor educator and coordinator of the school counseling program at Oregon State University. Kathy also recently served as the president of the Oregon School Counselor Association.*

*Gene Eakin is a former school counselor and supervisor for 23 years at Lebanon High School in Oregon. Gene is currently School Counseling Program Leader at Oregon State University where he has worked part-time or full-time since 1990. He also serves as an adjunct professor at Lewis and Clark College and Capella University.*

*career in law enforcement and perhaps some time in the U.S. Coast Guard. Kiley was always a solid student but is now failing two classes this quarter. Kiley no longer plays softball and has been seen with a new group of friends.*

How could motivational interviewing be useful in this situation?

## Solution Focused Counseling

**Solution focused counseling** or brief counseling was developed primarily by Insoo Berg and Steve De Shazer at the Brief Family Therapy Center in Milwaukee (Nichols & Schwartz, 2006). Like the motivational interviewing approach, solution focused counseling is characterized by the counselor in a collaborative and/or a one-down position. Davis and Osborn (2000) note, "the counselor assumes the role of the *student* and the student becomes the *teacher*. This means that in solution-focused counseling you, the school counselor, become the learner, and in turn, the student assumes the role of teacher or informant, telling you what the problem is and when a workable solution has been created" (p. 11). Using solution focused theory, students identify what works, discuss what has worked for them in the past, and discuss how they can construct workable solutions in the future.

### Techniques

Some techniques that are used in the solution focused model are counting on change, highlighting exceptions, the miracle question, the great instead, establishing measurable goals, and using scaling questions. All of the techniques associated with this model are forward-thinking and embrace a climate of openness to new possibilities.

Among other techniques, school counselors using the solution focused model employ curious and respectful listening skills, and carefully construct a change-oriented relationship that promotes student competence in understanding what changes have been or could be successful. Problems are clarified and specific goals are identified so that even the smallest change can be measured and used as a foundation to promote more change. Using the highlighting of exceptions techniques, students are asked to determine when the problem is not a problem or what circumstances keep the problem from happening (Legum, 2005; Patterson, 2009).

Changing the doing and/or viewing of the problem can also be powerful techniques that are used in this model. By paying attention to problems only, students may find themselves trapped in a cycle of defeating thoughts and behaviors. A shift in attention to solutions has the potential to break the cycle and allow new possibilities and ideas to emerge. Changing the doing of the problem is a behavioral technique that invites students to "do" something different in relationship to the problem and evaluate the positive and/or negative consequences of the change (O'Hanlon, 1999; Patterson, 2009).

By using measurable goals and scaling questions, counselors and students can view problems and their progress in creating or discovering solutions. If a situation has moved in a positive direction, why? Is it possible to do more to keep the positive momentum moving? In other words, do more of what works and do less of what does not (Davis & Osborn, 2000; Legum, 2005; O'Hanlon, 1999).

The miracle question invites students to pretend that a miracle occurred while they were sleeping and now the problem no longer exists. How would they know that the miracle happened? What are the signs of change? Are any of them happening right now? (Legum 2005).

### Theory into Practice

Schools are ideal environments for the use of solution focused counseling. Time away from instruction can have a detrimental effect on students and parents do not put children on buses every morning for them to participate in lengthy therapeutic activities designed to uncover unconscious drives. In addition, solution focused counseling can be characterized as a strengths-based theory, fostering in students a sense of mastery and independence (Legum, 2005).

### Practical Application

*Brent is in sixth grade and has come to you to talk about his test anxiety. He tells you that whenever Ms. Donnelly gives out a math test he starts to feel queasy, his palms get sweaty, and he can't remember any formulas or equations. You begin by asking Brent what exactly he wants to work on during this visit to your office. He says he wants to feel more confident about test-taking. You ask on a scale of 1 to 10 where Brent feels his confidence level is now about test taking, 10 being completely confident and 1 being not confident at all. Brent replies that he thinks he is at a 3 right now. You invite him to consider how he might move it to a 4 or a 5. You ask Brent if there was a time when his anxiety level was lower and why he thinks it was so. He replies that he felt more confident when he went to Ms. Donnelly's weekly extra-help sessions. He said he stopped going when after-school baseball practice started in the spring. He said he thinks he can talk to the coach and ask to be late once a week so he can go back to the extra-help sessions.*

How did solution-focused counseling help Brent?

## Choosing a Theoretical Approach

School counselors must be fully cognizant of which theoretical applications or dominant approaches are incorporated in the counseling process. School counselors who are confident in their knowledge, understanding, and application of theory will operate from a perspective that is compatible with their assumptions about student development progression, emotional well-being, and school appropriateness. The differential effectiveness of various approaches, a familiarity with a broad range of treatment systems (Seligman, 2001), and the melding of one's own knowledge and experiences in utilizing various theories has resulted in some clinicians choosing an eclectic or integrated approach. Taking an eclectic approach is a challenging choice; approaching treatment in an eclectic manner requires a solid foundation in knowledge and experience. School counselors do not always have the luxury of indefinite periods of time to work from a particular theoretical approach and sometimes choose to draw on more than one approach to work with students.

# THE PRACTICE OF COUNSELING SKILLS AND TECHNIQUES

Counseling is a continuous process, a series of stages that begins with exploration and investigation and terminates at an appropriate time when the client's (student's) goals are achieved. The stages are not necessarily sequential or discrete and overlap is common, but they offer a structure to help school counselors evaluate and monitor their level of skill and application of technique in the counseling process (Carkhuff, 1985; Corey, 2009; Egan, 1994; Gladding, 2009; Ivey, Ivey, & Simek-Morgan, 1993).

Stage 1: Establishing a Relationship

Stage 2: Setting the Tone in a Counseling Setting

Stage 3: Exploring the Issues

Stage 4: Setting Goals

Stage 5: Transitioning to Independence

## Establishing a Relationship

A strong relationship with a student is paramount to success in order to gain the commitment and willingness on the part of the student to establish and achieve the agreed-on goals defined by the counseling relationship. Relationship building starts with the initial contact between counselor and student. The relationship builds during the exploration of the issues that directly affect the student's state of mind, well-being, and motivation. The counselor's level of skill, selection of techniques, and theoretical orientation of the counselor influences the counseling relationship and ultimately the student's satisfaction and success.

Attending, an important counseling technique in the first stage, establishes the working relationship between client and counselee. The effective school counselor knows how to build rapport with students and considers all of the variables that influence a student's arrival at your door. Attending requires that the school counselor unilaterally focus on the student and avoid distractions and interruptions. Many students have learned to read adults and are highly intuitive and can easily recognize insincerity or lack of interest. Depending on their history and experiences, many students may come to counseling with resistance.

The counseling relationship can be affected by whether or not the student is referred by others or is a self-referral. Teachers and administrators may send a student to the counseling center and inadvertently or pointedly give the student the impression that they are going to see the school counselor for a disciplinary reproach, which creates a position of defensiveness and/or resistance to counseling. A teacher may send a student to seek remediation for problem or apathetic behavior. Appropriate referral approaches can be a staff development topic and increase the likelihood of relationship building and success. As a relationship begins to develop, consider the following:

- What is the student's motivation to engage in a counseling process?
- How does the student view the situation?
- Is the student open to learning new behaviors, motivated to seeking alternative solutions, willing to make a change?
- Does the student see how counseling can help?

Students may enter the counseling situation reluctantly or with no desire to change. Engaging students in the process of exploring options to change behavior is a constant challenge. Resistance to change and lack of commitment on the part of students to become engaged in their education are encounters. School counselors need to display unconditional acceptance and understanding to gain the confidence and trust of their young clients (Gladding, 2009). Accurately reflecting the students' feelings and capturing the content of what is shared facilitates the establishment of this trusting relationship. School counselors respond to the student in a manner that helps her or him integrate feelings, behaviors, and thought processing to influence the desired outcome or change.

When counseling is effective, then the school counselor directly affects the student's ability to maximize the educational process. The intentional counselor can generate multiple alternatives and approach a problem from many vantage points using a multitude of skills and personal qualities while adapting styles to individualistic needs and cultures (Ivey, 2010).

## Setting the Tone in a Counseling Session

School counselor behavior, skills, and techniques are carefully chosen to set a tone in the counseling session that will provide optimum opportunity for growth. Unconditional positive regard, active listening, attending, empathy, and congruence are considered by many in the profession as powerful tools in setting a tone conducive to client growth.

*Unconditional positive regard* is primarily rooted in respect and requires that the counselor accept the student in an open and respectful manner. This sets the tone for the student to reveal her or his thoughts in a manner that will not result in a judgmental response.

*Active listening* is the counselor's way of showing the student that she or he is paying close attention to everything that the child is sharing in the counseling session. Active listening clarifies the counselor's ability to confirm the nature of the problem or presenting issue (Carkhuff, 1985).

*Attending* is a way of behaving that attests to communication and understanding (Egan, 1994). The school counselor demonstrates by her or his physical behavior that psychological contact is established. Body position, eye contact, nonverbal encouragement, and a relaxed and open posture all contribute to the students' perception of the counselor's involvement.

*Empathy* is the counselor's ability to respond in a way that the student realizes that the counselor understands her or his frame of reference and point of view (Egan, 1994). A skilled counselor perceives the worldview as the student sees it and has the ability to communicate that understanding. Empathy involves the skills of perception and communication (Rogers, 1961).

*Congruence* displays genuineness and implies that the counselor is behaving in an open and honest manner (Rogers, 1980). There is no sense of artificiality about the manner in which the counselor is behaving. Congruence helps the student gain a sense of trust about the counseling relationship.

## Exploring the Issues

Frequently, the school counselor needs to help a student identify and clarify what has brought her or him to the counseling office in the first place. Depending on the developmental, cognitive, and social maturity level of the child, the process of exploring, identifying, and clarifying can be complex. School counselors need to be cognizant of moving too quickly or too slowly and making assumptions until the student reveals the problem. If the student defines the problem it increases her or his ownership—a necessary step if progress is to be made (Perls, 1969). There are a variety of techniques in the counselor's repertoire to help students illuminate the issues for themselves and you.

*Questioning* is both an art and a technique and must be appropriate for the developmental level of the child (Garbarino & Stott, 1989). Questioning is not an interrogation with a string of "why" questions. Interrogations lead to defensiveness and withdrawal. Rather, questioning is selectively used to enhance the counselor's understanding of what the student is communicating and to cause the student to self-disclose. As opposed to closed questions for which there is a "yes" or "no" response, open-ended questions support the conversation and engage the student as you are inviting her or him to talk.

*Focusing*, bringing the conversation back to the salient issues, is sometimes necessary when students stray away from the issues for too long. For some students the school counselor is the only adult in their life who provides undivided attention. For others, rambling in the conversation is a diversionary tactic to avoid the issue or potential conflict.

*Paraphrasing* is used to restate what the student has said by using almost the same wording but capturing the intent of both the content and the meaning. This technique offers the student an opportunity to review or reexamine both the content and the intent of the statement.

*Reflecting* helps the school counselor clarify the content of the student's statement. Reflecting means that the counselor synthesizes what was communicated and accurately shares this with the student, strengthening understanding, rapport, and communication.

*Exploring alternatives* assists the student in identifying courses of action prior to making a commitment to any one solution. This exploration can be done by the student or counselor gathering information, while at other times, it is the result of the student's participation in a formal decision-making process. Exploring alternatives helps students understand the necessity of gathering information and exploring options to make needed changes.

*Summarizing* offers the student a review of the thinking and processing that took place during the counseling session. Oftentimes the summary can "string together" or connect the multiplicity of issues, concerns, and explorations in a format that the student can understand and put into action.

Throughout the counseling process we constantly assess the student's ability to take control of the situation and make positive and constructive change. Students have minimal legal rights, little influence over the dysfunction in their family, and usually no control over the level of income in their household. However, with help, support, and confidence, they can learn to successfully overcome many of the obstacles they face at home and encounter in a school setting. As school counselors explore the issues that affect school success, so too they help their students identify barriers and challenges and address these in a plan of action.

## Setting Goals

Counseling helps students define for themselves what personal achievement and personal best mean for them and set goals toward this end. Counseling provides structure and a way of measuring the results of their efforts toward goal attainment. A course of action is mutually agreed on by the student and counselor and may involve negotiating and mediating. For most students goals need to be clearly stated, positive in nature, and approached in small increments. School counselors celebrate successes with students whether minuscule or huge.

## Transitioning to Independence

In the world of community-based organizations and mental health agencies, the term *terminating* the counseling relationship is often used. This is not as easily accomplished in a school setting. What will it take to maintain the appropriate level of support to ensure that the student can sustain the progress made to date and continue to grow in self-confidence and achieve self-efficacy? Although the student may no longer need to engage in frequent or scheduled counseling sessions, monitoring and evaluating progress is still needed. The continuity of a school setting facilitates the transition process for counselor and student as an abrupt termination of services would only be needed if the student leaves the school, parents refuse your involvement, or if there is some other interruption of the relationship.

How will you know that the student is ready to move on? A mutually developed transition plan will help the student assume independence and control. Students need to know that their counselor remains available even after the initial need has been reduced or eliminated (Corey, 2009; Corey et al., 1998). Because counseling is about change, it is necessary to make sure that the transition plan engages students in a process that can result in positive change, despite the situations and circumstances that envelop their day-to-day lives. The counseling process for the student was intended to make her or him personally stronger, make good choices, and assist the student in clarifying what she or he wants out of life, now and in the future. The transition plan will build on the student's coping and resiliency skills to continue progress despite environmental and societal influences.

## THE CHALLENGE OF COUNSELING INDIVIDUALS AND GROUPS IN SCHOOLS

Although the sphere of school counselor responsibility and influence has greatly expanded over the years, individual and group counseling in schools is not fully appreciated as an acceptable option to help students maximize the school experience. School counselors face limitations in the scope of counseling practice due to district policies and procedures, parental concerns, community values, time constraints, and sheer numbers of students. Faith groups may require an assurance that there is no encroachment on moral or ethical pressures that school-aged children experience.

Successful school counseling programs are designed and organized by counseling professionals who have a deep understanding of the factors that impinge on their ability to deliver individual and group counseling services to students. Through collaboration and teaming, school psychologists, school social workers, agency-based counselors, and school counselors can address the culture and norms and seek solutions as partners in prevention and intervention.

In addition to an in-depth knowledge and application of counseling theory, techniques, and process, schools' counselors must consider all aspects of diversity in their work with students to include gender, race, culture, religion, learning ability and disability, and sexual orientation. Appreciating diversity helps counselors to effectively develop a trusting relationship with students who bring a variety of different learning styles, cultural issues, attitudes, family pressures, and social mores and customs (ASCA, 2009; Holcomb-McCoy, 2004, 2007; Lee, 2007a).

As societal issues continue to grow in complexity and as peer pressure dominates the decision-making ability of most children, adolescents, and teenagers, educators and families alike turn to the school counselor for insight and assistance. Each student requires a different set of goals, presents a different set of challenges, and demands a different set of counseling skills and techniques (Sciarra, 2004). It is the school counselor who can make the difference in the lives of these students by supporting them as they cope with developmental and emotional challenges and by nurturing them as they achieve their goals and seek balance in their lives. This is the reason we choose the profession of school counseling.

## TECH TOOLS

When you become a school counselor, use the power of technology to maximize the grounding of your practice in counseling theory.

- Surf the American Counseling Association (ACA) website (www.counseling.org) to find out more about the various divisions and specialties within the counseling field.

- Establish an electronic forum with your colleagues to discuss strategies and techniques to help you do your job more effectively.
- Maintain an electronic journal of your applications of theory into practice.
- Use a database to categorize your practicum observations. Which theoretical approaches were most frequently used by school counselors?
- Construct "virtual" simulation activities for future role-play with students. Presentation software tools such as PowerPoint have easy-to-use graphics, sound, and animation that can help you capture students' attention more easily. Game-like simulations helps break down barriers and give students a comfortable and familiar medium to explore.
- Search websites of organizations such as the Association of Supervision and Curriculum Development or the National Association of Secondary School principals to learn more about models such as those proposed by William Glasser, Maslow, and others in school settings.

## Internet Resources

All Kids Grieve: www.allkidsgrieve.org

Children and Grief: www.aacap.org/publications/factsfam/grief.htm

Cinematherapy: www.cinematherapy.com

Connect for Kids: www.connectforkids.org

Crisis Communications Guide and Toolkit: www.nea.org/crisis

Family Policy Compliance Office: http://www2.ed.gov/policy/gen/guid/fpco/index.html

Helping Children Deal with Deployment: http://www.nasponline.org/resources/crisis_safety/parents-called-to-active.pdf

Internet concerns—Keeping children safe online: http://www.nasponline.org/publications/cq/cq342internetsafety_ho.aspx

Motivational Interviewing: http://www.motivationalinterview.org/

National Institute of Mental Health: http://www.nimh.nih.gov/index.shtml

National Institute on Alcohol Abuse and Alcoholism: http://www.niaaa.nih.gov/

National Institute on Drug Abuse: http://www.nida.nih.gov/

National Mental Health Information Center: http://mentalhealth.samhsa.gov/

National Center to Improve Recruitment and Retention of Qualified Personnel for Children with Disabilities: http://www.personnelcenter.org/

REBT information: http://www.rebt.org/

Solution Focused Brief Therapy Association: http://www.sfbta.org/

Substance Abuse and Mental Health Services Administration: http://www.samhsa.gov/

Talking with Children, Tips for Parents: www.nasponline.org

Tragic Times, Healing Words: www.sesameworkshop.org

William Glasser Institute: http://www.wglasser.com/index.php?option=com_content&task=view&id=13&Itemid=28

## *School Counselor Casebook: Voices from the Field*

### The Scenario Reviewed

Katie's dad abruptly left their home over the weekend. She has not heard from him for three days. Her second-grade teacher came to you to talk about the dramatic change in her behavior—she is withdrawn and cannot concentrate. How will you address her needs through individual counseling?

### A Practitioner's Approach

Here's how a practicing school counselor responded to the school counselor casebook challenge:

Katie is having great difficulty coping with the abrupt absence of her father. As she is only seven years old, Katie is lacking the skills she needs to deal with feelings of loss, sadness, and disappointment.

Before I met with Katie, I called her mom to see if she can offer any insight into why Katie was reacting as she is, perhaps gain insight as to her relationship with her dad, and gain permission to work with Katie and talk to her teacher. I also offered to help her mom find some resources to help them both, such as relevant books and family support groups.

I decided to use the person-centered theoretical approach (Rogers, 1961) with Katie. Through active listening and reflection, I focused on creating a positive environment where Katie felt comfortable expressing her feelings. I let her know that she was not alone in the situation and it was not her fault that her father left. Katie and I also discussed positive coping strategies or things she can do when she is feeling sad, such as talk to a friend, write in a journal, draw a picture, or play a game.

I provided Katie's teacher with strategies for how she can support Katie in the classroom and help all of the students understand the many different family situations that exist. For example, her teacher could read aloud books that portray different types of families, such as *Goodnight, Daddy* by Angela Seward.

Katie will continue to need ongoing support until she becomes more accepting of the situation at home and she and her mom establish a new lifestyle. I also need to work with Katie to prepare her just in case her father returned. To closely monitor how she is doing, I follow up with classroom observations as well as communicate frequently with her teacher to see how she is adjusting. I have ongoing communication with Katie's mom to maximize the home-school connection. Most importantly, Katie is aware that she can come talk to me anytime she has the need. We all want her to have a successful year in school as she also learns to cope with a very stressful and potentially traumatic situation.

*Tara Benevento has been an elementary school counselor for three years at the Roosevelt School in River Edge, New Jersey. Prior to becoming a school counselor, she was a teacher for three years and was invited to join Chi Sigma Iota, the Counseling Academic and Professional Honor Society as a master's student. Tara is also a member of the New Jersey School Counselor Association.*

# LOOKING BACK: SALIENT POINTS

### Counseling in the Complex World of Schools

Abuse, dysfunctional home environments, blended families, hunger, poverty, violence, harassment, bullying, peer pressure, and homelessness are just some of the issues and pressures students encounter and struggle with on a daily basis. Although many children have developed the coping and resiliency skills needed to survive and even thrive, a growing number develop emotional, social, and behavioral problems that necessitate intervention.

### Counseling Students: Purpose and Limitations

Counseling in schools is a complex helping process in which the counselor establishes a trusting and confidential working relationship. The focus of counseling in schools is on making positive change, goal setting, problem solving, decision making, and discovering personal meaning related to learning and development (ASCA, 1998). School counselors can assess the need for counseling services and establish clear goals with students to create benefits for all involved, including parents.

### Theoretical Underpinnings

Counseling theories provide a point of reference from which the counselor develops a personal perspective of human growth, development, and behavior. Counselors must recognize and choose the appropriate behaviors and strategies that best match their theoretical approach and philosophical orientation and select different theories and approaches according to the models used and the assistance that a student needs.

*Gestalt* theory emphasizes the present and supports the equation now = experience = awareness = reality.

*Person centered* theory focuses on the "core conditions" of genuineness, empathy, positive regard, and concreteness, all of which are considered universally essential to all helping relationships and the counseling process.

*Individual psychology* encourages the client to be well aware of her or his surroundings and environment and supports healthy development to overcome any feelings of inferiority.

*Behavioral counseling* works with the premise that all behavior is learned and that learning is effective in changing maladaptive behavior.

*Reality therapy* encourages the client to set realistic goals and take ownership of goals, thus accepting responsibility for choices in life and to obtain what she or he wants in the present and future.

*Cognitive behavior therapy* assists clients in being able to deal with life and accomplish personal and professional goals.

*Rational-emotive behavior* therapy focuses on helping people live balanced, productive, and more rational lives by limiting the demands that one makes on oneself.

*Existential theory* emphasizes the importance of examining anxiety, values, freedom, and responsibility to find meaning. The client uncovers life's meaning by doing a deed, experiencing a value, or by suffering.

*Motivational interviewing* seeks to support people's desire to change by maximizing their personal motivation for change while working with their ambivalence and resistance.

*Solution focused counseling* helps move people from a problem-centered approach to an approach that highlights solutions and times when the problem is not a problem.

### Acquiring Counseling Skills and Techniques

Counseling, like the other key elements of a school counseling program, is a process, a series of sequential stages that begins with exploration and investigation and ends when the goals are achieved. Many factors will influence the counseling process and the success of the client, and these include the skill, techniques, and theoretical orientation of the counselor

### The Challenge of Counseling in Schools

Counseling is one component of a school counseling program. It is paramount to counselor training, to interactions with students and other stakeholders, and to acquiring a professional identity. Specialized training in counseling is what differentiates the work of counselors from those who advise or guide.

## KEY TERMS

Counseling p. 31

Counseling process p. 31

Counseling theory p. 31

Gestalt theory p. 33

Person-centered theory p. 35

Individual psychology p. 36

Rational emotive behavior therapy p. 42

Behavioral therapy p. 43

Existential theory p. 47

Motivational interviewing p. 48

Solution focused counseling p. 51

## LEARNING EXTENSIONS/MAKING CONNECTIONS

1.  Reflect on the personal qualities that a school counselor should possess to successfully engage students in the counseling process. Which qualities do you need to further develop? How will you do this?

2.  How would you conduct a first counseling session with an elementary or middle school or high school student? What preparation needs to be done in advance? Outline the steps that you would follow.

3.  Reflect on your personal experience(s) with counseling involving yourself or someone close to you, in a school setting or in a private/agency setting. Consider the insecurities, anxieties, and

uncertainties faced when the process began. As a counselor in school, what can you do to engage the student early on in the session and alleviate some of her or his anxiety?

4. Create a theory summary chart for your personal use. The chart should have five columns: Theory, Summary, Goals of Therapy, Techniques, and Applications in the School Setting.

5. Name the theory from which each of the following techniques is derived. Give an example of a situation in which it could be used:

   a. Saying to the student/client: "You feel _____ because you _____ and you want _____."
   b. Expressing genuine confidence in the student and using encouragement.
   c. Asking the student/client to complete this sentence: I take responsibility for _____.
   d. Discussing the difference between friendly competition and "one-upmanship."
   e. Saying to the student/client: "How can you remove those self-defeating thoughts that are holding you back from doing better?"

# Counseling Practice in Schools

## CHAPTER OBJECTIVES

*By the time you have completed this chapter, you should be able to*

- articulate the multitude of counseling practices and applications in a school setting;

- define the multi-dimensions of counseling in schools including individual counseling, group counseling, and the school counseling curriculum;

- discuss the school counselor's role in gathering, interpreting, and presenting testing and assessment data;

- design opportunities to work with teachers on student development/behavior management issues;

- describe how to help students build resiliency and acquire the developmental assets.

---

## *School Counselor Casebook: Getting Started*

### The Scenario

You have just left your middle school improvement team meeting and your head is spinning. The primary topic of conversation was an increased number of reported incidents of bullying and harassment. Your principal suggested in front of all of the committee members that individual counseling for all of the students involved would be the perfect remedy.

You responded that individual counseling is only a small part of the solution and that using classroom lessons and group counseling are also effective and efficient ways to address a potential schoolwide problem. Before the meeting broke up, you reminded the group that alleviating bullying and harassment required a commitment from the entire faculty and staff if any positive change would be realized. With a personal caseload of more than 600 students, you are feeling pretty overwhelmed.

### Thinking about Solutions

As you read this chapter, think about how you will educate your principal to help her or him understand that individual counseling is not the only solution for intervention. Understanding that buying and harassment are systemic concerns, how might you get your colleagues involved? What options might you present to your principal?

---

## APPLICATIONS OF COUNSELING IN SCHOOLS

### The Starfish

There was a young man walking down a deserted beach before dawn. In the distance he saw a frail old man. As he approached the old man, he saw him picking up stranded starfish and tossing them back into the sea. The young man gazed in disbelief and watched as the old man carefully picked up the starfish, one by one, and gently tossed them back into the water. He asked, "Why do you spend so much energy doing what seems to be a waste of time?" The old man replied that the stranded starfish would die if left in the morning sun. "But there must be thousands of beaches and millions of starfish," exclaimed the young man. "How can you make a difference?" The old man looked down at the small starfish in his hand, and as he threw it to the safety of the sea, he said, "I just made a difference to this one."

—*Source unknown*

There was a time, and not too long ago, when it was expected that a school counselor would spend the preponderant amount of her or his time working with students, one at a time. Students who were in crisis or in trouble usually were sent to the school counselor. Like the starfish, the school counselor picked them up one by one, used the best counseling skills possible, and then set them back on their feet. The focus of attention was on individual intervention; however, with large caseloads the sphere of influence remained small. Energy was expended predominantly on those who sought assistance or with those students who were brought to the school counselor's office for immediate attention and needed intervention or crisis support. Counselors recognized that effectiveness was limited by time constraints; the ability to intervene and assist more students in this manner remained elusive.

School counselors know that much more needs to be accomplished than saving one "starfish" at a time by picking it up, supporting it, and placing it gently back into the sea. Is there an assurance that the starfish will not find its way back to the beach after being placed in the sea? How can we prevent the starfish from washing up on shore in the first place?

The transformed school counselor looks at the cause and effect that lie at the root of the problem. Why are so many starfish (or children) finding their way to our shores (our offices)? What is the fundamental cause of this dilemma? Oftentimes, the answers lie not with the individual student but in the systemic issues that cloud our schools and community. Why are so many students adrift or, worse, left to survive on their own? We must value the importance of working with some students one on one, but when we look deeply within our school system, we will discover that we can reduce and eliminate academic, career, and personal-social barriers by working parsimoniously and utilizing effective prevention and intervention methods.

*Counseling*, the term that defines our profession, is preeminent in the work of school counselors. Counseling is a helping process implemented by trained and credentialed personnel that involves a variety of strategies and activities that help students explore academic, career, and personal/social issues that can impede healthy development or academic progress (ASCA, 2005). Counseling skills and techniques underpin the ability of school counselors to lead, advocate, use data to contribute to school improvement, and team and collaborate. Counseling theory and technique hold a paramount position in training, in interactions with students and other stakeholders, and, most importantly, is the key indicator of one's professional identity. Specialized training in counseling differentiates the work of school counselors from those who advise or guide. Counseling and the counseling relationship is the foundation on which candidates are prepared to be school counselors in the university preparation programs.

The increased need for students to have counseling in schools and agencies has become more apparent as documented occurrences of children's personal, social, and emotional difficulties have been evidenced in violent, disruptive, and aggressive behavior (Likona, 2004; Lockwood, 2008; Luongo, 2000). Schools are a significant source of referrals of young people to mental health agencies for increasingly complex problems (Center for Mental Health in Schools, 2008).

## THE AMERICAN REALITY

Each young person is fully prepared for adulthood, with a supportive family and community, effective school, and high-quality health care.
The American Dream

- One out of 10 children has a serious emotional disturbance; more children suffer from psychiatric illness than from leukemia, diabetes, and AIDS combined.
- Only 20 percent of children who have emotional disturbance receive treatment.
- Emotional disturbance is associated with the highest rate of school dropout among all disability groups.
- Suicide is the leading cause of death among 15- to 24-year-olds.

Source: Engaging in the Next Steps, 2008. NYS Office of Mental Health, p. 3

Adolescent suicide rates continue to be a major concern for counselors working with adolescents, and suicide follows accidents and homicide as the third leading cause of death for youth (Children's Defense Fund, 2010). Homelessness, poverty, domestic and community violence, alcohol, and drug abuse all affect the mental health and well-being of our children (New York State Office of Mental Health, 2008). The lines have blurred between school and community with interrelated problems flowing back and forth.

> Research suggests that high-quality counseling services can have long-term effects on a child's well-being and can prevent a student from turning to violence and drug or alcohol abuse. High-quality school counseling services can improve a student's academic achievement. Studies on the effects of school counseling have shown positive effects on student's grades, reducing classroom disruptions, and enhancing teachers' abilities to manage classroom behavior effectively. High-quality school counseling services also can help address students' mental health needs. (U.S. Dept. of Education, 2002, p. 117)

In Chapter 2, key theoretical models were presented that can be applied to counseling situations in a school setting. Skilled school counselors select the appropriate theories that consider the age and mental and emotional maturity for students who present themselves in need of either individual or group counseling. Theoretical orientation(s) can influence the design and delivery of the entire comprehensive school counseling program from prevention and intervention (responsive) services to system support. Whether school counselors apply reality therapy, rational emotive behavior, or cognitive-behavioral theory, the growth and learning benefit to the student cannot be minimized.

For example, person-centered theory (Rogers, 1961) promotes the use of unconditional positive regard, which implies a deep and genuine concern for the individual. When utilizing unconditional positive regard, the counselor would create an environment that is safe and nonjudgmental in an individual, group counseling, or student planning session. School counselors can apply the same principle to the creation of a safe and respectful school culture and use system support to foster collaboration and teaming. In a classroom guidance setting, the school counselor ensures that every student's opinion is valid and that all contributions are welcome. This is just one example of applying theory in the larger context of the school counseling program and not treating activities as unrelated services.

The concept of a comprehensive program provides a philosophy and structure for the professional school counselor. The overall program is comprehensive in scope, preventative in design, and developmental in nature (ASCA, 2005). Counseling knowledge and theoretical orientation influence the selection of techniques, strategies, and approaches and informs practice across all the components of a comprehensive program. The ASCA National Model, which we will study extensively in Chapter 7, has an organizational structure and the delivery system is the quadrant under which counseling strategies, services, and activities align.

A counselor's insight and instinct are best supported by knowledge, skills, and experience that consider both the needs of the student and the presenting situation. School counselors who are secure in their knowledge and understanding of theory have the ability to transform theory and techniques into applications that provide for student growth and development. The application and integration of theory is not owned exclusively by "responsive services" or perceived as magic-wand waving. Theory into practice is thus more fully aligned with the mission of each school and supports each student's academic, career, and personal-social development.

By utilizing leadership, advocacy, teaming, and collaboration, school counselors work diligently to promote equity and access to rigorous educational experiences for all students. As social justice advocates, school counselors support a safe learning environment and work to safeguard the human rights of all members of the school community (Sandhu, 2000). School counselors address the needs of all students through culturally relevant prevention and intervention programs as a component of a comprehensive school counseling program (Lee, 2007a). Transformed school counselors can shift from the traditional individual remediation model to a proactive counseling process that places greater emphasis on skill building rather than deficit reduction (Galassi & Akos, 2007). Counseling in schools is then viewed as learning, as a problem-solving process, and as a developmental growth process (ASCA, 2005; Campbell & Dahir, 1997; Gysbers, 2006; Myrick, 2003b).

Counseling, equated with emotional well-being, is flexible in its approach and is applied to a wide variety of student academic, career, and personal/social needs. School counselors typically serve large numbers of students, parents, and teachers. Not every student needs counseling in the formal sense; it is critical to assess which students will benefit from the counseling relationships in a school setting (ASCA, 2005). Counselors become aware of individual student issues, concerns, needs, and problems through a variety of sources including student self-referral and referrals from faculty, family members, or other acquaintances of the student.

# THE MANY DIMENSIONS OF THE SCHOOL COUNSELOR'S ROLE

As discussed in Chapter 1, role confusion has prevailed as school counseling was equated predominantly with **individual counseling**; traditional school counseling practice has been perceived as reactive and remedial in comparison to the contemporary transformed and new vision approach, which is proactive and positive. Some schools of thought view counseling in schools as an opportunity for students to move from the negative emotions generated by involvement in certain situations to a focus on the positive emotions that could be generated by the same situation (Fredrickson, 2001). As counselors work with students on identifying the issues necessary to be more successful, decision making is often at the core of behavioral change because choices can often be overwhelming and peer influences play heavily in a child's ability to choose wisely and in her or his best interests.

Counseling also is used with individuals and groups to address issues such as grief, substance abuse, socialization issues, learning frustrations, interpersonal skills, stress, and behavior modification. Counseling services also are affected by many factors including the depth of counseling considered appropriate in a school setting (Geroski & Knauss, 2000). Each state has statutes that regulate the scope and parameters of counseling in the schools. Parents and community school boards can dictate guidelines regarding parental permission and the purpose and duration of counseling services (Baker & Gerler, 2008), and in some instances school boards have claimed that it is beyond the school's authority to provide mental health services in the schools (Kaplan, 1996). Specifically it should be noted that the American School Counselor Association National Model states that school counselors do not provide traditional therapeutic sessions but work with the presenting issues and problems from a developmental perspective to ensure the student's educational success.

School counselors always consider the reason for referral, the development stage and cognitive processing skills of the child, as well as cultural background and influences when selecting a theoretical approach or techniques. School counselors have an ethical obligation to make certain that students understand the difference between a school counseling activity and the purpose and nature of the counseling relationship (ASCA, 2010a). Counselors must also ensure that students understand the purpose of engaging in counseling as confusion or distress can result if a child is unsure as to why she or he has been called to the counseling center. Resentment of the reason for the referral can lead to student resistance to counseling. Counseling in schools often is equated with "having a problem" or "being in trouble," and the potential stigma on the student must be taken into consideration and eliminated. As the developmental age appropriateness of the student is considered, it is important that confidentiality is carefully explained in a way that very young students can understand. For older students, privacy and confidentiality is always a cause for concern (Remley & Herlihy, 2009).

Professional school counselors are responsible for a wide range of services and activities involving students, parents, teachers, administrators, and community members. In addition to individual counseling, services are delivered in groups, through classroom guidance lessons, in large assemblies, and through parent meetings and faculty presentations. With so many needs and limited time, a new school counselor could easily run randomly putting out one fire after another, which can lead to constant feelings of being overwhelmed and frustrated. Years ago Bilzing (1996) reminded us, "No more random acts of guidance." School counselors keep their focus by aligning their work to the goals of school improvement and student needs as revealed by data, observation, and family and faculty input.

## ASSESSING NEEDS: DESIGNING INTERVENTIONS

School counselors select counseling approaches that are aligned with the intervention and take developmental needs and cultural influences into account (Baker, 2008). Student interventions reside in the responsive services component of the delivery system in the comprehensive school counseling program, including the ASCA National Model (2005), which we will study in depth in Chapter 7.

Active listening skills, the utilization of developmentally appropriate interviewing techniques (Ivey & Ivey, 2010), and sensitivity to the presenting concerns are essential in the early stages of gathering information for an individual or group of students. To assess students' needs, school counselors consider at all times their social, emotional, cognitive, and physical development and how these influence the students' relationships with teachers, family, peers; school experience; and the students' strengths and talents (Orton, 1997). Utilizing both formal and informal methods of assessing an individual or group of students presenting concerns helps school counselors determine which is the most effective intervention to provide in a counseling context. Formal assessment can include appraisal instruments such as interest checklist, behavioral scales, and attitudinal measures; whereas informal assessments are the result of observation, conversations with teachers and parents, or reviewing a thought paper that a student may have written.

Using a variety of assessment tools, including a first or second interview with the student, provides the foundation to select the most appropriate intervention that will reflect the student's current developmental and maturity stage, personality characteristics, cultural influences, and current situation. For some students, individual counseling may be the most appropriate venue; for others, **group counseling** or participating in a classroom lesson might be the most appropriate option to initiate the counseling process with the understanding that flexibility is key to finding the most successful approach. In counseling, as in any situation involving human dynamics, no one approach will work for a multitude of students or situations.

### Individual Counseling

Many external and internal factors can affect a student's academic, career, and personal/social development. The wide range of complicated issues that face 21st-century school-aged children continues to increase as societal issues also become more complex. Professional school counselors know when a situation calls for individual counseling and also know when a serious issue requires an outside referral for a therapeutic intervention that would be outside the scope of practice of a counselor in a school setting. Counseling is an important component of the role of school counselors and it is through academic, career, and personal/social counseling that school counselors contribute to improving student success (House & Hayes, 2002).

Individual counseling is both a proactive and reactive response to student needs. The counselor explores a problem or topic of interest through a personal and private interaction with a student. This face-to-face meeting with a school counselor provides a student maximum privacy to freely explore ideas, feelings, and behaviors. School counselors convey in actions and words, trust and confidence, always considering the rights, integrity, and welfare of students.

School counselors can be challenged by which students need the benefit of individual counseling as well as how the scheduled session can fit into a student's busy day. The decisions as to which theoretical orientation is developmentally appropriate and best matches the student's presenting problem as well as monitoring the effectiveness of the counseling process present challenges (Cobia & Henderson, 2007). Establishing a relationship in an individual session helps the student understand the purpose of the session as many children have no understanding of the purpose of counseling. They may believe that it is because they are in trouble or that there is something terribly wrong with them. Children too are privy to adult and media commentary about the value of the counseling experience. Children also may perceive the counseling session as something that someone else—a parent or teacher—wants for them and thus are unmotivated or indifferent to the prospect of change. The end result may be different than for the student who initiates assistance with relationships, emotional balance, or behavior management.

In a **comprehensive school counseling program**, individual counseling is considered a responsive service and part of the delivery component. However, the experienced school counselor who is well skilled in individual counseling knows when this approach will be most effective and when alternatives such as group counseling or classroom guidance would best benefit the student's situation. It is also important to be able to explain the diversity of approaches to colleagues and administrators who may perceive individual counseling to be the only effective "remedy." When school counselors use individual counseling exclusively, they significantly reduce their ability to reach all of their students in a meaningful way.

## Group Counseling

Group counseling is an effective and efficient way for a counselor to deliver direct services to two or more students simultaneously who have common concerns or problem behavior. The discussions may be relatively unstructured or quite formal in focus with specified goals for each session. Group topics can range from common school success topics such as motivation to more dire topics such as anger management. Group counseling requires a high degree of complex counseling skills and techniques to manage and organize group sessions and facilitate appropriate topic and age group interaction.

Group members have an opportunity to learn from each other. Students can learn much from each other and group counseling can be perceived as developmentally appropriate as well as an effective pedagogical tool (Goodnough & Lee, 2004). They can share ideas, give and receive feedback, increase their awareness, gain new knowledge, practice skills, and think about their goals and actions (Greenberg, 2003). Students also gain insight from exploring their feelings, attitudes, and behaviors. Group counseling can reduce social isolation and build skills in peer relations to create a sense of belonging (Arman, 2000). Group counseling specifically engages the students in behavioral analysis, change, and adjustment.

Group counseling can proactively or reactively address problems, or it can be growth-centered, where general topics are related to personal and academic development as students can acquire and practice new behaviors while seeking feedback and in some instances approval from their peers. Group counseling can also teach students developmental advocacy and help them acquire the skills, attitudes, and knowledge that are associated with healthy youth development (Galassi & Akos, 2004b). School counselors also need to be cognizant to collaborate with teachers to set up groups.

### Applying Group Facilitation Skills

School counselors who have acquired the specialized skills associated with group counseling can also apply these to other school-based situations. The Association for Specialists in Group Work (ASGW, 2007) defined four specific group experiences: task groups, psychoeducational, group counseling, and group psychotherapy. These different forms of group work offer ample opportunities for prevention, intervention, and remediation. However, in a school setting counselors predominantly work with psychoeducational groups and group counseling.

The primary purpose of a psychoeducational group is to help students learn new skills and practice these skills in a safe and supportive environment, while group counseling, as explained above, offers students the opportunity, as in individual counseling, to address a behavior that the group members wish to discuss and develop the growth skills necessary to make a positive change. Psychoeducational groups tend to be more structured and content orientated while group counseling is more process oriented (Newsome & Harper, 2010). Evening parenting groups on skill-building topics and specialized tasks and knowledge-building groups for teachers are examples of using group counseling and process skills to provide system support services as part of the overall comprehensive school counseling program.

School counselors can also use their group counseling skills to work with teachers, administrators, parents, and community members to facilitate task groups such as a crisis-intervention team collaborating on a particular assignment. School counselors are highly skilled in group process and group dynamics and can bring this needed skill set "to the table" when faculty are debating important school-based issues around policy and practice. Using group work skills to help facilitate adult problem solving is an invaluable contribution to helping your school's administration and faculty meet their goals.

## School Counseling/Student Development Curriculum

The school counseling (guidance) or the student development curriculum (Dahir, 2009) is another form of a psychoeducational group experience and a component in the delivery quadrant of the ASCA model (2005). The **school counseling/student development curriculum** is a sequence of learning activities and strategies that address the academic, career, and personal social development of every student (Gysbers & Henderson, 2000). The student development curriculum promotes knowledge, attitudes, and skills through instruction in three areas: academic achievement, career development, and personal-social growth. The curriculum is planned, ongoing, has a scope and sequence, and is systematic with units of instruction aligned with the ASCA National Standards and input from school and community stakeholders. School counselors provide instruction tied to identified competencies that are outcome based and are articulated with the school's core academic curriculum (ASCA, 2005). The school counseling or student development curriculum is most frequently delivered through the following methods:

- Classroom Instruction: School counselors provide instruction, in collaboration with classroom teachers, staff, and/or other stakeholders, around topics such as motivation, getting along with others, goal setting, decision making, career and college planning, respecting self and others, peer pressure, career awareness, conflict resolutions, etc. Existing curricula such as Second Step, Steps to Respect, Bully Busters, Student Success Skills, and Positive Behavior Management may also be used as part of the curriculum.

- Interdisciplinary Curriculum Development: School counselors work in conjunction with staff to develop lessons that connect the academic content areas and the student development (guidance) curriculum. Examples may include organizational and study skills, test-taking strategies, community service, etc. Teachers and counselors can use literature to teach getting along with others and how to address conflict as many of the students' required readings have thematic relationship to personal and interpersonal relations. Ethics and decision making can align with science classes while history and geography classes provide the counselor with the ability to work with students on culture understanding. Math classes lend themselves to problem solving and using relevant polls and surveys to calculate, analyze, and visually display data. The possibilities are endless.

- Large-group activities: School counselors may use these settings such as grade-level meetings to provide information to students and then follow up with classroom activities or individual sessions. These can be most effective with older students such as eighth graders who are exploring high school options or teaching ninth graders how to get their Web-based career plan started. The effectiveness of this type of informational session resides in the type of follow-up that is scheduled.

The school counseling curriculum is not counseling in the pure sense; it is an import delivery mechanism in a comprehensive school counseling program. The classroom experience allows the school counselors to affect students' thinking and influence their choices. However, it does not have as a primary goal the development of the counselor-client (student) relationship, the trademark of counseling. The school counseling/student development curriculum is designed by the school counselor in collaboration with teachers and other specialists and connected to the school improvement goals. The curriculum is intentional with a specific purpose and goal in mind and is instructive and cognitive in nature. Classroom programs are most successful when they are developed as a result of data-driven decision-making and can demonstrate their effectiveness through measures of accountability.

School counseling curriculum can be used as a tool that supports the need for group and individual counseling. For example, a school counselor in a middle school may use classroom guidance lessons to "teach" students how to protect themselves from sexual harassment. The counselor might also need to visit the same class to process a classroom incident that involved the majority of the children in a sexual harassment incident. From the lessons delivered in the classroom and the observations of the counselor and the classroom teacher, some students may present themselves needing further support and intervention through group and individual counseling.

Counselors also need skill development to deliver student development curriculum including lesson design, assessment strategies, and classroom management techniques. New counselors without previous classroom teaching

## SCHOOL COUNSELING/STUDENT DEVELOPMENT CURRICULUM LESSON PLAN

Unit/Topic:

Title of Lesson:                               Grade:

ASCA Standard:

Competency:

School Improvement Goal:

Learning Objective(s):

Collaborators:

Materials:

Learning Activities:

Time Available for Lesson:

    Introduction:

    Activity:

    Conclusion:

Measurable Outcome:

Follow-up Plan:

experience can benefit from collaborating and teaming with more experienced professionals.

Utilizing a school counseling/student development curriculum is an effective and efficient way of abiding by the law of parsimony and allows for a large number of students to benefit from prevention and intervention strategies. It provides a forum to reach every child in your building and provide knowledge and skills around important topics. After the lesson(s) some students will need additional "reinforcement" or group counseling, whereas a few students may require one-on-one support through individual counseling. In classroom instruction teachers often deliver a whole-group lesson. Some students may need a small-group follow-up lesson; a few may need individual tutoring. A similar analogy can be used for the counseling process:

| | FROM CLASSROOM TEACHER | FROM SCHOOL COUNSELOR |
|---|---|---|
| All Students Receive ——> | Subject Classroom Lesson | School Counseling/ Student Development Curriculum |
| Some Students Receive ——> | Small-Group Remediation | Group Counseling |
| A Few Students Receive ——> | Individual Extra Help | Individual Counseling |

## APPLICATIONS OF TESTING AND ASSESSMENT

Since the onset of No Child Left Behind, the continued emphasis on **assessment and testing** significantly affects every member of the student population and is an important component of the work of school counselors (Wall & Walz, 2004). Frequently in the absence of a school psychologist, the school counselor is the only professional with a background in testing and assessment. It is not uncommon for school counselors to find themselves involved in situations that require different levels of assessment; they also must be prepared to administer tests and interpret the results. With the proliferation of students undergoing assessment, and testing for special education and/or 504 accommodations, school counselors must understand the nature and purpose of different tests and assess the data that accompany these decisions, especially if they are to act as competent advocates for students and their families (Guindon, 2003; Wall & Walz, 2004). It is also ethically important that school counselors communicate to colleagues, parents, and students that standardized test results are not the only indicator of student success; multiple measures of assessment are needed to understand the learning dynamics of the whole child.

Assessment involves gathering data and information, researching and interviewing, analyzing the variables, looking for patterns, and organizing the results in a way that has meaning for decision making and/or problem solving. School counselors can teach students how to conduct a self-assessment and self-awareness about their interests, achievement, aptitude, and motivation to help them further plan for their futures. Testing, on the other hand, is a subset of assessment for the purposes of selection or placement, checking for understanding of content, measuring cognitive ability, identifying personality traits, and discovering career preferences (Anastasi, 1992). Testing in PreK–12 schools is most frequently aligned with academic achievement. With the current demand for results, decisions regarding student and school performance are often based on test data (Guindon, 2003).

Testing and assessment have evolved over the years from an initial focus on vocational guidance in the early 1900s to the more complex processes of psychological appraisal and evaluation. The impact on school was more dramatic in the mid-1950s when the National Defense Education Act (NDEA) provided funding incentives to identify students with the aptitude to successfully pursue mathematics and science careers. The mandates of No Child Left Behind (2001) has placed undue pressure on schools for accountability of results as demonstrated especially by the proliferation of high-stakes testing from grade 3 to high school graduation. The law required state-developed annual assessments in grades 3 through 8 and additional high school testing is required for achieving a diploma. The results of high-stakes testing affected annual promotion from grade level to grade level as well as the rating of each school building, which determines each school's level of success in educating its students. The Blueprint for Reform (2010) continues the emphasis on standards-based instruction, outcome-based assessment, and teacher performance aligned with student results. With this continued spotlight on testing and results-based education, more than ever before school counselors often are assigned the coordination, administration, and interpretation of test results (Schmidt, 2007).

A test can only depict a moment in time; it is a snapshot of a performance. As advocates, school counselors can remind teachers, parents, and students too that a single test score does not provide enough information to make significant and important decisions. An ASCA position statement recognizes the use of standardized testing as one of a range of measures used to assess student performance and learning (ASCA, 2007).

There are many different kinds of standardized tests and descriptions that can be found in the *Mental Measurement Yearbook*, first published in 1938 by Oscar Buros. The 18th edition (Spies, Carlson, & Geisinger, 2010) contains reviews of more than 400 newly published or revised tests and is a comprehensive resource to identify and evaluate various types of instruments including psychological, critical thinking, personality, achievement, and school ability tests.

A variety of standardized tests are commonly used in a school setting and are categorized in the following ways: achievement, intelligence, aptitude, career, personality, and diagnostic. Definitions of each of these follow.

*Achievement tests* measure a student's knowledge of a subject or task; these tests are often normed, which means one can compare progress of an individual or group of students as compared to other individuals or groups. Achievement tests are teacher designed or standardized. Most often standardized tests are used to assess knowledge and growth, measure academic progress, and demonstrate progress in a particular subject or across the content areas.

*Intelligence scales* are used to evaluate intelligence and cognitive abilities. These tests are sometimes used to assess possible learning disabilities, developmental disabilities, psychoeducational evaluations for special education placements, and also to place children in gifted programs. The battery of cognitive tests measure fluid reasoning, knowledge, quantitative reasoning, visual-spatial processing, and working memory. Commonly used intelligence tests are the Stanford-Binet Scale (5th edition) and the Otis-Lennon School Abilities Test (8th edition).

*Aptitude or ability tests* are defined as a capability for a particular skill (Aiken, 2000). Single skills such as manual dexterity, spatial perception, gross motor coordination, or eye/hand coordination are tested either individually or in a battery comprised of several subtests (Guindon, 2003). The Armed Services Vocational Aptitude Battery (ASVAB) is an ability test to assess readiness for various military and civilian occupations. The Differential Aptitude Test (5th edition) is used in high schools and community colleges to assess career readiness and help individuals with their school-to-career transition.

*Career and interest inventories* help to determine a student's preference for specific activities or areas of interest. There are numerous interest inventories available for elementary, middle school, and high school students to help students gain career awareness and explore career opportunities. Some career interest inventories such as those developed by John Holland combine personality characteristics and temperaments in addition to a like or dislike scale.

*Personality tests* measure emotions, feelings, inclinations, individual characteristics, attitudes, and opinions (Conlon & Hansen, 2004); however, the uniqueness of the nature of individual personalities makes assessment difficult. The most widely used and researched instrument is the Minnesota Multi-Phasic Personality Inventory—A and B (MMPI-A and MMPI-B; Butcher, Dahlstrom, Graham, Tellegen, & Kraemmer, 1989), which has an adult and an adolescent version for youth ages 14–18. The MMPI-A and MMPI-B manuals stress that the purpose of the instrument is to differentiate among the various patterns of personality and emotional disorders (Butcher et al., 1989, p. 2).

Another widely used instrument, the Myers-Briggs Type Indicator, is based on the work of Jung. His theories suggest that differences in behaviors are related to the ways in which individuals prefer to perceive and the ways that they judge their perceptions. The Myers-Briggs is intended to help people understand their preferences and is used by counselors and school district administrators to better understand the dynamics of human interaction.

Other personality assessments are structured and projective in nature. School counselors generally do not administer tests such as the Rorschach Thematic Apperception Test (TAT) or House-Tree-Person Test (H-T-P) due to the additional specialized training required for administration and interpretation. A student in need of a complex personality assessment may be referred by the school counselor to the school psychologist or mental health professional specially trained to interpret the complex scoring and analysis procedure.

*Diagnostic assessments* are used to assess student ability and disability for learning problems, emotional disorder, and mental illness. Assessments are used to determine suicide risk, eating disorder behaviors, substance abuse, and violent tendencies. Psychologists, psychiatrists, and specially trained professional counselors use a variety of tools for diagnostic purposes. The *Diagnostic and Statistical Manual: Mental Disorder* (*DSM-IV-TR*) published by the American Psychological Association (2000) includes 13 major categories of mental disorders and addressed the role of culture in diagnosis and assessment. Understanding the scope of the *DSM-IV-TR* is an invaluable skill for school counselors and this knowledge informs their communication with other mental health care professionals.

As the use of testing is extensive, it creates anxiety and stress in students (Cheek, Bradley, Reynolds, & Coy, 2002; Helms, 2004). One of the common uses of testing and assessment is for classroom and grade-level placement. Tests results frequently are used to label students and grouping in instructional "tracks." High-stakes tests such as the SAT or the ACT are used for college admissions or, in 50 percent of the states, serve as an exit exam for high school graduation. Educators continue to debate the value of homogeneous (grouping of students of similar learning characteristics) versus heterogeneous (grouping of students with dissimilar learning characteristics) grouping and use testing as a vehicle for placement.

The accountability component of No Child Left Behind (2001) has placed an all-consuming emphasis on testing and assessment. With this increased significance also comes the need to more closely examine the larger perspective of assessment with respect for all aspects of diversity, taking gender, ethnicity, culture, and language into account as well (Baker, 2000).

Reasonable accommodations, modifications, and/or alternative assessments must be considered also for students who have limited English capability as well as for students with disabilities (ACA Task Force on High Stakes Testing, 2004). Test bias is almost impossible to totally eradicate; thus, it is important to use multiple measures of assessment (Gladding, 2009). School counselors have an ethical responsibility to look beyond the use of a single test score for decision making as well as to educate their colleagues to use multiple assessments, thus gaining a broader view of a student's potential and prognosis for success. No decision about a student's educational status (i.e., graduation, promotion/ retention, tracking, advanced placement, special education, postsecondary admission, etc.) should ever be unilaterally made on the basis of a single test score (ACA Task Force on High Stakes Testing, 2004).

Assessment goes far beyond paper-and-pencil tests. Observation must not be overlooked as a contributing element to any comprehensive assessment. Formal and informal observations conducted by school counselors and other education professionals offer the human dynamic and interactive component that cannot be gleaned from a paper-and-pencil diagnostic instrument. Observations in the classroom, on the playground, and in a multitude of situations offer insight into academic as well as social-emotional performance. The counselor, observing both behavior and verbal interaction, can look for patterns. Observations are often used in assessing students for learning and emotional disabilities.

Individual interviews of students also contribute to understanding behavior, thinking, and ways of responding. Careful attention must be given to crafting questions that provide thoughtful and insightful responses. Interviews remind us of the importance of adding the human dimensions to the reams of paper that often comprise a comprehensive assessment. This use of qualitative data helps gather a broader view of the individual, not limited to any one paper-and-pencil tool.

## Looking at Learning Styles

Every student tends to have a **learning style** that works best for her or him. Dunn and Dunn (1978) researched this topic extensively over the years. Dunn's Learning Styles Inventory (LSI) is a comprehensive approach for assessing a student's learning style preference. The Dunn and Dunn learning styles model consists of 21 elements classified into five stimulus strands. The elements included are the individual's (1) immediate environment (sound, light, temperature, and furniture/seating designs); (2) own emotionality (motivation, persistence, responsibility-conformity versus nonconformity and need for either externally imposed structure or the opportunity to do things one's own way); (3) sociological preferences (learning alone best, in a pair, in a small group, as part of a team, with either an authoritative or collegial adult, and with variety as opposed to patterns and routines); (4) physiological characteristics (perceptual strengths, time-of-day energy levels, and need for intake and mobility while learning); and (5) processing inclinations that are global/analytic, right/left, and impulsive/reflective (Honigsfeld, 2004). As a result of extensive research, learning styles inventories were developed for the different educational levels, elementary, middle school, high school through college level.

There is a plethora of information available of proven research validating the effectiveness of how teacher, student, and parent knowledge of one's unique learning style has helped to improve academic performance at all levels of education. Various studies have proven that if teaching strategies are guided by student and teacher knowledge of individual learning styles of students, academic improvement results (Burke & Dunn, 2003; Honigsfeld & Dunn, 2009; Lister, 2005). Based on the research, success has been documented when pedagogues administer learning style batteries, such as the Dunn and Dunn Learning Style Inventory (Dunn, Dunn, & Price (2003) to students and guide instruction, teaching strategies accordingly, academic performance improved. If the learning style of a student is appropriately identified, an effective form of differential instruction, curricula, and pedagogy can be developed to help our minority students succeed. Various educational leaders, such as Haycock (2001), Mubenga (2006), and LaRocque (2007), have taken this stance. This will help close the achievement gap between students of color and White students (Honigsfeld et al., 2009). Socially, such action will afford equal opportunities into college and the job market for all students. Society as a whole will become more competitive with other countries as a result of more trained, qualified individuals having received high-level educational preparation for the job market.

## Counseling with Style—Learning Styles, That Is!

For years, Ron Smith, elementary and middle school counselor in New York City, was curious about and intrigued by learning comprehension and began to observe and note patterns among struggling students. When it came to schoolwork and academic performance, some students just "didn't get it," especially among his minority students.

The statement was made based on informal observation in the different classrooms during instructional time. The teacher would ask the students to summarize in her or his own words key points of the lesson just presented. Some students had no difficulty explaining what was taught. However, at least one-third of the students could not explain the lesson, or the feedback they provided was not even close to the lesson presented by the teacher. On reviewing test scores for the unit presented in the observed classes, further validation revealed poor performance.

I decided to interview some of the students and had informed them earlier that I wanted to see how they well they did on the test. Most of the students who did not perform well on the test explained that they just "didn't get it!" To my surprise, I realized that even in my counseling lessons, which focused on building self-confidence/self-esteem, career planning, conflict resolution, and the development of positive character traits and social skills, that some students understood better than others. I realized that the bottom line was that one method of a teaching strategy does not work with every student.

Going back to observations from the students who stated they "just didn't get it," I collaborated with a teacher on a lesson about Harriet Tubman and the Underground Railroad during Black History Month. I presented the information the teacher had presented visually (showing diagrams of a path one might have taken through the Underground Railroad) and kinetically in which students acted out what they felt took place with the slaves as they tried to escape and make it through the Underground Railroad or drew a picture of what they thought took place. The students interacted with each other, corrected, or offered suggestions as to how they could better express ideas that were discussed from the unit. I used a familiar example of comparing the slaves' desire to move north to have a better life to the situation faced by many people from the Caribbean nations—that is the primary demographics of my school—to start a better life for their family.

To test this theory about learning styles further, I administered a learning styles inventory, *Learning Styles: The Clue to You* (Dunn & Burke, 1998), to a group of sixth graders. The inventory is specifically designed for middle school students. The analyses helped me to identify which learning style was best for the students tested. I shared the information with the students' teacher, parent(s), and the students and we worked together to develop appropriate teaching strategies and study skills catering to the students' specific learning styles. Different levels of academic improvement were noted

*(continues)*

after a few weeks. The parents, teachers, and students reported that the students had a better understanding of schoolwork assigned.

The success of this intervention can be attributed to involving key players of the educational community. Separate meetings were conducted with the teachers, parents, and full class with students as a part of a full-class guidance unit. Everyone shared the desire of having students perform better academically. Admittedly, some teachers felt differential instruction based on learning styles was too much work (about 23 percent) and did not participate in the study. Teachers of special needs students were most responsive (100 percent), mainly because the students' learning styles are used to guide development of their Individualized Education Plans (IEP). The parents were willing to try anything that would help improve their student's school performance. Many were seeking advice related to what they could do at home to help their child improve study habits. The guidance relating to a more personalized study plan was embraced by, and followed through by, 86 percent of the parents and students, and this was validated by feedback from both students and parents.

Educators are continually seeking techniques to help students improve academically. When a school counselor takes the initiative to help teachers and students best understand how they learn, student achievement improves. When the students stated "I get it now!" I realized firsthand the importance of incorporating learning styles into the teaching and learning process. I am using the same diversity of teaching strategies in my counseling groups.

School counselors can investigate various learning styles inventories that are available and help administrators and teachers determine if this is a direction that will help their students. By doing so, we have made a commitment to ensure that every child will succeed to the best of the child's ability. Teaching to their learning style can make that happen.

*Ronald Smith has been a school counselor for more than 17 years, 11 years in elementary school and the remaining years in a middle school. He serves as vice president for middle/junior high school on the Executive Board of the Guidance Chapter of the United Federation of Teachers in New York City and as an elected officer for the New York State School Counselor Association. His doctoral research is also on student learning styles.*

School counselors are not clinicians with expertise in diagnosis but rather developmental experts who gather information from a multitude of assessments and work with colleagues to determine the best educational setting for each child. School counselors gather, interpret, and present data comprehensively, ethically, and fairly at all times. Professional school counselors, in collaboration with other educators, also advocate for the following:

- Appropriate testing conditions and administration of standardized tests.
- Opportunities to retake a test when a student is unsuccessful in one administration.
- Opportunities to take comparable tests when a student is unsuccessful in one administration.
- The use of standardized tests norm-referenced with all student populations.
- Discontinuation of standardized tests that show socioeconomic or cultural bias (ASCA, 2007).

Using data gathered from observation can lead to schoolwide systemic changes as did Ron Smith as he helped teachers and himself differentiate instruction through the use of learning styles. Assessment and testing are valuable tools and resources when they are chosen wisely, administered carefully, and the results are used in ways that open the door for students to new and appropriate opportunities. The professional school counselor encourages multiple measures of assessment when life-influencing decisions are being made by students, educators, and parents (ASCA, 2007).

# THE IMPORTANCE OF UNDERSTANDING STUDENT DEVELOPMENT

One of the many challenges of working with children and youth is knowing when a particular behavior is developmentally appropriate (Vernon, 2004), and understanding developmental theory helps to better understand which theoretical approaches will work best with students at different ages, school levels, and stages of maturation. Children at the preK level will differ in their responses from children in the intermediate elementary grades. School counselors are specially trained as developmental specialists who are familiar with the different stages in which children are able to identify and recall feelings, develop logical thinking, accept responsibility for actions, and engage in simple and complex relationships. This knowledge helps the school counselors to design specific interventions for students at all grade levels across a broad span of activities, including individual counseling and classroom guidance lessons.

Using a developmental counseling and therapy-based consultation model, school counselors can assess how a teacher is conceptualizing a student's behavior, respond to the stress a teacher may feel connected to that behavior, and indirectly effect systemic classroom change (Clemens, 2007). The classroom teacher is the person most likely in a position to effect change in the classroom environment, and this can ultimately lead to behavior improvement for the students that the teacher is having the most difficulty with as well as improve the overall classroom climate and increased ability to learn for all students.

School counselors have expertise in student development and can assume an objective position to assess classroom dynamics. School counselors are in an ideal position to help teachers control their stress levels by exploring and experimenting with alternate ways of understanding and working with student behaviors. The school counselor can help the teacher make meaning of a specific situation and support them to rethink problematic situations around student behavior. Utilizing observation, knowledge of student development, behavior modification, and communication skills, the school counselor can collaboratively problem solve with the teacher whose expertise lies in pedagogy, their subject matter, and strategies for learning. Together, school counselor and teacher can identify best practices to help teachers create a dynamic and supportive learning environment.

## Developing Helping "Skills" with Teachers

Teachers can benefit from learning about counseling techniques to help develop better relationships with their students. Frequently, teachers are called on to resolve conflict and arguments among students, address emotional needs, identify children who are suffering from abusive situations, help them acquire resiliency skills, and guide students' physical, emotional, and social development. Teachers also meet with parents to resolve difficult situations as well as work collaboratively with grade-level and vertical teams.

As teachers must adapt to multiple roles in addition to the expectation of teaching and learning, they could benefit from acquiring "helping skills" to assist them in their role as caregiver, mentor, role model, surrogate parent, and authority figure (Kottler & Kottler, 2007). School counselors acknowledge the importance of helping teachers better understand student dynamics and behavior. It is also important for teachers to appreciate the many different ways that they influence children's lives as well as the complexity of student-teacher relationships that are built on mutual respect, trust, and understanding. Teachers are not trained as counselors, nor should they be counseling students. However, counselors can help teachers acquire enhanced communications skills and use foundational counseling techniques such as active listening, paraphrasing, reflecting, and using open-ended questions, which will result in stronger learning communities within their classroom (Kottler & Kottler, 2007). Students positively respond to teachers who show an interest in personalization, making connections, and responding to students as individuals. Not to be confused with the art and science of counseling, it is good pedagogy.

## Student Development and Resilience

When the school environment and culture are supportive and based on rigor and relationships, this creates the ideal environment to assist children, youth, and teens to identify how they develop their inner strength. Fostering **resiliency** requires instilling in students the attitude that suggests strengths are more powerful than problems (Benard, 2004; Henderson, 1996). Students have reported that they find school to be a consistently open and safe place (Devine & Cohen, 2007). Grotberg (1998) identified 15 key elements that are in a resilient youth's active voice (Table 3.1).

TABLE **3.1**
Key Elements of Resiliency

| I have | I am | I can |
|---|---|---|
| People around me | A person people can like and love | Talk to others about things that bother or frighten me |
| People who set limits for me | Glad to do nice things for others and show my concern | Find ways to solve problems that I face |
| People who show me how to do things right by the way they do things | Respectful of myself and others | Control myself when I feel like doing something not right or dangerous |
| People who help me even when I am sick, in danger or need to learn | Willing to accept responsibility for what I do | Find someone to help when I need it |

Additionally, researchers have noted that youth who have bounced back from adversity also develop a level of competence in affective and personal-social development (Benard, 2004; Devine & Cohen, 2007). School environments are most successful when they include a cadre of adults who build strong and significant relationships with youth. Dryfoos (1994) identified the following common elements of successful programs:

a. positive adult-youth relationships;
b. youth involvement in community and service opportunities;
c. an established vision of high expectations for students;
d. affective and academic skills building;
e. school and community collaboration to provide information and support services; and,
f. positive connecting strategies that involve adults, peers, activities, recreation, and learning.

Benard (2004) identified four protective factors: environment, family, school, and community, which can help each student assess her or his ability to cope, show determination, overcome, and succeed. As educators we must build caring relationships, set high expectations, and give students opportunities to participate and contribute to their school and community. A student's success depends on a caring and supportive environment. Teaching students the concept of resiliency, exposing them to positive role models, and developing mentoring programs can turn any student from "at risk" to "resilient." "Positive development and successful outcomes in any human system depend on the quality of the relationships, beliefs, and opportunities for participation" (Benard, 2004, p. 48).

These include a student's ability to

- use life skills;
- demonstrate perceptiveness;
- be self-motivated;
- persevere;
- show competence;
- have inner direction;
- have a sense of humor;
- build relationships;
- be flexible;
- have positive view of the future;
- develop a love of learning.

These protective factors bear a strong resemblance to the personal-social development competencies in the ASCA model (2005) and, whether viewed through the eyes of a school counselor or mental health provider, have similar objectives for youth growth and development.

## Acquiring the Developmental Assets

Building resiliency and acquiring protective factors is also about "asset" building. With the knowledge that healthy student development is at the core of school-community collaboration, the Search Institute in Minneapolis has conducted extensive research, identifying specific assets as the foundation of healthy development for young people. The 40 Developmental Assets (1997, 2007) are indicators of healthy, caring, and responsible students. Assets are internally and externally based and are reflective of the willingness of school and community to mentor, guide, and nurture children. Parental involvement is essential to asset acquisition and youth development. The four major categories of external assets (Table 3.2) focus on positive experiences that young people receive from the people and institutions in their lives.

A community's responsibility for its youth does not end with the provision of external assets. There needs to be a similar commitment to nurturing the internal qualities that guide choices and create a sense of centeredness, purpose, and focus. Indeed, shaping internal dispositions that encourage wise, responsible, and compassionate judgments is particularly important in a society that prizes individualism. The four major categories of the internal assets (Table 3.3) support a commitment to internal nurturing.

The **developmental assets** are the relationships, competencies, values, opportunities, and self-perceptions that are necessary for success in school, at home, and in the community. Research (Leffert & Scales, 1999) attributed performance and achievement to asset building. Students who reported acquiring 31–40 assets were more likely to achieve higher grades in school than students who reported acquiring 11–20 assets. Significant relationships were found among variables such as academic goals, grades, graduation success, and beliefs about the value of education with asset building (Leffert & Scales, 1999). Asset acquisition has also been linked to lower reported instances of substance abuse and sexual intimacy.

The Search Institute identified more than 20 assets that schools can most directly influence. At the top of the list are student engagement in school, achievement motivation, positive peer influence, youth programs, and safety (Benson et al., 1999). A caring school climate with clearly established and enforced guidelines coupled with the strength of parental involvement appeared to be at the foundation of developing successful learners and future citizens. The premise of asset building is grounded in the potential of the "power of one" (Lerner & Benson, 2002), which is the ability of one individual to heal, support, challenge, and change for the better the life of one young person.

Assets underscore the premise that students need to be prepared to face pressure and acquire skills to face the challenges of a world that with each day becomes more complex and complicated. Successful students acquire skills in coping, learning to adjust to new and different situations, and building resiliency skills to overcome barriers and obstacles that come their way whether these are academic, personal-social, career, or environmentally related.

Resiliency is the capacity to spring back, rebound, successfully adapt in the face of adversity, and develop social competence despite exposure to stress

TABLE **3.2**
External Assets

| Category | Asset | Description |
|---|---|---|
| Support | Family support | Family life provides high levels of love and support. |
| | Positive family communication | Young person and her or his parent(s) communicate positively, and young person is willing to seek advice and counsel from parent(s). |
| | Other adult relationships | Young person receives support from three or more non-parent adults. |
| | Caring neighborhood | Young person experiences caring neighbors. |
| | Caring school climate | School provides a caring, encouraging environment. |
| | Parent involvement in schooling | Parent(s) are actively involved in helping young person succeed in school. |
| Empowerment | Community values youth | Young person perceives that adults in the community value youth. |
| | Youth as resources | Young people are given useful roles in the community. |
| | Service to others | Young person serves in the community one hour or more per week. |
| | Safety | Young person feels safe at home, at school, and in the neighborhood. |
| Boundaries and Expectations | Family boundaries | Family has clear rules and consequences, and monitors the young person's whereabouts. |
| | School boundaries | School provides clear rules and consequences. |
| | Neighborhood boundaries | Neighbors take responsibility for monitoring young people's behavior. |
| | Adult role models | Parent(s) and other adults model positive, responsible behavior. |
| | Positive peer influence | Young person's best friends model responsible behavior. |
| | High expectations | Both parent(s) and teachers encourage the young person to do well. |
| Constructive Use of Time | Creative activities | Young person spends three or more hours per week in lessons or practice in music, theater, or other arts. |
| | Youth programs | Young person spends three or more hours per week in sports, clubs, or organizations at school and/or in community organizations. |
| | Religious community | Young person spends one hour or more per week in activities in a religious institution. |
| | Time at home | Young person is out with friends "with nothing special to do" two or fewer nights per week. |

Source: Reprinted with permission from Search Institute (1997, 2007), Minneapolis, MN: www.search-institute.org.

TABLE **3.3**
Internal Assets

| Category | Asset | The young person: |
|---|---|---|
| Commitment to Learning | Achievement Motivation | is motivated to do well in school. |
| | School engagement | is actively engaged in learning. |
| | Homework | reports doing at least one hour of homework every school day. |
| | Bonding to school | cares about her or his school. |
| | Reading for pleasure | reads for pleasure three or more hours per week. |
| Positive Values | Caring | places high value on helping other people. |
| | Equality and social justice | places high value on promoting equality and reducing hunger and poverty. |
| | Integrity | acts on convictions and stands up for her or his beliefs. |
| | Honesty | "tells the truth even when it is not easy." |
| | Responsibility | accepts and takes personal responsibility. |
| | Restraint | believes it is important not to be sexually active or to use alcohol or other drugs. |
| Social Competencies | Planning and decision making | knows how to plan ahead and make choices. |
| | Interpersonal competence | has empathy, sensitivity, and friendship skills. |
| | Cultural competence | has knowledge of and comfort with people of different cultural/racial/ethnic backgrounds. |
| | Resistance skills | can resist negative peer pressure and dangerous situations. |
| | Peaceful conflict resolution | seeks to resolve conflict nonviolently. |
| Positive Identity | Personal power | feels she or he has control over "things that happen to me." |
| | Self-esteem | reports having a high self-esteem. |
| | Sense of purpose | reports that "my life has a purpose." |
| | Positive view of personal future | is optimistic about her or his personal future. |

Source: Reprinted with permission from Search Institute (1997), Minneapolis, MN: www.search-institute.org.

(Leffert & Scales, 1999). Social competence, problem-solving ability, autonomy, and a sense of purpose and future are the individual traits and assets that resilient students carry as part of their middle school survival tool kit (Moe, 2001). Students who demonstrate characteristics of resiliency and acquire the majority of the internal and external assets are more likely to be successful throughout the middle and high school years (Search Institute, 1997, 2007).

# PERSONALIZING THE SCHOOL EXPERIENCE: ADVISORY PROGRAMS

Schools and society put much pressure on youth to grow up in perfect compliance and conformance with rules and structure that will lead to wonderfully perfect, successful lives. However, the mechanisms are not always in place to create an environment in which every child has a safety net, and the mechanism is in place to make sure no child is forgotten. Although some students can make it through the secondary school years without any personal connections, all students require a supportive environment, some more than others (NASSP, 2004).

> On any given day, I think every adolescent is at-risk in some way. How many schools approach such concerns with purposeful, planned, and progressive awareness-building, educational, and intervention strategies in place as opposed to trying to deny these realities or being caught in a reactive, crisis-oriented position? (Maine Commission on Secondary Education, 1998, p. 37)

High schools are often large and impersonal environments. Every teenager needs a significant adult in her or his life to support the challenges presented by school rigor, policies, and socialization pressures. Smaller, more intimate environments ensure that no child goes unnoticed and afford students the ability to make connections with adults. Here's one school's response to creating a personalized, more student-centered experience:

School counselors play important leadership roles in helping to develop and organize **advisory programs**. This is a powerful way to extend the student development curriculum into a schoolwide systemic program that involves all school personnel in a meaningful way and supports every student's ability to acquire the skills needed to succeed in the 21st century.

Advisory programs are an important component of the personalized school experience. Clarke and Frazer (2003) identified six developmental needs of students that can be addressed through personalization:

- Voice—the need to express their personal perspective;
- Belonging—the need to establish individual and group identities;
- Choice—the need to examine options and choose a path;
- Freedom—the need to take risks and assess effects;
- Imagination—the need to create a projected view of self; and
- Success—the need to demonstrate mastery (NASSP, 2004, p. 70).

Engaging students in the personalization experience allows each student to earn recognition. Advisory models provide opportunities for students to establish an identity and a mechanism for self-expression. School counselors can assume a leadership role in the organization and curricular development of an advisory model that emphasizes effective and life-skills instructional components.

Successful counseling practice relies not only on the skills of the counselor but also on the attitudes, knowledge, and skills that students acquire as a result of individual and group counseling, and classroom lessons. The

## MEET RANDY BOWEN: PERSONALIZING THE HIGH SCHOOL EXPERIENCE

As my school expanded and added a ninth, 10th, and now 11th grade to our middle school, we realized that we had to look at the advisory program that was firmly in place in the middle school. It was grade specific and encompassed lessons centered on the mental, social/emotional, college preparation, and the physical health of the student and the affect of these on the community. As with the middle school program, our new high school advisory would evolve out of the school mission and qualities we wish our students to have: respect for each other, respect for self, and respect for their community.

First, we examined the issues affecting the student body and their community. Students are faced with many pressures from parents, religious groups, school, peers, and the media. Educators across the country have realized that children will not learn if their minds are focused on something other than school. The next step was to secure the approval of administration. Schanfield (2010) states that "advisor buy-in will increase if the administration frequently—and publicly—agrees to support the program" (ASCA School Counselor, p. 22). Principals and assistant principals, on a daily basis, deal with the macro issues that arise in the school setting such as curriculum committees, various program initiatives, the safety of every student and staff member, discipline policy, and the learning environment. They also have to address the day-to-day micro issues such as student fights, peer pressure, and conflicts. Our administrators realized that an advisory program would assist with prevention as well as reinforce the important character skills we want our students to acquire to become successful and productive citizens. With permission in hand and continuous support, we were able to go to the next step and schedule 37½ minutes twice a week for a new high school advisory program.

As the transition from middle school to high school can be the difference between a successful student and a student who decides to drop out, we decided to focus on self-identity, organization, conflict resolution, healthy relationships, and resiliency for the ninth grade. In addition to the issues and topics that the faculty selected, our 10th graders worked on a special project in their advisory and were given the opportunity to help design certain features of the new school building we will be moving to. Empowering students in their community is so important and what better way to do this than giving students control over what the cafeteria will look like!

Getting started was a challenge, and in retrospect this was a direct result of the lack of collegiate-level training available for teachers as advisors. I used my experience in my former school along with looking at the skills our students needed to build on moving from middle school to high school to get our faculty to work on ideas, lessons, and units. While counselors are trained to handle groups including expectations, pace, and confidentiality, teachers are often at a disadvantage during advisory. It is so important to support the teachers taking on the advisor role, which is why we are currently working on providing professional development for advisors through consultation.

Our students had advisory throughout middle school, and they came in with their own expectations. Connecting the student's well-being with teaching results, academic achievement, testing success, and building relationships helped our teachers understand its importance. Setting aside time during grade-level team meetings was invaluable to discuss advisory curriculum and activities. The faculty identified an advisory liaison to work on curriculum for the entire ninth grade and communicate ideas, trips, and events. While I wouldn't call it the best program ever, we continue to work to strengthen it every school year!

It is essential that counselors are intimately involved in a school's advisory program, whether it is in the capacity of coordinator, advisor, researcher, etc. Some may suggest that the advisory system is a derivative of group counseling. Corey (2008) suggests that adolescents in a group learn to communicate with others, model their leader, explore reality, and learn their limits. I like to think of advisory as the big brother/big sister of education. Many students in the urban setting lack a strong home environment and learn mostly from television, radio, and peers. Their character traits such as integrity, honesty, and self-efficacy need to be developed especially for the students who may be the oldest without a strong adult figure in their life. Our students spend 1/3 of their day with us, 1/3 with their family, and 1/3 sleeping (hopefully). With caseloads growing, advisory allows the school counselor the opportunity to deliver student development/guidance lessons to every student in the building. As accountability for school counselors increases, advisory is an important tool that will help ensure that every student is prepared to be a productive citizen in society.

*Randy Bowen is a high school counselor at the Community Health Academy in Washington Heights, New York City. Randy has been a school counselor for three years working at the high school level and is dedicated and committed to advisory programs as way of involving more teachers in personalizing the school experience. Randy is a member of the American School Counselor Association.*

application of counseling in a school setting is most effective when faculty, administrators, and all student support personnel recognize the unique role that counseling plays in a school setting. School counselors can provide great insight and support to teachers and administrators around the issues of student development and behavior management. With the assistance of the school counselor, schools can establish themselves as personalized and supportive learning communities in which students grow academically and thrive in the affective development and become productive citizens and contributors to a global society.

# TECH TOOLS

When you become a school counselor, use the power of technology to maximize the efficiency and effectiveness of your counseling practice in schools.

- Use technology to help you create a simple survey to identify issues that students have or concerns of the faculty about students. Input the data into a spreadsheet; use charts and graphs and presentation software to share the results.
- Explore additional resources for yourself, your colleagues, and your students. Go to the American Psychological Association help center at www.apa.org/helpcenter/.
- Find out more about the work of the Search Institute and the 40 Developmental Assets. Go to www.search-institute.org/developmental-assets; use the use the Activity Generator and the Conversation Generator to get ideas fast.
- Review the ASCA website (www.schoolcounselor.org) to better understand how the national association serves members and makes resources available on a variety of counseling applications. Look at the resources available for school counselors, administrators, and parents. Find the websites for your state school counselor association and your local professional associations.
- National School Counseling Week (NSCW) takes place the first week of February. Search the Web for ideas and resources and use presentation software to present five tips to your faculty that can help them in their work with students. Use your school's electronic or traditional bulletin board to highlight a different message for each day.
- Check out the resources on http://resiliency.cas.psu.edu/ on Family and Youth Resiliency.
- Visit the National Middle School Association's website and read about advisory programs (www.nmsa.org/Research/ResearchSummaries/AdvisoryPrograms/tabid/812/Default.aspx). Work on a plan to develop a "we believe" statement with your colleagues for middle schools or high schools. The American Student Achievement Institute website has many suggestions to help you develop a K–12 advisory program (www.asainstitute.org/advisory/index.html).

---

## *School Counselor Casebook: Voices from the Field*

### The Scenario Reviewed

You have just left your middle school improvement team meeting and your head is spinning. The primary topic of conversation was an increased number of reported incidents of bullying and harassment. Your principal suggested in front of all of the committee members that individual counseling for all of the students involved would be the perfect remedy.

You responded that individual counseling is only a small part of the solution and that using classroom lessons and group counseling are also effective and efficient ways to address a potential schoolwide problem. Before the meeting broke up, you reminded the group that alleviating bullying and harassment required a commitment from the entire faculty and staff if any positive change would be realized. With a personal caseload of more than 600 students, you are feeling pretty overwhelmed.

## A Practitioner's Approach

Here's how a practicing school counselor responded to the school scenario:

As I stepped away from the meeting, I knew I would need to schedule an appointment to meet with my principal privately and spend some time talking about the extensiveness of the bullying problem and how to best address this issue. Given my responsibilities and the large number of students in our school, I realized that this could be a perfect opportunity for me to help her to mobilize everyone in the school around creating a culture that was bullying-free. It would have been inappropriate to verbalize my personal opinions in front of everyone after being given a directive at the meeting. She was so passionate about wanting me to resolve the problem through individual counseling that I realized that perhaps she is not aware of the additional strategies I can offer.

I realized that I need to plan a meeting with my principal and have an opportunity to talk about the differences between individual and group counseling, and which counseling practices could be most appropriate and effective to use with students who have been involved as bullies or victims. I would explain to my principal how a Rogerian, client-centered approach could be utilized to target behaviors and help empower students to change their outlook and actions in a group or on an individual level. Even more importantly, I wanted my principal to understand that not every student needs counseling but every student would benefit from prevention education to reduce and ultimately eliminate the number of incidents that appeared to be increasing.

Next, I would propose working with the teachers at each grade level to develop a curriculum that would include lessons on topics such as respect, friendships, resolving conflict, and cyberbullying. During our meeting I would present specific examples that help to strengthen the students' relationships while incorporating anti-bullying and harassment activities.

Principals have so many issues that they have to deal with on a daily basis and may not have the time to think through all the different solutions that will help make our school a more respectful place and reduce the bullying and student harassment. School counselors need to use all of their skills to apply a variety of counseling practices in a school setting. Bringing in specific examples, a clear-cut action plan, and a discussion about outcomes will help you when working with your principal to maximize your effectiveness as a school counselor.

Bridget Anderson has worked with middle school level students and has worked with elementary level students for the past five years. Assessing student needs every year and using data to show her results, Bridget has offered a new wave of services for elementary children through a variety of support groups including Banana Splits and other topically related groups.

# LOOKING BACK: SALIENT POINTS

## Applications of Counseling in Schools

Documented occurrences of children's emotional difficulties have escalated in large numbers of violent, disruptive, and aggressive behavior. Counseling skills and techniques underpin the way school counselors approach and apply skills in leadership, advocacy, and teaming and collaboration. School counselors cannot overlook its paramount importance in our training, in our interactions with students and other stakeholders, and, most importantly, to our professional identity.

## The Many Dimensions of the School Counselor's Role

Role confusion has prevailed as school counseling was equated predominantly with individual counseling; traditional counseling practice has been perceived as reactive and remedial versus proactive and positive. Professional school counselors are responsible for a wide range of services and activities involving students, parents, teachers, administrators, and community members. In addition to individual counseling, services are delivered in groups, through classroom guidance lessons, in large assemblies, and through parent meetings and faculty presentations.

## Assessing the Need: Designing Interventions

Counseling is equated with emotional well-being, is flexible in its approach, and can be applied in a wide variety of student academic, career, and personal-social issues. Every student benefits from prevention and intervention knowledge, attitudes, and skills that are presented in the classroom guidance lesson. Some students will need specific group intervention to help them acquire and practice the skills. Others may need one-on-one counseling intervention.

## Applications of Testing and Assessment

Testing and assessment are important components of the work of school counselors. Oftentimes, in the absence of the presence of a school psychologist, the school counselor is the only professional with a background in testing and assessment. School counselors, acting as advocates for their students, gather, interpret, and present data comprehensively, ethically, and fairly at all times.

## The Importance of Understanding Student Development

School counselors are especially trained as developmental specialists who are familiar with the different stages in which children are able to identify and recall feelings, develop logical thinking, accept responsibility for actions, and engage in simple and complex relationships. This knowledge helps school counselors to design specific interventions for students at all grade levels across a broad span of activities, including individual counseling and classroom guidance lessons.

*Student Development and Resilience.* Fostering resiliency requires instilling in students the attitude that suggests strengths are more powerful than problems. School counselors can help each student assess her or his ability to cope, show determination, overcome, and succeed.

*Acquiring the Developmental Assets.* The developmental assets are the relationships, competencies, values, opportunities, and self-perceptions that are necessary for success in school, at home, and in the community. Assets are internally and externally based and are reflective of the willingness of school and community to mentor, guide, and nurture children.

*Personalizing the School Experience: Advisory Programs.* School counselors play an important leadership role in helping to develop and organize advisory programs. This is a powerful way to extend the student development curriculum into a schoolwide systemic program that involves all school personnel in a meaningful way and supports every student's ability to acquire the skills needed to succeed in the 21st century.

## KEY TERMS

Individual counseling p. 68

Group counseling p. 69

Comprehensive school counseling program p. 70

School counseling/student development curriculum p. 72

Assessment and testing p. 74

Learning styles p. 78

Resiliency p. 82

Developmental assets p. 84

Advisory programs p. 87

## LEARNING EXTENSIONS/MAKING CONNECTIONS

1. Systemic involvement leads to systemic change. Reflect on the scenario at the beginning of the chapter. How did your suggested strategies shift the principal's focus from individual counseling to a broader spectrum of prevention and intervention activities?

2. Prevention is a critical component of every student's education. Proactive approaches to student issues can help to alleviate future pitfalls.

   You are concerned about the seniors in your caseload making a good transition to college life. You know that many students have difficulty adjusting the first year and that you have heard that the national dropout rate for first-year college students is approximately 30 percent. Students are beginning to receive their letters of acceptance and seem very excited about the independence that comes with leaving high school. There are still three months before they graduate.

   How can counseling strategies address these issues?

   How will you use the dimensions of counseling—classroom guidance, group counseling, and individual counseling—in your school setting?

3. Intervention may be necessary to deal with crisis or at-risk behaviors. *Remediation,* which is a term often equated with teaching and learning is about acquiring skills for learning new behaviors.

Several students in Mr. Bryant's third-grade class have gotten into trouble repeatedly for fighting on the playground. The class has developed a reputation for being full of trouble-makers. The majority of the students are concerned about how the other students and teachers in the school are talking about them. This situation has caused conflict in the classroom and Mr. Bryant has asked for your help.

How will counseling help to alleviate the problem? Who needs to be involved? How will you use the dimensions of counseling to intervene and prevent future occurrences?

4. The primary topic at the faculty meeting last week focused on a child abuse case that received national attention in a neighboring school district. Your middle principal called you and your colleague into his office after the meeting and strongly suggested that the two of you organize a counseling program for all 1,000 of your sixth, seventh, and eighth graders. You left your principal's office with a sinking feeling. How will you add this important activity to your already busy schedule? Who else can you involve and how?

5. Developing a school counseling or student developmental curriculum is a vehicle for advocacy for student success. Consider how a classroom program will further help your commitment to creating a supportive school environment. Educational and career planning are used to encourage a positive "mindset" for achievement and success for all students.

6. Often overlooked are the community-based organizations (CBOs) that specialize in prevention and intervention counseling and education on social issues and youth-related concerns. Go to your local yellow pages and identify 10 CBOs that can help support your school counseling program.

7. How would you go about presenting the 40 Developmental Assets to your faculty as a school-community initiative?

## CHAPTER 4

# School Counselors as Leaders

**Collaborative Leadership for the 21st-Century School**

**School Counselors as Collaborative Leaders**
Leadership as a Mindset
Personal/Social Consciousness Skills and Leadership
Principals as Partners
School Counselors and Power

**School Counselors Developing Leadership Skills**
Self-Awareness
Facilitative Communication

Team Development
Staff Development

**The Impact of the School Counselor as Leader**
Improving School Climates
Successful Instructional Programs
Developing High Aspirations in Students
Course Enrollment and Tracking Patterns

**Leadership: Rewarding but Challenging**

**Tech Tools**

**Looking Back: Salient Points**

## CHAPTER OBJECTIVES

*By the time you have completed this chapter, you should be able to*

- define educational leadership and types of leadership and power;

- describe the role of the school counselor as a leader in the school;

- explain the school counselor's role on the principal's (or school's) leadership team;

- describe how school counselors use leadership to holistically support academic, career, and personal/social development for every student;

- identify the behaviors of a school counselor as a leader, advocate, and collaborator to (1) change attitudes and beliefs; (2) contribute to successful instructional programs; (3) develop high aspirations; (4) influence course enrollment and tracking patterns; and (5) contribute to safe and respectful school climates.

---

## School Counselor Casebook: Getting Started

### The Scenario

In your school district, large numbers of students are classified and receive special education services. The school where you just started your counselor position seems to be especially entrenched in the practice of testing and placing students in special education as a natural intervention for students struggling academically. It has become an automatic practice to test a student for special education when a student is in danger of failing.

### Thinking about Solutions

As you read this chapter, think about how you as a school counselor would define your leadership role in this scenario. When you come to the end of the chapter, you will have the opportunity to see how your ideas compare with a practicing school counselor's approach.

---

## COLLABORATIVE LEADERSHIP FOR THE 21st-CENTURY SCHOOL

**Collaborative leadership**, also known as distributed leadership, is building and sustaining relationships to accomplish the seemingly impossible task of helping all students match ever-rising expectations (Rubin, 2009). Collaborative leadership entails collaboration among multiple parties such as community, parents, teachers, school counselors, and others for the development, acceptance, and achievement of goals that lead to academic success for all students (Adelman & Taylor, 2007; Bryan & Henry, 2008; Rubin, 2009). Leadership is increasingly recognized by businesses and educational institutions as too critical and too far-reaching to be the lonely domain of a sole designee (Adelman & Taylor, 2002; Hackman, 2002; Smith & Piele, 2006). In schools, collaborative leadership also has become an increasingly valued and shared phenomenon given the multiplicity of student needs. All community members with a stake in quality education are needed to bring their skills and talents to bear in support of students' academic, career, and personal/social success (American School Counselor Association, 2005; Bryan & Holcomb-McCoy, 2007).

Against the background of commonsense reasoning that "many minds are better than one," it is necessary to ask why shared leadership has struggled for acceptance and identity in K–12 schools. The answer is profound in its simplicity: Schools have not differentiated well between the concepts of administration and leadership (Lindahl, 2008, p. 299). That principals are the only figures who do or should behave as leaders is an assumption that is now widely disputed (Janson, Stone, & Clark, 2009). Collaborative leadership places the principal at the hub; however, this type of leadership is extended to other players including teachers, counselors, and community members. "Principals who develop collaborative cultures shift from being the person who sets the goals to being the person who sets up the conditions that allow others to establish goals" (Kohm & Nance, 2009, p. 68).

Collaborative leadership fosters a school culture or climate that contributes to learning outcomes for students as defined by the educational reform agenda (or school improvement agenda). Collaboration for the sake of collaboration alone will not heighten achievement and reduce inequities. When educators bring their talents to bear around the right initiatives in a collaborative culture, the opportunity for success is significantly advanced. According to Kohm and Nance (2009), "when teachers have many opportunities to collaborate, their energy, creative thinking, efficiency, and goodwill increase—and the cynicism and defensiveness that hamper change decrease" (p. 68).

School principals shifted their leadership focus from middle managers to instructional leaders to serve as collaborative problem-solvers around academic success issues. A similar shift is also occurring for school counselors since the American School Counselor Association (ASCA) developed a new school counseling model that emphasizes a leadership role with the ultimate purpose of casting a wider net and affected a greater number of students. "Leadership is exactly what the American School Counselor Association's National Model is about. The model is a guide for all school counselors, in all settings, and with all populations. It is a model that is flexible and adaptable to meet the unique needs of schools and students" (Schwallie-Giddis, Maat, & Park, 2003, p. 170). "National initiatives in professional school counseling make it clear that leadership is an essential skill for school counselors working in the 21st century" (Mason & McMahon, 2009, p. 107).

School counselors are exercising a central role in the collaborative culture toward educational reform (Bryan & Holcomb-McCoy, 2007). "Since school counselors are seen as having potential for leadership in educational reform and as advocates of student success, it is suggested that school counselors promote educational reform through leadership in partnerships between school, families, and communities" (Bryan & Holcomb-McCoy, 2004, p. 162). "School-family-community partnerships provide integral system support for the school counseling program and that school counselors, if involved in such partnerships, may better meet the personal/social, academic, and career needs of larger numbers of students" (Bryan & Holcomb-McCoy, 2007, p. 441). "School-family-community partnerships provide valuable system support services that help school counselors bridge cultural gaps among school, families, and communities, build educational resilience in children, and empower families" (Bryan & Holcomb-McCoy, 2007, p. 452). As valued partners in leadership efforts, school counselors are placing themselves squarely in the center of educational reform (Dollarhide, Gibson, & Saginak, 2008; Mason & McMahon, 2009; Scarborough & Luke, 2008).

## SCHOOL COUNSELORS AS COLLABORATIVE LEADERS

School counselors as leaders and critical change agents are key contributors to improving the conditions under which students learn (Amatea & West-Olatunji, 2007; Astramovich & Coker, 2007; Dahir & Tyson, 2010; Janson, Stone, & Clark, 2009; Walker, 2006). School counselors traditionally have been supported by the administration, faculty, and parents to assume the role of working with individual or small groups of students, educators, and parents. Educational reform demands have allowed school counselors to be viewed through a wider lens as the person who can make a difference in a child's life and as a leader who supports the same school improvement agenda that teachers, administrators, and all other educators must sustain (Adelman & Taylor, 2007; DeVoss, 2010a; Dollarhide, Gibson, & Saginak, 2008; Mason & McMahon, 2009).

The **school counselor as leader** joins forces with other educators and the larger school community to positively affect the opportunities students will have to be successful learners, to achieve high standards, and to become productive citizens (DeVoss, 2010a; Janson, Stone, & Clark, 2009; Mason & McMahon, 2009). Leadership for the school counselor is acting and fully participating as an integral part of the mission and function of schools, supporting each student, and enabling student success within the system. An in-depth examination of literature by Bryan and Holcomb-McCoy (2007) found that 18 partnership role behaviors are being promoted for school counselors, such as helping parents, family, and community members organize support programs for students, collaborating with community agency professionals, providing parent education workshops and seminars, collaborating with local businesses and industries, and conducting home visits to families (Bryan & Holcomb-McCoy, 2007, p. 441).

Leadership for school counselors is not administration or management. Many counselors already have the task of testing coordinator, an administrative task among many others that school counselors try to avoid or have reassigned. Leadership for school counselors does not mean being involved in managing the day-to-day life of a school such as overseeing the bus program, giving attention to the smooth running of the cafeteria program, evaluating teachers, or taking an active part in discipline. Rather, leadership for the school counselor is an exciting, powerful way to literally and figuratively wrap your arms around each student by influencing and collaborating with both the internal school community and the larger external community to break down institutional and environmental barriers to create the conditions that help students realize the potential of their lives (Cheek & House, 2010a; Clark & Stone, 2000a). Leadership is most easily carried out through collaboration with the significant people in the lives of students, i.e., teachers, administrators, family, and community members (Bryan & Holcomb-McCoy, 2004; Adelman and Taylor, 2007). When the principal takes a stand on important educational issues, she or he is perceived as a strong leader and an advocate for continuous school improvement. More frequently school counselors are exercising similar models and leadership behaviors (Erford & McCaskill, 2010). Counselors are change agents, a role made easier when they are seen as leaders in their schools. The more visible school counselors are in classrooms and working side by side with teachers, parents, and administrators, the more credible they become (Dollarhide, Gibson, & Saginak, 2008; Gibson, 2010).

## Leadership as a Mindset

Leadership for school counselors does not necessarily equate with membership on a **leadership team** such as a school improvement team, committee, or task force. Rather, leadership for school counselors is a mindset, a way of thinking about how you can affect student success. Although school committees, teams, and task forces are excellent vehicles for school counselors to extend their leadership efforts, school counselors can use their leadership influence with or without membership on committees. The counselor possesses a mindset for leadership, which means that the school counselor views her or his role as another person or additional set of eyes and ears looking for and identifying environmental and institutional barriers that stratify opportunities for student success. The **leadership mindset** means that the school counselor along with colleagues who embrace leadership view her or his position in the school as critical in supporting indicators of student success such as grades, attendance, discipline referrals, test scores, dropout rate, and student retention. This mindset can also affect conditions of learning such as school climate, the instructional program, and students' emotional well-being. Throughout this textbook, you will be introduced to practicing school counselors behaving as leaders, working with students individually, in small groups, in classroom guidance, and in their family/community/educational systems to help students be successful. Leadership as a mindset calls for school counselors to behave and act in collaborative, proactive ways to support all students. Membership on the school improvement team and other critical committees gives counselors a mechanism for their voices to be heard. Membership on the school improvement team, albeit not a necessity in the leadership equation, is highly desirable to facilitate your leadership efforts.

## Personal/Social Consciousness Skills and Leadership

As a school counseling candidate, you have an opportunity to develop and nurture those aspects of your personality that will enhance your ability to be a successful leader. School counselors are "people persons" and are drawn to the school counseling profession because of their strong personal/social consciousness skills. The school counselor as leader in the 21st-century school is someone who can "create a fundamental transformation in the learning cultures of schools" (Fullan, 2002). School counselors of today are called on to emphasize accountability, social justice, and systemic change and deliver these within a comprehensive developmental school counseling program that removes barriers to student success and addresses the academic, career, and personal-social needs of all students. This approach requires leadership skills. Leadership in today's schools requires vision, the ability to develop others, collaboration skills, the willingness to be accountable, and the ability to see the big picture (DeVoss, 2010; Erford & McCaskill, 2010). "Successful leaders tend to engage others with their energy and are, in turn, energized by the activities and accomplishments of the group" (Fullan, 2002, p. 15). An effective school counselor as leader has a moral purpose and a mindset for action (Fullan, 2002). As Charles Handy (2002) observed: "A worthwhile life ... requires that you have a purpose beyond yourself" (p. 126).

> In an attempt to distinguish leadership roles from administrative roles, some leader-ship schemas from the professional knowledge base may be of assistance....
> Crowther et al. (2002) proposed six ... arenas for teacher leadership:
>
> - Convey conviction about a better world.
> - Strive for authenticity in their teaching, learning, and assessment practices.
> - Facilitate communities of learning through organization-wide practices.
> - Confront barriers in the school's culture and structures.
> - Translate ideas into sustainable systems of actions; and
> - "Nurture a culture of success."
>
> (Lindahl, 2008, p. 302)

## Principals as Partners

School counselors working in partnership with principals and other critical **stakeholders** toward common goals enhance each other's influence and thus increase the school's leadership potential. Principals have one of the most difficult jobs in America (Rubin, 2009). The changing face of American society and the fact that schools reflect all the social issues of the larger society often result in unrealistic expectations on principals. Just a few of the tasks principals are called on to perform on a daily basis are the following:

- Be the instructional leader.
- Take responsibility for the success and failure of all students.
- Keep the school climate safe and conducive to learning.
- Run a fiscally responsible school and balance the budget.
- Evaluate, motivate, and support faculty and staff.
- Effectively work with parents and be able to tell the truth even when it is going to be tough for parents to hear.
- Hold the line with parents and maintain control of the school.
- Understand teachers', parents', and students' rights.
- Understand the role and function of every school employee from the bus driver to the superintendent.
- Monitor student progress and know the patterns of students' failures and successes.
- Attend to students' physical health, emotional well-being, and social growth.

- Keep the school site clean and well maintained.
- Be a master at public relations and public image.
- Know how to negotiate legal landmines.
- Be willing to take the responsibility for all that can go wrong when hundreds of people gather under one roof each day.

The issues in our schools today and their complexity demand that many hands work together and many minds come to the table to solve problems (Dahir, 2000; Fink & Resnick, 2001). Principals are more frequently seeking collaboration with a leadership team as autonomous leadership makes the job daunting (Lawson & Barkdull, 2000). Professionals cannot address the multifaceted needs of students and their families if they work in isolation (Anderson-Butcher & Ashton, 2004).

The expectations of leadership in the schools have changed dramatically since its inception (Lindalh, 2008). With the change in the philosophy of school leadership some leaders were rendered incompetent, although these same leaders at one point had matched the socially determined expectations of an exemplary leader. The social ground of leadership in schools shifted under them and these leaders did not shift with it (Fink & Resnick, 2001; Leithwood, Steinbach, & Jantizi, 2002). The "social ground" has shifted for all educators, including school counselors, and the profession is turning its attention to the development of leadership skills for school counselors and collaborative skills for sharing leadership with principals to equip these professionals with the tools needed in today's schools (Amatea & Clark, 2005; Janson, Militello, & Kosine, 2008; Janson, Stone, & Clark, 2009; Militello & Janson, 2007).

The principal and school counselor are increasingly engaging in a leadership partnership, demonstrating by their collaborative efforts a commitment to delivering optimum educational opportunities (Clark & Stone, 2000b; Janson, 2008). This spirit of cooperation between school counselor and principal will garner support for the school's counseling program, move forward the counselor's efforts to be viewed as a critical player in the school, and more importantly make a difference for students. The Eight Elements of Effective School Principal-Counselor Relationships evolved from a study Janson and Militello conducted in 2007. Janson and Militello investigated how school counselors and principals perceived their current professional relationships with each other (Janson & Militello, 2009). Eight themes emerged:

1. Mutual value. The principal and school counselor value each other's job responsibilities, tasks, and contributions to the school and its educational mission.
2. Open and reflective communication. The principal and school counselor are accessible and available to each other to discuss issues related to their individual and shared roles in the school, as well as issues relevant to the educational mission of the school.
3. Shared belief in interdependency. The principal and school counselor believe that many aspects of their individual roles cannot be accomplished without contributions from the other.

4. Trust. The principal and school counselor trust one another to support their own individual practices as well as their individual contributions to the shared educational mission of the school.

5. Collective enterprise. The principal and the school counselor share in facilitating the development of the common educational mission of the school.

6. Awareness of the other's repertoire. The principal and school counselor understand each other's scope of training and professional expectations and standards.

7. Purposeful and focused collaboration. The principal and school counselor collaborate with intention around specific goals and strategies related to the common educational mission of the school.

8. Stretched leadership. The principal and the school counselor share in leadership tasks and practices related to meeting the educational mission of the school. (Janson & Militello, 2009)

In 2009 College Board conducted a similar study titled "A Closer Look at the Principal-Counselor Relationship." The findings of this study show that the basic priorities of both principals and counselors were well-aligned.

- Principals and counselors both ranked communication and respect as the two most important elements in the principal-counselor relationship.

- Principals and counselors both saw time as being the biggest barrier to collaboration between them.

- Principals had a better match between their perceptions of how important an element is to a successful principal-counselor relationship and the extent to which they saw that element as being present in the principal-counselor relationships within their own schools. When elements were rated as important, principals tended to rate them as being more present than did counselors.

- When asked what one thing they would change that would lead to an improved principal-counselor relationship within their schools, both principals and counselors most frequently mentioned communication, followed by respect/understanding.

- Principals and counselors agreed that the most important activities for a counselor to engage in to improve student outcomes are helping to promote students' personal growth and social development and helping students with career planning.

- Although both principals and counselors agreed that supportive administrative tasks are less important for counselors to engage in to improve student outcomes, principals saw these tasks as taking up less of counselors' time than counselors said they took.

- Both principals and counselors saw state test scores as the area where gaps between subgroups most needed to be addressed in their schools.

- When asked about the roles of principals and counselors in education reform efforts, both principals and counselors most often said that the role of the principal is to be a leader and the role of the counselor is to be an advocate (Finkelstein, 2009).

**MEET MARY MORSETH: PARTNERING WITH HER PRINCIPAL TO REDEFINE HER ROLE**

Mary Morseth is a high school counselor in Minnesota. She was the advanced placement coordinator and administered approximately 750 exams in a 4-week period in May (2 weeks regular testing, 3 days late testing, 3 days special circumstances testing). Mary and her colleagues were working hard to increase the enrollment and rigor in AP, reduce retentions, and increase academic success and were making great strides. However, the AP testing was taking Mary away from some of her individual work with students as well as her leadership and systemic efforts to help more students access and be successful in rigor. Mary went to her principal and listed the four broad categories, specifics under each category, and the data she hoped to move and the students she intended to touch if given the month of May back. Her principal listened intently and then simply said, "You are no longer AP test coordinator."

## School Counselors and Power

School counselors have a number of natural entrées to promote leadership through power. **Power** is an opportunity for influence. Power types are defined below with examples of school counselors exercising the power they have by virtue of their job description, their preparation, and/or their penchant for advocacy, leadership, and social justice.

Growth toward leadership can be facilitated by the exercise of power. Authors have defined the power behind leadership roles in many ways (Leithwood, Begley, & Cousins, 1992). "Researchers such as Kipnis et al. were able to identify eight means of influence in the workplace (assertiveness, ingratiation, rationality, sanctions, exchange, upward appeals, blocking, and coalitions)" (Kipnis, Schmidt, & Wilkinson, 1980).

"Yukl and Tracey (1992) examined the effectiveness of each nine power tactics (rational persuasion, inspirational appeal, consultation, ingratiation, exchange, personal appeal, coalition, legitimating, and pressure)" (Elias, 2008). It is French and Raven's (1959) classic work that aligns most closely with the school counseling role. Following is a discussion of the congruence between French and Raven's dominant themes and the school counselor role with respect to (1) position power or legitimate power; (2) referent power or relationship power; (3) caring power; (4) transformational power or developmental power; (5) connection power; (6) reward power; and (7) technical, information, or expert power (French & Raven, 1959; Raven, 1965).

*Legitimate power*, often called **position power**, is when a power-holder has a genuine right to ask for compliance with a request (Elias, 2008). Legitimate or position power is power that comes from the authority invested in the job or position. In education, legitimate or position power has historically been assigned to superintendents and principals (Elias, 2008; Leithwood, Begley, & Cousins, 1992).

School counselors possess position power when they are placed in charge of committees such as the child study team, the Response to Intervention Team, or the Student Services Team, usually comprised of a school psychologist, social worker, and others who are working toward interventions for special needs students. Position power that comes with committee membership enables school counselors to exercise leadership on behalf of students. Other examples of position power for school counselors include leadership positions within their professional organization such as the American School Counselor Association, the teachers' union, or movement into district-level positions such as district supervisor for counseling.

*Referent or relationship power* is power that comes from positive relationships with others. The leader who relies on referent power hopes to influence through her or his positive relationships with others. **Referent power** greatly depends on the influence leaders have on followers through supportive behavior such as encouragement and recognition. Other additional aspects of leadership involve community building, working with others, facilitating, exercising good listening skills, and persuasion as the leader expresses concern about the vision and mission of the group. School counselors are in a unique position to focus on and develop relationships among members of the organization.

There are situations in which expert or referent power can take negative forms. For example, while a supervisor may possess superior knowledge, that does not necessarily mean that it will be put to use in a way that will benefit her or his subordinates. On the contrary, that supervisor's knowledge may be used in such a fashion (i.e., negative expert power) that strictly benefits herself or himself, resulting in resistance to the influence attempt. Negative referent power is said to occur when a supervisor who is disliked or not identified with by her or his subordinates attempts to utilize social power. In such situations, doing the opposite or ignoring what the supervisor requests is likely to occur (Elias, 2008).

School counselors because of their training in facilitative skills are likely to try to seek and explore the dynamics that exist among members of the organization, which in turn enhances referent power. This skill in understanding the dynamics of groups is an asset school counselors can capitalize on to help move the school agenda forward. School counselors need referent power to capture and profit from furthering their work as consultants, change agents, and systemic reformers.

*Caring power* relies on the passion of the individual and one's ability to relate that deep-seated caring to further one's mission and goals. Although closely related to referent power, caring power is different because of the influence that results even if the relationships are not optimal. The respect garnered for the school counselor who cares about the children in her or his charge can be used to optimize resources and opportunities for students. It is difficult to deny a passionate educator who is advocating for resources and opportunities to level the playing field of opportunity for all students. More than any other type of leadership power, school counselors can capitalize on caring power. School counselors as child advocates can use caring power to a maximum advantage in the leadership role. Caring power, often viewed as natural for a person who goes into the helping field of school counseling, serves the professional well especially in the role of advocate. Caring power centers on motivating students, supporting teachers, and assisting the administration. An example of this is a middle school counselor in an urban setting who was able to rally a local business to provide funds and people power for an after-school tutoring program to change the 32 percent failure rate of her eighth graders. Her caring power was apparent and caused people to respond generously with their time, talent, and money.

*Transformational or developmental power* is the ability to empower others. This power is about enhancing the individual and collective problem-solving capacities of organizational members (Leithwood, Begley, & Cousins, 1992). Transformational leadership occurs when the goals, vision, and motives of the followers are shaped and enhanced by the ability of the leader to empower others to be part of exercising a leadership role in furthering the collective mission of the school. School counselors have endless opportunities to exercise transformational leadership by establishing counseling programs whose purpose mirrors the mission of the school and exercising a leadership role to further that mission. The School Improvement Team (SIT) is where many school counselors are finding a voice for their transformational power. For example, if a determination is made by the SIT that the failure rate in the fifth grade is unacceptable, the school counselor, as part of the problem-solving or transformational leadership, may want to implement a mentoring program for students in danger of repeating the fifth grade.

*Connection power* is based on the school counselor's connections with others. Connections are defined as people of power or influence or people holding the key to something followers need or want. School counselors as a group may have no more or less connection power than most other educators and thus rarely rely on this type of power. However, school counselors can look for opportunities to have connection power especially with school board members, central administration staff, parent organizations, and others who are in a position to positively influence the future. Counseling organizations recognize the power of connection and in most states will seek connection power with legislators through "legislative days" in which counselors visit lawmakers and lobby for their causes. Much time, interest, and money are spent grooming a relationship to influence legislation. In particular, high school counselors recognize the power of connections when they start advocating for their students with admissions representatives. When counselors have been able to groom a relationship with select admissions representatives, they have connection power and are in a better position to be effective advocates. The opportunities to help students are endless when school counselors pay attention to and utilize the power of connections.

*Reward power* means you have the ability to lead through material or psychological rewards. Forms of reward power include praise, support, recognition, promotions, and monetary rewards. This power can influence and shape the behaviors of others. For school counselors who do not possess the power to give raises or other types of monetary rewards, referent or relationship power is an asset in achieving reward power. When the school counselor has the respect of the person she or he is praising or acknowledging, this can serve to shape behavior in the desired direction. For example, an elementary school counselor who is respected in her school developed a recognition program to enhance effective teaching called "spotlight on teaching." Every two weeks this counselor features a teacher who has been observed implementing an effective teaching technique. The teacher's picture is placed on a bulletin board with a write-up and is asked to briefly discuss her or his technique during the next faculty meeting. These spotlights (from someone the teachers respect) are effective in disseminating throughout the school a variety of successful techniques to enhance learning such as behavior management techniques.

*Technical, information, or expert power* is the power that one has because of specialized knowledge, information, or expertise. This power is bestowed on a leader by others because the leader can assist where the other members of the group have less skill or lack of skills. Individuals with this power can achieve goals based on their abilities or training. For example, school counselors enjoy a high degree of expert power by virtue of their specialized training in areas such as consultation, counseling, data analysis, and collaboration. Counselors can capitalize on their expert power to benefit students in their charge by providing information to teachers, parents, and others on topics that support students in areas such as interventions for special needs students, i.e., underachievers, Attention Deficit Hyperactivity Disorder (ADHD) students, or acting-out students. The special education qualifying criteria, postsecondary admissions information, and academic advising are just a few examples of areas in which school counselors exercise expert or informational power. Providing parents, students, and teachers with critical, timely information furthers a school counselor's leadership stance.

All of these various power types are important to understand as they can influence, support, or prove to be a barrier to effective leadership. Effective use of power equates to an successful leadership style, and like other educators, school counselors need to develop an effective leadership style. The higher the comfort level, the more the school counselor will exercise leadership and increase one's opportunities for positively affecting the lives of the children in their charge. The development of leadership means capitalizing on the "natural power" in addition to the "groomed power" that school counselors have by virtue of training, professional development, and a penchant to be helpers.

# SCHOOL COUNSELORS DEVELOPING LEADERSHIP SKILLS

Developing leadership skills is neither an event nor acquired in a professional development opportunity but occurs during a long and conscientious process in which you continually reassess how your progress, gaps, victories, and deficits align with the leadership needs of your students. Over the years, it has been our observation that school counselors who are effective leaders developed their leadership skills through attention to the following four areas: self-awareness, facilitative communication, team development, and staff development.

## Self-Awareness

Developing leadership skills starts with a personal analysis of your current strengths and weaknesses. From the self-knowledge gained, you can begin to develop a style of leadership that can grow and be enhanced. Leadership development is less daunting if you begin by focusing on your strengths. Working from a position of strengths will allow for creativity and excitement as you acquire greater self-knowledge and skills.

There are many techniques to help you understand your leadership strengths such as examining your behavior in prior leadership roles and using feedback from colleagues and friends as an opportunity to grow. Examining prior leadership roles is a great place to start the self-awareness process. Follow these steps to help organize this effort.

1. Think back to a time when you were in any leadership role—large or small, professional or personal (professional usually refers to a paid position and personal refers to a nonpaid position). An example of a personal leadership position could have been taking charge in organizing your team's tennis matches, being your child's Girl Scout leader, or taking on the task of leading the July 4th celebration in your neighborhood. This position may have been an appointed one such as the guidance department chairperson, an elected one such as a school board member, or a position entirely dependent on your ability to influence others.
2. Take this leadership position and examine how you proceeded to make policy, shape behavior, organize work, and/or set and meet goals. In other words, examine your "way of work" in the leadership arena.
3. From this leadership experience, make a list of the skills, competencies, and dispositions you brought to the leadership role. Reflect on the approaches that were the strongest for you and the areas where the comfort level was lowest and the success weakest.
4. Turn some time and attention to the strong areas and consider how these areas promoted success and how the weak areas detracted or hindered success. Consider what you would do differently in the future. Write a plan of action for a future leadership role that builds on your successes and minimizes your weaknesses or grows them into strengths.

## Facilitative Communication

Another approach to self-analysis of your leadership strengths is to reflect on any feedback you have been given by employers, coworkers, or people in your personal life as to how you interact with others. Leadership depends on personal relationships, and informal and formal feedback can help illuminate areas of strength and weaknesses.

The facilitative skills for school counselors, primarily for use in individual counseling sessions, are also valuable in developing a successful leadership style. By using facilitative communication in your leadership interactions, you can enhance your ability to influence others. In Chapter 2 you learned about counseling techniques and facilitation skills. These skills can contribute to good communication in leadership, a key ingredient for success. Throughout your preparation program you will build and increase your skills in reflecting, paraphrasing, clarifying, and questioning.

1. *Reflecting*—when the leader responds by capturing the meaning beyond the expressed words. Responding to the speaker with a high degree of sophistication lets the speaker know that she or he has not only been heard but more importantly has been understood because the listener has reacted to unexpressed meanings or feelings. Sometimes the listener reacts and misses the intent of the speaker. This is generally not a major drawback as the speaker knows the listener is trying to understand at a deeper level the concerns or expressions of the speaker.

2. *Paraphrasing*—when the leader uses active listening to repeat in summary what was communicated. Paraphrasing can be a powerful communication tool when used judiciously to reinforce to others that they have been heard. When a leader pays attention to verbal and nonverbal behavior and communicates this to others by paraphrasing, it is a relationship builder. The difference between reflecting and paraphrasing is that paraphrasing usually just captures the words and gives back to the speaker a succinct response that captures the main meaning. Reflecting captures the meaning behind the words.

3. *Clarifying*—when the leader helps others in the school bring to focus ambiguous meaning. Clarifying helps the speaker define and refine thoughts, motives, feelings, and actions by the carefully chosen words of the listener.

4. *Questioning*—gathering information by carefully choosing open-ended questions, which in turn gives the speaker the chance to convey information, feelings, understanding, etc. Open-ended questioning invites the speaker to talk whereas closed questions are less facilitative and reduce the speaker to answering "yes," "no," or responding with a word or two.

Three examples of dialogues follow demonstrating the need of **facilitative responses** on the part of a school counselor: (1) a teacher who is resisting a principal mandate that all teachers must seek consultation with the Pre-referral Assistant Team before her or his students can be considered for a special education referral, (2) a consultation exchange between the school counselor and a mathematics teacher about Samantha, his student, and (3) an exchange between the school counselor and Samantha.

### Facilitative Responses with a Resistant Teacher

As the school counselor you have tried to explain to a resistant teacher the benefits and purpose of the Pre-referral Assistance Team (a team that tries to help teachers with students instead of going right to Special Education), but the teacher continues to resist using this team and insists on skipping over this step.

> *Teacher:* "I really think it is insulting that I have to go before a pre-referral team before Jim [the student] can be tested for special education. I have tried everything and if I say Jim is not going to make it in regular education then I think that should be enough. I have been in the classroom for 32 years and I have never before had to beg my way into getting a student into special education. Who knows a student better than the classroom teacher?"

> *School Counselor:*

> Reflecting: "This change in SE procedure has you reeling."

> Paraphrasing: "You believe you should be able to make a recommendation for SE as has always been the procedure."

> Clarifying: "You are struggling to avoid what you believe is an unfair change in procedures."

> Open Question: "Would you talk more about why this procedure is so offensive to you?"

> Closed Question: "Would you give the Pre-referral Assistance Team a try?"

> Interpreting/Analyzing: "You really think it is second-guessing and questioning a teacher's competence and judgment to insist that all students come before the Pre-referral Assistance Team."

### Facilitative Responses in Teacher-Student Conflict

Mr. Jefferson, a seventh-grade mathematics teacher, and Samantha, one of his students, are at odds.

> *Teacher:* "I have tried to work with Samantha but her attitude makes it so difficult. She never turns in any assignments and she makes it impossible to help her or correct her on anything as she will refuse to communicate when you try to talk to her. I really have tried but I am at the end of my rope with her. I don't know if she can do the math as I never get any work from her. She may need a lower level math class."

> *School Counselor:*

> Reflecting: "You are really frustrated with Samantha."

> Paraphrasing: "You are at a loss as to how to get Samantha to complete her work."

> Clarifying: "There are two issues working here. You are stumped as to what to try next with Samantha and you are considering the possibility that the work may be too hard for her."

Open Question: "Can you describe a time when Samantha responded positively?"

Closed Question: "Do you want me to move her from your class?"

Interpreting/Analyzing: "I suspect the math class is too challenging and that Samantha needs to stay for after-school tutoring."

Interpreting/Analyzing: "Samantha is a strong personality and it is a well-known fact that you expect a great deal from your students. If you agree, we can have a three-way conversation to try to resolve the stand-off between you and Samantha."

*Student:* "I want to try to succeed in that class but Mr. Jefferson has it in for me and no matter what I do he is going to make sure I fail. I really do try but then I think why bother, it is no use. I was doing my work but he would not help me when I did not understand so I quit."

*School Counselor:*

Reflecting: "You are really discouraged about your math class."

Paraphrasing: "The conflict with your teacher has caused you to stop trying."

Clarifying: "You are struggling to figure out how to salvage your math class but the answer is not apparent right now."

Open Question: "Can you describe the last incident of conflict between you and your teacher?"

Closed Question: "Are you asking to drop this class?"

Interpreting/Analyzing: "I think your troubles are only partly with your teacher as I suspect you have found the subject matter too challenging."

Interpreting/Analyzing: "Both you and Mr. Jefferson are strong personalities. The trouble lies in the fact that you are having a test of wills and neither of you will budge an inch."

As is true in a counseling and consultation role, lower-level questioning in the leadership role is best used sparingly or avoided. The facilitative responses outlined above are in hierarchical order from most facilitative, which encourages conversation and problem solving, to least facilitative. The first four facilitative skills encourage the student and teachers to continue to talk so that the school counselor can more successfully guide them toward a resolution. Interpreting and advising are low-level skills as they often shut down communication especially if the recipient feels she or he is being judged or misunderstood. In the leadership role exercised by school counselors, interpreting and advising are sometimes necessary and appropriate. Facilitative communication skills have helped school counselors in their leadership role to become more effective communicators, an asset of leaders of influence.

## Team Development

Prior to becoming a school counselor, develop your team-building skills by practicing with a real team, perhaps on a class project. The best place to start for team building is to tackle a project for which you are passionate as this will fuel your energy and enthusiasm. For example, maybe you are interested in developing a bully-proofing program because you know that too many students are afraid while at school. The likelihood of success will be greater when you are working on something that you feel compelled to affect. Your enthusiasm will likely be infectious to the rest of your team members. Develop your team with Hackman's (2002) principles in mind. Hackman (2002) found five areas of consideration that made for effective teams:

- Is the team a real team or a team in name only?
- Does the team have a compelling direction for its work?
- Is the structure of the team designed to enable rather than impede teamwork?
- Does the team operate within a supportive environment?
- Does the team have expert coaching? (p. 31)

Hackman (2002) advised that your team should contain no more than six members and that bringing together people who only get along is not necessarily always best. Also, Hackman (2002) cautions that group leaders cannot assume that individual and group skills will evolve on their own but will need grooming and attention. Your facilitative communication skills will be effective in supporting group cohesiveness. Start with a small project and carefully grow your skills and increase your leadership so that you can enjoy a high-profile, powerful role that makes a difference for your students.

## Staff Development

School counselors who seize opportunities to stand before the faculty, parents, students, and community stakeholders and deliver presentations are exercising a particularly powerful leadership role. Learning to be comfortable with presentations is a matter of practicing. Presentation software such as PowerPoint from Microsoft is a great medium that is easy to learn, and it makes presenting more comfortable because you have an outline to cue your content. The appendix of this textbook (see text's website) provides an easy-to-follow outline of how to develop a PowerPoint presentation. In Chapter 5, staff development will be discussed in more detail.

# THE IMPACT OF THE SCHOOL COUNSELOR AS LEADER

In the remaining sections of this chapter are four specific areas that demonstrate how school counselors behave as members of the school's leadership team. Examples illustrate how practicing school counselors and other stakeholders collaborate to demonstrate leadership and advocacy. You will "meet" school counselors who will help translate these leadership concepts into the day-to-day reality of school counseling. The four areas that follow are not all-inclusive but provide the tip of the iceberg as examples of opportunities to exercise a leadership role that can translate into greater opportunities for students. Operationalizing leadership means taking a closer look at (1) improving school climates, (2) successful instructional programs, (3) developing high aspirations, and (4) course enrollment and tracking patterns.

## Improving School Climates

School counselors continually scan the school landscape, alert to recognizing an unhealthy school climate and promoting a safe environment that supports opportunities for all students to get a good education. School climate will be a major topic of discussion in Chapter 11. However, in order to demonstrate advocacy in action and to operationalize how these skills play out, let us now examine how a school counselor can advocate for change in an unsafe school climate. It has been shown that bullying adversely stratifies educational opportunities for students and establishes a hostile and dangerous climate for the bullied. Countless school counselors have promoted a safer, more inclusive school climate by initiating or supporting bully-proofing programs.

If a school counselor suspects that bullying is taking place, those suspicions can be confirmed or eliminated by examining the discipline referrals for conflicts, bullying, and/or aggressive behavior. Bringing in resources to tackle the problem of bullying and conflict resolution is a good leadership activity for a school counselor. By establishing a committee comprised of critical stakeholders such as Parent Teacher Association (PTA) members, goals can be set to reduce the number of discipline referrals that involved fighting, name-calling, verbal harassment, and other forms of bullying. Collaboration can come from many areas. Classroom teachers can follow through with activities suggested in the guidance lessons delivered by the school counselor. The teachers can implement various conflict resolution strategies, such as teaching the students to identify bullying behavior and charting it as a class, until they extinguished the behavior. The principal can provide leadership and support for all facets of the program. The art, music, and physical education teachers and the media specialist can establish lessons and activities in concert with school-wide efforts to eliminate bullying. Local businesses can provide volunteers as well as incentives for classes to reduce their bullying behavior. All of these efforts provide the school counselor with leadership opportunities to reduce the bullying in schools and create a safer, more respectful school climate.

## Successful Instructional Programs

How can the school counselor successfully affect the instructional program? Through the collaborative efforts of the school counselor, the principal, and other key stakeholders, the school instructional program can be strengthened. Conducting staff development for teachers and parents in such important areas as educational planning, motivation, student appraisal, interventions, and diversity issues demonstrates school counselors leading and teaming to play a unique role in fostering understanding and cooperation among the school community. Student leadership training, cooperative discipline, classroom management, study skills, and postsecondary admissions procedures are areas that have long been influenced by school counselors. The ultimate goal of staff development is to collaborate to provide support to teachers through information, interventions, modeling, and encouragement (Lewis & Bradley, 2000). The opportunities for affecting the instructional program are limitless.

One middle school counselor decided to try to address some student behavioral issues that frequently frustrated parents and teachers by organizing a Parent/Teacher Forum. She conducted a needs assessment and identified the most frequently occurring problems and concerns of educators and parents in her school such as Attention Deficit Hyperactivity Disorder (ADHD), lack of study skills, underachievement, aggressive/defiant behavior, and substance abuse. Each year, this school counselor hosts a one-night fair in which parents and teachers are able to choose three different presentations by local experts.

Helping teachers understand and use tests to maximize learning for students is another area in which school counselors can affect the instructional program. Teachers receive critical information in the form of test results. Analyzing and interpreting these test results and sharing the results in such a way that they can be used to benefit the instructional process is a powerful way to support students. Therefore, if school counselors can help increase students chances of doing well on the Preliminary Scholastic Achievement Test (PSAT) then their future chance to be admitted to the college of their choice and to get scholarship dollars will soar. Much controversy surrounds high-stakes standardized testing in this country and it is understandable that school counselors may want to avoid involvement. However, standardized tests are a fact of life; and it is through these tests that opportunities are advanced, such as who will have access to higher education and benefit from the resulting economic rewards that correlate with postsecondary education. Testing also affects who will get college credit for a high school course and who will be promoted to the next grade, thus reducing the risk of becoming a dropout.

## Developing High Aspirations in Students

School counselors working along with other key stakeholders can help students develop high aspirations rather than waiting for aspirations to emerge. Improving student motivation is an area in which school counselors can have tremendous influence. For example, by helping students understand their choices and the full meaning of those choices, school counselors can positively effect students' desire to stretch and strive academically (Stone, 1998). Students need to understand the logic and interrelatedness of the curriculum with the consequences of academic choices. Devising ways to clearly communicate to students and their parents that academic choices widen or narrow future options and opportunities is a central task of all school counseling programs (Amatea & West-Olatunji, 2007; Carnevale & Desrochers, 2003a; Daggett, 2003). The academic advising role includes

## MEET ROBERT (BOB) TURBA, WHO IMPROVED AN INSTRUCTIONAL PROGRAM

Bob, a high school counselor in a college preparatory magnet school in Florida, established a relational database in the guidance office using information from the school's student information system. The guidance department ordered the Preliminary Scholastic Aptitude Test (PSAT) scores on disk and imported these scores, along with all information the students provided on the PSAT application, into the database. The students' biographical information and their PSAT scores were paired with their mathematics and language arts teachers. Reports that contained their students' PSAT results on verbal, math, and writing scores and the answers that the students gave for each question were given to each math and language arts teacher. The teachers were also given the correct answers and a class set of unused PSAT booklets. The teachers used this information and reviewed the test questions and answers. Teachers held sessions with the students and helped the students to understand their incorrect answers. In this way, students (especially 10th graders) were able to understand more about the PSAT, its format, and how they could maximize their scores for the Scholastic Aptitude Test for which the PSAT is considered a precursor and how to improve their 11th-grade PSAT scores. This is an example of a counselor being able to affect the instructional program by providing teachers with critical information about their students. Since all students in this school system take the PSAT, all students' learning and instruction were affected by this proactive approach. It is ideal but not necessary that counselors know how to set up a relational database. If a counselor understands the power of data to inform teaching, she or he can find the person in the school district who can disaggregate the information so that teachers receive the information for their particular students. This approach to helping students gives considerable credibility to this counselor and helps students learn and acquire more scholarships. For example, the class of 2009 had 317 students and 77 of them were recognized by the National Merit Scholarship programs, i.e., the Merit Program, the Achievement Program for African American students, and the Hispanic Recognition Program. Seniors were offered over $10.2 million in merit scholarships. One hundred forty-four members of this class were offered at least one merit scholarship, and 80 percent earned a Florida Bright Futures scholarship. These impressive results were due in no small part to Bob's leadership in helping students raise their PSAT and SAT scores (www.stantoncollegeprep.org/Stantonian/StantonianSummer09.pdf).

informing students of appropriate courses to take that match their aspirations, helping them understand the interrelationship between curriculum choices and future economic success, and showing them that financing a higher education is possible.

"In our world, knowledge is the capital and the premier wealth-producing resource, making the process of education the ultimate supplier of power" (Drucker, 1989). Although over a decade old, Drucker's statement has even more meaning today. The most basic and significant mission of schools is helping youth develop into productive adult citizens who will effectively contribute to society. Adults of tomorrow need adequate preparation to function intelligently in their social, civic, and work worlds. With rapid changes that are occurring in the workforce, tomorrow's schools have a tremendous responsibility to prepare today's students to become productive workers in an ever-increasing global economy (Carnevale & Desrochers, 2003a. To this end, helping students understand the relationship between academic preparation and career development is paramount (Akos, Lambie, Milsom, & Gilbert, 2007; Carnevale & Desrochers, 2003a). This can be done by sharing statistics with students about the impact education has on lifetime salaries (Hoyt & Wickwire, 2001). The sharing of this information may encourage a higher degree of motivation and understanding of course relevancy. Giving specific, up-to-date information on what jobs and accompanying skills/training are required in the workforce will in turn contribute to students' understanding of the interrelatedness between what they do in school and future economic opportunities. Employment statistics will serve as a blueprint for students who are trying to build a future or who need encouragement to do well in school. Students will realize that their success in school is connected to future opportunities available to them. This type of information sharing is something that can begin in elementary school and can continue as a regular part of the school counselors' role in career and educational planning leading to higher aspirations (Murrow-Taylor, Foltz, McDonald, Ellis, & Culbertson, 1999).

Bryan (2009) conducted a study in which students clearly suggested that school counselors can have a positive impact on their college choices, aspirations, and rate of applying to college. College plans of low-income students and students of color (e.g., African American and Latino/Latina students) are more likely to be influenced by their high school counselors. Research suggests that students are influenced by their perceptions of others' (e.g., school counselor, parents, close relatives, teachers, peers) educational aspirations for them (Bryan et al., 2009).

Uwah, McMahon, and Furlow (2008) conducted a study to investigate the relationship between perceptions of school belonging, educational aspirations, and academic self-efficacy among a sample of African American male high school students. "Although students' perceptions of being liked by others and their general impression of membership may be valued, results from this study suggest that those feelings do not positively influence participants' academic self-efficacy. Students may require more than casual or passing acknowledgments from members of the school community or the perception that they are well liked in order to believe that they can succeed in school...." These findings suggest that being targeted and directly invited to participate may be especially meaningful to African American males, and without that invitation, these students may feel liked without feeling academically competent.

## MEET THE HIGH SCHOOL COUNSELORS OF JACKSONVILLE, FLORIDA, WHO DEVELOPED HIGH STUDENT ASPIRATIONS

An example of school counselors taking a leadership role in helping students develop high aspirations can be found in the high schools in Jacksonville, Florida, where each student is informed as to available financial aid and scholarship opportunities through a districtwide program, "Bringing Economic and Career Opportunities Nearer" (BEACON). The school counselors in this district annually collaborate with the supervisor of guidance to train and place approximately 100 volunteers into the 21 high schools of the district to deliver individual advising sessions about how to access financial aid and scholarships for postsecondary education. Harvey Harper, a volunteer, is one example of the many committed people who have helped countless students gain greater hope in financing a postsecondary education. Harvey has been volunteering each year in the program since its inception in 1991. Electronic Personal Education Planning is available through FACTS.org, Florida's online student advising system. Rising ninth graders can plan courses with an emphasis on an area they would like to explore. Students can select one of four graduation plans: a college preparatory plan, which meets state university admissions and Bright Futures Academic and Medallion Scholarship requirements; a career-preparatory plan, which will prepare them for a career and meets the requirements for a Bright Futures Gold Seal Vocational Scholarship; a plan that covers college and career preparation, which prepares students for both options; and the standard high school diploma plan, which meets the high school graduation requirements.

## Course Enrollment and Tracking Patterns

School counselors in collaboration with other members of the leadership team are ideally situated to positively affect **course enrollment and tracking patterns**. School counselors can operate professionally as "door openers" when they understand how tracking and course taking can further or hinder opportunities for the students in their schools. School counselors can influence enrollment patterns and implement academic safety nets for students who are willing to attempt rigor. Course selection contributes to furthering or hindering educational opportunity. Teachers, parents, administrators, students, and school counselors can choose course assignments that significantly narrow or widen future opportunities. Furthermore, students are making decisions that are inconsistent with their future goals. "Just over a third (34%) of students who entered ninth grade in public schools left school with both a regular diploma and the abilities and qualifications required even to apply to a four-year college. The situation is particularly bad for minority students. Only 23% of African-American students and 20% of Hispanic students left school college-ready, compared with 40% of white students" (Greene & Winters, 2005, p. 9).

A study by Stone (1998) examined the mathematics placement of the ninth graders of one large urban school district. An analysis of the 1,611 ninth graders who scored in the upper quartile on one of three mathematics subtests revealed that placement in higher-level mathematics differed for upper quartile students depending on where the student went to school. In this school district, a student's future opportunities were stratified based on the course enrollment patterns exercised by the educators and community of each school (Stone, 1998).

School counselors can also find leadership opportunities in professional organizations. The American School Counselor Association (ASCA) is the national organization for school counselors. It is the opinion of the authors of this text that it is important for school counselors to become members of their local, state, and/or national professional organizations. Membership in professional organizations gives one a collective voice legislatively; provides a multitude of professional development opportunities to include print materials, workshops, and conferences; and will increase your enjoyment of your work as you build relationships with your fellow professionals. Professional stagnation is less likely when one challenges oneself by the most current and effective practices and information brought to you by professional organizations.

## LEADERSHIP: REWARDING BUT CHALLENGING

Leadership is not easy. Hold firm in your leadership role and, in the words of Trish Hatch, co-author of the ASCA model (2003), "don't blink." Leaders are not always popular, and with leadership comes the understanding that the decisions made and the positions advocated for may naturally result with someone disagreeing. Hold steady and move with conviction toward the goals of the school's mission and the school counseling program and keep a clear eye on what you are trying to accomplish for the students. This will result in garnering respect and reducing resistance. Leadership is difficult but rewarding. Seize the challenge and embrace it as an opportunity to grow as you figure out how to negotiate the school terrain. Success will be yours. Refuse to fail.

> **Success**
> When we think of failure
> Failure will be ours.
> If we remain undecided
> Nothing will ever change.
> All we need to do
> Is want to achieve something great
> And then simply do it.
> Never think of failure
> For what we think,
> Will come about.
> (Maharishi Mahesh Yogi)

## TECH TOOLS

When you become a school counselor, use the power of technology to maximize the efficiency and effectiveness of your leadership.

- Query databases to answer questions about course enrollment patterns. Order tech-generated information to support changes in course enrollment patterns such as The College Board Report on PSAT results that Bernadette Willette gathered to garner support for initiating Advanced Placement classes.
- Assist the instructional program by providing student achievement data in a way that is most advantageous for students, such as the work Bob Turba did by disaggregating PSAT scores by teacher.
- Use tech tools such as discussion lists, email messages, and websites to increase communication and the exchange of critical and timely information. For example, some counselors have weekly electronic newsletters that are sent via email. Counselors are increasingly collaborating via discussion lists.
- Regularly seek a spot on the faculty meeting agendas to deliver an 8 to 10 minute bullet-point PowerPoint staff development presentation as a part of your role as a member of the leadership team.
- Consider using spreadsheets to help you keep track of a number of important clusters such as students who have completed a career plan, parent conferences, classes who have received classroom guidance, etc. Spreadsheet programs have the capability of generating summary data and graphs so that you can include these in your end-of-year report about your program's progress toward student outcomes.
- Establish electronic support groups and supervision groups with other counselors so that collaboration can help you do your job more efficiently and effectively.

---

## *School Counselor Casebook: Voices From the Field*

### The Scenario Reviewed

In your school district, large numbers of students are classified and receive special education services. The school where you just started your school counselor position seems to be especially entrenched in the practice of testing and placing students in special education as a natural intervention for students struggling academically. It has become an automatic practice to test for special student education when a student is in danger of failing.

## A Practitioner's Approach

Here's how a practicing school counselor responded to this school scenario:

Although I am fairly new in this position, I realize that the teachers are referring students for testing because they may not have the strategies and interventions that could help struggling students when the familiar methods fail to provide results. As a school counselor leader, it is my responsibility to see why this is common practice and to develop and support options that would benefit the students and teachers. I would speak to my principal and offer to investigate why our school has such a high referral rate for special education. I am aware that many students are referred for comprehensive evaluations but are not eligible for special education services and may need other supports from their teachers in the classroom. As my principal is the instructional leader, I don't want to step on his toes but I do want to offer my help as someone who may look at the situation differently than the classroom teachers.

The first step would be to form a student support team consisting of myself, the principal, the school nurse, any other professional who works with the student, and the teachers of the referred students. Our team would meet to discuss students who are struggling and, most importantly, we would brainstorm strategies and interventions to target areas of concern. The team would also guide teachers in data collection on these students and help them to graph progress. When students are referred for special education testing, looking at data is important. If a team were to be assembled and periodically review the data collection on students, we would clearly see the patterns, determine which interventions are working, and provide more appropriate referrals. I would propose to the team that we would meet every six weeks to review the students who were referred to the student support team. If the student continues to struggle and the teacher has implemented all the interventions and strategies suggested by the team, the team could then agree to move the student to the next phase of the special education referral process.

When teachers are given the tools needed, such as strategies and interventions for specific areas of concern, they are able to help students become more successful. Leaders identify the issues and design plans and collaborate to make the appropriate changes. Teachers also need support from counselors who can help them look at the underlying issues that are causing failure or lack of success or they may continue to refer students to special education testing if for no other reason than because they are at a loss for how to help these struggling students succeed. As a school counselor, I can take the initiative and lead and guide teachers toward more appropriate referrals and to help develop processes in the school building that will make this possible. The students and teachers will both succeed and my work will contribute in a powerful way!

Michelle L. Brantley, EdS
Head Counselor
Ocee Elementary School

# LOOKING BACK: SALIENT POINTS

### Collaborative Leadership for the 21st-Century School

Leadership is becoming an increasingly valued and shared phenomenon at the school level. Leadership in schools of the 21st century entails collaboration among multiple parties for the development, acceptance, and achievement of goals that lead to academic success for all students. A multiplicity of student needs requires all stakeholders to bring their skills and talents to bear in support of students' academic, career, and personal/social success. Leadership is group authority, responsibility, and expertise, and leadership teams change according to the activity or need.

### School Counselors as Leaders

Leadership for the school counselor is fully participating as an integral part of the mission and function of schools, supporting every student to be a successful learner, and enabling student success. Leadership for school counselors requires joining forces with other educators and the larger school community to positively affect the opportunities students will have to be successful learners and to achieve high standards. Leadership means entering into partnerships to demonstrate commitment to help the principal and other internal and external stakeholders deliver critically important tasks to support student learning.

### Developing Leadership Skills

Leadership development is less daunting when a counselor begins with personal strengths. Working from a position of strength will allow for creativity and excitement in the venture.

### Facilitative Communication for Effective Learning

Good communication is a key ingredient in successful leadership. School counselors who use high-level facilitative skills such as reflecting, paraphrasing, and clarifying can capitalize on these skills and enhance their ability to influence others.

### The Imperative to Move to a Leadership Role

The students we are educating today are different from the students we educated yesterday, and the students we educate tomorrow will be different from those of today. School counselors cannot practice traditionally when faced with the reality that students will be a more diverse group in the future. Educators who are not changing with the times are actually losing ground, because those who are committed to change have difficulty keeping pace. Educators are faced with the need to prepare all students for a society that will be unlike any that has come before us. The school counselor as part of the leadership team can join forces with others to ensure that all students have access to the information and experiences that will allow them to influence the society of the future. This leadership team is ideally situated to advocate for all students by providing the support necessary to obtain the best possible education as the gateway to greater social and economic opportunities for students' futures.

### The Impact of the School Counselor as Leader

School counselors can become members of the leadership team formally but this is not necessary. Leadership is a mindset and a way of work for school counselors who will join forces with other educators to assume and exert leadership within their schools and communities. The school counselor as educational leader establishes a vision and belief in the development of every child. Opportunities for leadership are plentiful. School counselors can view themselves as natural allies with the school's leadership team and look for opportunities to develop and implement their special leadership skills to maximize their effectiveness in the promotion of success for all students.

## KEY TERMS

| | |
|---|---|
| Collaborative leadership p. 96 | Connection power p. 105 |
| School counselor as leader p. 98 | Reward power p. 105 |
| Conflict resolution p. 99 | Transformational or developmental power p. 105 |
| Leadership mindset p. 99 | Technical, information, or expert power p. 106 |
| Leadership team p. 99 | Clarifying p. 108 |
| Stakeholders p. 100 | Facilitative responses p. 108 |
| Power p. 103 | Paraphrasing p. 108 |
| Position power p. 103 | Questioning p. 108 |
| Caring power p. 104 | Reflecting p. 108 |
| Referent or relationship power p. 104 | Course enrollment and tracking patterns p. 116 |

## LEARNING EXTENSIONS/MAKING CONNECTIONS

1. Which of the types of power described do you use most and why? Which type of power do you least prefer and why?

2. Using the points presented throughout the chapter, describe a leader whose style you admire and for whom you respond positively. Explain why you appreciate this leadership approach.

3. Find two counselors who have operationalized leadership in one or more of these areas: (A) changing attitudes and beliefs; (B) influencing the success of instructional programs; (C) developing high aspirations; and (D) changing course enrollment patterns. Interview these counselors and then write up your findings to include a brief description of what they did and your reaction as to whether or not their activities reached a large number of students. Was their activity an efficient use of time? What impact did the activity have on the success of the students?

4. Leadership opportunities for school counselors are all around us. Imagine that you are a practicing school counselor. How do you envision exercising a leadership role in your new school?

5. Describe your leadership style. What are your strengths and weaknesses?

6. The principal is a key partner in enabling school counselors to exercise a leadership role and in delivering an effective school counseling program. Name six to eight strategies you will employ to develop a partnership with your principal.

7. How did Bob Turba change the instructional program for his school? Why was his approach effective?

8. Describe Mary Morseth's advocacy. What personal attributes and skills do you believe Mary needed to have the influence she did with the teachers of her school?

9. Discuss how the school counselors of Jacksonville, Florida, are raising aspirations rather than just attending to aspirations as they emerge.

# School Counselors as Advocates

## CHAPTER OBJECTIVES

*By the time you have completed this chapter, you should be able to*

- describe how school counselors work as advocates and describe areas in which school counselors are having success as an advocate;

- identify the personal/social consciousness skills needed for advocacy;

- understand the ethical imperative for school counselors to behave as advocates;

- begin the process of developing your own plan for behaving as an advocate;

- describe research and accountability measures that reveal areas of inequities in schools and the need for school counselors to advocate;

- understand how technology and staff development skills can help you in your advocacy.

---

## School Counselor Casebook: Getting Started

### The Scenario

Three of your sophomores complained to you, their counselor, about not being able to enroll in any Advanced Placement (AP) courses in their junior year. They did not score high enough on the ninth-grade standardized test last year. The policy in the handbook clearly delineates the criteria. All three of the students really want to take AP courses and are certain they will be able to handle the work.

### Thinking about Solutions

As you read this chapter, think about possible solutions. Is there a role for you in this situation? What would you do? When you come to the end of the chapter, you will have the opportunity to see how your ideas compare with a practicing school counselor's approach.

---

## THE ROLE OF SOCIAL ADVOCACY IN SCHOOL COUNSELING

**Advocacy** in the counseling world involves "identifying groups of people who might benefit from increasing their own strength" (Lewis, Lewis, Daniels, & D'Andrea, 1998, p. 25). Groups of people for whom policy, procedures, and practices adversely stratify their opportunities have been referred to as "socially devalued populations" (Lewis et al., 1998). Because individuals in these socially devalued groups typically have limited power and little say about things that happen in their families, schools, workplaces, and/or communities, they frequently come to believe that they are not valued by others (Hipolito-Delgado & Lee, 2007; Smith, Reynolds, & Rovnak, 2009). "Social advocacy implies questioning the status quo, challenging the rules and regulations that deny student access, protesting changes...that decrease opportunities for the under-represented" (Osborne et al., 1998, p. 201). Problems that individuals face can often be traced to the system(s) in which they live, work, and play. Some examples of these systems are families, work environments, social agencies, the legal system, neighborhoods, educational institutions, and many others. The origins of problems and impediments to effective decision making often lie not in individuals but in an intolerant, restrictive, or unsafe environment (Lee, 2007a). It is generally acknowledged that individuals' situations can lead to poor academic performance; indeed, many students who underachieve and drop out are also pushed out by unchallenging and unsupportive school experiences (Bill and Melinda Gates Foundation, 2006). The practice of counseling is more complete and effective when the counselor helps students and their families negotiate the systems that affect their lives or when the counselor creates change in the system. Changing systems increases counselor effectiveness in multiple ways.

> Unfortunately for the youth of marginalized communities, their educational experience also includes an indoctrination into oppression (Howard, 1999; Potts, 2003; Smith, 2000). For example, the experiences of communities of color are generally not accurately portrayed in American curricula. Instances of racism and injustice are silenced and the contributions of communities of color to American society are ignored (Loewen, 1995; Martinez, 1995; Potts, 2003; Smith, 2000). Furthermore, students of color do not hear of the greatness of their cultures (Potts). American students collectively do not learn how centuries of racism and classism have contributed to the existence of privileged classes and oppressed classes. Within this context, students from marginalized communities are taught from an ethnocentric, monocultural perspective that may cause them to question their ability and the worth of their culture (Howard, 1999; Loewen, 1995; Potts, 2003). (Hipolito-Delgado & Lee, 2007, p. 327)

## THE SCHOOL COUNSELOR AS AN ADVOCATE

A school counselor as advocate feels compelled to survey (scrutinize) the internal and external school landscape to identify the barriers that are impeding student success and to collaborate to create the conditions necessary for all students to be successful in their academic, social, emotional, career, and personal development (Singh, Urbano, Haston, & McMahon, 2010; Stone & Dahir, 2011). Educational-reform leaders are increasingly focusing on the school counselor as advocate and **change agent** (Bemak & Chung, 2008; Cheek & House, 2010a; Singh et al., 2010). School counselors are ideally situated to serve as conduits of information and practices to promote a **social justice agenda** (Fields & Hines, 2010; Galassi, Griffin, & Akos, 2008; Lee & Rodgers, 2009). School counselors who have strong personal/social consciousness skills and understand equity issues are contributing to a global society in which students who have not traditionally been served well in the past have a chance to acquire the skills necessary to unconditionally participate in a 21st-century economy (Stone & Dahir, 2011).

School counselors help members of a school family become inspired to consider greater possibilities for their students and to usher students toward these possibilities (Cheek & House, 2010a; Fields & Hines, 2010; Galassi & Akos, 2004; Stone & Dahir, 2011). Advocacy for the school counselor is helping all students to realize the American Dream of an optimum and quality education (Lee & Rodgers, 2009). Because counselors care about students a great deal, they motivate other critical stakeholders to build systems that widen students' opportunities. Conversely, school counselors look for those systems that impede success and inspire, instruct, and incite others to eliminate these obstacles.

School counselors have been engaged in advocacy for years, especially with individual students, but their role is expanding to include advocating for social justice and challenging oppression on a wider scale (Lee & Rodgers, 2009).

School counselors assuming social action and social intervention roles are generally extended permission, both spoken and unspoken, to take on the social challenges of a student's community or home environment. Even the toughest educators often give school counselors support when they ask for help for a particular student.

Counselors who understand issues affecting equity and opportunity are changing systems that continue to adversely stratify opportunities, influencing attitudes and beliefs regarding equitable practices, providing attention to equity and access issues, and securing resources designed to improve opportunities (Stone & Dahir, 2011). Counselors bring expertise to social problems for individuals, communities, and the wider society in proactive, socially critical behavior and the skills needed to strategically challenge the status quo in systems where inequities impede success. School counselors are specialists in helping change human behavior. For example, the preparation school counselors receive in communication skills and interpersonal relationships provides them with tools to help change hostile school climates to productive learning environments for every student (Chen-Hayes et al., 2011).

## Advocacy and the Achievement Gap

A primary focus for the school counselor as advocate is to become the voice for those students for whom educational opportunity has traditionally been adversely stratified, especially low-socioeconomic students and minority students (Bemak & Chung, 2008; Chen-Hayes, Miller, Bailey, Getch, & Erford, 2011; Lee & Rodgers, 2009; Singh et al., 2010). Martin (1998) described the school counselor advocate as one who possesses proactive, socially critical behavior and skills needed to strategically challenge the status quo in systems where inequities impede students' academic success. "All students, regardless of their cultural background and heritage, deserve equal access to a quality education. Anything less than that, for any child, is a grave educational injustice" (Lee, 2001, p. 257). The school counselor as an advocate raises aspirations, nurtures dreams, and empowers students to become their own advocates. School counselors have a critical role to play in supporting brighter futures for all students, especially for those traditionally underserved such as minorities, those in lower socioeconomic groupings, and those persecuted because of their sexual orientation (Singh et al., 2010).

### Empowerment

Learned helplessness or situational helplessness can be affected when counselors work with individuals to help them feel empowered. McWhirter (1997) defines this empowerment:

> the process by which people, organizations, or groups who are powerless or marginalized (a) become aware of the power dynamics at work in their life context, (b) develop the skills and capacity for gaining reasonable control over their lives, (c) which they exercise, (d) without infringing on the rights of others, and (e) which coincides with actively supporting the empowerment of others in their community. (p. 12)

The concepts of empowerment and advocacy provide the basis for the role of counselor as a social change agent. Empowerment is a complex process that encompasses self-reflection and action, awareness of environmental power dynamics that may affect psychosocial development, and the development of skills to promote community enhancement (McWhirter, 1997). Any counselor with a belief in the possibility of a better world develops a sense of social responsibility. Part of such a counselor's philosophy should be a commitment to social change within a larger context beyond schools and her or his role as a catalyst for such change (Lee & Rodgers, 2009). "Empowering students can be done by working with students on self-advocacy tools in the classroom, in small groups, or individually. Empowering examples include...facilitating groups on bullying or peer mediation" (Ratts, DeKruyf, Chen-Hayes, 2007, p. 92).

## CHARACTERISTICS OF AN EFFECTIVE ADVOCATE

Interpersonal skills, communication, empowerment, leadership, and advocacy skills are areas where many counselors excel, and these are the critical skills needed to address the social and economic issues that challenge our global society. Although advocates need heart and a passion to help students, this section also examines the skills needed to be an advocate.

School counselors have a willingness to listen, a quality that makes strong advocates. Advocacy for all students requires a high level of caring for students, parents, and fellow educators. Generally speaking, these qualities are often present in people who seek the school counseling profession. School counselors do not like to see students' opportunities limited and want to create a shared vision of the possibilities for students beyond their current realities. It is good that school counselors generally come to the profession with the personal quality of caring because, according to Kottler (2000), preparation programs in counseling, law, and medicine cannot possibly do justice to the development of caring and compassion.

School counseling candidates usually have strong personal/social consciousness and a desire to be a voice for students who are under-represented or not considered part of the mainstream. School counseling students are often risk-takers as advocacy often involves taking an unpopular position.

## MEET TAMMY DODSON: A HEART FOR ADVOCACY

Tammy Dodson, School Counselor of the Year finalist for the American School Counselor Association, has a heart for advocacy. During the school year Tammy's administration and security guards were constantly complaining about a group of eight tough girls who were continually being disruptive in the commons areas and the classrooms. Tammy volunteered to run a group with these girls and recruited a counselor who was a member of the district's equity parent group to co-facilitate. During the first meeting she began to question the wisdom of bringing these girls together as a fistfight almost ensued. However, the group went uphill from there. After 10 weekly meetings, there was a dramatic difference in these young women. Their attendance, grades, and discipline referrals improved. The group had a celebration and each girl was allowed to invite one teacher. There wasn't a dry eye in the room as administrators and teachers celebrated the new road these girls had found for themselves with the help of Tammy. Later, the administration asked Tammy what she had done with the girls to get such great results. As Tammy explained, "I couldn't really show them a gold standard curriculum that I used. I told them that we listened, held them accountable, taught them it was okay to have educational goals and how to set them, raised the bar once they met their goals, and acknowledged them for their accomplishments and they responded."

Qualities appreciated in school counselors are sensitivity to the needs of students, genuine positive regard for others, compassion, flexibility, understanding, empathy, insightfulness, and emotional stability. Can one be taught to be a passionate advocate? "Each of us can be encouraged to access that part of us that is most compassionate and caring" (Kottler, 2000, p. 3). It is not enough to know how to use technology for advocacy, to have skills to disaggregate and aggregate data, to understand how to negotiate the political landscape, to recognize inequities, and to establish connections to influence change. Without deeply held beliefs about students and their need for a voice, without a willingness to be a passionate advocate, skills alone will not move the profession in the right direction. The school counselor of the 21st century must negotiate bureaucratic systems and be willing to be labeled an idealist.

School counselor advocates are risk-takers, sometimes taking on causes at the displeasure of colleagues or others (Lee & Rodgers, 2009). The role of advocate can be uncomfortable as it sometimes carries controversy, conflict, and personal risk. However, it is also a rewarding role school counselors embrace because it calls on them to champion the causes of equity, justice, and inclusion. To maintain their effectiveness and influence, school counselors exercise caution and political astuteness by negotiating the pitfalls and landmines in the political landscape. Conversely, fear of falling into disfavor does not paralyze the school counselor from fully exercising an advocacy role. School counselors are often the voice of advocacy when no one else will be.

To be outstanding advocates for all students, professional school counselors and their colleagues must understand their own biases, recognize potential harm when dealing with culturally diverse students and parents, and be open to change in personal worldviews. (Chen-Hayes et al., 2011, p. 114)

There was a simple job that Everybody wanted done and Anybody could do.
But Everybody thought Somebody should do what Nobody would.
So Nobody did what Everybody wanted, and thought Somebody should,
even though Anybody could. (Anonymous)

School counselors benefit from giving themselves permission and a pat on the back to be an idealist and an optimist. The school counselor/optimist, far from being the proverbial Pollyanna who relies on goodness, puts effort and skill behind the idealism. The optimists who bring skills to the fight for **systemic change** and believe in students and their abilities will sometimes have to steady themselves before the cynics, who will quickly point out that "we have tried that before" and "your ideas won't work." The dispirited cynics are found everywhere, pointing out how students are hopeless and the situation is dire, but the tenacity of school counselors most often allows them to stay focused. The cynics may have been spirited fighters for students at one time. Acknowledge them, respect them, work with them or, if need be, work around them, but don't succumb to the negativity. The cynics may even respect you for all you do for students and wish they still had the will.

## THE ETHICS OF ADVOCACY

Advocacy is an ethical imperative for school counselors. ASCA's Ethical Standards for School Counselors (2010) states in A.1.b., "Professional school counselors are concerned with the educational, academic, career, personal and social needs and encourages the maximum development of every student."

Advocacy is also a legal imperative. Chapter 6 covers court cases that give legal muscle to counselors to advocate on behalf of their students (e.g., *Davis v. Monroe County Board of Education*; *Sain v. Cedar Rapids Community School District*; and *Eisel v. Montgomery County Board of Education*).

The ethical obligation school counselors have to advocate for their students is complex and not without controversy as to whether or not advocacy is an ethical imperative. Kitchener's five moral principles—beneficence, nonmaleficence, loyalty, justice, and autonomy—are most often applied by counselors when in the throes of an ethical dilemma. However, we believe the moral principles also provide a fitting lens through which to view the concept of advocacy as an ethical obligation and are presented here in the context of social advocacy as an ethical imperative.

*Beneficence* or to "do good" means to continually seek ways to groom opportunities for student success. Exercising an advocacy role is one of the most ethical behaviors a school counselor can practice, as will be examined in greater detail later in this chapter.

*Nonmaleficence*, or "above all do no harm," implores school counselors to consider the impact of their action or lack of action to determine if potential harm will result. If a school counselor cannot be certain that an action will "do good," at least one is to be confident in the knowledge that it will "do no harm." Nonmaleficence requires that one is vigilant as to motives, biases, and prejudices that knowingly or unwittingly guide individual behaviors.

*Loyalty* in advocacy means remaining steadfast in the efforts to make systemic change and for individuals and groups of students. Loyalty is trying to make an impact for all students, not just the top 5 percent who are most at-risk. School counselors can figuratively "wrap their arms" around all students through advocacy when a school counselor implements a systemic change that involves every student. If there is a bullying problem in your school that affects more than 70 percent of the students, and despite resistance you are able to team with others to deliver an effective prevention program, then you are being loyal to your students and advocating on their behalf.

*Justice* means treating equals equally but treating unequals unequally in direct proportion to their relevant differences. In other words, we avoid a one-size-fits-all educational system and we look at each individual and her or his unique needs. Justice means that when we treat students differently we need to be able to justify to ourselves and to others why we acted as we did. Why did we choose to advocate for some students in certain situations and not for other students who appear to have the same circumstances? How are these students or their circumstances different to allow us to be there for one individual or group of individuals but not another? Did one group need us more because it has had fewer advocates in the past? Did one group need us more because we knew that its voices were weaker than others who on the surface may appear to have an equal voice? School counselors have to wisely choose their advocacy battles, and this sometimes means making tough decisions about which causes we tackle.

Promoting *autonomy* is a delicate balancing act for school counselors because our students are minors and in a school setting, resulting in a combination that requires loyalty to the minor that also extends to the parents of the minor. The advocacy role can help us promote autonomy in many ways. For example, the goal of a career guidance program should be to empower every child to become her or his own advocate. Career counseling for all students closes the **information gap**, a gap that enables some students to make informed decisions while others wander aimlessly through their school experience never understanding the connection between academics and their future. School counselors can work to promote students' autonomy, understand and apply childhood development principles to help them, and equip them with as much "armor" as possible to support their full development.

## THE IMPACT OF ADVOCACY ON STUDENTS, THE SCHOOL, AND THE COMMUNITY

School counselor advocacy contributes to furthering educational opportunity. The school counselor as advocate is ideally situated to affect important areas such as helping students access and succeed in rigorous academics, creating a safer school climate, and helping students and families understand and widen their opportunities.

## Advocating for Systemic Change

What does systemic change mean? Systemic refers to the organizational policies, procedures, and/or practices of a school or school district. The literature on systemic change frequently cites a shared vision to guide change, leadership capable of driving the change, research on which to build change, professional development and other opportunities for learning to implement and sustain the change, organizational arrangements to support change, and strategies to implement change (Lee & Rodgers, 2009).

As a part of the leadership team effort to drive change, school counselors think systemically by examining the institutions in which they work to identify both those practices that negatively affect students and should be eliminated and those systems that positively affect students and should be replicated or expanded. Through systemic change school counselors reach many more students (Ratts, 2008; Stone & Dahir, 2011). With systemic change, school counselors look beyond developing their school counseling program as an isolated entity of the school to that of understanding the context in which their program is embedded. For example, does your school have a policy that automatically fails students if they are absent a set number of days? This policy has an adverse effect if implemented without considering individual student circumstances. The counselor can advocate for a change in this policy or, in other words, affect systemic change.

Poor learning is frequently explained by enumerating the barriers such as poverty, crime-ridden neighborhoods, lack of parental support, and lack of motivation that students bring to school rather than the **systemic barriers** that schools and districts place before students (Williams & Noguera, 2010). Educators are turning their attention toward the system and the damage done there. "We take the children who have less to begin with, and then systematically give them less in school, too. In fact we give these children less of everything that we know makes a difference" (Haycock, 2001, p. 1). "[L]ow-income children are most likely to attend schools offering the poorest quality of teaching from the least experienced teachers" (Amatea & West-Olatunji, 2007, p. 81). To become a school counselor/advocate, study the systems, practices, and ideologies that negatively and positively affect student success so that you have the knowledge to assist in adapting or replicating those systems.

Inequality of funding represents the largest stratification in the American educational system. The children of the economically advantaged attend better-funded schools, while children in poor communities receive substantially less funding for education (Potts, 2003; Rothstein, 2004; Smith, 2000). Less funding represents diminished access to the most qualified teachers, fewer teachers overall, fewer professional school counselors, and diminished art, music, and special programs. These limited resources hurt the quality and depth of education received by students of lower socioeconomic status (Rothstein, 2004). Within any particular school, children of marginalized communities are likely to be overrepresented in special education, remedial education, lower ability groups, and vocational tracks (Potts, 2003; Rothstein, 2004). "The consequence of this educational experience could potentially impede educational advancement. Additionally, lack of college preparation makes it more difficult for marginalized students to attain the educational capital necessary to reach the upper rungs of socioeconomic status" (Hipolito-Delgado & Lee, 2007, pp. 327–28).

School counselors are infusing principles and practices in school counseling that are being used in school reform and connect their programs to the school's mission for the purpose of supporting students to be successful (Bemak & Chung, 2005). The role of the school counselor as an advocate involves looking at the individual student as well as examining the systemwide inequities and practices.

Educational reform and societal changes are compelling reasons for school counselors to join forces with other educators and use their influence to eradicate systems and ideologies that have the potential to negatively affect students (Amatea & West-Olatunji, 2007; Hipolito-Delgado & Lee, 2007). Helping to examine institutional and environmental barriers so that these obstacles can be eliminated will in turn create alternatives and opportunities for the people who have not enjoyed the full advantage of an equal opportunity education. There are systems and practices both communitywide, districtwide, and school-site based that stratify opportunities for students and the results are reflected in the data presented in *Working in 21st Century Schools*. School counselors collaborating with other educators can take action to identify, eradicate, and/or replace those policies and practices that have marginalized groups in our society (Lee & Rodgers, 2009; Ratts, DeKruyf, & Chen-Hayes, 2007).

What are some of these systems that impede student success? The following list poses just a few policies, practices, and procedures that may hinder students. What can you add to this list of possible systemic barriers?

- Giving the best teachers to the most capable students in the most rigorous courses in the most affluent schools.
- Tracking students into coursework based on test scores.
- Focusing most of the school counseling program goals on the top 5 percent of the students or the 10 percent of students most at risk for failure.
- Shifting unsatisfactory educators to the schools with the least parental involvement.
- Encouraging only select students in certain categories to take the Preliminary Scholastic Achievement Test (PSAT).
- Expecting teachers who have poor classroom management skills to improve in absence of support.
- Supporting students with career and **academic advising** only when they seek the counselor's help.
- Having a 27 percent average absenteeism rate without a strategic plan to address the problem.
- Having a 42 percent failure rate for the ninth graders without safety nets such as alternative schedules, summer school, and tutoring.

- Automatically assessing students for special education when they fail a grade.
- Having a 36 percent failure rate in algebra without academic safety nets.
- Focusing on the demands of the most vocal parents while ignoring the needs of the silent majority.
- Not placing students into higher level academics based on a brief scheduling contact in which the student says she or he does not want to be in the higher-level academics.

Bernadette Willette is a systemic change agent who skillfully changed her school's practice of not offering Advanced Placement courses. This practice was borne of the belief that the students in this school did not need higher-level academics. Bernadette felt that the status quo adversely stratified opportunities for the students in her school and she quietly and respectfully went about changing attitudes and beliefs, considerably widening opportunities for these rural, low-socioeconomic students who had traditionally accessed postsecondary opportunities in dismal numbers.

Another example of systemic change comes from Paul, a high school counselor who has watched with dismay as large numbers of his ninth graders were retained. Paul observed that there were no significant interventions for students between their first year as a ninth grader and the year they repeated

## MEET BERNADETTE WILLETTE, SYSTEM CHANGE AGENT

Bernadette Willette, a high school counselor in Maine, changed attitudes and beliefs. Bernadette's rural, low-socioeconomic school did not offer any Advanced Placement (AP) courses. These AP courses are important because students who take them are challenged to take college courses in high school, and if they obtain a certain AP test score at the end of the AP courses they can receive college credit from most universities and colleges. The consensus at Bernadette's school was that AP offerings were not necessary as the students were not aspiring to go to college. Bernadette decided to tackle this belief by arming herself with data from the College Board organization, which administers the AP program. With data and research, Bernadette demonstrated to teachers the correlation between the PSAT scores of many of their current and former students and predicted success in AP courses. Faced with the fact that many of their students' PSAT scores predicted success and the realization that these students would now graduate without ever having the opportunity to take AP courses, these teachers made the commitment to offer AP courses in the future. Bernadette Willette in her leadership role identified attitudes and beliefs that were adversely stratifying students' opportunities and advocated to make a systemic change that will benefit many students in the future. Her school offers three AP courses with plans for two more in the near future. This collaborative leader changed attitudes and beliefs (Stone, 2003).

ninth grade. Paul gathered data on all the interventions and learned that there were few, infrequent, and disjointed attempts at assistance. Armed with the information he collected, Paul mobilized other educators to implement a tracking system for these students and to provide summer interventions to include mentoring, tutoring, and contacts by school officials. Paul's advocacy skills enabled him to implement a systemwide change that included safety nets for the students at his school.

### Changing Attitudes and Beliefs

A leadership effort among school counselors, principals, teachers, other educators, and community members is particularly crucial in changing attitudes and beliefs about student success and students' abilities to learn. School counselors as human relation experts can affect the beliefs and attitudes of teachers and administrators regarding widening opportunities for students.

The school counselor collaborating with other educators can help foster a vision and belief in the development of high aspirations in every child. The school counselor, who believes that all children should be supported to be successful in rigorous academic coursework, will act in ways that demonstrate this belief while influencing other educators (Stone & Clark, 2001). For example, if a school counselor advocates for students to have access to rigorous coursework and then helps to establish safety nets such as tutoring and mentoring to support the success of these students, then the counselor has acted in a way that demonstrates a belief that all students can be supported to be successful.

The preparation school counselors receive in communication skills, interpersonal relationships, problem solving, and conflict resolution gives them a vantage point in promoting collaboration among colleagues. In a collaborative leadership model, the roles of principals, teachers, and school counselors are interchangeable, allowing them to work together to change attitudes and beliefs in each student's ability to learn and in improving instruction and providing support in the classroom. Bernadette Willette is a systemic change agent and a counselor who understands the value of collaborative leadership.

## Advocating for Individual Students

Advocacy for early prevention and systemic interventions should focus on all students. Changing the system to meet the needs of individuals rather than trying to have the round-peg individual fit into a square hole is a large part of advocacy. We change systems to make a difference for every individual in that system. Advocacy requires us to give some individual students more help to right an injustice against them, improve their condition, or provide an opportunity.

## Advocating for Your School Counseling Program

School counselors who know how to advocate for their program are less likely to be saddled with responsibilities that are extraneous to the goals of

## MEET SEJAL PARIKH: AN ADVOCATE FOR INDIVIDUAL STUDENTS

An example of changing systems while also working with individuals can be found in the work of Sejal Parikh, an urban elementary school counselor. Sejal suspected that there were an inordinate number of discipline referrals in fourth grade and she tested her observations by gathering school data on discipline referrals. She found that for the previous year discipline referrals increased each month until there were 30 suspensions for the month of May. Sejal brought this information to the administration of the school who gave her time on the faculty meeting agenda to discuss the information. In a presentation, Sejal demonstrated with charts and graphs the discipline and suspension rates for each month. The teachers were alarmed because they had no idea so many students were out of school on a daily basis. The next hour was spent with the teachers, administrators, and Sejal brainstorming and strategizing to find ways of reducing or eliminating suspensions and the attendance problem. Sejal established as one of her school counseling program goals to deliver classroom guidance lessons on conflict resolution and to work with individual students who were most in danger of being suspended. Sejal brought her skills and her programs' objectives to bear on changing discipline and suspension rates by establishing a daily behavior management program for the most at-risk-of-suspension students with daily brief contact to check on their progress. Here is an example of a counselor identifying a problem through observation, corroborating her observations with real data, developing a plan with the faculty and other stakeholders, and implementing that plan with good results. The discipline referrals for fourth grade went from 19 in February to 7 in April.

---

school counseling. Behaving as an advocate demonstrates that school counselors can carry out a program curriculum just as English, mathematics, and science teachers implement their curricula. Having a plan in mind assists school counselors to assess the needs of the school and develop program strategies around those needs. This is vitally important to the success of the school counseling program. Keeping calendars and placing your weekly schedule on your office door is a way to advocate. A schedule that shows non-counseling duties such as hall monitoring helps convey the message to other educators that some vital contact time with students is being lost. If extraneous duties are suggested, then the school counselor can present the schedule and ask for help in problem solving what to take out to comply with the request. Advocacy is educating legislators, school board members, parents, administrators, and teachers about the school counseling program. Advocacy for the school counseling program is joining a professional organization that provides school counselors with a legislative voice.

### Advocating for Social Action in the Wider Context of Community
#### Families and Institutions of Society

Counselors can be agents of social change in the wider community by helping students and families develop the strength and the strategies needed to advocate for themselves in relationship to other institutions in society. For example, counselors can provide information, resources, or teach families how to do the following:

- Use legal aid to get delinquent child support for their families.
- Negotiate city hall to force a landlord to make needed repairs on a dwelling.
- File for financial aid assistance so they can go back to school.
- Get job training.
- Find free medical help.
- Find counseling services for their children.
- Get special services for their academically challenged child.
- Find mentors and tutors for their children.
- Access social services for elderly parents.

A counselor who is an agent of social change can rally families to write legislators to push for changes in laws that adversely affect them and to lobby lawmakers for their rights. Political action, voicing their concerns, overcoming reticence to advocate for themselves, and other such proactive steps usually result in families who are better able to shake helplessness and exercise more control over their own destiny.

#### Service Learning

School counselors can encourage involvement of students in service learning and also address some of the social problems, issues, and injustices of their larger community. The tragedy of September 11 resulted in many school counselors taking the time to advocate for tolerance and cultural acceptance while arguing against labeling our Muslim neighbors as dangerous.

## ADVOCACY SKILLS

Advocacy to support students involves specific skills, not just a philosophical orientation to function as an advocate. It is important that counselors learn how to bring about change. Simply suggesting that counselors be change agents without helping them grow in acquiring the specific skills needed for educational advocacy is unlikely to produce positive effects for students, schools, or counselors.

### Use of Technology for Advocacy

One of the most powerful skills acquired in school counselor preparation and inservice programs is technology. School counselors use technology advances to offer better services to students and with a concerted effort have enhanced and changed forever the way they support teachers and foster student development (Hayden, Poynton, & Sabella, 2008).

Martin (1998) described technology as a critical tool in advocacy, explaining that counselors must learn to use technology in monitoring student progress, addressing student career planning, and in acquiring and accessing the data needed to inform the decision-making of individual students and of the entire school. "School counseling technology . . . could be conceived as a study and ethical practice of facilitating the academic, personal/social and career development of students by creating, using, and managing appropriate technological processes and resources" (Sabella, Poynton, & Isaacs, 2010, p. 609). School counselors who understand equity issues and have the technological skills to aggregate and disaggregate student information have critical, powerful skills that allow them to act as advocates in identifying and eliminating school practices that deter equitable access and providing opportunities for student success in higher-level academics. Through the use of technology, the school counselor/advocate can identify broad systemwide practices that deter access to rigorous coursework as well as uncover inequitable situations for individual students. Using school district data obtained from a school's student information management system, school counselors can manage and monitor patterns of enrollment and student success.

Technological skills are needed by school counselors in their role as social advocates to support students' academic achievement. Technology enhances the counselor's role in advocacy, and in certain situations, the advocacy task can only be accomplished through the use of technology such as looking at course enrollment patterns. "Today's students have changed the way they learn and today's counselors must change the way they communicate on behalf of student academic success. . . . If learner outcomes can be better achieved through technology, it is incumbent that counselors adapt their strategies accordingly" (Casey, 1995, p. 34). Many school counselors have student management systems or databases available within their schools or districts that contain student biographical information as well as scheduling, attendance, discipline, and test history data. This information is extremely useful when working with students as the database contains information such as attendance, test scores, current grades, past academic performance, etc. The information in these systems can be exported to relational databases to provide more flexibility and increased accessibility to more student information. Student data management systems can be accessed with varying degrees of ease depending on the school system. Some school systems go so far as to give administrators laptops and at the touch of a mouse are able to access data that other administrators wait weeks to acquire. However, when advocating for the needed information, know what to ask for and go after this information with steady insistence. If it is not available, ask for a program to be written to provide you with the necessary information to make informed decisions for your students. By using student information management data, assurances are built into the system that no student is left out of the picture. This provides equity in analysis as well as in access to opportunities, and it also guarantees that no group of students will be left out of calculations. "Technology can be used as a tool for advocacy.... Computer technology impacts how school counselors disseminate information.... Information provided on the Web site can help promote 'public awareness about the role and functions of a school counselor' "(Van Horn & Myrick, 2001, p. 125)."

---

## MEET THREE COUNSELORS WHO USE TECHNOLOGY AS AN ADVOCACY TOOL TO CLOSE THE INFORMATION GAP

Lack of access to guidance services means academic counseling at critical junctures will be weak or nonexistent; a travesty for our students. School counselors are helping to close the information gap despite high caseloads. Meet three counselors who represent hundreds of school counselors who are exercising advocacy by offering their academic and career counseling to more students through technology. Shawna is a hypothetical student, but through her case you can see how these three counselors reach hundreds of "Shawnas" in their caseloads through technology.

Shawna, a 12th grader, is seeking advice on careers, and she starts her search with the help of the school counselor who assists her in completing a career inventory on the computer in the school counseling office. Shawna receives immediate feedback linking her results to national organizations where she gets up-to-date information on the career and discovers trends in employment, salary, and other useful information. An example can be found at Career Mosaic at www.careermosaic.com. After narrowing her choice of careers, Shawna conducts a college search linking her career choices to college majors. Shawna compiles a list of colleges that interest her and decides to apply to four of the colleges that she discovered with her search. Shawna then applies online to these colleges, searches the virtual college catalog for all information about the college, and even interfaces with students attending the college and majoring in the same field. Shawna applies online for all the state scholarships and meets all the deadlines, and searches for other financial assistance. Shawna was able to take her parents' financial information and do an online financial need estimation form that indicated the expected family contribution for a year of college expenses. An example of a site where this can be done is the Financial Aid Information Page, www.finaid.org, and an example of a scholarship search site is FastWeb at www.fastweb.com. Finally, Shawna linked to the Free Application for Federal Student Aid (FAFSA) website and completed an online FAFSA, receiving her results in 48 hours. With a little help from her counselor, Shawna began and finished a career, college, scholarship application, and financial aid search without leaving the computer. The strategies above were contributed by Bob Turba, Penny Studstill, and Nan Worsowicz, school counselors and supervisors.

## Advocacy through Staff Development

One of the principles of systemic change in education is to advocate for opportunities for staff to practice new skills, gather new information, or learn new behaviors. School counselors can have a significant role in this by contributing to staff development opportunities. The best educational practices or changes will become daily practice if the faculty has been properly educated and equipped.

Challenges exist in delivering staff development but there are strategies to help ensure success and gain support from administrators, teachers, parents, and other stakeholders. Getting the input of teachers before planning a staff development activity is a smart approach as top-down planning is rarely welcomed by participants. Collaborative planning is the optimum way to proceed and furthers success more than just initially seeking input. Collaborative planning is time-consuming, but the results are worth the investment when the staff development activity proposed has the potential for affecting students.

## Recommended Steps When Advocating for Change

Here are seven steps you can use to approach any advocacy situation, regardless of the change you are attempting to effect.

1. *Identify the problem.* Informally identify a situation in your school that you believe to be an obstacle or problem. Test your hypothesis by gathering data to illuminate the problem. Is the problem multidimensional? What is the scope of the problem? Who is affected by the problem?

2. *Gather additional information.* Determine what additional information one needs to know in examining the problem. How will this information be gathered? Can you gather the information through informal conversations, formal interviews, surveys, and/or tapping into the student information management system?

3. *Identify the stakeholders.* Who needs to be involved in addressing this problem? Who are the stakeholders that need to come together to address the problem? Is there already a vehicle or forum in place such as the school improvement team to help address the problem? With the help of the stakeholders, identify the internal and external community members who must be involved in addressing the problem.

4. *Research the advocacy history of the problem.* What has already been done by others in your school to address the problem? What can you learn from these previous efforts? Is there research from other school sites on strategies to address the problem?

5. *Identify the institutional and/or environmental barriers contributing to the problem.* Analyze the barriers. Are the barriers systemic in nature, easy to remove, complicated, etc.? Identify those who would bring conflict or resistance to efforts to implement the strategies the collaborators have identified as needed. From where does the resistance originate? Should you tackle trying to change the resistance or in this situation should you just move through, around, or over it?

6. *Develop an action plan.* In concert with the other principal stakeholders, develop an action plan to address the problem. The action plan consists of stakeholders identifying proven strategies that they would feel qualified to implement, and if the stakeholders are open, you can assign strategies. A timeline for completion of strategies and an interim check of progress would be a helpful part of the action plan.

7. *Set goals and develop* **accountability** *measures.* How will you evaluate the effectiveness of your advocacy program? Does the program have a timeline? Determine the goal of the program and set interim targets as you steadily move toward improvement. Decide in advance how you will measure achievement of those goals.

---

## *Advocacy in Action*

You can best learn the steps to advocacy by working through an exercise using a hypothetical example. We will provide an example and insert information at various points in the exercise. Use what you have learned so far—and some imagination—to fill in the information we have left blank.

*In this example you are using data to advocate for students and your school counseling program. As a member of the leadership team of the school, you are in step with the mission of your school to affect the academic achievement of your students. You want to be another set of eyes and ears ferreting out problem areas and addressing them. You continually hear from teachers that there is an attendance problem but none of them are able to give you specific information about the problem.*

1. *Identify the problem.*
   Using Step 1, you have identified attendance as a problem area for your school and your data gathering has revealed that

   32 percent of absences at the school are for fifth graders;

   71 percent of these students are boys; and

   51 percent of the absences happen on the first day back after a weekend or holiday.

2. *Gather additional information.*
   After additional research using Step 2, you have found that bullying is a serious problem in fifth grade and that many students are avoiding coming to school because they are being bullied. On Mondays the rate of absence is aggravated by bus delays, parents and children who have problems getting started on Mondays, etc.

3. *Identify the stakeholders.*
   Who needs to be involved in addressing the problem of bullying? How might they be brought to the table?

   _____

   _____

   _____

4. *Research the advocacy history of the problem.*
   What may already have been done by others to address the problem of
   bullying? What can be learned from these previous efforts? Is there
   any research on addressing the problem?

   _____

   _____

   _____

5. *Identify the institutional and/or environmental barriers contributing to
   the problem.*
   What institutional and environmental factors might constitute barriers
   to solving the problem of bullying at this school?

   _____

   _____

   _____

6. *Develop an action plan.*
   What will be the specific strategies of your school counseling program
   to reduce bullying, and therefore absenteeism, for the fifth-grade boys?

   _____

   _____

   _____

7. *Set goals and develop accountability measures.*
   How will you evaluate the effectiveness of your school counseling program to reduce bullying, and therefore absenteeism, for the fifth-grade
   boys? Does the goal have an interim target to reach as you steadily
   move toward improvement? Does the target have a timeline?

   _____

   _____

   _____

## GUIDING PRINCIPLES OF EFFECTIVE ADVOCACY

1. Be a calculated risk taker. You must be politically astute to live to "play
   the game" another day. But at the same time being too conservative or
   paralyzed by the fear of possibly bringing disfavor on yourself or being
   overly concerned about protecting yourself will keep you from exercising
   an advocacy role to the extent to which you are capable. Your students
   need you to be their voice when no one else will.
2. Believe you can make a difference and relentlessly, respectfully, and collaboratively pursue your advocacy role. Just as it is the salesperson's responsibility to make a sale, the CEO's responsibility to monitor the profit
   margin, and the nurse's responsibility to make certain the right medicine is
   administered, think of advocacy as your responsibility and make it happen.
3. Believe in your students. Don't allow yourself or others to sidetrack your
   efforts at advocacy with the "bless their hearts" syndrome. Students need

our empathy, but our sympathy only serves to hinder us from challenging and causing students to better their situation. Empathy will help us empower students and support them to achieve despite their sometimes dismal options.

4. Advocacy is difficult and we should be willing to take advantage of opportunities to be kind to ourselves and celebrate our successes, however small.

5. Stay the course. Don't accept failure. As school counselors we must believe we can affect change. "Those who entertain the possibility of losing are only a doubt away from its reality" (author unknown).

# TECH TOOLS

When you become a school counselor, use the power of technology to maximize the efficiency and effectiveness of your advocacy.

- Use technology to help you develop four-year career plans for students. Help students become their own advocates for their future career plans by helping them learn to use the Internet for career tasks such as interest inventories, identifying job clusters, and finding higher education institutions that offer preparation in the job cluster or specific job that they are interested.

- Identify through technology school practices that deter equitable access and opportunities for student success, such as who has access to higher-level classes.

- Provide staff development using PowerPoint presentations so that teachers and administrators can acquire new skills, gather new information, or learn new behaviors. A 10-minute presentation during weekly faculty meetings can strengthen your position as a member of the leadership team.

- Set up computer conferences for your students who are experiencing personal/social/emotional problems. In a friendly, inclusive electronic environment the medium is largely neutral and student participation may increase.

- Set up videoconferencing so that students who do not have the benefit of visiting college campuses can virtually tour campuses and meet with the admissions representatives.

- Develop discussion lists for parents, students, and school counselors to exchange information needed to advocate for students.

- Develop email mentor or tutor programs so that older students, business partners, and community agency members can mentor or tutor students. For example, if the absenteeism for chronic offenders happens on Mondays, then schedule your email mentoring for Mondays.

- Have computers in the school counseling office for mentorship, career advising, etc. Find businesses and community members to donate them and help them stay up and running.

- Benefit from collaborating with your fellow counselors who have established websites that offer critical timely information from scholarship resources to eating disorders. Some examples of sites are http://wiseman-tech.com/guidance and www.cyberguidance.net.

- Build the potential of students to participate in the 21st-century economy by helping all students have access to technology.

---

## School Counselor Casebook: Voices from the Field

### The Scenario Reviewed

Three of your sophomores complained to you, their counselor, about not being able to enroll in any AP courses in their junior year. It seems that they did not score high enough on the ninth-grade standardized test last year. The policy in the handbook clearly delineates the criteria. All three of the students really want to take AP courses and are certain they will be able to handle the work.

Here's how a practicing school counselor responded to the school scenario:

As a counselor, one of the most vital roles we play for our students is to be their advocate. When presented with concerns from several students about a school policy that is preventing them from accessing AP courses, despite their goals, aspirations, and hard work, I would want to take action immediately. To present an educated request, I would take a methodical and thoughtful approach.

I first need to find out how and by whom the school policy was determined. I would want to know who the stakeholders are and how they arrived at this policy. This would help me to understand the perspectives of those involved so that I can approach the topic in the most constructive manner possible. The more I can show that I understand the rationale behind my colleagues' intentions, it may be easier to get them to talk with me. After gathering adequate background information, I would collect information about the academic accomplishments of my students. I might also do the following:

1. Ask other counselors if they have students in similar situations (power in numbers).
2. Find research that supports the value of student access to AP courses.
3. Seek out research about the concerns with high-stakes testing (since the ninth-grade test score seems to be what is preventing these students from accessing the courses).

My final step in advocating for a policy change would be to meet with the person or people who have the power to change the policy. I would be careful to make sure I followed the appropriate protocol. With my principal's permission, I may ask the students involved to join us for part of the meeting and to provide their own "testimony" about why they want to take the AP courses.

*(continues)*

While on the surface many issues might seem straightforward to us as counselors, we have to keep in mind that we rarely have the power to act in a vacuum and make decisions about school policies. We also might not know the background that went into determining a policy. Therefore, we have to do our homework so that we can be the best advocates possible and make those necessary changes in the "system" that will benefit our students.

Amy Thompson is a college and career counselor at the secondary level and past president of the Illinois School Counselor Association (ISCA).

# LOOKING BACK: SALIENT POINTS

### The Role of Social Advocacy in Counseling

School counselors who understand issues affecting equity of opportunity can help change systems that continue to adversely stratify students' opportunities. The school counselor who behaves as a social change agent provides a high-profile, powerful role and increases her or his effectiveness in multiple ways.

### School Counselors as Advocate

The preparation school counselors receive in communication skills and interpersonal relationship development facilitates their effectiveness in advocacy for both individual students and for systemic change. Social action and social intervention are readily available roles as counseling is generally perceived by administrators, parents, and teachers to be a natural fit for advocacy.

### Personal/Social Consciousness for the School Counselor as Advocate

School counselors do not merely master the nuts and bolts of counseling but have the heart and soul needed to advocate for their students. School counselors who serve as social activists are risk-takers with a sensitivity to the needs of students, genuine positive regard for others, compassion, flexibility, understanding, empathy, insightfulness, and emotional stability.

### The Ethics of Advocacy

Advocacy is both a legal obligation and an ethical imperative for school counselors. The five moral principles of beneficence, nonmaleficence, loyalty, and the promotion of autonomy and justice serve as a context for framing ethical behavior.

### Advocacy Impacts Students, School Climates, Systems, the School Counseling Program, and Communities

Counselors as systemic change agents are able to affect all students in their case loads when they change or improve the policies, procedures, or practices in the school that are hindering students. School counselors as advocates examine and intervene in the environment to promote an emotionally and physically safe school that supports equal opportunities for all students to get a good education. Other systems in which students have to move, such as home and the wider community, are also of concern to school counselors.

### Advocating for Social Action in the Wider Context of Community

School counselors who have a strong sense of social responsibility often seek to be agents of social change in the wider community by helping students and families develop the strength and the strategies needed to advocate for themselves. School counselors are encouraging involvement of students in service learning and are also addressing some of the social problems, issues, and injustices of their larger community.

### Skills for Advocacy

A philosophical orientation to function as an advocate is important but is of little use in isolation of the specific skills needed by advocates. Using technology and providing staff development are two of the advocacy skills examined throughout this textbook.

## KEY TERMS

Advocacy p. 124

Change agent p. 125

Social justice agenda p. 125

Systemic change p. 129

Beneficence p. 129

Nonmaleficence p. 130

Loyalty p. 130

Justice p. 130

Autonomy p. 130

Information gap p. 130

Systemic barriers p. 131

Academic advising p. 132

Accountability p. 140

## LEARNING EXTENSIONS/MAKING CONNECTIONS

1. Interview a practicing counselor about three or four systemic practices, policies, or procedures that they believe enhance students' ability to be successful and three or four systemic barriers to students' success. Discuss how you would try to address these barriers.

2. Think about your time as a student in a school or your work with any school. Can you describe the course assignment or tracking procedures of the school? In other words, who decided what procedures were used for determining who gets in the blue bird or the red bird group, Spanish I, or AP Calculus? What data are used in these decisions?

3. If you were given 15 minutes at the next faculty meeting for a staff development presentation, what topic would you like to deliver that would make a difference for students? What data would you use? How would you use technology to deliver this topic?

4. Your principal is desperately trying to raise the dismal 70 percent daily attendance rate, one of the areas of accountability for principals in the district. Using this example, discuss the role the school counseling program can have in helping the principal positively impact this data.

5. Chose four of the following topics and write a two-paragraph response.

- Collaborating with Stakeholders to Make Systemic Change.
- Using Data as an Advocacy Tool.
- Connecting School Counseling to School Reform.
- Achieving Access and Equity for All Students.
- Surviving Financial Crises through Accountability.
- Building Multicultural and Diversity Skills for All School Personnel.
- Creating a Climate Sensitive to Diversity and Cultural Differences.
- Challenging and Changing Attitudes and Beliefs.
- Using Technology to Support Your Advocacy Role.

6. Discuss all the ways you can think of that Bernadette Willette affected her school's students, parents, teachers, administration, and community. Why was her approach effective?

## CHAPTER 6

# Legal and Ethical Issues for School Counselors

## CHAPTER OBJECTIVES

*By the time you have completed this chapter, you should be able to*

- understand the difference between ethics and the law;
- identify the steps in making ethical decisions;

- discuss privacy, confidentiality, and privileged communication;

- understand the Family Education Rights and Privacy Act;

- identify the components of negligence and apply negligence and malpractice to cases involving school counselors;

- apply informed consent and confidentiality to group work;

- discuss principles established by court cases that have implications for school counselors' work;

- advocate for students' rights and respect parental rights.

---

## *School Counselor Casebook: Getting Started*

### The Scenario

Your colleague is planning to conduct group counseling for the students in your school this semester. The four areas of concern that your colleague wants to address are for students (1) who have been a victim of incest, (2) whose parents are experiencing a divorce, (3) who have a history of aggressive or violent behavior, or (4) who are underachievers. Your colleague has asked the teachers to recommend students and also prepared an announcement for homeroom. This situation is making you uncomfortable.

### Thinking about Solutions

As you read this chapter, consider how you would answer your colleague's questions. How might you caution her from an ethical perspective? When you come to the end of the chapter, you will have the opportunity to see how your responses compare with the advice a practicing school counselor would give to your colleague.

---

## PROFESSIONAL ETHICS

All school counselors are governed by the **American School Counselor Association (ASCA) code of ethics** (see text's website for the ASCA code of ethics). When a school counselor joins ASCA, she or he agrees to abide by the ASCA Code of Ethical Standards. This professional relationship strengthens the case of the counselor (assuming she or he was within the bounds of ethical behavior as interpreted in standard of practice). Nonmembers are also held to the **standard of care** outlined in the ethical codes. "The problem is that non-members diminish their standard of care and professionalism as there is no tangible evidence that they honor or ever agreed to abide by ethical standards and therefore will have a tougher time defending themselves in a court of law" (J. Cook, assistant director of ASCA, personal communication, September 9, 2010).

**Ethics** are the customs, mores, standards, and accepted practice of a profession (Corey, Corey, & Callanan, 2010). Ethical standards are an attempt by the profession to standardize professional practice for the purpose of protecting students and also to protect the school counselor. "ASCA specifies the principles of ethical behavior necessary to maintain the high standards of integrity, leadership and professionalism among its members" (ASCA, Preamble, 2010). Ethical standards or codes are guides and have to be interpreted in context as there are few right or wrong answers in absence of the real situation in which a counselor may find herself or himself. Knowing and following your profession's code of ethics is part of being an ethical practitioner, but these codes do not make decisions for you (Corey, 2009). Ethical standards guide us to meet the needs of individual situations but are rarely appropriate for rote application as it is the context of the dilemma that matters. It is only the school counselor in consultation with other professionals who can determine how to apply a code to further the best interest of the student. Ethical standards do not hold the answers to our specific ethical problems, but coupled with help from our professional colleagues, the standards do provide guidance. Ethical standards "provide self-appraisal and peer evaluations regarding school counselors' responsibilities to students, parents/guardians, colleagues and professional associates, schools, communities and the counseling profession" (ASCA, Preamble, 2010).

Ethical standards are the ideal to which school counseling professionals should aspire while **laws** are the minimum standard society will tolerate (American Counseling Association, D.1.e, 2005a). Take time to read the codes and discuss them with colleagues. This may sound unrealistic as time is always in short supply for school counselors, but we cannot afford to be ignorant of the ethical standards in a profession that is responsible to minors. With this responsibility comes the imperative to know what ethical actions would be for the reasonably competent professional.

The ASCA ethical standards matter. Even when a legal infraction has not occurred the codes can be used as evidence when a school district is trying to determine whether or not to retain an employee. The codes can show that the school counselor adhered to the norms of the profession or stepped outside the boundaries of what the reasonably competent school counselor would do.

## Ethics, the Law, and Administrative Hearings

"Although following the law is part of ethical behavior, being an ethical practitioner involves far more" (Corey, 2009, p. 39). In a situation where the law and ASCA's ethical standards may be in conflict, the professional must attempt to resolve the conflict in a reasonable manner. Counselors must make their clients aware of the conflict and their ethical standards (Cottone & Tarvydas, 2007).

The court case of *N.C. v. Bedford Central School District* (2004) demonstrates a conflict between legal and ethical principles. A child was sexually abused at the hands of an older cousin. The parents expressed a need to keep the details of the abuse private because further trauma might ensue if his peers or other members of the community learned of the abuse. However, the social worker and school counselor discussed the abuse in a professional child study team meeting attended by school site and district-level educators. The communications took place so that the educators could adequately determine the student's need for Exceptional Student Education. The parents sued the social worker and counselor for breach of privacy, but the court said the facts provided no basis to infer that these professionals were engaging in gossip; rather, they were involved in professional communication that occurred in a professional setting, and all individuals had a significant interest in communicating about the student's sexual abuse history. Therefore, the court found that the defendants' interest in professional communication for the student's benefit outweighed the student's and the parents' rights to privacy (*N.C. v. Bedford Central School District*, 2004). The court found that the educators acted legally, but in your opinion, did they act ethically? Could the school counselor have handled this information in a way that did not leave the parents feeling that their **privacy rights** had been disregarded?

The legal system requires that you behave as the reasonably competent professional would. If faced with a lawsuit would you pass the "Standard of Care" test? Standard of care is the benchmark the courts use to determine the actions of the reasonably competent professional school counselor. The operative word is *reasonable*. The courts are not asking for extraordinary care, only reasonable care. The ethics of the profession help school counselors aspire to exceptional care but the courts do not demand this level. The message to you is to know your ethical standards and abide by them, exercise skill and care in every action you take as a professional, and wrestle with dilemmas you face by applying the ethical decision-making model explained in the next section.

If a school counselor is cleared of wrongdoing, legally the school district still has recourse in an administrative hearing to dismiss the counselor. In a 2004 case, a teacher was cleared in a criminal case for allegedly sexually abusing one of his female students. The school board subsequently voted to dismiss him based on the same incident. In a school district, unlike criminal trials where prosecutors must overcome the much higher reasonable doubt standard to secure a conviction, school boards may rely on substantial evidence to terminate employees (Shapiro & Stefkovich, 2005). Additionally, evidence is permitted in school district hearings that is not permitted in criminal trials. For example, the results of a polygraph test showing deception were allowed in the school district hearing; however, it was inadmissible in Virginia criminal courts. The board also considered the discovery of pornography on the school counselor's school computer deemed inadmissible in the court hearing because it was not possible to determine who had downloaded the material (Shapiro & Stefkovich, 2005).

School counselors hold themselves to a high standard. We are rarely the subject of lawsuits. Educators in general are less and less the subject of lawsuits even though the perception is otherwise. "Even though various special interest groups have contributed to skewed perceptions, objective research reveals that K–12 education litigation, in terms of published court decisions, have gradually continued to decline since the 1970s; the outcomes have continued to favor school district defendants; and the outcomes of the student suits, which are of primary concern to school counselors, have shifted significantly further in favor of district defendants" (P. A. Zirkel, personal communication, December 1, 2008).

## An Ethical Decision-Making Model

In reviewing ethical decision-making models, it was discovered that most fit well with work involving adults, but when considering students some key components needed to be measured. The following suggested steps for ethical action (Stone, 2001) have been created by incorporating the principles set forth by a number of authors as such those represented in the American Counseling Association's (2005a) ethical codes as well as others such as Corey, Corey, and Callanan (2010) and Alexander and Alexander (2010). For school counselors, Steps 1, 4, 5, and 6 were added to the traditional ethical models and Step 2 was clarified to give importance to rumors and hearsay, which can contain vital truths in school settings. The traditional models include: examine the facts, review the relevant ethical guidelines, identify the nature and dimensions of the problem, consult or seek supervision, consider possible and probable courses of action, examine the good and bad consequences of various decisions, and implement your course of action. Because of the unique nature of counseling in schools, we must also add these steps: identify your emotional reaction, consider parental rights, consider the setting, and consider the student's chronological and developmental levels. These additions were made as it is critically important to remember that ethical considerations are context specific. Because our clients are students in a setting called school, this means that parental rights, students' developmental and chronological age, and our own emotional reactions to dilemmas carry additional weight and meaning. Although the model is presented sequentially it will rarely be a sequential deliberation when you are in the throes of an ethical decision-making process.

1. *Identify the emotional reaction.* It is important to keep in the forefront of your mind your first reaction to the problem. What did you immediately want to do to help this child? This emotional reaction is important because it helps us protect and guard our students' confidences. We don't act on the emotional reaction without considering the other ethical decision-making steps; because we care about students, we don't want to discard the emotional reaction.
2. *Examine the facts.* Take the necessary steps to gather the facts separating innuendos, rumors, hearsay, and hypotheses. However, in school settings we cannot rule out the hearsay or rumors as this is often how school counselors discover the truth about situations that involve their students.
3. *Review the relevant ethical guidelines.* Ask yourself whether your code of ethics offers a possible solution to the problem. Remember to apply the ethical standards using judgment not in a routine or emotional manner as you consider the uniqueness of your dilemma.

4. *Consider parental rights.* You must consider the rights of parents to be the guiding voice in their children's lives, especially in value-laden decisions. Serious and foreseeable harm is not necessarily an uplifted knife when you are talking about a minor in a setting called school and parents' rights to be informed and involved when their children are in harm's way.

5. *Consider the setting.* You must consider the dilemma in the context of the school setting. Ethical dilemmas in a school, a setting designed for academics, take on a different meaning than ethical issues in other contexts. Students come to school for academic instruction and when they enter into the personal emotional arena we cannot discount that this will carry obligations to other educators and to parents.

6. *Consider the chronological and developmental levels.* How does the student's developmental level affect the dilemma and how you will approach it? This step is critical, yet it has been left out of decision-making models. It matters how old a child is and how the child demonstrates her or his ability to make informed decisions.

7. *Identify the nature and dimensions of the problem.* Consider the basic moral principles of autonomy, beneficence, nonmaleficence, justice, and loyalty (Kitchener, 1986) and apply them to a particular situation. It may help to prioritize these principles and think through ways in which they can support a resolution to the dilemma. K. S. Kitchener (1986) was one of the first to apply the virtues of autonomy, beneficence, nonmaleficence, justice, and fidelity to ethical decision-making. Her evaluation model is discussed in depth in Chapter 5 and will be discussed in brief here.

   *Autonomy* refers to promoting students' ability to choose their own direction. The school counselor makes every effort to foster maximum self-determination on the part of students. *Beneficence* refers to promoting good for others. Ideally, counseling contributes to the growth and development of the student, and whatever counselors do should be judged against this criterion. *Nonmaleficence* means avoiding doing harm, which includes refraining from actions that risk hurting students. *Justice or fairness* refers to providing equal treatment to all people. This standard implies that anyone—regardless of age, sex, race, ethnicity, disability, socioeconomic status, cultural background, religion, or lifestyle—is entitled to equal treatment. *Loyalty or fidelity* refers to staying connected with students and being available to students to the extent possible. School counselors often carry heavy caseloads and loyalty takes on a different dimension than what an agency counselor might consider as loyalty. Loyalty for the school counselor does not necessarily mean that we have 50-minute sessions once a week with our students. Staying loyal may include connecting with students by encouraging them to stop by before and after school, visiting them at the bus loading zone, or stopping briefly by a student's classroom. All of these activities further the virtue of loyalty or fidelity in spite of the barriers of caseloads, time constraints, and roles.

8. *Consult.* Always discuss your case (without identifying the student if this is appropriate) with a fellow professional, preferably a supervisor, to help you illuminate the issues. In the throes of an ethical dilemma it is sometimes difficult to be as thorough or to see all the issues when caught up in the dilemma. This is the one step that we must always follow.

9. *Consider possible and probable courses of action.* In this process of thinking about many different possibilities for action, it is helpful to write down the options and also to discuss options with another person.

10. *Examine the good and bad consequences of various decisions.* Ponder the implications of each course of action for the student, for others who are related to the student, and for you. List the good and bad consequences of each decision.

11. *Implement your course of action.* Go forward with your decision after you have considered the previous steps. Regardless of your decision, risk follows, but you made the best decision based on the advice and information you had at the time. School counselors cannot practice risk free but we can reduce our risk and raise our support for students by using ethical reasoning.

## THE COMPLICATIONS OF CONFIDENTIALITY IN THE CONTEXT OF SCHOOLS

What mitigating factors do school counselors consider when wrestling with the difficult dilemma of **confidentiality**? School counselors must consider not only students' rights but also parental rights when approaching the issue of whether to protect or breach confidentiality. Parents are continually vested by our courts with legal rights to guide their children (*Bellotti v. Baird*, 1979; *H. L. v. Matheson*, 1982). School boards and administrators adopt policies that counselors are ethically bound to obey. Teachers, informed regarding children's special needs and circumstances, are in the best position to affect positively a child's life during school and often beyond the school day. The ASCA ethical standards dictate that school counselors have a primary obligation and loyalty to students. All of these issues contribute to the complex nature of working with minors in schools (Remley & Herlihy, 2009). The setting in which school counselors work defines the student–school counselor relationship.

Confidentiality, found in Standard A.2 and Standards B.1 and B.2 of the American School Counselor Association (ASCA) Ethical Standards for School Counselors (revised August 2010), gives us guidance. However, the nature of confidentiality makes it the most complex of all the legal and ethical issues that school counselors face and, therefore, each of the confidentiality ethical standards are addressed in the case studies that are presented later in the chapter. The ethical standards that address confidentiality and parental rights are repeated here and a brief discussion follows the ethical standards.

**A.2. Confidentiality Professional school counselors:**

a. Inform individual students of the purposes, goals, techniques and rules of procedure under which they may receive counseling. Disclosure includes the limits of confidentiality in a developmentally appropriate manner. **Informed consent** requires competence on the part of students to understand the limits of confidentiality and therefore, can be difficult to obtain from students of a certain developmental level. Professionals are aware that even though every attempt is made to obtain informed consent it is not always possible and when needed will make counseling decisions on student' behalf.

This ethical standard or code instructs professional school counselors to give informed consent to the counselee of the purposes, goals, techniques, and rules of procedure under which she or he may receive counseling at or before entering the counseling relationship. The meaning of *confidentiality* is given in developmentally appropriate terms and helps the student understand that school counselors will try to keep confidences except when the student is a danger to self or others, the student or parent requests that information be revealed, or a court orders a counselor to disclose information.

**A.2. Confidentiality Professional school counselors:**

c. Recognize the complicated nature of confidentiality in schools and consider each case in context. Keep information confidential unless legal requirements demand that confidential information be revealed or a breach is required to prevent serious and foreseeable harm to the student. **Serious and foreseeable harm** is different for each minor in schools and is defined by students' developmental and chronological age, the setting, parental rights and the nature of the harm. School counselors consult with appropriate professionals when in doubt as to the validity of an exception.

This code protects the confidentiality of information received in the counseling relationship as specified by federal and state laws, written policies, and applicable ethical standards. Such information is only to be revealed to others with the informed consent of the counselee, consistent with the counselor's ethical obligation. In a group setting, the counselor sets a high norm of confidentiality and stresses its importance, yet clearly states that confidentiality in group counseling cannot be guaranteed.

Loyalty and a sense of obligation to students are at the heart of our profession. The school counselor must provide a safe and secure environment in which trust can be established and maintained. Without the assurance of confidentiality, many students would not seek help. Counselors must keep confidential information related to counseling services unless disclosure is in the best interest of students, or is required by law.

**B.1. Parent Rights and Responsibilities Professional school counselors:**

a. Respect the rights and responsibilities of parents/guardians for their children and endeavor to establish, as appropriate, a collaborative relationship with parents/guardians to facilitate the students' maximum development.

c. Are sensitive to diversity among families and recognize that all parents/guardians, custodial and noncustodial, are vested with certain rights and responsibilities for their children's welfare by virtue of their role and according to law.

B.2. **Parents/Guardians and Confidentiality** Professional school counselors:
a. Inform parents/guardians of the school counselor's role to include the confidential nature of the counseling relationship between the counselor and student.

Parents send their children to school for curriculum instruction and when children's emotional needs are being addressed by school counselors, conflict can result between parents' right to know what is happening in their child's life and a student's right to privacy (Linde & Stone, 2010; Remley & Herlihy, 2009; Wheeler & Bertram, 2008). School counselors face a dual responsibility to their minor students and to the students' parents. The challenge of protecting their students extends beyond "students" to include the parents of minor students.

## Students' Rights and Responsibilities

The legal status of minors is complicated. Remley and Herlihy (2009) emphasize in their writings that because students are minors, they are not legally able to make their own decisions, and although they have an ethical right to confidentiality, the legal right belongs to their parents or guardian. Minors are emancipated or free from parental or guardian control when they reach the age of 18, enter the military, marry, or the Circuit Court declares them emancipated (Alexander & Alexander, 2010).

Students' rights and responsibilities are far-reaching and differ by states (consult your state's statutes). However, in most states there are similar student responsibilities while on school grounds or under school supervision. Students must avoid unlawful activity, including sexual behavior, drinking alcohol, gambling, using dangerous drugs or tobacco, and causing damage or injury to persons or property. Infractions may result in suspension, expulsion, or financial restitution. Students and their parents or guardians are liable for damages they cause to persons or property of the school district, and for all property such as books that have been lent to them and not returned (FL§ 1006.42).

## Parents' Rights and Responsibilities

In addition to the points already discussed, parents have the right to be the guiding voice in their children's lives in value-laden decisions. **Family Educational Rights and Privacy Act** (FERPA, 1974), a federal law that governs the disclosure of information from **educational records**, gives parents the right to talk to teachers and school administrators about their children, to see their children's educational record, and to decide if their child will participate in a questionnaire, survey, or examination regarding a parent's personal beliefs, sex practices, family life, or religion. FERPA allows parents to request that information that they believe to be inaccurate or misleading be purged from their child's educational record (FERPA, 1973).

## Community Standards and School Board Policy

How school counselors address ethical problems depends in large part on the culture and/or standards of the community. The message here is to understand the culture and the prevailing written and unwritten standards of the community, school district, and individual work site and behave sensitively toward the culture and consistently with **community standards**.

A school counselor who acted on her religious values became the center of a court case in *Grossman v. South Shore Public School District* (2007). Based on her religious beliefs, Grossman discarded board-approved literature on contraceptives and ordered replacement literature on abstinence. Grossman also prayed with students on at least two occasions. The superintendent recommended nonrenewal for Grossman's contract, explaining that she was not a "good fit" with the school based on her religious practices. Grossman stated she believed her contract was cancelled because her views on abstinence and prayer aroused the district's religious hostility. How do you think the court ruled?

The 7th U.S. Circuit Court of Appeals barred Grossman from pursuing her claim, instead rendering the opinion that the district had a legitimate right to be concerned about Grossman's conduct. The court removed the issue of religious discrimination based on Grossman's Christianity. The court concluded that it was Grossman's conduct, not her beliefs or the expression/exercise of them, that caused the dismissal. School authorities have a right to control the school district curriculum and, equally, to control the policies of guidance counselors and other staff (p. 1099).

Ethics are situational. A school counselor's ethical behavior is determined in part by the school, district, and community standards. Further, school boards establish policy based on community standards and needs, and if we accept employment in a district we are agreeing to abide by the written and unwritten rules of the school district. Counselors have to understand the threads that comprise the community's fabric to discern how to behave ethically in a particular environment.

### Confidentiality and Privileged Communication

Although all school counselors have a confidentiality responsibility, their relationships with students are rarely privileged. In most states, school counselors do not have **privileged communication**, which is given in state statutes to the clients of certain professionals such as lawyers and psychiatrists. A few states grant partial privilege that protects a counselor's students by securing their confidences except when required by a court of law to breach those confidences. Full privilege communication renders the counselor incapable of testifying to information related in confidence. The school counselor's ethical responsibility to keep confidential almost all communications with students is complicated because of the school setting.

## ETHICS AND GROUP WORK IN SCHOOLS

The legal and ethical complexities of working with minors in schools require that school counselors remain vigilant as to the rights and responsibilities of students and their parents and the implications of these rights on their work. A school counselor's **multiplicity of responsibility** in a setting designed to deliver academic instruction complicates the legal and ethical world of school counseling. These complications are acutely present in the personal counseling arena of group work because other students are present to hear possible discussions of the private world of students and their families.

## Confidentiality and Informed Consent

Working with minors in groups requires that school counselors must come from the posture that whatever is said in a group will be repeated. We are risking the emotional safety of students when we expect developmentally maturing students to respect confidentiality. The ASCA ethical standards tell us that confidentiality cannot be guaranteed in a group.

> (ASCA) A.6.c. Establish clear expectations in the group setting, and clearly state that confidentiality in group counseling cannot be guaranteed. Given the developmental and chronological ages of minors in schools, recognize the tenuous nature of confidentiality for minors renders some topics inappropriate for group work in a school setting.

Because we cannot guarantee confidentiality in groups, even adult groups, we avoid putting risky faith in minors in a social setting called school. Minors often change friends and loyalties and with this fluid behavior there is the danger of a student gaining attention, seeking revenge, or just thoughtlessly and without malice revealing another student's personal pain. For every group we form, regardless of whether the topic is as innocuous as School Success Skills or as value-laden as Children of Alcoholics, Children in Divorce Situations, or Victims of Date Rape, it is imperative that we remind ourselves that confidentiality will be breached. We must continually ask ourselves, "Will the potential emotional cost to students and their families be worth any gains that we may accomplish?"

Competence, voluntariness, or voluntary participation, and knowledge are necessary elements if students are to give us informed consent to participate in a group. Are middle schoolers able to understand that they will be discussing a sensitive topic and their private revelations may be repeated in the halls and locker rooms? An adolescent may developmentally be unable to understand the ramifications of discussing painful personal information in the presence of other students.

## Appropriate Topics for Group Work in Schools

Are there topics that are not appropriate for group counseling in a school setting? For example, can we adequately address in groups in schools tough therapeutic issues such as eating disorders that are resistant to change even in residential treatment programs and other specialized settings designed to tackle eating disorders? In classroom guidance lessons we can tackle the issue of body image and nutrition for the benefit of all students, but there are some topics that can't be adequately addressed in schools.

## Adequacy of Counselor Skills for Group Work

It is unrealistic for members of the school and larger community to expect that we should have all the skills and knowledge necessary for group work with the myriad of serious clinical topics many of our students face. For example, agency counselors who spend considerable time and training focusing on self-mutilating students often find trying to affect change in these students to be a daunting responsibility.

Schools' counselors work to shore up and support all students to be successful learners. While students with serious emotional issues often cannot learn if their needs are not met, it is unfair and unrealistic of the school and wider community to expect that the school counselor has the depth of skill and the privilege of time to be a mental health expert for the myriad of serious problems and dysfunctions presented by students. Many school counselors are becoming managers-of-resources, reaching beyond the walls of their school to reposition mental health support into their schools or to develop a mechanism for helping students find support outside their schools. It isn't that the school counselor is less talented or competent than colleagues in an agency or community setting, it is that the needs are bigger than can be managed by the school counselor alone. The mental health needs of our youth must become the responsibility of the larger community as we work desperately to give all students the gift of becoming a successful learner. More information about working with groups is available in the Voices from the Field section of this chapter.

# WORKING THROUGH CASE STUDIES

There are court cases, state and federal legislation, ethical standards, and school board policy that inform our practice. Following are hypothetical and real cases addressing case notes, educational records, parental rights, negligence, suicide, letters of recommendation, sexually active students, group work, negligence in academic advising, abortion counseling, and sexual harassment. Working through these cases will illuminate principles of law and practice that we can apply to our daily work.

## Counselors' Case Notes or Sole Possession Records

*You have been seeing Stephen for individual counseling for three months. You have received a request from Stephen's mother, who is incarcerated in another state, for copies of all school records. His mother has also asked for your case notes. Are you legally required to provide her with education records? Must you provide her with your case notes?*

Noncustodial parental rights are often misunderstood. FERPA (1974) makes it clear that both parents have equal access to education records. Even incarcerated parents, parents who have refused to pay child support, and abusive parents have rights to education records under FERPA (1974) unless there is a court order expressly forbidding a parent to have education records. Must case notes be sent also?

The American Counseling Association (1997) has helped clarify whether school counselors' case notes are education records. Case notes to be exempt from education records must be "sole possession records." Not all of the information collected and maintained by schools and school employees about students is subject to the access and disclosure requirements under the Family

Education Rights and Privacy Act (FERPA, 1974). One of the five categories exempt from the definition of "education records" under FERPA is records made by teachers, supervisors, counselors, administrators, and other school personnel that are kept in the sole possession of the maker of the record and are not accessible or revealed to any other person except a temporary substitute for the maker of the record."

The exemption of **sole possession records** from the definition of education records is narrow and specific. To be considered sole possession records, written case notes must meet three requirements: (1) the information must be a private note that is created solely by the individual possessing it; (2) the information must be a personal memory aid; (3) the information must not be shared or accessible to any other person except the individual's temporary substitute. Case notes will only qualify for the sole possession exemption if they record personal observations about the behavior of students or conclusions the counselor has drawn on the basis of interactions with a student or others. Linde explains that exemptions include "personal notes, reports to Child Protective Services for abuse or neglect, and in some states, reports from law enforcement agencies regarding students' arrests for reportable offenses" (Erford, 2011a, p. 85).

## Rights for Non-custodial Parents

*Rouel, a 14-year-old student, occasionally seeks your help with relationship issues with her mother. Rouel's parents are divorced and generally at war over everything including how best to raise Rouel and her sister. Rouel describes her mother as being very strict and closed off. Rouel, who lives with her mother, sees her father almost every weekend. A teacher expressed concern that lately Rouel's grades have been plummeting, she seems to have lost interest in her studies, and she rarely smiles or engages in conversation with others. All these behaviors are in marked contrast to how Rouel usually behaves. After meeting with Rouel you believe you need to involve her parents. Rouel begs you to call her father instead of her mother. It is Friday and Rouel explains she is going to her father's home right after school. You believe Rouel's mother will be enraged that you contacted Rouel's father. Can you consult Rouel's father without seeking permission or notifying her mother, the custodial parent?*

School counselors can find guidance in the court case *Page v. Rotterdam-Mohonasen Central School District* (1981). John Page had visitation rights for his fifth-grade son Eric but repeated requests to the school district to provide him with educational records went unheeded. Mikado Page, Eric's mother, sent a statement to the school (at what was believed to be the school's request) explaining that she has legal custody of Eric and that she did not want John Page to have Eric's education records, participate in teacher-parent conferences, or in any way engage in the educational progress of Eric. When the matter landed in court, the court found that John Page was not trying to alter custodial rights but simply participate in his son's educational progress. The court found that school districts have a duty to act in the best educational interest of the children committed to their care, which means providing educational information to both parents of every child fortunate to have two parents interested in her or his welfare (Huey & Remley, 1988; *Page v. Rotterdam-Mohonasen Central School District*, 1981). Parents, whether or not they have legal custody, do not have to give up their rights to be psychological guardians. The court concluded that in the event of the death of one parent "it would be disastrous for the welfare of a child if an uninformed and ill-prepared parent were suddenly cast into a custodial role upon the occurrence of such a misfortune."

## Negligence and Malpractice Involving Suicide

*You have been told by a student that her friend Rolando is threatening suicide. When you call Rolando in she vehemently denies it and scoffs at the idea that she would ever harm herself. You are convinced and you drop it without discussing it with anyone. Is there an ethical or legal dilemma?*

The law of **negligence**, which composes a large part of the law of torts, involves injury or damage to another through a breach of duty owed to that person. Four elements must be present for negligence. First, a duty must be owed by one person to another. Until the *Eisel v. Montgomery County Board of Education* case, courts consistently found that school counselors did not owe a duty to their minor students to prevent suicide. The *Eisel* case changed the way school counselors must look at suicide prevention. The second element that must be present in a negligence case is that the duty that was owed was breached. The third element is that there must be sufficient legal causal connection between the breach of duty and the injury, and lastly, injury or damages must be present (Weaver, Martin, Klein, Zwier, Eades, & Bauman, 2009).

The Maryland Court of Appeals in *Eisel v. Montgomery County Board of Education* (1991) determined that school counselors had a duty to notify the parents of a 13-year-old student of suicidal statements she made to fellow students. Nicole Eisel apparently became involved in Satanism and told several friends and fellow students of her intention to kill herself. Some of these friends informed their school counselor of Nicole's intentions, and this individual in turn informed Nicole's counselor. The two counselors questioned Nicole about the statements and she denied making them. Neither the parents nor the school administrators were notified about these events. Shortly thereafter, in a public park away from the school, the other party to the suicide pact shot Nicole and then herself (*Eisel v. Montgomery County Board of Education*, 1991).

The court cited as critical the *in loco parentis* doctrine, which means the school counselors were standing instead of the parents. *In loco parentis* brings a legal responsibility or special duty to exercise reasonable care to protect a student from harm. The court concluded that "school counselors have a duty to use reasonable means to attempt to prevent a suicide when they are on notice of a child or adolescent student's suicide intent" (*Eisel v. Montgomery County Board of Education*, 1991). The court in *Eisel* broke new ground and found a **special relationship** sufficient to create a **duty of care** when an adolescent in a school setting expresses an intention to commit suicide and the counselor becomes aware of such intention. Pursuant to this duty of care and in light of the slight burden on the counselor in warning the parents, future cases that follow *Eisel* are likely to hold counselors negligent for a failure to warn parents of suicidal intentions of students (*Eisel v. Montgomery County Board of Education,* 1991). Linde states, "While this case is legally binding only on professional school counselors in Maryland, it has become the standard used in subsequent cases. For example, a federal circuit court in Florida made a similar ruling in 1997 in *Wyke v. Polk County School Board,* and several other courts are following suit. But courts in other states have rejected the Eisel decision and have found in favor of the school systems" (Erford, 2010, p. 89)

Courts in other states have refused to impose liability in these kinds of cases, primarily because of state laws granting immunity to public schools and their employees. In *Killen v. Independent School District No. 706* (1996), the Minnesota Court of Appeals applied the immunity doctrines to a student suicide case. Under the doctrine of official immunity, "a public official charged by law with duties that call for the exercise of judgment or discretion is not personally liable to an individual for damages unless the official's actions are wrongful or malicious."

The facts of the case were as follows: a ninth-grade student killed herself at home with a gun retrieved from her parents' basement. A school counselor warned Jill's parents that she had expressed suicidal thoughts and recommended counseling, but the allegation was that the school counselor did not share information that the student had made other, more specific suicidal statements. The court in Killen held that a school's decision not to create a suicide prevention plan was a protected, discretionary action, or rather inaction. Because it was the result of a conscious decision not to implement a policy, it was protected. Therefore, the school could not be held liable for failing to prevent a student's suicide, despite having four direct reports of the student's suicidal intent over a period of months.

All of the cases that imposed liability, however, involved employees who failed to notify parents that their children had written or talked to others about killing themselves (Portner, 2002; Simpson, 1999). The Code of Ethics for the American School Counselor Association explicitly permits disclosure when there may be "serious and foreseeable harm" to the student or others (ASCA, 2010, A.1.c). In addition, the Seventh Circuit Court of Appeals has ruled that a school district lawfully can punish a counselor for failing to report a student's "suicidal tendencies." Whether you believe a student is serious about suicide or not, the expression of **suicidal ideation** is a cry for help. It is never advisable to ignore a suicide threat. Adolescents who are threatening suicide are too volatile or fragile to be ignored.

## Letters of Recommendation

*Emily is applying to a competitive university and your letter of recommendation will be a critical part of her admission application. Emily's ninth-grade year was dismal academically. She confided in you that she was being physically abused by her boyfriend during ninth grade but she ended the relationship after seven months. Emily has been a stellar student since her sophomore year and is not the same person who allowed herself to remain in an abusive relationship. You are considering explaining all of this in your letter of recommendation in hopes that Emily will only be judged based on what she has done since leaving this abusive relationship. Legally and/or ethically can you include this information in a letter of recommendation?*

School counselors conscientiously work to behave legally in writing letters of recommendation and find their guidance primarily in Family Education Rights and Privacy Act (FERPA, 1974), the federal statute protecting parents' and students' rights regarding educational records. Some of the ethical considerations involving letters of recommendation are (1) letters and confidential, sensitive information; (2) writing letters for problem students; and (3) supporting weak students.

### Confidentiality and Letters of Recommendation

In an informal survey of more than 800 school counselors, the overwhelming majority reported that they would never put sensitive, confidential information in a letter of recommendation without student and parental permission (Stone, 2010a). However, in Emily's case counselors report that they would not include this information with or without Emily's permission. Even when it comes to confidential information that would benefit a student, counselors would rather secure the student's permission to include an invitation in the letter to call the counselor to discuss the student's special circumstances.

Legally, school counselors can include anything in a letter that is common knowledge and observable (Fischer & Sorenson, 1996), such as "Kennard has never let the fact that he is wheelchair bound keep him from being an active and high-profile school leader, engaged in numerous school activities such as. . . ." However, best practice is to always get a student's consent. It is best practice to leave out sensitive, confidential information or, if in your judgment it is important to include the information to benefit the student, then secure student and parental permission to relay what they may not want known.

### Writing Letters for Problem Students

Counselors report (Stone, 2010b) that if they cannot write a strong letter of recommendation, then they prefer not to write a letter at all. A response to the student such as "I am not a good choice as you would get a stronger letter from someone who knows you better" will send the message that their letter would not be helpful.

### Writing Letters for Weak Students

Counselors are skilled at advocating for their weak students who deserve a chance. Counselors know how to focus on students' assets without bending the truth, skirting the major issues, or in any way painting a false picture. As one school counselor said to an admissions representative, "Let me tell you what you can't learn about Roger from his application and transcripts. Roger has been on this long cultural journey and has developed survival and problem-solving muscles that can never be measured by standardized tests or grades. Roger has demonstrated he is an astute and determined person who has aspirations and ambitions that will make your university proud to have admitted him. For example, Roger has taken care of three siblings. . . ." Counselors often focus on life skills when a standard approach to recommendation letters will not help a student (Stone, 2010b).

## Negligence in Academic Advising

School counselors have a legal responsibility to exercise care in fulfilling their professional responsibilities as they too can be charged with malpractice for failure to render competent services in carrying out the duties of their profession.

*Bruce Sain, a senior in Cedar Rapids, Iowa, had talent as an all-state basketball player. In 1996, he was awarded a five-year basketball scholarship to Northern Illinois University to start as a first-year student. In the summer prior to his first year in college, Sain was notified in a letter that he did not meet the National Collegiate Athletic Association (NCAA) regulations for incoming first-year athletes at Division I schools. Sain fell one-third credit short in the required English credits because his one-third English credit in Technical Communications was not on the list of classes his high school submitted to the NCAA for approval. Sain's family filed suit against the Cedar Rapids School District citing the school district as negligent and the school counselor, Larry Bowen, as guilty of negligent misrepresentation in his role as an academic advisor (Parrott, 2002; Reid, 2001; Sain v. Cedar Rapids Community School District, 2001). How did a scholarship opportunity for Bruce Sain turn into shambles and how did Larry Bowen find himself at the center of a lawsuit?*

Sain was dissatisfied with his second trimester English course and asked Bowen to place him in another English class. Allegedly, Bowen suggested Technical Communications and explained to Sain that it was being offered at the school for the first time but that the Initial Eligibility Clearinghouse would approve the high school course and that he would have no problem with his NCAA eligibility. The summer following his graduation, the NCAA Clearinghouse declared Sain ineligible because technical communications was not on the list of approved NCAA eligibility courses for Sain's high school (*Sain v. Cedar Rapids Community School District*, 2001; Zirkel, 2001a). With his scholarship offer voided, Bruce Sain turned to the courts to claim **negligent misrepresentation** against Bowen for erroneously telling Sain that he was safe to take Technical Communications (*Sain v. Cedar Rapids Community School District*, 2001). It was never implied or expressed that it was the school counselor's responsibility to submit courses for approval but rather that it was the school counselor's responsibility to give proper academic advice.

The lower court rejected Sain's suit, but on appeal, the Iowa Supreme Court remanded the Sain case back to the lower court to be tried (*Sain v. Cedar Rapids Community School District*, 2001). The case was settled out of court for an undisclosed amount of money.

It is important to note that the Iowa Supreme Court did not find for guilt or innocence but left that to the lower court to decide. However, in the school counseling profession we pay attention to this case because the Iowa Supreme Court found that the claim of "negligent misrepresentation" had merit and should not have been dismissed by the lower court. The majority opinion for the Iowa Supreme Court said that school counselors are liable for providing information to students about credits and courses needed to pursue post–high school goals (Parrott, 2002; Reid, 2001; *Sain v. Cedar Rapids Community School District*, 2001). The allegedly erroneous advice given by the counselor was equated to negligent misrepresentation in professions such as accounting and the law and others whose business requires that they give accurate and appropriate information (Zirkel, 2001a). The court has determined that school counselors have a similar business relationship of giving accurate advice to students when the student has a need to know. The court explains that just as accountants and lawyers stand to gain financially from giving accurate advice, so do school counselors as that is what they are paid to do. Therefore, negligent misrepresentation can be applied to the school counselor–student relationship when erroneous advice means a student loses a lucrative scholarship. The Iowa Supreme Court says this is a classic case of negligent misrepresentation (*Sain v. Cedar Rapids Community School District*, 2001; Zirkel, 2001a).

The court acknowledged that the ruling could have a "chilling effect" on academic advising by school counselors. However, the court cautioned that the ruling should have limited effect as negligent representation is confined to students whose reliance on information is reasonable (such as, Does this course meet NCAA eligibility?) and that the school counselor must be aware of how vital the information is to the student. This explanation was intended to comfort school counselors and to keep them from overreacting to the principles outlined by the Sain case (*Sain v. Cedar Rapids Community School District*, 2001).

The following are recommendations for avoiding negligence in the role of academic advisor:

1. Educate yourself to the extent possible in the areas needed for competent academic advising and check your facts as often as appropriate. With care you will be able to demonstrate that you tried to keep yourself abreast of critical information. Ask for professional development from your school district, counseling organizations, and/or literature in the area of academic advising.
2. Manage resources and equip selected professionals to be a key component in the career and academic advising roles. For example, the coaches can be in charge of advising students about NCAA regulations.
3. Publicize widely academic information for all students and parents. Newsletters, form letters, and email discussion lists can all help you in the advising role and demonstrate that you are proactively trying to disseminate critical, timely information.
4. Require that students and parents sign off when they have been given critical timely information. For example, when you give seniors their

personal credit check for their remaining graduation requirements, have them sign off an acknowledgment that they have been told and understand what they need to do.

5. Consult. You never stand alone unless you fail to consult with others who are in a position to help you.

## Negligence in Abortion Counseling

*You have been working with a young woman who finds herself pregnant and unwilling to carry the pregnancy to term. You live in a state where a student can secure an abortion without parental involvement. She is asking for your support as she wrestles with the abortion decision. She wants your help in finding an abortion clinic and in finding financial assistance to pay for the abortion. She has asked you to go with her when she has the procedure. What are your ethical and legal obligations in this situation?*

The legal and ethical complications of working with minors in schools pose daily dilemmas and never more so than in **value-laden** issues such as abortion counseling usually involving a family's religious beliefs, values about sexual conduct, privacy rights, freedom of choice, parental rights to be the guiding voice in their children's lives, and other rights. Respecting students' confidences requires school counselors to balance the rights of minors with the rights of their parents (Huss, Bryant, & Mulet, 2008). Legal rulings and the ASCA codes for ethical behavior offer suggestions and guidance in the complexities of confidentiality. However, it is ultimately the responsibility of the school counselor to determine the appropriate response to the individual student who puts their trust in the security of the counseling relationship.

Under what circumstances will a counselor be held liable for giving abortion advice? In *Arnold v. Board of Education of Escambia County* (1989), Jane and John, two high school students, filed suit along with their parents against the School District of Escambia County, Alabama, alleging that the school counselor, Kay Rose, and the assistant principal, Melvin Powell, coerced and assisted Jane in getting an abortion. Further, the accusation was that Powell and Rose hired the two students to perform menial tasks to earn money for the abortion. John, the father of the baby, and Jane claimed that their constitutional rights were violated including involuntary servitude and free exercise of religion. The parents claimed that their privacy rights were violated when they were not informed by the school counselor and assistant principal that Jane was pregnant and when school officials urged the students not to tell their parents. The trial court dismissed the suit and plaintiffs appealed (*Arnold v. Board of Education of Escambia County*, 1989; Zirkel, 2001b).

The 11th Circuit Court of Appeals partially reversed the decision of the trial court and found Jane's privacy claim and both students' religious claims as worthy of further consideration by the courts. If Jane and John's religion prohibited abortion and Rose and Powell coerced Jane and John to proceed with Jane's abortion, then their constitutionally protected right of freedom of religion was violated and the court remanded the case back to the trial court to be heard (Zirkel, 2001b).

In fact finding, the trial court established that Jane visited a physician who confirmed she was pregnant and provided her with abortion information on her request. John and Jane told Hill that they did not want their parents to know about the pregnancy as they were not supposed to be seeing each other and that Jane left home because she was being abused by her stepfather. Hill presented various alternatives but the students rejected all alternatives except abortion including consulting with their parents. Rose reported the alleged abuse by the stepfather to the Department of Human Resources who sent a representative to meet with Jane. The representative urged Jane to consult with her mother and offered alternatives such as foster care and adoption but when Jane rejected all alternatives, she assisted Jane in trying to get financial assistance and Medicaid. Jane and John said they felt pressured by Rose when she asked them how they planned to care for the baby and where they were going to take the baby. During the process of discovery, Jane admitted that these were good questions, that she alone made the decision to have an abortion, and that she was not coerced by Rose or Powell. The trial court concluded that the students were not deprived of their free will, had chosen to obtain an abortion, had chosen not to tell their parents, and that there was no coercion on the part of school officials. The principles established by the 11th Circuit Court of Appeals have implications for the school counseling profession, i.e., coercion by school officials in private matters is unconstitutional (*Arnold v. Board of Education of Escambia County*, 1989; Zirkel, 1991, 2001b).

More recently, in *Carter v. Hickey* ("ACLJ Lawsuit," 1999), a Pennsylvania court ruled that the school district is obligated to issue and enforce a directive banning school personnel from encouraging, assisting, aiding, or abetting a student in obtaining an abortion. In a lawsuit filed in U.S. District Court, the American Center for Law and Justice (ACLJ), a public interest law firm founded by TV evangelist Pat Robertson, asserted that a high school guidance counselor usurped the parents and circumvented their privacy rights by failing to divulge the pregnancy while coercing their 16-year-old daughter into having an abortion despite her misgivings about the procedure. ACLJ affiliate attorney Joseph P. Stanton said parents Howard and Marie Carter had a right to "familial" privacy under the same Fourteenth Amendment protection that formed the basis of the 1973 Supreme Court ruling that established abortion rights in *Roe v. Wade* (Hull & Hoffer, 2001). The school district settled with the parents out of court for $20,000.

Counselors in the course of fulfilling their job responsibilities can assist students with these value-laden issues if they are competent to give such advice and if they proceed in a professional manner. "Counselors during the course of their professional responsibilities may assist students with value-laden issues such as abortion if they are competent to provide this advice and proceed in a professional manner" (Cottone & Tarvydas, 2007, p. 180).

Can school boards adopt policy forbidding school counselors to discuss with their students information about contraception, abortion, or sexual activity? School boards can (and some do) adopt policy forbidding counselors to address certain topics or instructing them to immediately call parents if such topics are brought up by their students. Counselors are urged to be well educated regarding school board policies. "Some schools can and do adopt policies that forbid counselors from addressing certain topics and instruct the counselor to immediately contact parents if specified topics are brought up by students" (Cottone & Tarvydas, 2007, p. 180).

In absence of a school board policy expressly forbidding you to discuss abortion, school counselors can discuss with students their options. The caveat is that school counselors must be ready to defend themselves that they behaved as the reasonably competent professional would have. Coercion and imposing one's values on a minor student must be avoided to dodge liability for negligence.

The following are recommendations for avoiding negligence in a situation like those just described:

1. Know your school board policies.
2. When working with minors on value-laden issues it is especially important to consider the chronological and developmental level of the minor to determine whether intervention is needed and how much is required. To promote the autonomy and independence of minors is to decide if they can continue on the path they have chosen without interference or should some level of intervention or breach of confidentiality be exercised. Primary to the counselor's ethical decision-making is the seriousness of a minor's behavior in the framework of their developmental milestones and the minor's history of making informed decisions (Stone, 2001).
3. Consider the impact of the setting. Parental rights are more complicated when the minor is in a school setting as parents send minors to school for academics, not for personal counseling. Therefore, when a minor seeks counseling in a value-laden area such as abortion, which may affect a parent's religious beliefs and/or rights to be the guiding voice in their children's lives, consideration must be given to parents (Isaacs & Stone, 1999).
4. Encourage students to involve their parents in these value-laden difficult dilemmas such as abortion. Use all your skillful techniques to help them make the decision to involve their parents such as offering to be with them when they tell their parents.
5. Consider diversity issues. Each ethical dilemma must be made in context and must consider a minor's ethnicity, gender, race, and sexual identity.
6. Consult with a supervisor and/or respected colleague, examining the good and bad consequences of each course of action, striving to minimize the risk to the student while respecting the inherent rights of parents. It is ethical, lawful, and beneficial to inform and consult with supervisors and colleagues. Consult again after you implement your course of action to process the results and strengthen the probability of making more appropriate decisions in the future (Stone, 2010a).
7. Know your own values in sensitive areas such as abortion and understand the impact of those values on your ability to act in the best interest of your student. Professionals know they cannot leave their values out of

their work but they understand when those values can interfere. Refer students to a colleague when you can no longer be effective (Stone, 2001).

8. The professional school counselor would never provide referrals to birth control clinics or agree to take a counselee for any kind of medical procedure, especially one as controversial as abortion (Stone, 2002).

## Sexual Harassment

*Fourteen-year-old Regina is subjected daily to sexually suggestive remarks by a group of boys in the hallway near her math class. Regina has started to come to math class late to avoid the taunts and jeers of the boys. Regina's math teacher, Ms. Lopez, unaware of the situation, has sent Regina to the office for tardy slips but without effect to change her behavior, and now Regina is in danger of being suspended. Ms. Lopez, sensing that something unusual is happening to her conscientious student-turned-truant, asks you the school counselor to talk with Regina. You begin to learn the truth of Regina's misery when she confides about the harassment. Regina describes her embarrassment and her attempts at coping by "laughing it off," "avoiding them," "taunting back" (which she said only made her feel more dirty), or "dressing in really baggy clothes." She begs you not to tell anyone as "it [the harassment] will only get worse." Must you report the sexual harassment to the administration of your school? Can you keep Regina's identity confidential? Can the school administration keep Regina's identity confidential when confronting the perpetrators?*

Through the case of Regina, let's explore the legal muscle school counselors have been given to advocate for Regina and other victims of sexual harassment including males and the most vulnerable students for abuse, gay and lesbian students. The National Women's Law Center (2007) recently addressed the issue of sexual harassment in schools. They found that "83% of female and 79% of male students in grades 8 through 11 had been sexually harassed at school in ways that interfered with their lives. One third of the surveyed students—20% of boys and 44% of girls—said that they fear being sexually harassed during the school day" (p. 1).

Regina fits the profile of the harassed student: self-blame, self-doubt, using avoidance techniques, and wanting to be free of the harassment but enduring it rather than risking being victimized twice when students find out she is a "snitch," "nark," or "informant." The impact sexual harassment has had on Regina's education and the lengths she will go to to avoid the harassment underscore the seriousness of sexual harassment. Once regarded as harmless peer interaction deemed to be flirtatious or playful, sexual harassment is now widely understood to be destructive, illegal, and adversely affecting a student's education (Stone, 2001).

A Supreme Court ruling, *Davis v. Monroe County Board of Education* (1999), has given sexual harassment a prominent place on the national agenda and has established that public schools can be forced to pay monetary damages for failing to address student-on-student sexual harassment. Sexual harassment can no longer be ignored or given cursory attention by school districts as Davis demands action against known sexual harassment (*Davis v. Monroe County Board of Education*, 1999).

The *Davis* case involved L. Davis, a fifth-grade girl who repeatedly during a five-month period reported sexual abuse behaviors by G.F. to her teachers and principal but to no avail. The abuse continued. L. was unable to concentrate on her studies (her previously high grades dropped) and her father found a suicide note. Mrs. Davis, who had also reported the abuse on more than one occasion to the educators of the school without redress, finally filed a complaint with the Monroe County, Georgia, Sheriff Department and G.F. pled guilty to sexual battery. Mrs. Davis then filed a $1,000,000 lawsuit under **Title IX**'s prohibition of sex discrimination in schools (*Davis v. Monroe County Board of Education*, 1999). The Supreme Court's 5-to-4 ruling in favor of Mrs. Davis emphasized a stringent standard stating that the harassment must be known to educators and must be "so severe, pervasive, and objectively offensive that it can be said to deprive the victim of access to the educational opportunities or benefits provided by the school" (*Davis v. Monroe County Board of Education*, 1999, n.p.).

The *Davis* case clearly encourages more protection against sexual harassment and gives school counselors legal muscle to exercise an advocacy role to assist individual victims and to help establish a respectful school climate. With 80 percent of students experiencing sexual harassment and fewer than 10 percent of that number reporting the harassment to an adult at school, it is obvious that there is a need for students to have a safe confidential place to report harassment (American Association of University Women Educational Foundation, 2001).

Must you report the sexual harassment to the administration of your school? School counselors are required by law to report the sexual harassment to school officials. "A school has notice if a responsible employee 'knew, or in the exercise of reasonable care should have known,' about the harassment" (U.S. Department of Education, The Office of Civil Rights, 2008). Once Regina confided that she was being harassed, this constituted notice and triggered the school counselor's legal requirement to report the harassment and the school's responsibility to take corrective action (U.S. Department of Education, The Office of Civil Rights, 2008).

Can you keep Regina's identity confidential? The **Office of Civil Rights** (OCR) promotes protecting confidentiality, understanding that breaching a student's confidences will often discourage reporting of harassment, an already horrific problem in many schools. If your school has a procedure or policy in place in which the victim is identified on the report, then your advocacy role can spark change in this practice. Reporting is critical! Identifying the victim is not. The school counselor will need to educate Regina about the legal requirement to report the sexual harassment and, if appropriate, encourage Regina to allow her identity to be known to support addressing sexual harassment. However, the OCR does not require that educators breach confidentiality just to ensure that the perpetrators are disciplined; rather, they require that educators have to address the harassment, and this can take many forms.

Can the school administration keep Regina's identity confidential when confronting the perpetrators? OCR realizes that withholding the name of the victim may interfere with the investigation and infringe on the due process rights of the accused. In the context of each situation, school counselors and school administrators will need to wrestle with the difficult decision to honor an alleged victim's request for confidentiality, yet to take "effective action to end the harassment and prevent it from happening again to the victim or to others" (U.S. Department of Education, Office of Civil Rights, 2008, p. 10). A student's request for confidentiality should be respected even if this hinders the investigation. The school should make every effort to address the harassment in another way, but sometimes the investigation and the discipline of an individual perpetrator must be sacrificed to protect the victim. Regina's confidentiality needs might outweigh the need for disciplinary action against the accused. If disciplining the individual perpetrator is not possible without revealing Regina's identity, then other strategies might have to be employed, such as a schoolwide sexual harassment workshop, a student survey that tries to determine the prevalence of harassment, and classroom presentations. Techniques such as positioning a teacher in the hall during class changes where the teacher can observe and report the harassment is preferable to a peer report where the identity of the victim can be surmised. Depending on the seriousness of the harassment and the age of the victim, the identity of the victim may have to be revealed as a last resort.

Students will not report harassment and risk being victimized twice. Students need assurances that everything possible will be done to protect their identity. The case of Regina is a small snapshot of the problem and remedy to protecting sexual harassment victims. School counselors can be instrumental in helping to heighten the awareness of the sexual harassment problem, assist in helping to establish a safe school climate, and advocate for protection of a student's privacy rights in reporting harassment. School counselors can be a source of strength for the individual student who needs help in confronting and dealing with sexual harassment. The legal and ethical complications of working with minors in schools continue to pose daily dilemmas and never more so than in sexual harassment issues. Respecting students' confidences can send a message that the school counseling office is a safe place to report sexual harassment.

Two other cases involving school counselors give us guidance. In *Plamp v. Mitchell School District* (2009), the student brought claims against the school district contending that she notified her counselor that her teacher was sexually harassing her and the counselor did nothing to put an end to his inappropriate behavior. The student claimed that the school district was responsible under Title IX, but the court ruled that for the school district to be liable in this case the student would have to show that she reported the incidents to "appropriate persons" who could address the alleged discrimination and institute corrective measures. The court ruled that a counselor does not qualify as an "appropriate person" and therefore ruled in favor of the district. Best practice would be for the school counselor to always report to the administration sexual harassment as suggested by *Sexual Harassment: It's*

*Not Academic,* a publication of the Office of Civil Rights (OCR). Protecting the identity of the victim to the extent possible is best practice according to the OCR.

In *L.W. v. Toms River Regional Schools* (2007), the school district was sued based on the New Jersey Law Against Discrimination. A student claimed that he was subject to discrimination for years based on his sexual orientation, and when he brought the issue to his school counselor, the counselor responded by telling him to "toughen up and turn the other cheek." The counselor did not inform the principal of the allegations and did nothing further to address the situation with the students who were harassing the plaintiff. The court ruled that a school district will be liable for such harassment where the school administration or its agents or employees knew or should have known of the harassment and failed to take effective measures to stop it. The plaintiff was awarded $50,000, due in part to the school counselor's failure to take measures to stop the harassment.

## Child Abuse Reporting

School counselors are ethically, morally, and legally responsible to report suspected child abuse. Some states and school districts have policies that require that a child abuse report is funneled through a designee in the school, which could be the principal, but educators can't give away their obligation to see that abuse is reported if they see signs of child abuse. State statutes vary slightly in language, but the meaning is generally the same and reads similarly. Educators and counselors are mandatory child abuse reporters, which means they

- have an absolute duty to report;
- do not have to be certain—suspicion is enough to establish a duty;
- have a duty that is not discretionary; it is inextricably clear;
- have an obligation to report within a certain time frame (see your state statute);
- are protected in most states, since good-faith reporting is assumed (see your state statute);
- do not have to give their names as part of the school report;
- understand that there is not a statute of limitations on child abuse reporting.

Most states require the reporter to make an oral report within a reasonable period of time to a designated protection agency (i.e., Child Protective Services [CPS]). A definition of reasonable period of time to report ranges from 24 hours up to 7 days depending on the state statute (Fischer, Schimmel, & Stellman, 2010).

Once you have a suspicion of abuse, the next step is to file the report. The information reported to CPS generally includes the following: (a) the name, address, and gender of the child; (b) the name and address of the parent, guardian, or caretaker; (c) the name and age of any other children/adolescents living in the home; (d) the child's condition, including the nature and extent of the injury; (e) an explanation of the injuries as given by the child; (f) any information regarding the presence of weapons, alcohol/drug abuse, or other factors affecting the social worker's safety; (g) actions taken by the reporter, such as detaining the child; and (h) any other information the reporter believes may be helpful in establishing the cause of injuries and/or protecting the child (Crosson-Tower, 2009; Fischer et al., 2010).

Child abuse cannot always be definitively identified. What constitutes child abuse? What's the difference between "bad parenting" and abuse? Some cases are simple as the evidence is apparent, irrefutable, and conclusive. Other cases are occasions to weigh the facts and the specific considerations of each case. It is the gray area that is worrisome. Being a mandated reporter requires judgment. Deciding what is a preponderance of evidence and what extenuating circumstances need to be considered is truly an ethical conundrum. In matters of family and the sanctity of the home, due process of thought is needed. Decisions around neglect, mental and emotional harm, and threat almost always move into areas of judgment and degrees. There are no easy answers. Individual perceptions and personal beliefs will influence choices. Being directed by law to report means being aware and alert to the potential of abuse, then deciding its presence.

School counselors must be willing to identify and also acknowledge the signs of abuse and be brave enough to take action, knowing that there is tremendous support for them in the law and their ethical codes. School counselors can also admit that there is fear associated with reporting abuse but are reminded that their feelings of fear as an adult are magnified greatly for abused children who have no control over their situation. These are our most vulnerable citizens and good judgment and courage to care for them is our mandate. However, err on the side of caution; when in the throes of the struggle and when you cannot erase your doubt, make the call.

## CONTINUING YOUR PROFESSIONAL DEVELOPMENT

This chapter is an introduction to a few of the most common and/or crucial legal and ethical areas that affect the work of school counselors. For more detailed information, it is suggested that you become a member or maintain your membership in your professional organizations, attend all legal and ethical workshops presented in your area, read literature on the subject, and consider taking a university course when seeking opportunities for professional development requirements or when renewing your certificate. Workshops and courses help you develop sensitivity to ethical decision making that is difficult to accomplish using reference materials alone. Always remember to consult, consult, consult. You never stand alone legally and ethically if you seek guidance from your fellow professionals.

## TECH TOOLS

When you become a school counselor, use the power of technology to maximize your chances of behaving legally and ethically.

- Visit the ACA, ASCA, and other professional websites and bookmark their links to ethical codes and standards so that you will have a ready reference of resources and laws at your fingertips to support your work and to help you continue to behave legally and ethically. Grow a library of websites that can help you do your work.
- Reduce the risk of negligent misrepresentation and malpractice by learning to regularly consult specific sites that you might need in your work such as the NCAA clearinghouse site, the Department of Education site, and your state department site.
- Advocate that your school district establish an electronic newsletter so that critical, timely legal information can be passed to all interested persons.
- Encourage your school district to subscribe to legal search engines such as Lexis. Sites such as these will allow you to submit key words, and every time a law is passed or a court case is heard that includes those key words, you will be notified via email.
- Selectively and carefully identify and publicize respectable agencies and organizations that offer websites, information dissemination, and chat rooms that can serve as support for students who might not otherwise seek help, such as sites for students wrestling with sexual identity issues.
- Audio/visual equipment can heighten professional development activities. Counselors can have a library of DVDs or online videos such as tapes on the *Eisel* court case, the *Davis* case, etc., and have teachers check these tapes out for viewing (possibly for a reward such as credit toward certificate renewal).

---

## School Counselor Casebook: Voices from the Field

### Getting Started: School Counselor Casebook

One of the three counselors in your school will be conducting three small groups this semester. The first group will be for students whose parents are newly divorced or are going through a divorce, the second will be for students who are chronic referrals for aggressive or violent behavior, and the third will be for students who are not getting their class work or homework completed. Your colleague comes to you and asks your advice on her choice of topics for these groups. She also asks you if she should get written or oral parental permission before beginning any of the groups.

Here's how a practicing school counselor responded to the school scenario:

Your colleague is planning to conduct group counseling for the students in your school this semester. The four areas of concern that that your

*(continues)*

colleague wants to address are for students (1) who have been a victim of incest; (2) whose parents are experiencing a divorce; (3) who have a history of aggressive or violent behavior; and (4) who are underachievers. Your colleague has asked teachers to recommend students and also prepared an announcement for homeroom. This situation is making you uncomfortable.

It is important that my colleague and I come to consensus about what is the best approach to support our students. We agree that our challenge is to identify students who need counseling; however, the content and purpose of the proposed topics need to be considered carefully. Group counseling increases the vulnerability of students because confidentiality cannot be guaranteed. Because the school counselor works with minors, you need to get written parent permission for participation, including a statement of confidentiality. This statement explains that confidentiality cannot be guaranteed in a group. We can begin to plan our group sessions by defining the purpose, goals, techniques, and rules of procedure for group counseling.

It is important that my colleague and I carefully discuss the appropriateness of the topics and whether or not groups should be formed. I am most troubled by asking teachers to identify incest victims. Sending a request for this information does not protect the child's privacy and the sensitive nature of incest. School counselors are not therapists and incest is well beyond the scope of our practice in school.

Identifying students who have a history of aggressive or violent behaviors is also a major concern. In planning our counseling program, we can work together to study the campus discipline data to see the patterns of behavior, number of incidences, and recidivism. We can collaborate with the administrators and teachers to institute a conflict resolution or anger management program that would have a positive impact on all students. If experiencing a divorce has affected a student's academic progress, this group may be an effective intervention. However, we need to be careful about confidentiality regarding divorce and how this group supports the academic mission of the school.

Asking teachers to recommend students who need academic support and may benefit from study skills in group is a good opportunity to support academic instruction. This approach allows us to collaborate with teachers about students who have been inconsistent and need encouragement.

As school counselors, we need to safeguard our students as minors and be cautious about asking for personal, sensitive information that may be harmful. Group counseling makes confidentiality challenging, so this increases our professional role in being ethical and ensuring the protection of students who have sensitive issues that may not need to be revealed in a public setting.

Brenda Melton is a past president of the American School Counselor Association.

# LOOKING BACK: SALIENT POINTS

## Professional Ethics

All school counselors are governed by the American School Counselor Association code of ethics. Ethics are the customs, mores, standards, and accepted practice of a profession. Ethical standards are the ideal to which school counseling professionals should aspire while laws are the minimum standard society will tolerate.

## An Ethical Decision-Making Model

The ethical decision-making model offers a framework within which to grapple with ethical dilemmas. The traditional ethical decision-making models include the following: examine the facts; review the relevant ethical guidelines; identify the nature and dimensions of the problem; consult or seek supervision; consider possible and probable courses of action; examine the good and bad consequences of various decisions; and implement your course of action. Because of the unique nature of counseling in schools, we must also add these steps: identify your emotional reaction; consider parental rights; consider the setting; and consider the student's chronological and developmental levels.

## The Complications of Confidentiality in the Context of Schools

School counselors must consider not only student rights but also parental rights when working legally and ethically in schools. Parents are continually vested by our courts with legal rights to guide their children. School boards and administrators adopt policies that counselors are ethically bound to obey. Teachers, informed regarding children's special needs and circumstances, are in the best position to affect positively a child's life during school and often beyond the school day. All of these issues contribute to the complex nature of working with minors in schools.

## Student's Rights and Responsibilities

Tension exists between a child's right to privacy and the parent's right to be the guiding voice in their children's lives. Generally, the younger the child, the more rights are vested in the parents. Students must avoid unlawful activity and infractions may result in suspension, expulsion, or financial restitution.

Parent's Responsibilities and Rights. Parents have the right to guide their children's lives in value-laden decisions. FERPA (1973) gives parents the right to talk to teachers and school administrators about their children, to see their children's educational record, and to decide if their child will participate in a questionnaire, survey, or examination regarding a parent's personal beliefs, sex practices, family life, or religion.

Community Standards. How we address ethical problems will depend in large part on the culture and/or standards of the community. Ethics are situational and depend on the values of the larger community.

Confidentiality and Privileged Communication. All school counselors have a confidentiality responsibility and in a few states, school counselors are granted partial privilege that protects students by securing their confidences except when required by a court of law to breach those confidences.

# KEY TERMS

ASCA code of ethics and standards of practice p. 148

Standard of care p. 148

Ethics p. 149

Privacy rights p. 150

Confidentiality p. 153

Informed consent p. 154

Serious and foreseeable harm p. 154

Family educational rights and privacy act (FERPA) p. 155

Educational records p. 155

Community standards p. 156

Privileged communication p. 156

Multiplicity of responsibility p. 156

Case notes or sole possession records p. 159

Negligence p. 160

*in loco parentis* p. 160

Special relationship p. 160

Duty of care p. 160

Suicidal ideation p. 161

Negligent misrepresentation p. 163

Value-laden p. 165

Title IX p. 169

Office of civil rights p. 169

# LEARNING EXTENSIONS/MAKING CONNECTIONS

1. Find the addresses of the following websites on the World Wide Web and follow the directions below:

   - Read the NBCC Webcounseling Standards.
   - Order online from the Office of Special Education Programs, the publication *Early Warnings, Timely Response: A Guide to Safe Schools* and read it.
   - Explore the site for the Office of Special Education Programs (online). Under IDEIA 2004, find general information and become comfortable with the law. Using all the information you have gathered, discuss the implications for school counselors.
   - Go to the ASCA website and read the code of ethics. Discuss the sections of the ethical standards that you found to be the most important, the most ambiguous, and the least helpful.

2. Discuss the ethics of academic advising.

3. Study the standards of the community where you hope to be a counselor by interviewing at least five of the following people: local clergy, business owner, parent, teacher, principal, guidance counselor, other educator, public employee, elementary student, middle school student, high school student, or staff member of a school. Write a two-page report detailing your perspective of the community standards of the area.

4. A school counselor's responsibilities extend beyond the minor student client to the parents or guardians of that student. In a two- to three-page reaction paper, discuss how the school setting determines our responsibilities to parents and what impact those responsibilities have on the school counselor's work.

5. Prepare a 15-minute staff development presentation appropriate for a faculty meeting highlighting a topic of legal or ethical concern such as child abuse reporting.

# Implementing the ASCA National Model

## CHAPTER OBJECTIVES

*By the time you have completed this chapter, you should be able to*

- discuss the school counseling reform movement that led to the development of the ASCA National Standards for School Counseling Programs (1997);

- discuss the connection between comprehensive school counseling programs and school improvement efforts;

- identify the three domains of the ASCA national standards;

- explain comprehensive, developmental, and results-based school counseling programs;

- understand how to implement the ASCA National Model.

---

## *School Counselor Casebook: Getting Started*

### The Scenario

When the current junior class was polled at the beginning of their ninth-grade year, 90 percent of the students responded that they were planning to enter college or some form of postsecondary education. Three years later, as you and your colleagues review the junior class transcripts, only 27 percent of the students are enrolled in the kind of academic coursework that would widen their options to include college. What do you see as your role to help students see the connection between academic performance and enrollment in college? How can delivering a comprehensive program based on the ASCA National Model help?

### Thinking about Solutions

As you read this chapter, think about having a comprehensive standards-based program in place that could start with your ninth graders as soon as they enter high school. Think about how the foundation of your program, and the delivery, the management, and accountability systems can show how the comprehensive program is making a difference. When you come to the end of the chapter, you will have the opportunity to see how your ideas compare with a practicing school counselor's approach.

---

## MOVING THE PROFESSION FORWARD

**Comprehensive school counseling** programs are promoted nationally as the way of work for the 21st-century professional by the American School Counselor Association, the 50-state school counseling association affiliates, and by the associations that support and have an interest in the work of school counselors. Since the early 1990s, the majority of state school counselor associations have used elements of the comprehensive and/or developmental process as the underpinning for program design, delivery, and evaluation. The publication of the American School Counselor Association's National Model (ASCA, 2003, 2005, 2012) emphatically shifted practice from acts of service to a structured and outcome-based program, while simultaneously integrating the transformed school counselor skills as the process to promote the content. The ASCA National Model and the multitude of subsequent state spinoffs have had a far-reaching impact on the way of work of every counselor in every school and on every student they serve.

The **ASCA National Model** suggests that school counselor commitment to school improvement, a willingness to use data to address equity, and a social justice approach are essential mindsets to succeed with 21st-century students (Stone & Dahir, 2007). It is no longer sufficient for a school counselor to step back feeling emotionally satisfied or emotionally drained at the end of the school day; the school counselor must be able to articulate how her or his program is contributing to student success. This requires the need to rethink and redesign a "program" to document practice, use data to inform and design individual-student, school-based, and systemic services, and accept the mindset that maintaining the status quo is no longer an option.

How is this different from the days of old? It was not too long ago that school counselors focused on delivering services to those in need, those in crisis, or those who sought out the school counselor delivered primarily through individual counseling. The question "What do school counselors do?" continues to frustrate the field (Beale, 2004). There are varying opinions as to what the school counselor's role and service delivery should be (Burnham & Jackson, 2000).

## NATIONAL STANDARDS ACROSS AMERICA: AN AGENDA FOR EQUITY

The changing status of children and families, the needs of the workforce, the dynamics of the economy, and our interrelationship with the global community have, for the past 20 years, challenged the educational community. The demands on schools for higher student achievement and the reallocation of educational resources were noted as necessary to prepare the next generation of Americans with the computational, literacy, technical, and learning skills needed to be productive participants in tomorrow's economy (Annie E. Casey Foundation, 2008; Tang & Erford, 2010). Reform measures for results and accountability became the basis for political platforms (DeVoss, 2010a; Lunenburg & Ornstein, 2008; Owings & Kaplan, 2000; Tang & Erford, 2010). Pressure for improvements in public education came primarily from politicians and representatives of business and industry. As a result, **national standards** across the content areas were mandated as the solution for educational reform (McDivitt, 2010).

Since the publication of *A Nation at Risk* (1983), the education and business communities and the public and private sector regularly deliberated the expectations of American public education. GOALS 2000: Educate America Act of 1994 was the impetus to challenge the American educational system to use standards as the foundation for curriculum development across all of the academic disciplines. At the heart of the national debate about education is simply what's working and what's not in public schools. The school improvement agenda of the No Child Left Behind Act (2001) evolved from the decades-old educational reform movement that is rooted in *A Nation at Risk* and then to America 2000 (1990), and its reauthorization as Goals 2000. Phrases such as *higher academic achievement, increasing student potential, rigorous academic preparation,* and *accountability* have become commonplace in every community across the nation.

As the academic disciplines moved forward to develop statements of what "students should know and be able to do" (National Education Goals Panel, 1992) the intent was to transform American education (Darling-Hammond, 1992; Eisner, 1993; McDivitt, 2010; Wiggins, 1991.) As each discipline sought to raise educational achievement to a new level of excellence, this was translated into the development of standards-based education in 49 of the 50 states but not without controversy and concern for equity and equal educational opportunity for every student. All aspects of the educational system were affected from public policy to curriculum and instruction, teaching and learning, assessment, and accountability and continue to be so impacted today as the National Governors Association Center for Best Practices (NGA Center) and the Council of Chief State School Officers (CCSSO) released a set of state-led education standards, the Common Core State Standards (2010), to provide a consistent, clear understanding of what students are expected to learn, so teachers and parents know what they need to do to help them.

As the academic disciplines grappled with the pressures of educational reform, commissioned reports of national significance such as Keeping the Options Open (1986) and High Hopes Long Odds (Orfield & Paul, 1994) praised school counselors for the work they do and condemned them for what they didn't do. The Commission on Pre-college Guidance and Counseling (1986) proposed a comprehensive set of recommendations that identified the ways in which guidance and counseling can contribute to increasing student potential and the number of students pursuing postsecondary opportunities. Disturbing issues raised in these documents included the accusation that school counselors were gatekeepers perpetuating the accepted rules and systematic barriers that caused inequities between achievers and non-achievers based on race and socioeconomic status (Chen-Hayes, Miller, Bailey, Getch, & Erford, 2011; Hart & Jacobi, 1992).

As school counselors continued to work doggedly to deliver a constellation of **responsive services** to at-risk students in need of counselor intervention, the majority of American educators were focused on improving student achievement. Little research existed to connect counseling to student achievement; therefore, the few studies that did mention school counselors gained little national attention (Brown & Trusty, 2005a; Whiston, 2002). Traditional school counseling research examined the school counselor role, analyzed time and tasks, and explored the impact and significance of intervention and prevention activities (Borders & Drury, 1992; Johnson, 2000). Without clearly connecting the practice of school counseling to student achievement, the school counselor remained conspicuously absent in the conversations that centered on reform efforts to promote higher levels of student success.

# THE EVOLUTION OF THE ASCA NATIONAL MODEL

Concerned that school counselors were being viewed as peripheral to the school reform agenda, ASCA took a leadership role recasting school counseling as an integral component of the educational system (ASCA, 1994; Dahir & Stone, 2007; Perry, 1991). It became vital to show how school counselors contribute to preparing students to meet the increasingly complex demands of society and the workforce.

Concurrently, organizations that had an interest in the work of school counselors such as the Education Trust (1997, 2009a, 2009b) defined a new vision for school counseling that emphasized leadership, advocacy, use of data, and a commitment to support high levels of student achievement. School counselors were encouraged to shift their focus from the delivery of a menu of student services to providing a structured and programmatic approach for counselors to address the needs of all students (Gysbers & Henderson, 1994, 2006, 2012).

To move this agenda forward, three important ideological transformations were necessary for school counselors to do the following:

1. Shift the focus from the role of the school counselor position to the impact of the school counseling program on student achievement. Counselors would share the concerns and goals of other education professionals.
2. Look at their work from an "all students" perspective. No longer would it be enough for *some* students to profit from counselor services; every student would benefit from the school counseling programs.
3. Develop programs to support student developmental growth and academic achievement, improving results by affecting the system and show their commitment as powerful allies in school reform (Clark & Stone, 2000b; Dahir, 2004). School counselors would be seen as partners in school improvement, concerned with every student's ability to access a quality education.

As depicted in Table 7.1, school counselors, embracing the law of parsimony (Myrick, 2003b), have shifted their focus from a *some students agenda* to an *every student agenda* that assures the acquisition of skills and knowledge and equity in educational opportunity (Walsh, Barrett, & DePaul, 2007).

## TABLE **7.1**
### From Position to Program to System

| From Position | To Program | To System |
|---|---|---|
| Affecting Some Students | Affecting Every Student | Affecting the System to Affect Every Student |
| Advocacy for students on an as-needed basis | Advocacy to ensure that every student benefits from a program that emphasizes academic, career, and personal-social developmental growth and learning. | Advocacy to ensure that school district policies and practices fairly and equitably provide educational opportunity to every student. |

## The National Standards for School Counseling Programs

In response to GOALS 2000: The Educate America Act, the ASCA Governing Board committed to the development of the national standards, following the lead of the academic disciplines that were in the process of creating their own national standards (ASCA, 1994; Dahir & Stone, 2007). The National Education Goals Panel (1994) described program content standards as those that specify what students should know and be able to do; thus, the ASCA Governing Board followed suit and determined that development of school counseling program content standards would likewise define what students should know and be able to do as a result of participating in a school counseling program (Campbell & Dahir, 1997).

ASCA believed that standards would motivate the school counseling community to identify and implement goals for students that were deemed important by the profession, clarified the relationship of school counseling to the educational system, addressed the contributions of school counseling to student success, and served as the "single most legitimizing document in the [school counseling] profession" (Bowers, Hatch, & Schwallie-Giddis, 2001, p. 17).

A major research study was undertaken in 1995 to analyze relevant school counseling and educational reform literature and to review existing school counseling program models developed at the state level. Two thousand ASCA members were surveyed to assess the level of support for standards development and offer opinions about their content (Dahir, Campbell, Johnson, Scholes, & Valiga, 1997). The survey findings (Dahir et al., 1997) revealed that school counselors strongly supported national standards and believed that standards could help school counselors define program goals, a professional mission, and would raise expectations of practice. The ASCA National Standards were a historic landmark that gave direction to a profession floundering for a unified identity and role in school reform (Erford, 2011c, p. 44).

## Key Areas of Student Development

The study confirmed the continued importance of the three widely accepted and interrelated areas of student development and nine standards emerged from the research: **academic development, career development,** and **personal-social development** (Campbell & Dahir, 1997), which offered school counselors, administrators, teachers, and counselor educators a common language that also is readily understood by colleagues who are involved in the implementation of standards across other disciplines. The hope was that the standards would provide counselors, administrators, and the general public with an understanding of what school counseling programs should contain and deliver (McDivitt, 2010).

The concept of standards was not new to the school counseling profession. Standards for Guidance and Counseling Programs (ASCA, 1979) outlined the administrative structure, resources and facilities needed, and presented evaluation guidelines. The document did not suggest program content or methods of delivery, but promoted consistency in practice as counseling programs were adapted to the individual school's mission.

Similar to the academic subject standards, ASCA determined that the school counseling standards would define what K–12 students should know and be able to do as a result of participating in a school counseling program (Campbell & Dahir, 1997). The National Standards for School Counseling Programs (ASCA, 1997, 2004) tied the work of school counseling programs to the mission of schools and encouraged school counselors to assume a leadership role in school reform (Dahir & Tyson, 2010). The ASCA believed that national standards would

- create a framework for a national model for school counseling programs;
- identify the key components of a school counseling model program;
- identify the knowledge and skills that all students should acquire as a result of the K–12 School Counseling Program; and
- ensure that school counseling programs are comprehensive in design and delivered in a systematic fashion to all students (Campbell & Dahir, 1997, p. 5).

As our educational systems continue to look at new paradigms for improving the teaching and learning process, so too the leadership of ASCA is looking at refining the language of the national standards to reflect what

TABLE **7.2**

National Standards for School Counseling Programs

| Domain | | Standard |
|---|---|---|
| Academic | A | Students will acquire the attitudes, knowledge, and skills contributing to effective learning in school and across the lifespan. |
| | B | Students will complete school with the academic preparation essential to choose from a wide range of substantial postsecondary options, including college. |
| | C | Students will understand the relationship of academics to the world of work and to life at home and in the community. |
| Career | A | Students will acquire the skills to investigate the world of work in relation to knowledge of self and to make informed career decisions. |
| | B | Students will employ strategies to achieve future career goals with success and satisfaction. |
| | C | Students will understand the relationship between personal qualities, education, training, and the world of work. |
| Personal/ Social | A | Students will acquire the knowledge, attitudes, and interpersonal skills to help them understand and respect self and others. |
| | B | Students will make decisions, set goals, and take necessary action to achieve goals. |
| | C | Students will understand safety and survival skills. |

Source: Sharing the Vision: The National Standards for School Counseling Programs (Campbell & Dahir, 1997, pp. 17–19).

21st-century students need to know and be able to do (see Table 7.2). Along with the three domains, constructs such as student motivation, relationships, self-knowledge, and social consciousness are under consideration, as well as plans to design metrics that would assess student proficiency of the skills and knowledge as part of the revision process.

## Student Competencies

Expectations of specific student accomplishments or outcomes as a result of participating in a standards-based school counseling program are written in terms of student competencies. **Student competencies** support the goals of the national standards, guide the development of strategies and activities, and are the basis for assessing student growth and development. Competencies represent the specific knowledge, attitudes, and skills that students can acquire to support their academic, career, and personal-social success. The 122 ASCA student competencies are arranged in the three domain areas and provide the pathway to achieving the nine standards.

In addition to age-appropriate and developmental needs, there are many sources that influence the selection and/or design of student competencies. State, district-level, and building-site comprehensive school counseling programs often include specific competencies or outcomes that are aligned with the school's or system's mission statement and the academic or curriculum standards, and are categorized according to elementary, middle, or secondary levels. Annually, each school's improvement plan may identify the competency expectations by grade levels consistent with developmental expectations and local needs and priorities.

Competencies guide the development of the program content for student growth and achievement in the academic, career, and personal-social domains is an integral part of individual planning, guidance curriculum, responsive services, and system support (Gysbers & Henderson, 2006, 2012). Competencies may be organized developmentally by school level and thus inform the sequence of strategies and activities, reflecting local school system issues, priorities, and concerns. As students struggle in assuming responsibility for their educational plans, career goals, and personal behavior (Wittmer & Clark, 2007), the standards and competencies help each student to take responsibility for her or his academic development, career preparation, and personal-social skills to successfully transition from grade level to grade level and to the next phase of life after high school.

As a result of standards development, ASCA joined the ranks of the academic disciplines by providing a content framework to better define the role of school counseling programs in the American educational system. The national standards became unifying elements identifying school counseling as a discipline (Martin & Robinson, 2011).

## Comprehensive, Developmental, and Results-Based School Counseling Programs

Although interpretations may vary, there is historical consensus that comprehensive, developmental, and **results-based school counseling** programs are systematic in nature, sequential, clearly defined, and accountable (ASCA, 2003, 2005, 2012; Cobia & Henderson, 2007; Galassi & Akos, 2004b; Gysbers & Henderson, 2006, 2012; Johnson & Johnson, 1991, 2001; Stone & Dahir, 2011). Similar in presentation to other educational programs, the components include student outcomes or competencies, activities to achieve the desired outcomes, professional personnel, materials, resources, and a delivery system. Connecting school counseling to the total educational process and the need to involve all school personnel is essential (Stanciak, 1995). Comprehensive, developmental, and results-based school counseling programs share common goals, are proactive and preventive in focus (Borders & Drury, 1992; Cobia & Henderson, 2007), and assist students in the acquisition of lifelong learning skills by

- providing developmental as well as prevention and intervention programs;
- measuring student and program growth; and
- taking into consideration the rapidly changing nature of society, pressures on education from business and industry, and how these affect every student's need to acquire academic, career, and personal-social growth and development.

# UNDERSTANDING COMPREHENSIVE SCHOOL COUNSELING

The concept of the comprehensive program was developed by Gysbers and Moore (1981) and refined over the past 20 years by Gysbers and Henderson (2006, 2012) to redirect "guidance" from an ancillary set of services delivered by a person to a program intended to reach all students and affect every aspect of a student's education. When guidance and counseling is conceptualized, organized, and implemented as a program it places school counselors in the center of education and makes it possible for them to be active and involved (Gysbers, 2001, p. 103). To operationalize the overall goals of the school counseling program, the comprehensive model has a conceptual framework that addresses content, organization, and resources as well as organizational structure, which was adopted by the ASCA Model (2003, 2005) from the seminal work of Norm Gysbers.

## The Developmental Approach

The developmental progression of student affective growth preK–12 can be nurtured through school counseling. This approach incorporates human growth and development theory (Erickson, 1963; Kohlberg, 1984; Piaget, 1952) by considering the progressive needs of students consistent with the stages of growth and learning. Recognizing that all children do not develop in a linear fashion according to a certain timetable, a focus on the developmental progression of student growth preK–12 is essential. Therefore, **developmental school counseling**

> is for all students, has an organized and planned curriculum, is sequential and flexible, is an integrated part of the total educational process, involves all school personnel, helps students learn more effectively and efficiently, and includes counselors who provide specialized counseling services and interventions. (Myrick, 1997, p. 48)

Myrick's (2003b) developmental approach emphasized programs for all students, the importance of using an integrated approach involving all school personnel in the delivery of "guidance activities," and a guidance curriculum that is sequential, age appropriate, planned, and organized. Thus, the school counseling program must include age-appropriate and sequential learning experiences to deliver the national standards and competencies to every student. The program is an integrated part of the total educational process, involves all school personnel, helps students learn more effectively and efficiently, and includes counselors who provide specialized counseling services and interventions (Myrick, 2003b).

### The Results-Based Approach

Results-based guidance is also a competency-based approach. Developed by Johnson and Johnson in the 1980s, it emphasized a total pupil services approach with the student as the primary client (Johnson & Johnson, 1991, 2002). This approach also emphasized the importance of students acquiring competencies to become successful in school and in the transitions from school to postsecondary education and/or employment. At the center of the results-based approach is accountability to the student and to the building administrator (Johnson, Johnson, & Downs, 2006). As a result, management agreements between the principal and individual counselor are a means of measuring accomplishments. School-based issues, counselor-principal agreements, data and results, and accountability guide all counselor action and activity (Johnson & Johnson, 1991, 2002, 2003).

Comprehensive programs are organized and structured and place an emphasis on providing every student with a school counseling experience. They are grounded in developmental theories and are an assurance that student competencies and strategies are organized "stage and age" appropriate to the learner. These developmental stages aid in the identification of counseling theories and techniques that are the most effective with the age and cognitive and emotional development of the student taken into consideration. Most importantly, comprehensive school counseling programs recognize the importance of aligning school counseling with the mission and purpose of schools.

## UNDERSTANDING THE ASCA NATIONAL MODEL

To expand on and integrate the national standards into a comprehensive framework that addressed the "how" of school counseling (Erford, 2011c, p. 45), the American School Counselor Association (ASCA) developed the ASCA National Model (ASCA, 2003, 2005, 2012) to assist school counselors in designing comprehensive programs that are aligned with the mission of schools and support the academic success of every student. The ASCA National Model (2003) integrated the three widely accepted and respected approaches to program models, i.e., comprehensive (Gysbers & Henderson, 2000, 2006, 2012), developmental (Myrick, 2003), and the results-based approach developed by Johnson and Johnson (2001, 2003). Using the national standards as the foundation for program content, the ASCA Model offers a standards-based approach to school counseling that proactively responds to school reform and is intentional in its support of every student's academic, career, and personal-social development. Most importantly, the ASCA Model incorporated into its framework the themes of leadership, advocacy, collaboration, systemic change, and use of data, which were foundational to the work of the Transformed School Counseling Initiative at the Education Trust (Martin & Robinson, 2011, p. 11). The ASCA Model helps to forward the Transforming School Counseling Initiative (Education Trust, 2009a) by doing the following:

- Pointing counselors in the direction of improving academic achievement and eliminating the achievement gap. School counselors connect academic, career, and personal-social development to improving achievement for all students.
- Connecting school counseling to each school district's mission and the goals of school improvement. School counselors are encouraged to become leaders and systemic change agents to help ensure that no student is left behind.
- Providing school counselors with the tools to develop school counseling programs that include student competencies/outcomes based on national standards (ASCA, 2005; Dahir & Campbell, 1997), aligned with Common Core State Standards, and district standards which include measurable student learning outcomes.
- Encouraging school counselors to use data to assess student outcomes. School counselors use school-based data to understand the current situation in their school building and district and work collaboratively toward the goals of school improvement.

The outside frame of Figure 7.1 represents the Transformed School Counselor skills (Education Trust, 2009a, 2009b) of leadership, advocacy, collaboration, and systemic change that every school counselor needs to help every student succeed. The inside of the graphic depicts the four interrelated quadrants that are the essential components of successful and effective comprehensive school counseling programs (ASCA, 2005, 2012).

The ASCA National Model contemporized the school counseling foundation, management, and delivery systems and added an accountability component that aligned the program with the expectations of 21st-century schools (Myrick, 2003a). The ASCA Model provided the "the mechanism with which school counselors and school counseling teams design, coordinate, implement, manage, and evaluate their programs for students' success." This "framework for the program components, the school counselor's role in implementation, the underlying philosophies of leadership, advocacy, and systemic change" (ASCA, 2003, p. 165) is now clearly articulated.

The ASCA Model offers an inclusive approach for school counselors to design, coordinate, implement, manage, and evaluate their programs. The Model encourages the school counselor's role in implementing and promoting the underlying philosophies of leadership, advocacy, and systemic change and

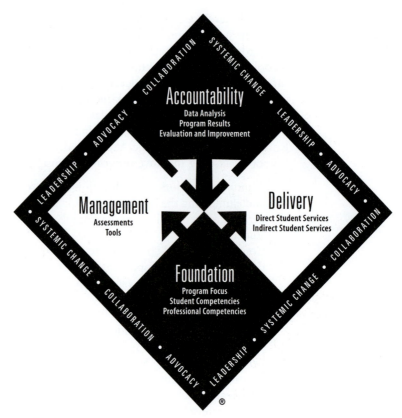

FIGURE **7.1** Transformed School Counselor Skills and the ASCA Model
Source: ASCA National Model (2012, 3rd edition)

challenges school counselors to respond to the question, "How are students different as a result of the work of the school counselor and the school counseling program?" No matter how comfortable the status quo or how difficult or uncomfortable change may be, every school counselor must work diligently to support every student's quest for success. The ASCA National Model directs school counselors toward a unified, focused professional school counseling program with one vision and one voice (ASCA, 2005, 2012).

## Working from a Program Perspective

Working from a programmatic perspective helps counselors to move theory into practice, responds to the needs and goals of the entire school community, and uses data to inform decisions. School counselors coordinate the objectives, strategies, and activities of a comprehensive school counseling program to meet the academic, career, and personal-social needs of all students (ASCA, 2005, 2012). Once the school counseling program has an organization and structure like the mathematics or science curriculum, it is no longer ancillary but an integral component directly linked to student achievement and school success.

## MEET ERIC SPARKS: MOVING A DISTRICT FORWARD ONE "CARAT" AT A TIME!

Implementing a comprehensive school counseling program had been the goal for school counselors in the Wake County (NC) Public School System for many years. The introduction of the ASCA National Model clearly defined that goal and set the district standard for what a school counseling program would achieve.

The district leadership team and I began by developing a three-year plan to implement the new model. Each year, school counselors were introduced to additional components of the model so that, within a few short years, the school would have a fully implemented program. At each stage, the school counseling team received recognition for their accomplishments through the "carat system" of ¼, ½, ¾, or full carat implementation. Once a school achieves full carat, the program is ready to apply for the Recognized ASCA Model Program (RAMP), ASCA's national recognition program.

Building district buy-in for the model was critical for success. The model was presented to stakeholders such as school board members, district-level staff, and principals, and these presentations were just as important as providing training to school counselors. To implement the most effective program, school counselors needed the support of education leaders who understood that school counselors have a vital affect on student achievement.

Intensive training in some areas of the model was needed to help school counselors feel comfortable with implementation. District counselors already had great school counseling skills, but understanding and using data to make decisions was new to many. While incorporating data took some time, school counselors were constantly reminded of the goal to spend more time with school counseling activities and less time with non-counseling activities. By developing training and support for accessing, reviewing, and collecting data, school counselors were able to incorporate the use of data into their program in ways that supported their school counseling program rather than detracting from it.

As a result of the district plan and the work of many dedicated school counselors, school counseling programs throughout the district documented results including improved promotion and attendance rates, decreased discipline referrals and suspensions, and increased participation rates in advanced and Advanced Placement courses. In addition, 32 schools have received the RAMP award from the American School Counselor Association.

*Eric Sparks is a former high school counselor and the director of school counseling for the Wake County Public School System (North Carolina) where he works with approximately 360 school counselors serving 144,000 students. He has trained school counselors and administrators across the country on the American School Counselor Association (ASCA)* National Model: A Framework for School Counseling. *Eric served as president of the American School Counselor Association (ASCA) and the North Carolina School Counselor Association (NCSCA).*

When building administrators, faculty, parents, and community members have substantial input into the development of the school counseling program, there is a willingness to assist in the implementation. Implementing a comprehensive, developmental, results-based program requires the following:

- Establishing a school counseling advisory committee of faculty, administrators, and representatives from all key stakeholder groups.
- Determining priorities to meet the identified student needs.
- Developing student competencies based on the national standards, school data, and student needs.
- Analyzing current services and activities and link these to the national standards and student competencies.
- Identifying gaps in the program to address needs and develop strategies.
- Securing the commitment of all teachers, administrators, and counselors to assist in program delivery.
- Building the program based on the four quadrants of Foundation, Delivery, Management, and Accountability.

## Looking at the Four Quadrants

## The Foundation System

School counselors create comprehensive school counseling programs that focus on student outcomes, teach student competencies and are delivered with identified professional competencies (ASCA, 2012). The vision and mission statements guide the development of an effective comprehensive school counseling program while the national standards and student competencies guide and support student development in academic, career, and personal-social domains. The foundation provides and serves as the solid ground on which the rest of the program is built. Beliefs, philosophy, and behaviors are inextricably related. What school counselors believe about students, families, colleagues, and community can strongly influence their approach to their work. The foundation addresses the *what* of the program, the content and beliefs about what every student should know and be able to do (ASCA, 2012, p. 21).

### The Mission Statement

The mission describes the purpose for the school counseling program, is aligned with the school's mission, and publicly commits the counselor's intent to provide every student with the skills needed to become lifelong learners and productive members of society. The mission statement promotes collaboration with colleagues to ensure that every student fully benefits from the educational opportunities offered in each school system. School counselors are reminded to align their work with their school's mission statement, which is a public proclamation about student success.

## The Delivery System

The Delivery quadrant offers the methods that show *how* to deliver an effective school counseling program. The scope of the program may differ across grade levels; thus, the variation of delivery methodology is adjusted to meet developmental needs. For example, in elementary schools, the curriculum and group counseling activities are utilized more frequently than at the secondary level. Gysbers and Henderson (2000, 2006, 2012) offered a model for distributing the time allotment of each delivery component across grade levels. The challenge lies in the school counselor's ability to deliver a program that is balanced and blends the four delivery methods: individual student planning, responsive services, school counseling curriculum, and system support.

By carefully examining current practice and student needs revealed by school improvement data, school counselors can determine the amount of time they need to spend on each of the key areas: School counselors provide services to students, parents, school staff and the community through Direct and Indirect Services. Direct services are in-person interactions between school counselors and students.

- **School counseling core curriculum**
- **Individual Student Planning**
- **Responsive services**

Indirect services are a result of the school counselors' interactions with others including referrals for additional assistance, consultation and collaboration with parents, teachers, other educators and community organizations.

Each of these delivery components has a specific purpose in the comprehensive school counseling program.

### Individual Student Planning

Successful students learn to take ownership of their academic, career, and personal-social development. Individual student planning provides opportunities for students to plan, monitor, and evaluate their progress. Activities can include but are not limited to working with students to establish and monitor goals, develop a career plan, commit to behavioral goals, create an educational plan, and apply testing and assessment information to present and future plans. The planning process personalizes the educational experience and helps students to develop a pathway to realize their dreams.

Individual student planning consists of ongoing, systematic activities that assist students with planning, managing, and monitoring their academic, personal-social, and career and employability goals. These activities are counselor directed and delivered on an individual or small-group basis. Each student is provided with the information, encouragement, and support needed to work toward her or his personal goals. Parents and/or guardians are frequently included in these activities.

### Responsive Services

When school counselors proactively address student-related concerns such as peer pressure, resolving conflict, family relationships, personal identity issues, substance abuse, motivation, and achievement challenges, they deliver responsive services. Included in responsive services are interventions necessary to help students succeed; these include individual and group counseling, consultation, referrals to community agencies, crisis intervention and management, and prevention activities. The impetus for response and intervention can be dominated by crisis, school building and faculty concerns, parental trepidations, community concerns, and student requests. Responsive services can also proactively address concerns including peer pressure, resolving conflict, family relationships, personal identity issues, substance abuse, and motivation, and prevent situations from occurring. Implementation strategies can include the following:

1. Individual or Small-Group Counseling: Counselors counsel students with identified needs/concerns or students who request counseling. This is an opportunity to discuss/clarify needs and guide therapeutic intervention. The school counselor must act ethically at all times in accordance with the ASCA Ethical Standards (2010a) and federal, state, and local laws and policies with respect to confidentiality, suspected cases of abuse, and threats of harm or violence.
2. Consultation: Counselors work collaboratively with students, parents, teachers, and community members to develop a broad base of support and help for students.
3. Referrals: Counselors consult with and make referrals to community agencies to assist students facing personal crisis outside the scope of the school counseling program.
4. Crisis Counseling: Counselors provide short-term prevention and intervention counseling and support to students and school staff dealing with crisis.
5. Crisis Prevention and Crisis Management Plans: Specialized plans guide school prevention, intervention, and management of crisis response. Staff crisis training establishes readiness to meet student/school needs in emergency situations.
6. Schoolwide Prevention and Intervention Programs: Counselors collaborate with all faculty, students, staff, and community-based organizations to expand responsive service outreach.
7. Student Support Services Team: Counselors collaborate with school-based professionals such as the school psychologist or social worker to plan interventions for the academic, social, and emotional needs of students in need.

### School Counseling/Student Development Curriculum

The school counseling/student development curriculum is a sequential, standards-based instructional program designed to assist *all* students to acquire, develop, and demonstrate competence in three content area domains: academic, career, and personal-social development. The involvement of school faculty and administration is essential for effective and successful curriculum implementation. In most circumstances, the curriculum is intended to serve the largest number of students possible and this is accomplished through large-group meetings and classroom presentations. The curriculum gives attention to particular issues or areas of concern in the school building or district such as eliminating bullying, conflict resolution, or raising aspirations.

Curriculum design requires building a scope and sequence that help to define and clarify the topics and competencies taught at each grade level and articulate what students should *know, understand,* and be able to *do* as a result of the curriculum. The student development curriculum can be delivered through classroom instruction in which *school* counselors design, teach, and assess the impact of standards-based lessons and presentations that meet the academic, career, and personal-social developmental needs of each student; or through *large-group instructional activities and presentations* that convey information in a variety of ways by offering group activities, workshops, assemblies, and meetings to accommodate student needs and interests.

Counselors provide information, knowledge, and skills to students through developmental and sequential lessons. In most circumstances, school counseling curriculum is designed to serve the largest number of students possible through large-group meetings, classroom presentations, and advisory programs. The curriculum gives attention to particular issues or areas of concern in the school building or district such as conflict resolution. School counselors often collaborate with teachers, student support services personnel, and community specialists to deliver the curriculum which can be aligned with Common Core State Standards.

Presented on the next page in Box 7.1 is an activity that shows the relationship of the academic development national standards to school improvement. This scenario is a familiar one, especially for school counselors who work with high school students.

This is an example of how to integrate the national standards in a meaningful and purposeful experience for students that supports school improvement goals. Success is not only about individual student skills; it is also demonstrated by drawing a direct line to the goals of school improvement and moving school data in a positive direction. Through teaming and collaboration strategies with a classroom teacher two purposes are served: (1) to encourage student affective growth with an emphasis on self-knowledge, motivation, taking responsibility, goal setting, and self-monitoring; and (2) to contribute to the improvement of English language arts and communication skills in both verbal and written forms.

As you can see from the sample activity, the shift to a standards-based school counseling program has the most impact when it is aligned with the educational initiatives underway in your school system or building.

### System Support

School counselors, when engaged in system support, offer ongoing sustenance to the school environment by actively participating in school-based activities when delivering the comprehensive school counseling program. Involvement in system support sends a strong message to the faculty that the school counselors are committed to achieve the system's goals and mission. System support demonstrates the degree to which the school counseling program is aligned with the school district's priorities and state and federal school improvement mandates.

System support usually consists of indirect services that are not delivered directly to students. For example, chairing the school improvement team, coordinating student service volunteers, and facilitating the school peer mediation program are examples of proactive ways services connect school counseling to the school's mission. System support also provides school

## BOX **7.1**

### *Standards Into Practice*

*Activity:* Classroom guidance session and follow-up appointments to meet in small groups
*Domain:* Academic Development
*Standards:*

A.  Students will complete school with the academic preparation essential to choose from a wide variety of substantial postsecondary options, including college.
B.  Students will understand the relationship of academics to the world of work, and to life at home and in the community.

*Competencies:* Students will

- Establish challenging academic goals.
- Identify postsecondary options consistent with interests, achievement, aptitude, and abilities.
- Understand that school success is the preparation to make the transition from student to community member.
- Understand how school success and academic achievement enhance future career aspirations.

*Level:* High School
*Targeted Population:* 9th, 10th, and 11th graders
*Purpose:* The purpose of this activity is to help high school students develop a plan of study and update it each year to reflect their educational (academic and career) goals.
*Delivery Method:* Classroom Lesson and Individual Student Planning
*Activity Summary:*

1.  Present a classroom session to review course selection planning materials, graduation requirements, career pathways information, and other relevant materials.
2.  The school counselor schedules follow-up appointments to meet in small groups with every student to discuss course selection to support educational and career goals; review current academic progress; and share any potential obstacles to or concerns about achieving these goals.
3.  The parent/guardian/caretaker of every student is invited to participate in a follow-up individual or small-group meeting.
4.  In collaboration with the classroom teachers, students monitor their progress on their educational plans and share their thoughts on each quarter's progress through reflective writing.
5.  Students needing additional support or intervention self-refer or are referred by the teacher to the school counselor for individual sessions.

*Materials Needed:* Annual educational program planning worksheets that include academic and career goals; student transcripts; achievement, aptitude, and/or college entrance test scores; interest surveys, career portfolios, and course selection materials.
*Results-based Data:* The results of this activity will show the following:

- One hundred percent of the 9th-, 10th-, and 11th-grade students will actively participate in the design of an educational plan that supports their academic aspirations and career goals.
- One hundred percent of parents/guardians/caretakers will be invited to participate in the educational planning process.
- Targeted efforts will result in an increase of 25 percent in parent participation from last year.

*Connection to School Improvement:* Student course changes and drops are reduced by 25 percent.
*Data:*

- Student participation and buy-in to this process reduces course failure by 25 percent.
- Seventy-five percent of the students show academic improvement at the end of the school year as a result of self-monitoring their progress and connecting academic success to future career goals.

counselors with multiple opportunities to act as leaders and advocates by facilitating discussions around school improvement, examining data that may be affecting success of some groups of students, and assisting with professional development and inservice activities for the faculty. Indirect services include professional development to faculty, serving on school committees, and coordinating safe school initiatives and are essential to effect systemic change and support the "new vision" of **transformed school counseling** (Erford, 2011c; Ripley, Erford, & Dahir, 2003).

Coordination of services involves managing resources and planning and connecting activities and services to goals of the counseling program in the school. For example, hosting an advisory committee helps to inform the program's direction and provides a sounding board for discussion about what is working, what needs to change, and how the comprehensive school counseling program can better support student success.

## The Management System

Effective programs require strong organization and effective management. The management component of the ASCA Model addresses the *when* (action plan and calendar), the *why* (use of data), the *who*, and *on what authority* (advisory council) the school counseling program is delivered. The ASCA National Model suggests the following key elements to manage the program.

### Principal–Counselor Collaboration

Collaborative agreements are established annually between school counselors and the building administrator. The counselor(s) produce and present yearly a document that prioritizes school counseling, timelines, and the implementation plan; the principal then reviews the document and arrives at consensus with the school counselor as to how students, services, and activities are assigned. These decisions should be made based on site needs and data analysis. The agreement delineates counselor responsibilities, program implementation, and methods of accountability, and it offers a timeline for when these activities will occur.

When the principal and school counselors meet, collaborate, and agree on program priorities, implementation strategies, and the organization of the counseling department, the entire program runs more smoothly and is more likely to produce the desired results for students. Thus, the management agreement is a public statement to all stakeholders and demonstrates the commitment of school counselors and administrators to collaborate on an annual statement describing what the counselors hope to accomplish in the coming year.

### Advisory Council

An advisory council helps to solicit school and community support to inform the program's direction, provide a sounding board for discussion about what is working and what needs to change, and discuss the ways in which the comprehensive school counseling program can better support student success. An advisory council assists in the development of the school counseling program by annually reviewing program goals and results and making recommendations for improvement. It provides a forum for open dialogue between schools and community and the perspective of community and parental expectations for the counseling program.

Council membership should reflect the community's diversity and can include school staff, parents, school board members, and student, business, and community representatives. Members selected must share an interest and enthusiasm for the school counseling program and representation could consider including the following stakeholders:

- Teachers
- Parents
- School counselors
- Administrators
- Community members (non-parent)
- Business/Industry/Labor leaders
- School board member
- Student(s)
- College (two- and four-year) representatives
- Community-based organizations
- Counselor educator

### Use of Data

Monitoring student achievement data helps to ensure that all students have equity and access to a rigorous academic curriculum that identifies academic gaps. Counselors suggest systemic changes in policy and procedures to improve student performance. The use of data to effect change within the school system is integral to ensuring students' success. School counselors should be proficient in the collection, analysis, and interpretation of data and monitor student progress through the collection of three types of data:

1. Student achievement data, which can include standardized test scores, GPA, graduation rate, promotion/retention rates, etc.
2. School improvement data, which can include course enrollment patterns, discipline referrals, suspension rates, attendance rates, parent/guardian involvement, participation in extracurricular activities, etc.

3. Student competency data, which can include percentage of students with a four-year plan, percentage of students participating in job shadowing, and percentage of students achieving the competencies as determined by the faculty.

### Action Plans

Planning is necessary to detail annual program activities that show how the desired results will be achieved. Action plans usually contain the following:

- Domain areas, national standards, and school improvement goals
- Student competencies and descriptions of the activity
- Curriculum/materials being used in the activity
- Time lines
- Methods of evaluation
- Measurable outcomes
- Person(s) responsible
- A description of the students involved

### School Counseling Program Assessments

A school counseling program assessment self-study helps to determine the degree to which the school counseling program is being implemented and is in alignment with the ASCA Model. Results provide information on the current state of the school counseling program, identify gaps and/or implementation challenges, and help the counselors plan for the following school year.

### Use of Time

Gysbers and Henderson (2012) offered specific recommendation for time distribution and suggested that school counselors spend 80 percent of their time in direct service to students and 20 percent in indirect services and program management. While the amount of time counselors should spend delivering services in each component area may vary according to the individualized needs of each school, the ASCA provides its recommendation in Table 7.3.

### Calendars

Calendars (district, departmental, and individual) are integral to maintaining a comprehensive counseling program because of the specificity in terms of activities, actions, and events. An annual district calendar articulates the delivery of the various elements that comprise the program. Developed by the leaders of the district's school counseling program, it allocates time for curriculum development, individual student planning, responsive and intervention services, and system support. When a calendar is developed and published, teachers, administrators, students, and families are aware of the scope and extensiveness of the activities of the school counseling program.

An annual school counseling department calendar follows the district calendar. The school counseling departments in each of the district's

TABLE **7.3**

Sample Distribution of Total School Counselor Time within the Delivery System Component

| Delivery System Component | Elementary School % of Time | Middle School % of Time | High School % of Time |
|---|---|---|---|
| Guidance Curriculum | 35%–45% | 25%–35% | 15%–25% |
| Individual Student Planning | 5%–10% | 15%–25% | 25%–35% |
| Responsive Services | 30%–40% | 30%–40% | 25%–35% |
| System Support | 10%–15% | 10%–15% | 15%–20% |

Source: ASCA National Model; adapted from Gysbers, N. C., & Henderson, P. (Eds.). (2000). *Developing and managing your school guidance program* (3rd ed.), Alexandria, VA: American Counseling Association.

elementary, middle, and high schools construct calendars that align with the building calendar. This calendar is set up by month and by grade levels for the entire year for each school. Counselors list activities or themes to be delivered and specify how collaboration with school, district, family, and community stakeholders will occur. Yearly calendars also include quarterly grade reporting dates, state assessments, college entrance exams, orientation, graduation, as well as ongoing activities such as respect days, wellness days, career fairs, college expos, and other special events for students and their families.

Calendars ensure involvement. When stakeholders are aware of activities and services, the probability of their decision to become involved or participate increases. Calendars are also significant public relations tools and are public statements of the variety of services and activities offered both during the school day and in extended hours and/or weekends.

The management quadrant reminds us of the importance of organization and building a cadre of support for comprehensive school counseling. Although the program is coordinated by school counselors, many activities are shared by the entire staff and require a collaborative approach. These can include the following:

- Planning and organizing tasks
- Action plans around specific school issues
- Organizing activities with teachers about program operation
- Publicizing activities and events

## The Accountability System

Counselors who do not add to the bottom line are considered superfluous (Martin, 2002).

Accountability provides evidence of program accomplishments or student gains as a result of intentional efforts by the school counselors

(Hart & Jacobi, 1992). School counselor accountability intentionally contributes to closing the achievement gap and meets the goals of school improvement. Accountability answers the question *what* is the result of these efforts. School counselors are often challenged to demonstrate the effectiveness of the school counseling program in measurable terms. The ASCA National Model (2005, 2012) encourages school counselors to collect and analyze data, use data-driven decision making, use evaluation methods focusing on student achievement, and contribute to the school and system improvement goals. By using their specialized training in group process, collaboration and teaming, and data analysis, school counselors demonstrate how the school counseling program moves school improvement data in a positive direction.

## MEET DR. BARBARA DONNELLAN AND THE COUNSELORS OF THE LINDENHURST UNION FREE SCHOOL DISTRICT

There was a clearly defined need to enrich and expand the nature, quality, and frequency of counseling services and ensure that the school counseling department was a key player to put our district on a clear path to improved student achievement. Our department's new three-year comprehensive school counseling plan became a blueprint for change and supported the vision and goals of the school board and administration.

The counselors shared a common belief that the majority of their students are qualified and motivated to attend college on graduation. The general community, however, did not share these expectations. To promote change in this core belief the counselors at both middle school and high school developed approaches, programs, and activities that kept the school community focused on preparation for college!

Their collaborative strategies included the following:

- Parent meetings with speakers from both local and more distant four-year colleges at both middle and high school levels
- College awareness days where teachers and staff wear apparel from the colleges they attended
- College of the month bulletin board at the high school
- Increased emphasis in all contacts with students on college preparation course selection
- Guidance Advisory Board agenda items to address college preparation
- Students with disabilities have been encouraged to advocate for themselves with regard to college and to apply to testing agencies to use their test modifications on college admissions tests
- Students with financial need have been assisted to seek fee waivers on college admissions tests and on Advanced Placement exams to expand participation in these programs

*(continues)*

- Counselors have sought to further their relations with college admissions personnel through campus visits and extended college tours whenever feasible
- We established a system to monitor our data so that we could provide our administration and community with the results of focused and intentional strategies.

Our community has responded so positively and supports the belief that college attendance is an important priority for our children. The counselors have worked hard to get the word out about the importance and availability of a college education for our district's children. "Information is power!" We closed the information and now the opportunity gaps! Incidentally, in tough economic times we increased our four-year college-going rate from 47 percent to 55 percent during the past two years.

*Barbara Donnellan, EdD, is the director of counseling services for the Lindenhurst Union Free District. A former high school counselor, her focus is on delivering comprehensive programs. She serves as an adjunct professor and is a regional governor for the New York State School Counselor Association.*

### Using Data

Data present the picture of the current status of student needs and achievement issues and corroborate the development of practices that can lead students to higher levels of success. Data inform, confirm progress, and reveal shortcomings in student performance (Stone & Dahir, 2004). Annual school report cards publicize critical data elements such as attendance, demographics, graduation and postsecondary planning rates, and standardized testing results. These can be monitored and analyzed longitudinally and show how the work of school counselors affects student achievement. You will have the opportunity to use MEASURE, a six-step accountability process that moves school counselors from a "counting tasks" system to aligning the school counseling program with standards-based reform (Stone & Dahir, 2011) in Chapter 8. MEASURE enables school counselors to demonstrate how they are accountable for results and contribute to student achievement.

A programmatic approach to school counseling places school counselors in a valuable position to affect the instructional program and contribute to every student's achievement through collaboration and teaming with teachers, student support personnel, and parents. Utilizing the ASCA National Model (2005, 2012) offers a blueprint for school counselors to

- establish the school counseling program as an integral component of the academic mission of school;
- provide for equitable access to school counseling services for all students;
- identify through the national standards and competencies the knowledge and skills that all students should acquire as a result of the K–12 school counseling program; and

- assists with annual performance evaluation based on the standards of practice expected of school counselors implementing a comprehensive school counseling program.

# THE TRANSFORMED SCHOOL COUNSELOR'S KNOWLEDGE AND SKILLS

Comprehensive school counseling programs facilitate the *new vision* of the school counselor (DeVoss, 2010a; Martin & Robinson, 2011). In contrast to past decades, today's school counselors additionally are expected to transform their practice to motivate students to meet the expectations of higher academic standards, and to contribute to closing the achievement, opportunity, and information gaps. An effective school counselor possesses the attitudes, knowledge, and skills to provide the direct and indirect components of the school counseling program. Successfully delivering the ASCA Model (2005, 2012) utilizes counselor skills and competencies based on the Transforming School Counseling initiative (Education Trust, 2009b). To accomplish this, the school counselor must possess a solid knowledge of what she or he needs to know and be able to do to serve as a student advocate, provide direct and indirect services, and ascribe to the belief that all children can learn and achieve.

Transformed school counselors build on the traditional practice of services and extend their skills to deliver comprehensive school counseling programs that are standards-based and data driven. These skills, in the transformed context, are briefly reviewed in Table 7.4.

*Counseling.* Counseling in schools is the process of assisting a student in understanding, assessing, and making a change in behavior for the

## TABLE **7.4**
### Traditional and Transformed Practice

| The Practice of the Traditional School Counselor | The Practice of the Transformed School Counselor |
|---|---|
| • Counseling<br>• Consultation<br>• Coordination | • Counseling<br>• Coordination of services<br>• Consultation<br>• Leadership<br>• Social justice advocate<br>• Collaboration and teaming<br>• Managing resources<br>• Use of data<br>• Technology<br>• Systemic change agent |
| Service-driven model | Systemic and programmatic model |

Source: Adapted from Transforming School Counseling Initiative, Education Trust, 1997.

purpose of advancing self-awareness and understanding, increasing self-efficacy, and improving or enhancing relationships with others. As a result of the counseling process, students learn to make decisions to further improve their ability to achieve academic, career, and personal-social success in school.

*Coordination of Services.* Counselors serve as a liaison between teachers, parents, support personnel, and community resources to facilitate successful student development. School counselors secure the appropriate and necessary services and supports that are essential to every student's ability to achieve.

*Consultation.* The school counselor exchanges and shares information and knowledge with parents/guardians, teachers, and the community to assist each student in her or his academic, career, and personal/social development. Consultation helps parents and teachers process problems and concerns, acquire more knowledge and skill, and become more objective and proactive.

*Collaboration and Teaming.* School counselors, as education professionals, join teachers and school administrators to improve student success and achievement through a collaborative approach to developing strategies to deliver a comprehensive program.

*Leadership.* A comprehensive program is a proactive response to school improvement. School counselors, empowered in the restructuring process within their school systems, establish a foundation for affective education and competency-based learning. The school counselor serves as a leader as well as an effective team member working with teachers, administrators, and other school personnel to make sure that each student has an equitable opportunity to succeed.

*Advocacy.* The school counselor advocates for the elimination of significant performance gaps among students from different economic classes, genders, races, or ethnic groups.

*Managing Resources.* Counselors identify, access, and coordinate the resources within the school and community that are necessary to support school success. The school counselor helps families, parents, guardians, and/or caretakers identify their children's needs and provide the information and assistance to access resources.

*Use of Data.* Data-driven results are the key to linking school counseling programs to improved levels of student achievement. Measurable success resulting from this effort can be documented by an increased number of students completing school with the academic preparation, career awareness, and personal-social growth essential to choose from a wide range of substantial postsecondary options, including college (Education Trust, 2009a, 2009b).

*Use of Technology.* Technology tools help school counselors access and analyze data that depict the current situation of student achievement. Technology also helps school counselors monitor improvements in school climate and other student-related school factors as a result of implementing a comprehensive school counseling program.

*Systemic Change Agent.* School counselors have an ethical responsibility to examine and act on the systemic issues in their schools that stratify students' opportunities. With change comes opportunity and access for all.

ASCA and the Education Trust have called for a shift in the role of the professional school counselor from that of service provider to one of promoting optimal achievement for all students (Clark & Stone, 2000b; Martin, 1998; Stone & Dahir, 2006). School counselors can "become the academic conscience of the school, insuring that the school remains focused

---

### MEET DR. ROSE PAOLINO: LEAVING NO STUDENT BEHIND AT WEST HAVEN HIGH SCHOOL

Year after year, it became apparent that the ninth-grade class encompassed the most failures, with approximately 40 percent failing one or more academic classes. Why? As you may surmise, there are many underlying issues to student failure. As school counselors we know that a student's social/emotional development is first and foremost to academic success.

It was very timely that ASCA's National Conference offered many breakout sessions on the failure rate of ninth graders. I thought, wow, this is not just a West Haven High School epidemic, it is national. With attendance at as many "Save the Freshman" breakout sessions as possible, I was fortunate to stumble on a presentation by a school counselor in Rhode Island who showcased their "Counselor of the Day" Program, which fostered the goal of reducing suspension rates. Their model could easily be duplicated, and thus, collaboration began with their lead counselor.

Immediately after the conference I met with my principal and provost (who is in charge of the discipline for students) and enthusiastically presented the program we had to have. We discussed the position of the counselors rotating on a daily basis as "Counselor of the Day" for what we named our Counselor Student Intervention (CSI) program. The program focus would be on student behavior, attendance, and academics.

After a meeting with the counselors, my vision became our vision. Three years after the initial stages of developing a comprehensive program and analyzing the various components, West Haven High School counselors realized that the personal/social aspect of their program needed a change. We were determined to be leaders and remove ourselves from our offices into the mainstream of the school culture, and launch the CSI Program.

CSI was introduced at the first faculty meeting of the year, with complete administrative support. Our goal as a school counseling department was to provide a leadership role and a vehicle for systemic change in the area of academics and personal/social responsibility. Data collection was based on student referrals from administration and teachers, follow-up on

*(continues)*

interventions by school counselors, evaluation from teachers, and final report card data. The CSI program readily became a proactive approach to reducing in-school suspensions and a watchful eye for academic failure. Teachers and administrators were utilizing the program and counselors were viewed as more than just staff who change schedules. It helped administrators, teachers, school counselors, and the rest of the staff work together to build positive relationships with students.

Just one year after the implementation of the CSI program, in-school suspensions were down by 14 percent and academic failure was decreased by 7 percent. This past year the impact continued with a decrease in academic failure. The reduction in the suspension rate had a direct correlation on the increase in promotion rate for ninth graders. The initiation of the program prompted the school as a whole to become cognizant of the ninth-grade failure rate and has since instituted the team approach for all ninth graders. This team approach has fostered more academic success for all ninth-grade students.

We felt so validated with accolades from the Board of Education, the school and district administration, and a presentation at the next ASCA National Conference. As we transformed our way of work, using data-driven practice truly helped us become systemic change agents.

*Rose Paolino, EdD, worked as a middle and high school counselor before becoming the chair of the middle and high school counseling departments in the West Haven school district. Under her leadership the West Haven comprehensive program was recognized by the Connecticut School Counselor Association (CSCA). Dr. Paolino served as president of the Connecticut School Counselor Association in 2006–07.*

on student achievement and accepts responsibility for student outcomes" (Hart & Jacobi, 1992, p. 49). It is imperative that school counselors play a proactive role in identifying and responding to complex academic, social, and personal issues on a daily basis. As the pressures on schools to raise the bar of academic performance persist, school counselors can take a front and center position to identify and rectify barriers that inhibit closing the achievement and opportunity gaps.

## MEETING THE CHALLENGES OF SCHOOL IMPROVEMENT

A hundred years of school counseling evolution have taught us that planned change is not happenstance (Krumboltz & Levin, 2004). Schools, as political and social institutions, are steeped in traditional practices that are both effective and ineffective. School counselors must be ready, willing, and able to embrace change as also must be their counterparts who represent the academic disciplines. Systemic change among school counseling professionals is essential before it is expected that school counselors will systemically change schools.

School counselors must act on their belief systems, not merely talk about them. Action means that social justice drives leadership; data drives program; and program drives role. Caseloads do not decline when there is no evidence that the investment of dollars has yielded any change in the bottom line. There is no luxury of time or dollars to wait for the educational system to wake up and value the work of the professional school counselor. Thus, change in the external world's perception about the effectiveness of school counseling will come about when evidence is produced that speaks to the language of principals who must meet adequate yearly progress. The ASCA National Standards, Transforming School Counseling, and the ASCA National Model are nonessential items in the school district operating budget unless these initiatives, intertwined as they may be, are used as intended and support the bottom line of education, i.e., improved student achievement.

The ASCA National Model requires school counselors to act as leaders, social justice advocates, data-informed practitioners, collaborators and team players, managers of resources every day and at all times. School counselors can no longer work in isolation, and comprehensive school counseling program goals and objectives must be aligned with the building and district school improvement plan. The strategic interventions that are focused on improving school report card data will demonstrate the effectiveness of school counseling and provide evidence. When the data show results, it is time to commit to a planned and focused campaign to educate administrators, teachers, school personnel, parents, students, and community as to the contributions of the school counseling program. Communities can then see that school counseling programs do produce the results they are demanding and that school counselors desire the same levels of success and positive results as do parents, teachers, and administrators. When comprehensive school counseling programs are linked directly to the mission of the school, they promote and enhance the learning process and are an integral part of the total school program.

ASCA (2003, 2005, 2012) has advocated that school counselors establish their identity and clearly articulate and define the role that school counseling programs play in promoting student achievement and educational success. New vision (Education Trust, 2009a, 2009b) school counselors work intentionally with the expressed purpose of reducing environmental and institutional barriers that impede student academic success (Education Trust, 2009a, 2009b). School counselors are challenged to demonstrate account-ability, document effectiveness, and the promotion of school counseling's contributions to the educational agenda (Stone & Dahir, 2011), and they are in a unique position to exert a powerful influence (Clark & Stone, 2000b; Stone & Dahir, 2011). The contributions of school counseling can support every student's progress through school to help each emerge more capable and more prepared than before to meet the challenging and changing demands of the new millennium.

The 21st century presents an array of challenges and opportunities for school counselors to renew their practice and respond to the climate of school reform. Voices from the profession have called for a shift in the role of the professional school counselor from that of service provider to one of promoting optimal achievement for all students (Dahir & Stone, 2007; Tang & Erford, 2010). Advocacy, leadership, teaming and collaboration, and use of data are essential components of the repertoire of skills that a contemporary school counselor employs in today's schools (Education Trust, 2009b). The school counseling profession has taken hold of the present and the future. No longer will the work of school counselors be defined by the perception of others. Comprehensive, developmental, results-based national standards-based school counseling programs have established our presence and will define our future.

# TECH TOOLS

Use the power of technology to learn more about the ASCA National Model.

- Create a spreadsheet to align your current school counseling activities and strategies with the national standards.
- Use a mapping tool to identify standards, competencies, delivery methods (individual student planning, responsive services, guidance curriculum, and system support), and activities for all services delivered in your school. This will help you identify gaps.
- Showcase the national standards and competencies that you are delivering to your students on your school counseling website. Parents will be pleased to see that the priorities that you have for your program meet national expectations.
- Create a checklist for your students of the competencies that they will acquire this year as part of your school counseling program. Show them how they can keep the checklist of their knowledge and skills in their school counseling portfolio.
- Subscribe to an ASCA and/or your state association's school counselor discussion list to help you identify best practices for comprehensive school counseling program implementation.
- Go to http://nces.ed.gov/nceskids/ and use the graphing section to show student growth and achievement in academic, career, and personal-social development standards. Use the graphs and charts as part of your parent and staff newsletters. If you are looking for more of a challenge try using Excel or Lotus for more "sophisticated" presentations.

## Internet Resources

ASCA: www.schoolcounselor.org

K–12 Counseling and Guidance: www.educationatlas.com/k-12-counseling-and-guidance.html

State School Counseling Legislation: www.schoolcounselor.org/content.asp?contentid=538

# School Counselor Casebook: Voices From the Field

## The Scenario Reviewed

My colleagues and I were shocked to see that our juniors had lost their focus on the goals they had set during their ninth-grade year. We had met all of our ninth graders as they started their high school careers. We talked with them and their parents about the future and what is required to meet the ultimate goals of high school curriculum. We also introduced options for after high school including a four-year university, two-year community college, a technical school, military career, or employment to help us best understand what the parents and students desired. Now, we realized that we had not checked on their goals since early on in their high school career to see where the students were.

We realized that it was time to make a change. We decided to take a careful look at our state's comprehensive model and reframe our work to reach our goal for the students. Under the *Delivery* system, we utilized individual student planning to ensure each student has an educational and career plan so we can monitor every student's progress throughout her or his academic career. The plan can be updated every year when we meet with each student. By doing this, you accomplish several things. You can sit down with them and go over their academic schedule and grades. You can talk with them about where they are in their studies and get an idea if anything has changed. You get some "face to face" time in a world where they may feel alone and scared. Most importantly, you also get the opportunity to know them a little bit. Not just as a student, but also as a person. In doing this, you provide the students with the opportunity to have a hands-on approach to their education. They can decide what to do while giving you the opportunity to monitor and make sure they are doing what they need to do to accomplish the goals they have in mind . . . even if those goals change every year.

Next we decided to develop a college and career readiness *guidance curriculum,* which we would begin now for our current juniors but we now realize how important it is to start with the ninth graders. We looked at the *Foundation* of our program and selected the standards and competencies that would keep us on target. The *Management* system reminded us to build a timeline while the *Accountability* quadrant of the model would help us monitor student data to show us whether or not our program initiatives have an impact.

Organizing our program around the comprehensive model will make a difference to keep our students focused and on track for the goals they set for themselves.

Steven Lay had five years of experience as an elementary school counselor before moving to the high school five year ago. Steven has been the recipient of a Tennessee Gold Star Award for three years for his work demonstrating accountability and using data. He presents frequently at state and local conferences and helped to institute the Tennessee Model for Comprehensive School Counseling in the Rutherford County school system.

### Websites for Comprehensive School Counseling

At the following websites, you'll find the domain areas, competencies, links to lessons, and other tools. Make sure you search your school counselor association to find your state's model and resources.

> North Carolina Public Schools: www.dpi.state.nc.us/curriculum/guidance/
>
> Orange County Public Schools, FL: https://www.ocps.net/cs/services/student/guidance/Pages/default.aspx
>
> Los Angeles County, Office of Education: www.lacoe.edu/dsss/
>
> Lee County, Florida: http://studentservices.leeschools.net/
>
> Montgomery County Public Schools, MD: www.montgomeryschoolsmd.org/departments/studentservices/counseling/
>
> Wisconsin Comprehensive School Counseling Model: www.dpi.state.wi.us/sspw/scguidemodel.html
>
> Rhode Island Framework for Comprehensive K–12 School Counseling Programs: www.rischoolcounselor.org/RIFramework_web.pdf
>
> Connecticut Comprehensive School Counseling Program: www.sde.ct.gov/sde/lib/sde/PDF/DEPS/Special/counseling.pdf
>
> Tennessee Model for Comprehensive School Counseling: www.tnschoolcounselor.org/tnschoolcounmodel.pdf
>
> Montana School Counseling Association: www.mtschoolcounselor.org/MT_School_Counseling_Program_Model/Introduction.html
>
> Virginia School Counselor Association: www.vsca.org/index.html

## LOOKING BACK: SALIENT POINTS

### Moving the Profession Forward

The school counseling profession applied the language of educational reform and school improvement to school counseling programs. Educational programs were about student growth, learning, and results. Students were the focal point, not the role of the teacher. Therefore, it was imperative that school counselors change the focus from position to program, i.e., from the role of the school counselor to the effect of the school counseling program on student achievement and school success. The publication of the American School Counselor Association's National Model (ASCA, 2003, 2005, 2012) shifted practice from acts of service to a structured and outcome-based program while simultaneously integrating the transformed school counselor skills as the process to promote the content.

### National Standards across America: An Agenda for Equity

Educational leadership across the nation sought to determine and define what was meant by standards. Issues surrounding standards have been the focal point of national education conferences and publications. The debate continues to this day as to whether standards-based education will ultimately result in a better-educated and better-prepared student who can succeed in a global society.

## The Evolution of the ASCA National Model

ASCA developed the ASCA National Model (ASCA, 2003, 2005, 2012) and uses an integrated approach to the three widely accepted and respected approaches to program models, i.e., comprehensive, developmental, and result-based models. The ASCA Model has contemporized the Foundation and Philosophy, Management Systems, and Accountability sections to align with the expectations of 21st-century school counseling.

## The National Standards for School Counseling Programs

Concerned about the absence of school counseling in Goals 2000 and the increasing importance of standards and assessment, the ASCA Governing Board committed to the development of the National Standards for School Counseling Programs (1994). The intent of this effort was to motivate the school counseling community to identify and implement goals for students that were deemed important by the profession, clarify the relationship of school counseling to the educational system, and address the contributions of school counseling to student success in school.

## Comprehensive, Developmental, and Results-Based School Programs

Comprehensive, developmental, and results-based school counseling are frameworks for the development, implementation, and evaluation of systematic school counseling programs. The characteristics are similar to other programs in education such as student outcomes or competencies, activities to achieve the desired outcomes, professional personnel, materials, resources, and a delivery system. These approaches have clear goals and include an organized and sequential curriculum.

## Delivering a Standards-Based Program

The national standards represent what a school counseling program should contain and provide to every student. The national standards are based on the three widely accepted and interrelated areas of student development as described in the counseling literature and research: academic, career, and personal/social development.

## Student Competencies

Competencies are the pathway to documenting and demonstrating student growth and progress development to the achievement of the nine standards and represent the knowledge, attitudes, and skills that students need for academic, career, and personal/social success. The competencies are incorporated into a comprehensive, developmental school counseling program, which emphasizes early intervention and prevention as well as responsive counseling services.

## The Transformed School Counselor's Knowledge and Skills

Today's school counselors additionally are expected to transform their practice to motivate students to meet the expectations of higher academic standards, and to contribute to closing the achievement, opportunity, and information gaps. An effective school counselor possesses the attitudes, knowledge, and skills to provide the direct and indirect components of the school counseling program.

### Meeting the Challenges of School Improvement

Change in the external world's perception about the effectiveness of school counseling will come about when evidence is produced that speaks to the language of principals who must meet adequate yearly progress. The ASCA National Standards, Transforming School Counseling, and the ASCA National Model are nonessential items in the school district operating budget unless these initiatives, intertwined as they may be, are used as intended and support the bottom line of education, i.e., improved student achievement.

## KEY TERMS

Comprehensive school counseling p. 178

ASCA national model p. 179

National standards p. 179

Responsive services p. 180

Academic development p. 182

Career development p. 182

Personal-social development p. 182

Student competencies p. 184

Results-based school counseling p. 184

Developmental school counseling p. 185

Individual student planning p. 191

System support p. 191

Student development curriculum p. 192

Transformed school counseling p. 195

## LEARNING EXTENSIONS/MAKING CONNECTIONS

1. Reflect on the scenario presented in the beginning of this chapter. What competencies would be most helpful for students in your school to acquire to intervene with bullying and prevent future occurrences? How can the national standards help to "bully proof" your school?

2. The PTA has invited you to explain the school counseling program at an open meeting. The PTA president has explained that the members seem to be supportive of the counseling program but really don't understand it. Prepare an outline of the key issues that you would explain in your 30-minute overview.

3. You are in the process of rethinking how counseling services are delivered in your school. You and your colleagues know that many students are rarely seen by the school counselors. You decide to meet with your principal and discuss how using the ASCA National Model would help to improve the quality and effectiveness of school counseling services in your school. Your principal has scheduled a meeting with you and your colleagues. What key issues should be brought up at this meeting? How will you get your principal to support a shift from a service-driven model to a program-based model?

4. Your leadership team is supporting the school counselor's decision to implement the ASCA National Model over the next two years in your building. How will you determine where to begin? How will you develop competencies that reflect the needs of your students and school?

5. You are meeting with the social studies teachers in your building about collaborating on classroom activities. Select one standard and develop a collaborative activity that supports one of the social studies standards or curriculum goals. How will you measure the success of the activity?

## CHAPTER 8

# Accountability and Data-Driven Decision Making

## CHAPTER OBJECTIVES

*By the time you have completed this chapter you should be able to*

- describe the components of a data-driven, accountable school counseling program;

- understand the power of data in delivering an effective school counseling program;

- define critical data elements and measurable outcomes for student success;

- analyze, synthesize, and disaggregate data to examine student outcomes and to identify barriers, successes, areas of weakness, etc.;

- establish accountability measures for a data-driven school counseling program;

- assess measurable outcomes for counseling programs, services, activities, interventions, and experiences;

- use school-based data to support decision making to design effective school counseling interventions and to support all students to be successful learners;

- identify critical data elements;

- know how and where to acquire data;

- identify steps to move critical data elements and to demonstrate your contribution;

- identify challenges and opportunities.

## ACCOUNTABILITY: SUCCESS, NOT SURVIVAL

Test scores are down, attendance is not improving, postsecondary enrollment rates are stagnant, and the end of year failure rate for students in grades 4, 8, and 9 is over 35%. Our children are slipping through the cracks in standards based reform. The school counselors of this district work very hard. The annual report shows that you delivered 2300 classroom guidance lessons, conducted 180 groups, and made innumerable individual contacts with student and parents. We applaud your efforts but we need you to go one step further. Add to your tally of services how your efforts made a difference in our district's report card data? We face a dire budget next year and we have to justify the continuation of funding for each educator. We know your school counseling programs are making a difference in our students' academic achievement. Help us add to your time-on-task numbers impact data that show that your school counseling programs contributed to students' academic achievement.

*(A school board member discussing the budget allocations for the next school year)*

---

## *School Counselor Casebook: Getting Started*

### Impacting Academic Achievement

Washington Middle School is a school in need of improvement. The state department of education has put the school on notice to improve eighth-grade reading and math scores and the average daily attendance rate for their entire student body. Everyone in the building has been asked to participate in committees to develop plans to improve both attendance and achievement. You, the counselor, volunteered for the accountability committee and offered to design a plan that would monitor attendance data, deliver targeted interventions, and hopefully improve the bottom line. What type of plan would you implement?

### "Thinking About Solutions" heading?

At the end of this chapter you can see how your approach compares to a practicing school counselor's solution.

---

This all-too-real challenge from the district school board is an example of what your future profession is being called on to do: show how the school counseling program influences the **critical data elements** that are sometimes called the school's report card data. Everyone in a school setting is accountable for student success and that includes school counselors as well as students, parents, and the community at large (Curry & Lambie, 2007; Dahir & Stone, 2009; Duffy, Giordano, Farrell, Paneque, & Crump, 2008; Sink, 2009).

School board members, administrators, and others who are charged with making tough decisions about spending are asking all members of the educational community for an accounting of their contributions to student achievement (Duffy et al., 2008; Sink, 2009; Whiston, 2002). The allocation of school resources is expected to produce a return on the investment and no educator is above accountability. Failure to show the impact of our work on school report card data places us at risk of being viewed as a fiscally irresponsible use of resources especially when education is competing at all levels for limited funding (Whiston, 2002).

Accountability governs the 21st-century school. School counselors are more frequently illustrating the influence and effects of their programs through the use of data. However, with the best of intentions, school counselors have not successfully documented that students have been more successful in schools as a result of their actions and interventions. In recent years school counselors have begun to scrutinize the relationship between personal accountability and student performance by working to acknowledge the importance of data-driven analysis of the school counselor's profession (White & Kelly, 2010). Sharing accountability for student success with stakeholders is a driving force for transforming and reframing the work of school counselors across the nation (ASCA, 2009a; Duffy et al., 2009).

It is in the spirit of preparing you to be ready to connect your program to school improvement and student success that this chapter offers concrete images of the "how to" of accountability. Rather than waiting for others to determine how your school counseling program will demonstrate accountability for student success, you can enter the field with a strong understanding of accountability. A data-driven approach to building your program will help garner support and secure your position as a valued player in school improvement (Sink, 2009; Studer, 2006; Van Velsor, 2009). Your school counseling program aligned with the educational enterprise is data driven, proactive and preventive in focus, and assists students in acquiring and applying lifelong learning skills.

> Accountability means demonstrating that something worthwhile is happening. In a public school setting, this principle may be manifested in procedures used to show that taxpayers are getting their money's worth. In such situations, the counselors are challenged to develop evaluations of their efforts (Baker, S. B., & Gerler, E. (2008), p. 31).

## ASCA STANDARDS AND THE NATIONAL MODEL FOR ACCOUNTABILITY

The development of the National Standards for School Counseling Programs was an important first step in engaging school counselors and stakeholders in a national conversation about program effectiveness and accountability.

The **ASCA National Model** (ASCA, 2008) was written to guide the design and implementation of school counseling program models nationwide, bringing to the school counseling program the imperative to align with the mission of schools and to demonstrate this alignment through accountability (Galassi, Griffin, & Akos, 2008; Myrick, 2003a). The standards and ASCA model helped the profession develop a common language to describe their work and contributions to accountability (Galassi et al., 2008).

The ASCA National Model for School Counseling Programs (ASCA, 2008) reinforces the importance of delivering a comprehensive, developmental, and results-based program that considers local demographic needs and the political climate of the community.

The Accountability quadrant of the ASCA Model speaks to the importance of having an accountability system and an organizational framework that answers the question, "How are students different as a result of the school counseling program?" (Johnson & Johnson, 2001). In the ASCA Model as in school counseling initiatives of the past decade, the shift has moved from answering the question "What do school counselors do?" to the question "How are students different because of what the school counselor does?" By collecting and using data, school counselors link the effectiveness of the program to student success (Luck & Webb, 2009). The ASCA National Model challenges school counselors to accept accountability as a means to demonstrate the program's impact in measurable terms. When the school counseling program goals are aligned with the mission of the school, it is inevitable that student achievement will improve as a result of the efforts of school counselors (ASCA, 2008). Accountability, as presented in the ASCA Model, links the work of school counselors to student success.

## Accountability Defined

Accountability is "the techniques by which citizens and their elected representatives control the activities of those who administer, teach, and serve in public schools and other institutions of youth development.... In education 'accountability,' as described here, requires schools and other public institutions that prepare our youth to pursue the goals established by the people and their representatives through democratic processes, and to achieve these goals to the extent possible by using the most effective strategies available" (Rothstein, Jacobsen, & Wilder, 2008, p. 1).

How does school counseling fit into this idea of accountability being a shared responsibility for student learning? School counselors up until recently escaped the accountability imperative because their work mainly focused on addressing individual issues and concerns related to social and personal development for the fraction of the school population that was perceived as the most talented or the most at-risk. The school counseling profession responded that counseling is a personal relationship and that it is impossible to measure a counselor's effectiveness or evaluate a series of services (Schmidt, 2007). Poverty, special needs, giftedness, exceptionality, and highly selective college counseling were some of the issues that required significant counselor involvement and fueled the cliché that 20 percent of the students commanded 80 percent of the school counselors' time. Before accountability, school counselors were viewed as working in a "support" role removed from what happens in the instructional arena of schools, and their work appeared only marginally related to teaching and learning. For these and other reasons, school counselors were not held to the same accountability standards as teachers, administrators, and other educators. Yet, for more than 20 years the professional literature was replete with calls for increased measure of counselor accountability (Dimmitt, Carey, & Hatch, 2007; Gysbers & Henderson, 2006).

## Surveys, Time-on-Tasks, and Results Based

Methods traditionally used for assessing needs and evaluating school counseling programs are being supplemented or replaced by accountability methods required of administrators and faculty (Whiston, 2002). Needs assessments, surveying, time-on-tasks, and results based are still used with good results by the profession; however, student impact data are becoming the required accountability method for all educators. For example, the concept of identifying areas of need by surveying stakeholders is a positive step but far from sufficient to increase success for every student. Looking at data to see who is failing multiple subjects, repeating for the second time, absent frequently, or in the office for frequent fighting is an essential step in identifying areas of need for focused attention.

## MEET KELLEY COX

Kelley is a school counselor in Jacksonville, Florida. Kelley targeted sixth graders to raise the overall grade point average (GPA). Kelley made frequent individual contact with 14 students deemed to be critical and developed academic improvement plans with a large number of sixth graders. She delivered classroom guidance lessons so all students would learn test-taking strategies, study skills, how to figure their GPA, learning styles, etc. She had focused small groups with those critically in need of raising their GPA or risk failing. Kelley collaborated with teachers to develop plans to help students make up work or acquire extra-credit work. Parent contact was frequent, attendance was closely monitored, and grade-level meetings spent part of the time focusing on the efforts to shore up all sixth graders. The average GPA for sixth-grade students in the second nine weeks was 2.9 and it rose to 3.1 by the end of the third nine weeks. This may seem minor but longitudinally the grade point averages for sixth graders dipped sharply the third nine weeks. The collaborative efforts not only kept this from happening but actually raised the overall GPA.

Compiling **time-on-task** activities such as how many classroom guidance lessons were conducted, how many students were seen individually, and/or how many small groups took place effectively contributes to an understanding of how school counselors spend their time (Myrick, 2003b; Scarborough, 2005; Sink, 2009). Tallying services delivered is a fairly straightforward accountability process and sends an important message that hundreds of students are being served by the school counseling program (Gysbers & Henderson, 2001; Scarborough, 2005). In the school board scenario at the beginning of the chapter the numbers presented to the school board attested to the hard work of the school counselors of the district and they were lauded for it. However, it is like the school board member said: "[W]e need you to go one step further. Add to your tally of services how your efforts made a difference in our report card data." This counting of services delivered is soft accountability (data) and school board members want to know how our work is affecting student success data such as attendance rates, discipline referrals, grades, and postsecondary going rates. Time-on-task, while accounting for how our day is being spent, is incomplete when used as the only method of accountability (Dahir & Stone, 2009; Green & Keys, 2001; Gysbers & Henderson, 2001; Lapan, 2001; Sink, 2009; Whiston, 2002).

Another approach sometimes used to document success is called "results based" accountability. For example, a school counselor may report time-on-task information such as 20 percent of every day is spent in career and academic advising, including helping students understand financial aid information for postsecondary education. A counselor may take it a step further and report results-based data with the information that 60 percent of the student population can identify financial resources for postsecondary education. Taking it a step further, the school counselor could report that 48 percent of the senior class filled out the Free Application for Federal Student Aid (FAFSA); we have now moved into a **data-driven school counseling** program that reports movement of critical data elements. Stakeholders, especially school board members, administrators, and teachers, understand the significant difference between reporting how the time is spent and reporting the academic outcomes for students, and they want the student impact data (Green & Keys, 2001; Lapan, 2001; Walsh, Barrett, & DePaul, 2007). The results of the school counselors' efforts show that more students were willing to take a step forward toward continuing their education after high school. Each year the data-driven school program would set a higher goal so that the next year the goal might be to move from 48 percent to 58 percent for the number of students completing the FAFSA.

Another example of results-based accountability is giving a posttest to determine if students learned from the conflict resolution classroom guidance lesson and can now identify a conflict resolution technique. As an aspiring school counselor, if this were your program, how would you move from a posttest or **results-based accountability** to assessing the impact of your conflict resolution efforts on impact data? This "one step further" requested by the school board member would be to describe how your students are more successful in school because they are participating in your conflict resolution program. Impact or critical data would be that the number of discipline referrals for fights and conflict went down by 9 percent. These impact data are stronger and support the position that our school counseling programs move critical data elements. Unlike student impact data, time-on-task (42 classroom guidance lessons) and results based (91 percent of students identified a conflict resolution technique), while helpful, do not resonate as powerfully with legislators, school board members, principals, and other stakeholders as saying, "the school counselor implemented a conflict resolution program and as a result contributed toward reducing the discipline referrals by 9 percent and raised our attendance rate from 78 percent to 83 percent during a four-month period."

The school counseling profession is building on the great work that has been done in the past with time-on-task and results-based data and is moving in the direction of impact data. This progression is demonstrated in another example. In our profession groups such as divorce groups are in place to help remove emotional barriers to concentration and learning. Stakeholders' questions are quickly becoming, "Were the students in the divorce group suffering academically? If so, how did the divorce group positively affect these students' academic achievement? Were you able to reduce their absenteeism, raise their test scores, or improve their grades?"

It is an accepted premise in your chosen profession that supporting a student's personal and emotional needs during the experience of parental divorce can help this student stay focused and succeed academically. However, beyond counting the number of divorce groups we conduct, can you demonstrate accountability? How would you show that the divorce group was an intervention needed to improve a student's academic success?

As a result of the work in the divorce group these students were more successful in school. Each participant's grade point average went up over the previous marking period and collectively the group had 12 fewer absences. Stakeholders now understand when you say you ran three divorce groups during the year and all participants improved their grade point averages and 20 of the 22 students had fewer absences.

If you conduct a series of conflict resolution classroom guidance lessons, what will be your accountability measure? If you answered that you would look to see if the classes that had the series of six classroom guidance lessons reduced the number of discipline referrals, then you are reporting accountability data that have meaning and merit for stakeholders. You have nothing to fear in seeking a data-driven school counseling program. Even if the data do not move in a positive direction, you are speaking the language of the critical stakeholders, garnering support for your program, helping students be more successful, and changing your program based on learning about what does and does not work.

## ACCOUNTABILITY SUPPORTS EQUITY

On a daily basis, issues of equity and access to opportunity lie at the school counselor's door. In many respects, school counselors hold the key to student success and are ideally situated to identify policies and practices that stratify student opportunity (Dahir & Stone, 2003; Kachgal, Romano, & Peterson, 2001).

School counselors have unknowingly and without malevolent intent regulated students' futures and narrowed opportunities by determining course selection and course placement process (Martin, 2004). For years, large numbers of poor students and students of color were consigned to limited

### MEET CHRISTA MUSSA: DISAGGREGATING DATA TO ADVANTAGE STUDENTS

Meet Christa Mussa, Arizona School Counselor and past president of the Arizona School Counseling Association. Christa tackled the absenteeism problem at her school. When she disaggregated the data she found that 44 students missed 18 or more days of school the previous year. She wanted to know if she currently had chronic absentees and she ferreted out the 21 students who were stuck in the same pattern with chronic absenteeism. By gathering stakeholders to help, and implementing and developing successful strategies, Christa was a major player in helping decrease the number of students missing 18+ days of school by 66 percent. She continued her work after the first marking period and subsequently reached all but one student. When praised about her accomplishment Christa said, "Yes, but there is still that one." You get the feeling that the determined Christa will never rest on her laurels. Christa knows about systemic change and also about reaching individual starfish.

options after high school (Haycock & Hines, 2006). For the first time in history, schools are being held accountable for the achievement of all groups of students. According to Kati Haycock, director of the Education Trust, "school counselors are ideally positioned to serve as advocates for students and create opportunities for all students to reach these new high academic goals" (The Education Trust, 2003, para. 5). "The research couldn't be more clear, compelling and consistent. Students need highly-qualified teachers and a high-level curriculum to be successful in the world of work and postsecondary education," said Stephanie Robinson, principal partner with the Education Trust. "School counselors are in a unique position to make sure that all students have access to these resources" (The Education Trust, 2003, para. 7).

School counselors can decidedly affect two of the major contributors to the achievement gap: (1) low expectations, specifically the pervasive belief that socioeconomic status and color determine young people's ability to learn; and (2) the sorting and selecting process that acts as a filter, denying access to rigorous course content to students because of low expectations (Haycock & Hines, 2006; Martin, 2004). Measurable success resulting from an effort to widen educational opportunities can be documented by an increased number of students completing school with the kind of academic preparation, career awareness, and personal/social growth essential to choose from a wide range of substantial postsecondary options, including college (Education Trust, 1997).

When school counselors are part of the accountability system, they can effectively identify and rectify issues that affect every student's ability to achieve at expected levels (Brigman, Campbell, & Webb 2007). Closing this gap in student performance is what educational reform is all about. The use of demographic and **performance data** makes it possible to determine how policies and practices are affecting issues of equity for every student, identifying results, and informing decision-making.

The work of school counselors can challenge the pervasive belief that socioeconomic status and color determine a young person's ability to learn and seek to eliminate the sorting and selecting process that acts as a filter denying access to rigorous course content (Martin, 2004; Stone & Hanson, 2002). School counselors, acting as agents of school and community change, can create a climate where access and support for rigor is the norm. In doing so, students who we have traditionally underserved have a chance of acquiring the skills necessary to unconditionally participate in the 21st-century economy (Martin, 2004).

School counselors as leaders, advocates, and collaborators, promoting equity and a social justice agenda, purposely behave in a manner that promotes entitlement to quality education for all students. They do this by contributing to the creation of a school climate where equitable access and high standards are the norm. If you are a school counselor/social justice advocate, your practice will look for ways to influence systemwide changes that lead to the following:

1. The delivery of a well-defined, data-driven counseling program that attends to issues of equity, access, and support services.
2. The routine use of data to target and enroll underrepresented students into rigorous courses.

## MEET VICTORIA FELIX

Victoria is a high school counselor in Jacksonville, Florida. Victoria conducted a data-driven accountability effort targeting the sophomore AVID students who had earned a D or F in any of their classes. AVID is a 4th-through 12th-grade system to prepare students in the academic middle for four-year college eligibility. It has a proven track record in bringing out the best in students and in closing the achievement gap. AVID stands for Advancement Via Individual Determination (Advancement Via Individual Determination, 2010).

At the end of the fall semester of 2009–10 (end of second quarter) 32 of the 68 AVID students had a D or F in one or more of their classes. Through a variety of strategies such as focused conferences with teachers about individual students and how to help them, frequent parent contacts, classroom guidance lessons, individual conferences with students, after-school sessions, focused reading materials, college admission counselors presentations, and cross-curricular projects, only 12 out of 68 students still had a D or F after one nine-week period (end of third quarter) representing a 30 percent reduction. Was this change by accident? Not hardly. One dedicated focused school counselor said, "I can make a difference" (V. Felix, personal communication, September 26, 2010).

3. The initiation, development, coordination of intervention systems designed to improve the learning success for students who are experiencing difficulty with rigorous academic programs.
4. The use of data to identify and analyze areas of success for replication and **institutional** and **environmental barriers** impeding student success.

Data help you fight more effectively for equity for your students. Data educate and demonstrate where the inequities are and the patterns of failure that need to be changed.

# BUILDING A DATA-DRIVEN SCHOOL COUNSELING PROGRAM

In God we trust, all others bring data

*(Dr. Eddie Green, Interim Deputy Superintendent,
Division of Educational Service, Detroit Public Schools)*

What does it mean to build a school counseling program around critical data elements that are important to legislators, school board members, superintendents, administrators, teachers, and parents? There are multiple ways in which a school counselor as part of the leadership team can use data to support students and remove barriers and develop a school counseling program around critical data elements. Data paint a vivid picture of a school and its students. Data draw a depiction of achievement patterns, successes and failures in teaching, equity issues, and overall effectiveness of the school to support successful learners. Data can help us understand the national picture, district picture, but more importantly, are the data for the individual school (Gysbers & Henderson, 2001; Isaacs, 2003; Stone, 2003). These school site data can help the school counselor determine goals for the school counseling program. A school counseling program built around data means use of numbers rather than assumptions or perceptions. Data, such as enrollments in college prep courses, graduation rate, retention rates, special education placements, attendance, grades, and standardized test scores, reveal a telling story of achievement patterns, equity issues, career and college connections, and overall effectiveness of the schools (Dahir & Stone, 2003; Martin, 2004).

School counselors as part of the leadership team, who understand the power of aggregated and disaggregated student information, can focus their work on those areas particular to their school so their allocation of time, attention, and resources will be judiciously spent to achieve the most desired results for their school's report card data (Martin, 2004; Stone & Dahir, 2004). If a school counselor builds her or his school counseling program around the identified needs of the school, she or he will hit the mark because these needs are decided on by the internal and external critical stakeholders of the school. For example, if one of the areas stakeholders identified as a need is the poor promotion rate for third and fifth graders, then the school counseling program can highlight this one area for the school counseling program and, as part of a collaborative team, develop strategies to move these data in a positive direction. Far better to build a program based on identified needs of the school than an arbitrary determination of what should be the focus of the program based on a preconceived idea of the direction the program should take. The school's data were generated by the students who stand before the school counselor every day. Therefore, it is the data about these students that are the focus of a data-driven school counseling program. Let's meet counselors who have established data-driven school counseling programs.

## MEASURE Framework for Accountability

MEASURE is an acronym that stands for Measure, Elements, Analyze, Stakeholders-Unite, Results, and Educate. It is a simple five-step model for doing accountability work. Let's look at a hypothetical counselor, Cynthia, in a real situation in many of our schools. Cynthia suspected that there were many suspensions at her school. Cynthia tested her observations by gathering school data on suspensions and found that for the previous year suspensions increased each month until there were 30 suspensions for the month of May. She brought the information forward to the administration, who gave Cynthia time on the faculty meeting agenda to bring this information to the faculty and allow them time for discussion. In a PowerPoint presentation, Cynthia graphically demonstrated suspensions and other attendance data. The teachers were alarmed as they had no idea that so many students were out of school on a daily basis. The next hour was spent with the teachers, administrators, and Cynthia brainstorming and strategizing to find ways of reducing or eliminating suspensions and the attendance problem.

Cynthia established as one of her school counseling program goals to work with students who are in danger of suspension and/or chronically absent. Cynthia brought her skills and her program objectives to bear in trying to change suspensions by establishing a daily behavior management program for the most at-risk of suspension students with daily brief contact to check on their progress. At the end of each day, Cynthia quickly visited classrooms of two grade levels where most of the at-risk-for-suspension students were concentrated. As part of a token economy program she checked the daily progress of these students and culminated her check each week with a brief visit to the school counseling office for students who met their goals. Cynthia added conflict management to her classroom guidance list because in her research she found that fights generated a large percentage of the suspensions. Cynthia initiated an outreach program by bringing in mentors to work with the students who had the most discipline referrals and were most at-risk for suspension. Additionally, she had these students serve as mentors to younger students in the school.

Cynthia used data to identify a systemic problem. She brought the problem to the attention of the faculty and together with these educators collaborated to make positive change. Cynthia is establishing a data-driven guidance program based on hard data that identify the needs of her school. Cynthia does not rely on perceptions to establish her guidance program nor does she bring a one-size-fits-all guidance program to her school. Cynthia as part of the leadership team for her school has established a program that contributes toward moving the school's data in a positive direction.

## MEET OLCAY YAVUZ: CHANGING SYSTEMS IMPACTING LIVES

A model example of engaging high school students and preparing them for college has been developed by Olcay Yavuz, a school counselor at the Paterson Charter School for Science and Technology in Paterson, New Jersey. The 2000 Census shows that less than 9 percept of the population holds a bachelor's degree or higher and more than 19 percent of families are below the poverty level, with a median household income of $32,778. Paterson also has a largely African American (33 percent) and Hispanic (50 percent) population. Given these demographics, this student support program is a vital component for the successful transition from high school into college. Olcay Yavuz counseled 80 seniors in 2009–10, and as of February 3, 2010, all 80 have college acceptances.

Paterson faculty and staff have opened many doors for students. When Olcay started at Paterson, less than 40 percent of the students were even applying to college. The dramatic change has come about because of a number of school counselor–led efforts that Paterson offers. Strategies include teamwork that involved many levels, such as principal support by paying teachers and subsidizing SAT prep materials, English teachers enhancing essay development, and bringing in on-site college admissions counselors and career and college advising. Between 2008 and 2009, student participation in college-related activities has experienced huge increases. Participation in activities such as SAT-prep programs has increased from 2 students to 20 students; SAT tutoring participation has increased from 6 students to 56 students; seniors attending college fairs have increased from 4 students to 80 students; senior participation in Instant Decision Day increased from 5 students to 70 students; and home visits increased from 6 visits to 85 visits. These results are a concrete example of what every student support program can accomplish. Olcay is but one of thousands of counselors who are closing the informational and opportunity gaps and heavily influencing the achievement gaps (Stone, 2010b).

## 2008–10 Counseling Department Data Summary

| College Guidance Related Activities | 2008–09 | 2009–10 |
|---|---|---|
| • of seniors who have been accepted into four-year programs | 6 | 57 |
| • of seniors who have been accepted into two-year programs | 42 | 15 |
| • of seniors who have been accepted into vocational and trade schools | 2 | 7 |
| • of seniors who have been accepted into National Guard | 1 | 2 |
| • of seniors who did not apply to college | 30 | 0 |
| Amount of estimated total earned scholarship | $40,0000 | $2,500,000 |
| • of sent applications | 40 | 370 |
| • of organized instant decision days | 0 | 11 |
| • of SAT prep after-school tutoring sessions | 7 | 58 |
| • of students who participated in SAT tutoring sessions | 8 | 49 |
| • of Saturday full SAT practice test | 0 | 8 |
| • of seniors who took SAT | 20 | 79 |
| • of juniors who took PSAT in October | 4 | 65 |
| • of colleges invited | 2 | 13 |

*(continues)*

| College Guidance Related Activities | 2008–09 | 2009–10 |
| --- | --- | --- |
| • of parent college awareness workshops | 0 | 3 |
| • of senior college awareness workshops | 1 | 4 |
| • of career search workshops | 0 | 2 |
| • of college fairs | 0 | 4 |
| • of seniors who participated in college fairs | 4 | 80 |
| • of Armed Forces invitation | 0 | 4 |
| • of seniors who participated in instant decision day | 5 | 70 |
| • of home visits | 6 | 87 |
| • of organized career fairs | 0 | 1 |
| • of classroom guidance activities | 1 | 7 |
| • of counselors and school administration meetings | 3 | 21 |
| • of counselors and teachers meetings | 4 | 19 |

### Olcay's Systemic Changes

- Institutionalized collaboration among schools to improve the promotion rate for ninth grade.
- Changed practice so that every counselor and administrator will disaggregate data on a regular basis to see which students need more attention.

---

## MEET JIM MACGREGOR: HAMMERING AWAY AT THE ACHIEVEMENT GAP

Jim MacGregor, steward of equity and access, persevered until all students in Pike High School in Indianapolis, Indiana were supported with access to algebra and safety nets such as double mathematics periods and tutoring. Jim looked around his school and saw inequity. Jim decided that he would advocate for greater opportunities for his students. He set about widening opportunities and for six years persistently hammered away at the system until he significantly affected the achievement gap. Jim MacGregor is a hero. This quiet, unassuming, self-effacing counselor has affected thousands of lives by giving students the opportunity to access and be successful in higher-level academics. The data show Jim's results. Jim does not know the meaning of the words "it can't be done." Jim did not do anything that you and I, as school counselors, would not want to do.

Jim raised students' aspirations by implementing a career awareness program for every student in the school to help them see the interrelationship between postsecondary education and their future economic opportunities. Jim involved parents in academics by helping them see that their children's future would be severely handicapped if they did not participate in the rigorous courses that prepare them for postsecondary options. These parents became supporters for changing the academic expectations for the whole student body. Jim advocated for a systemic change in course enrollment patterns to support more students to access higher level academics. Using data and anecdotal information about student success in higher-level academics, Jim was able over time to successfully change attitudes and beliefs about widening opportunities for higher-level academics. Jim affected the instructional program by using disaggregated test results so that teachers had better information about student weaknesses, he led large- and small-group sessions on motivation and problem solving, used software for four-year plans to track every student from ninth grade so that course selections were in writing and matched students' aspirations, and established a mentoring program. For a complete list of his strategies see Stone and Dahir (2004).

### Jim's *MEASURE of Success*
#### Students graduating with college core:

|                  | 1994  | 2000 |
|------------------|-------|------|
| White            | 62.5% | 78%  |
| African American | 26.7% | 66%  |

*College core meant completing 40 specified semester credits.

|          | 91–92 | 95–96 | 00–01 |
|----------|-------|-------|-------|
| ALG 1&2  | 71    | 94    | 99    |
| GEO      | 66.1  | 83    | 96    |
| ALG 3&4  | 55.4  | 63    | 65    |
| Pre-CAL  | 31.5  | 39    | 46    |
| CAL 1&2  | 11    | 20    | 20    |

**During the time Jim was at Pike the demographics changed for this large urban school of 2,492 students:
1989—66% White/Non-Hispanic, 30% African American, 4% Other.
2000—39% White/Non-Hispanic, 51% African American, 10% Other.

*(continues)*

### Jim's Systemic Changes

- The approach to transitioning between middle and high school became a state model for Indiana.
- The school district added counselors and funded counselors to work in the summer based on their success rate in helping students complete higher-level mathematics.
- Double mathematics periods were implemented.
- Change in attitudes and beliefs on the part of teachers, all other educators, and community members about opening higher-level academics to all students.
- The district superintendent and other central office decision-makers developed an awareness and appreciation for what could happen when there is a counselor-led data-driven focus on ratcheting up academics for all students.

Jim moved to Florida in 2002 and continues to make a difference. See two of his email communications that indicate this systemic change agent is not resting on his laurels.

From: Jim MacGregor
Sent: Thursday, June 10, 2010 3:45 PM
To: Martin, Pat; Stone, Carolyn
Subject: Caught a big one!

It has been a focused effort the last couple of years to increase the number of students taking the PSAT. In 2009 we administered 1180 PSAT's to juniors, but in 2010 we plan to administer it to 3019. Pat Martin gave me a challenge about how we are going to encourage the low scorers to keep going and to continue their efforts to get to college. Our Community College always tells us that if their students complete the remedial courses that there is no difference in their quest to attain a degree compared to those who do not need remedial courses. We [the four counselors] intend to prepare all 9000 ninth through eleventh graders for the test and tell them why they are taking it and that they can still get a college degree despite a low PSAT score. We are working on Pat's other challenge: to increase the % of Black and Hispanic males in challenging courses.

Jim MacGregor
Counselor
Secondary Education

From: MacGregor, Jim
Sent: Wed 4/27/2005 7:08 PM
To: Stone, Carolyn; pmartin@collegeboard.org
Subject: AP enrollment

I have just been able to obtain our AP enrollment for next year. Thought you might be interested. Our AP enrollment took a big jump for next year.

This year our total AP enrollment is 155. Next year it is 423. Our AP Exam order increased for this year. Last year 114 kids took 166 exams but for this year 170 kids will take 394 exams.

My school is around 70% Hispanic and over 50% free and reduced lunch. [a post script April 2006: 740 AP exams given! (up from 129)—Now 56% free and reduced lunch and 47% of students in AP are on Free and Reduced Lunch]

Jim MacGregor
Counselor
Secondary Education

---

## Critical Data Elements

Data inform. The school board challenge clearly tells us that presenting summary data on time and task is not enough. Needs assessments or surveys that describe thoughts, opinions, desires, or requests of students, faculty, or parents will not bring us to the bottom line of demonstrating the impact of school counseling on students. Accountability requires systematically collecting, analyzing, and using critical data elements to show improvement with positive changes as results. Examining demographic and performance data makes it possible to determine how policies and practices are affecting issues of equity for every student, identify results, and inform decision-making. Data can help us look at student progress and results, inform, challenge our thinking, determine the need for systemic change, confirm progress, and reveal shortcomings in student achievement.

Critical data elements are those pieces of information that are important to all stakeholders, e.g., attendance, demographics, graduation and postsecondary planning rates, and standardized testing results. Closely examining critical data elements that identify the needs of your students and the schoolwide issues that cloud success is the first step to inform and guide the development and construction of an accountable school counseling program. With data, school counselors are able to paint a picture of the current situation in the school for students and can begin to document their successes and failures.

Many school counselors have databases available that contain biographical information as well as scheduling, attendance, discipline, and test history. This information is useful in itself when working with students about any of the information contained in the database, such as attendance, test scores, current grades, and past academic performance. By using data on the entire school population, assurances are built into the system that no students are left out of the picture when viewing the data (Martin, 2004). This provides equity in analysis and guarantees that no group of students will be left out of critical calculations for a data-driven school counseling program (Stone & Turba, 1999).

## What Are Some Examples of Critical Data Elements?

### Measures of Achievement

Test results

State exams such as the Florida Comprehensive Achievement Test

Preliminary Scholastic Achievement Test (PSAT)

Scholastic Achievement Test (SAT)

ACT

ASVAB

Standardized achievement tests such as the CTBS, Iowa Tests, Stanford Achievement Tests, NAEP, etc.

Number of credits taken per year

Retention rates

Drop-out rates

Postsecondary enrollment (four-year-college, community college, apprenticeship, career and technical, military training)

Grade point averages

Rank in class

The following are areas that do not are not "measures of achievement" but affect achievement:

Course enrollment patterns that demonstrate commitment to high achievement

Numbers of National Merit/Achievement Semi/Finalists

Enrollment in Honors, AP, IB, or college-level courses

Enrollment in general, remedial courses

Exceptional student education screening and placement

Gifted screening and enrollment

Alternative school enrollment

*A quick look at data alone does not tell the whole story. It is important to disaggregate all critical data elements and look at them in terms of gender, race/ethnicity, socioeconomic status, and perhaps by teacher to shed light on areas of success or areas in need of attention.*

There are other data elements that can inform the work of school counselors such as **demographic data** of the internal and external community.

Demographics of the Internal and External School Community

Entry and withdrawal information

Ethnicity

Gender

Number and type of discipline referrals to include suspension rate

Attendance rate

Single Family Situations

School geographic areas

Free/Reduced-price lunch students and other available socioeconomic measures

## Disaggregated Data

**Disaggregating data** or separating out the data by ethnicity, gender, socioeconomic status, grade level, or teacher assignment (see Figure 8.1) is important in the study of student performance and in examining equity issues. This disaggregation of data makes it possible to determine how policy and practices affect issues of equity as counselors work toward closing the gap in student opportunities and achievement.

Often the discussion will be centered around what data elements you don't have instead of examining the data you are able to obtain.

When looking to create change, it is important to know what areas need the most attention. For some, the evidence may reveal itself, while for others, key questions must be asked and data must be utilized to obtain the answers. Presented here are easy steps for analyzing data that will help identify areas of interest and, therefore, will assist in creating change. Once the data are brought together in a story, they can be used to inform, provoke, and persuade those individuals who may not be open to change (Martin, 2004).

An important place to begin is to remember that simple kinds of data analysis can go a long way; complex statistics is not the best way to present

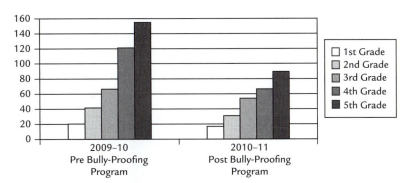

FIGURE **8.1** The Impact of a Bully-Proofing Program on Discipline Referrals Disaggregated by Grade Level

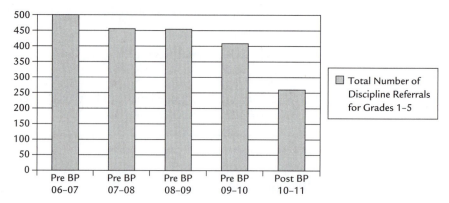

FIGURE **8.2** Total Number of Discipline Referrals Each Year and the Impact of the 2010–2011 Bully-Proofing (BP) Program

data to others. Start with simple statistics such as averages and percentages. Then disaggregate or "slice" that piece of data into different units. For example, if the average score on an achievement test is 149, look to find out what the scores were for each ethnicity (The Education Trust, 2001).

Next, look for data as they relate to time. This process will add yet another dimension to the data by adding longitudinal elements. For example (see Figure 8.2), when looking at test scores, also look at the scores over a period of time to compare how they are changing.

In Figure 8.3 the school counselor is comparing mathematics assignment by ethnicity and Figure 8.5 is a chart cross-tabulated by the rigor of high school curriculum by the race of college entrants. Finally, cross-tabulate the data or "dice" them by comparing two sets of disaggregated data. Compare not only the scores of students across different ethnicities, but also compare them with other variables such as the classes in which they are enrolled.

Cross-tabulation can be obtained by following these easy steps. Ask questions that will lead you to the data you are looking for: (1) What are you trying to measure (e.g., college completion rate)? (2) What is the first

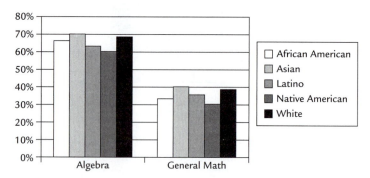

FIGURE **8.3** Graph of Cross-Tabulated Data

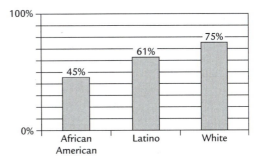

FIGURE **8.4** Postsecondary Completion Rates by Ethnicity

characteristic to be used to divide these data into groups (e.g., race)? (3) What is the second characteristic to be used to divide these data into groups? For example, it could be divided by high school curriculum. The answer to question two produces results in Figure 8.4. When the answer to the third question is added, Figure 8.5 is the result.

Remember you do not have to know and use the technology to disaggregate data, but if you understand the power of data and know the right questions to ask, then you can get others to help you with the technology piece or provide the disaggregated data for you. School counselors do not have to fear using data if they are not comfortable with the technology.

## MEASURE: A SIX-STEP ACCOUNTABILITY PROCESS

Revisit the case presented at the beginning of the chapter and also the lament from the school board member. To illustrate the school counselor's work with accountability, let us look at the data element that the case and school board stated was a challenge—improving postsecondary enrollment rates. But first, let's learn the steps to approach moving these data in the right direction. MEASURE stands for Mission, Elements, Analyze, Stakeholders-Unite, Results, and Educate. MEASURE is a six-step accountability process that helps school counselors demonstrate how their programs affect critical data, those components of a school report card that are the backbone of the accountability movement

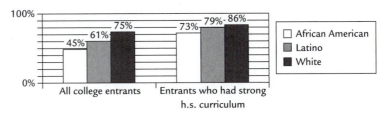

FIGURE **8.5** Cross-Tabulated by Race and High School Curriculum

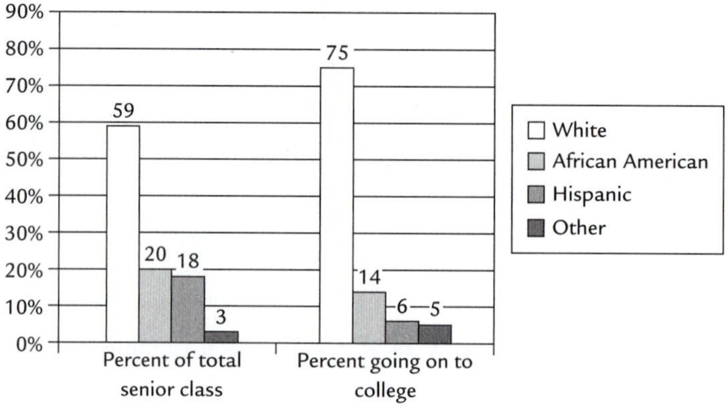

FIGURE **8.6** What do the data tell us?

(Dahir & Stone, 2004). Implementing MEASURE is an easy way to connect to the school leadership team and demonstrate that you are helping to drive data in a positive direction (Dahir & Stone, 2010). MEASURE will help organize your efforts and show your results. MEASURE is a way of using information to target critical data elements, such as retention rates, test scores, postsecondary going-rates, and to develop specific strategies to connect school counseling to the accountability agenda of today's schools (Dahir & Stone, 2004).

Through MEASURE it is possible to look at what we do in a manner that shows the direct impact of the work of school counselors on student success. Not only is it possible, but it is probable that you are already looking at, thinking about, and analyzing much of the information that comes across your desk every day. Think about all those questions that came to mind when you looked at your elementary school building's report card this year. How did you feel about the high school profile when the data were compiled? Did they meet your expectations? Were you confused when you saw the huge number of eighth-grade failures at the end of the school year that meant summer school or retention for so many of your students? These questions and others are all about student achievement, school improvement, and accountability for results. Incorporating accountability measures into your school counseling program will provide insight as to how we can share in the responsibility to widen educational opportunities for every one of our students.

Let's learn how to use the six steps by using a common goal for school districts to improve the postsecondary going rates. MEASURE: Mission, Elements, Analyze, Stakeholders-Unite, Results, Educate.

## Step One: <u>M</u>ission
### *What Do I Need to Do?*
Connect the design, implementation, and management of the school counseling program to the mission of the school and to the objectives of the annual school improvement plan. Student achievement and success in

rigorous academics is at the heart of every school's mission statement. School counselors ask how every aspect of their program supports the mission of the school and contributes to student achievement.

---

## *School Mission*

Connect your work to your school's mission in keeping with the ASCA or your state's comprehensive school counseling model.

The mission of our school is to promote the conditions necessary so that each student experiences academic success. Each student will have the coursework required to choose from a wide array of options after high school.

---

### Step Two: <u>E</u>lements
#### *What Do I Need to Do?*

As a member of the school's leadership team, identify and examine the critical elements of the available data that are important to your school's mission. School counselors play a pivotal role in this process as they work collectively with all stakeholders to focus on areas of concern for student success. Critical data elements usually can be found on the school's district or building report card. School systems routinely collect and store academic and demographic data in a retrievable form. Let us assume that the number of students in your school district going on to postsecondary educational institutions is not what it should be. The critical data element then might be the postsecondary going-rates for your school district, which have been holding steady around 50 percent for the last five years.

---

## *Current Critical Data Element*

What critical data *element* are you trying to affect? (Examples include grades; test scores; attendance; promotion rates; graduation rates; postsecondary-going rate; enrollment into honors or AP courses, special education; discipline referral data; etc).

What is the *baseline* for the data element? What is your *goal*?

Fifty percent of our students access postsecondary education (college and other educational opportunities after graduation).

---

### Step Three: <u>A</u>nalyze
#### *What Do I Need to Do?*

Analyze the critical data elements to determine which areas pose problems. Analysis will determine the institutional or environmental barriers that may be impeding student achievement and adversely influencing the data elements. School counselors can initially determine which elements to tackle first and which elements the school counseling program can move in a positive direction to specific targets. A quick look at data alone does not tell the whole story. It is important to disaggregate the critical data elements on which you are focusing and to look at them in terms of gender, race/ethnicity, socioeconomic status, and perhaps by teacher to shed light on areas of success or areas in need of attention. The analysis will reveal how far away the data are from your school improvement goal.

---

Analyze the data element. You can use percentages, averages, raw scores, quartiles, or stanines. You can aggregate or disaggregate the data to better understand which students are meeting success. You can disaggregate by gender, race, ethnicity, socioeconomic status, or in a multitude of ways to look at student groupings.

| Baseline: Where is this data element currently? | Goal: Where do you want the data element to be in a year? |
|---|---|
| Fifty percent of our students access postsecondary education. | We want a 5 percent increase in the postsecondary going-rate. |

---

What other information do you need to know? Which student groups are represented in the 50 percent accessing postsecondary schooling? Which students comprise the 50 percent not accessing this option? Disaggregate the data to answer these and other questions. You can disaggregate data in a number of ways: gender, ethnicity, socioeconomic status, home location, teacher or counselor assignments, course-taking patterns, feeder schools, etc. This information can be gathered through the student information management system, school report card, etc.

Assume you are a high school counselor and these tables represent your graduating class last year. What do these tables tell you? What else do you need to know about these data? How will the school counseling program contribute toward positively improving these critical data elements and connecting the work of school counselors to better results for students?

The data revealed (among other important things) that of the 50 percent of your students seeking postsecondary education, the majority, or 34 percent, came from one particular feeder middle school where all students were assigned to algebra classes in eighth grade and were supported with mentors and tutors to be successful. The feeder middle school practice to place every student in algebra is a positive practice that could be replicated by the other feeder school.

## Step Four: Stakeholders-Unite: Identify Stakeholders to Help and Unite to Develop an Action Plan
### What Do I Need to Do?

Identify stakeholders to become part of a team to be involved in addressing the movement of the critical data elements. All concerned members of the internal and external school community should be included. Determine how to secure their commitment and who will bring them together. If possible, use an existing school action committee. Accountability for school counselors is about collaborating with other stakeholders and avoiding tackling issues in isolation. Examples of stakeholders are the following:

| Internal Community | External Community |
|---|---|
| Principal | Parent |
| Teacher | Business representative |
| School board member | Faith representative |

### What Do I Need to Do?

Unite with stakeholders and develop and implement strategies to move critical data elements in a positive direction. The team will:

1. define targeted results;
2. decide what information is needed and how to gather it;
3. determine the strategies to move the data;
4. identify skills and resources needed and assign responsibilities to appropriate stakeholders; and
5. develop a timeline and a way to assess interim progress and final results.

With your stakeholders, begin to develop and implement an action plan that contains strategies, a timeline, and responsibilities to move the postsecondary going-rates to 55 percent. The table below gives a high school example of stakeholders and strategies that could be used to increase postsecondary going-rates. Similar tables can be created for middle and elementary school based on the target results from Step Three.

| Stakeholders | Strategies |
|---|---|
| | Beginning date: September of this school year<br>Ending date: June of this school year<br>*School counselors, as managers of resources, join existing groups of stakeholders, such as the school improvement team, or bring other stakeholders and resources into the task of creating and implementing an action plan.* |

*(continues)*

| Stakeholders | Strategies |
|---|---|
| | *Strategies are developed that will change systems as well as affect individual students and targeted groups of students.* |
| | *Affecting systems means (1) replicating successful programs and interventions, (2) identifying barriers that adversely stratify students' opportunities to be successful learners, and (3) developing strategies to:* |
| | • *change policies, practices, and procedures* |
| | • *strengthen curriculum offerings* |
| | • *maximize the instructional program* |
| | • *enhance the school and classroom culture and climate* |
| | • *provide student academic support systems (safety nets)* |
| | • *influence course enrollment patterns to widen access to rigorous academics* |
| | • *involve parents and other critical stakeholders (internal and external to the school), etc.* |
| | • *raise aspirations in students, parents, teachers, the community* |
| | • *change attitudes and beliefs about students and their abilities to learn* |
| School Counselors | • Implement a career awareness program for every student in the school to help each see the interrelatedness between postsecondary education and her or his future economic opportunities. |
| | • Advocate for a systemic change in course enrollment patterns to support more students to access higher-level academics. |
| | • Use data and anecdotal information about student success in higher-level academics to try to change attitudes and beliefs about widening opportunities for higher-level academics. |
| Teachers | • Social studies teachers have students research their career goals and project how their career paths fit with economic trends and the business climate. |
| | • English teachers have students write essays for scholarships. |
| | • Mathematics teachers integrate financial aid calculations into lessons. |
| Administrators | • Provide professional development for the faculty on raising aspirations. |
| | • Orchestrate collaboration with feeder schools to see how to replicate the practices that are proving successful in raising aspirations. |

| Stakeholders | Strategies |
|---|---|
| School Psychologists | • Provide additional group and individual counseling to high-risk students on motivation and problem solving. |
| School Social Workers | • Work with parents and caretakers on teaching students the importance of attendance for school success. |
| Clerical Staff | • Monitor student progress in submitting applications for postsecondary admissions.<br>• Organize group meetings between the counselors and the students who are not submitting information in a timely manner to postsecondary institutions. |
| School Clubs | • Invite community leaders to talk about career opportunities and the education and skills needed to be successful in the work environment.<br>• Help close the information gap by sponsoring awareness activities regarding postsecondary opportunities. |
| Parents | • Assist in establishing a tutoring program.<br>• Create a phone chain to call parents to remind them of important school events. |
| Volunteers | • Work with individual students on the power of financial aid to affect their future. |
| Business Partners | • Assist in establishing a mentoring program.<br>• Provide site visits to their businesses.<br>• Help organize and participate in career fairs. |
| Community Agencies | • Assist in establishing a mentoring program.<br>• Run evening and Saturday programs with school personnel for parents and students on raising aspirations, homework help, technology awareness, etc. |
| Colleges and Universities | • Host "College for a Day" programs for elementary and middle school students.<br>• Offer diagnostic academic placement testing to 10th and 11th graders.<br>• Provide targeted interventions for underrepresented populations. |

## Step Five: Results
### What Do I Need to Do?

If the targeted results were met there is still reflection and refining to do. Did the results of everyone's efforts show that the **interventions and strategies** successfully moved the critical data elements in a positive direction? If so, reassess your efforts to develop your next steps toward continuous school improvement, including any changes in the school counseling program.

If the targeted results were not met, the next step would be to reanalyze and refocus the efforts to determine why the interventions were unsuccessful in moving the data in a positive direction. Identify the components of the effort that worked. Reanalyzing means replicating what is working and developing new or different strategies for what did not work. Based on your analysis determine what changes need to be made to the school counseling program to keep the focus on student success. We can't hold fast to programs and strategies that do not help our students become more successful learners. There is too much work and too little time to accomplish all that needs to happen for our students. A school counselor recently was lamenting, "What if I find that my conflict resolution program did not really impact the discipline rate [it did with a 54 percent decrease]." If the program had not made a difference we would have to rethink investing so much time and energy. In other words, if the horse is dead, get off!

---

Results: Restate your baseline data. State where your data are now. Did you meet your goal?

Restate baseline data: We had 50 percent postsecondary going-rates.

Results (data now): We have 56 percent postsecondary going-rates.

Met Goal: Yes____x____ No ____

Yes, the goal was not only reached but exceeded! Postsecondary going rates grew by 6 percent.

### Questions to consider as you examine results and revise your MEASURE:

Which strategies had a positive effect on the data?
Which strategies should be replaced, changed, added?
None should be replaced, changed or added at this time.
Based on what you have learned, how will you revise Step Four, "Stakeholders-Unite?"
For now all stakeholders worked well so no modifications will take place.
How did your MEASURE contribute to systemic change(s) in your school and/or in your community?
The MEASURE increased postsecondary going rates, which contributed to the systemic change within the school.

It is always necessary to reanalyze and refocus to determine whether you met your targeted results. If the targeted results were met, set new targets, add new strategies, and replicate what was successful. If the postsecondary rates increased by only 2 percent and thus fell short of the targeted results, it will be necessary to refocus efforts to determine which strategies were successful and which need to be replaced or revised. Stakeholders can then determine which efforts worked well and which strategies need to be modified, adjusted, or perhaps changed altogether. The next steps will be to revise the action plan for the following year and to continue to move the critical data elements in a positive direction.

Look at that high school profile now! Now 56 percent of our students are accessing postsecondary opportunities, slightly better than the goal of 55 percent. What did we learn from this process?

- Critical data element analyses helped us focus our efforts.
- Districtwide systemic change issues must begin in elementary school.
- Stakeholders across all levels were willing to share responsibility for moving critical data elements.
- Changes in data clearly demonstrated the intentional focus of the school counseling program on improving the postsecondary going-rate.
- Collaborative efforts made the changes happen.
- The school counselors' commitment as key players in school improvement was well established and acknowledged.
- Strategies delivered K–12 positively moved this data forward.
- Measurable results showed how the school counseling program worked to increase the postsecondary going-rate through a systemwide focused effort.

## Step Six: Educate Others as to the Results
### What Do I Need to Do?

Disseminate to **internal** and **external stakeholders** the changes in the targeted data elements that show the positive impact the school counseling program is having on student success. Publicizing the results of an effective school counseling program is a vital step in the accountability process and key to garnering support for your program. This can be a time to celebrate success and recognize and applaud your partnerships. Through this education, stakeholders will have a deeper understanding about the contributions of the school counseling program focused on student achievement. School counselors will be seen as partners in school improvement and have demonstrated a willingness to be accountable for changing critical data elements. Because of these efforts, school counselors are viewed as essential to the mission of our school. An example of a report to the school community follows.

### Systemic Changes and Other Interim Data

As you work together with the other stakeholders toward meeting your goals you will have interim success stories that are both anecdotal and hard data.

You will implement systemic changes. Capture these successes and note them on your report card.

When you tackle delivering a data-driven school counseling program, you become a systemic change agent affecting policies and procedures that will widen opportunities and empower more students to be successful learners. If the system is working optimally then a MEASURE would not be necessary; we can't drive data without changing systems. So, when you are gathering stakeholders and developing strategies, make certain you implement a MEASURE that intentionally tackles systemic barriers. Give yourself credit for affecting systems.

*Affecting systems means (1) replicating successful programs and interventions; (2) identifying barriers that adversely stratify students opportunities to be successful learners; and (3) developing strategies to do the following:*

- *Change policies, practices, and procedures*
- *Strengthen curriculum offerings*
- *Maximize the instructional program*
- *Enhance the school and classroom culture and climate*
- *Provide student academic support systems (safety nets)*
- *Influence course enrollment patterns to widen access to rigorous academics*
- *Involve parents and other critical stakeholders (internal and external to the school), etc.*
- *Raise aspirations in students, parents, teachers, the community*
- *Change attitudes and beliefs about students and their abilities to learn*

---

**MEASURE**

Mission, Element, Analyze, Stakeholders-Unite, Results, Educate,
A Six-Step Accountability Process for School Counselors

**Name and Address of School:**

**Principal:**

**Name of Counselor(s) Leading the Initiative:**

**Enrollment:**

**School Demographics:**

Caucasian/Non-Hispanic
African American
Hispanic
Asian/Pacific Islander
Native American
Multi-Racial
Free-Reduced lunch
English as Second Language
Exceptional Student Education/Special Education

### *Practice What You Have Learned*

It is your turn to complete a MEASURE. Take one of the three scenarios below and fill in the blank MEASURE.

1. *You are collaborating with the leadership team at your school to improve a 79 percent daily attendance rate at your school.*
2. *You are collaborating with the leadership team at your school to improve a 71 percent promotion rate.*
3. *You are collaborating with the leadership team at your school to reduce discipline referrals.*

---

## *Step One: Mission*

### Mission

Connect your work to your school's mission in keeping with the ASCA or your state's comprehensive school counseling model.

Your school or department's mission statement is:

---

## *Step Two: Element*

### Element

What critical data *element* are you trying to affect? (Examples include grades; test scores; attendance; promotion rates; graduation rates; postsecondary-going rate; enrollment into honors or AP courses; special education; discipline referral data; etc.)

What is the *baseline* for the data element? What is your *goal*?

Element:

Baseline:

Goal:

## *Step Three: Analyze*

Analyze the data element. You can use percentages, averages, raw scores, quartiles, or stanines. You can aggregate or disaggregate the data to better understand which students are meeting success. You can disaggregate by gender, race, ethnicity, socioeconomic status, or in a multitude of ways to look at student groupings.

The Baseline Data revealed:

## *Step Four: Stakeholders-Unite*

Stakeholders-Unite to develop strategies to affect the data element.
Beginning Date:
Ending Date:

| Stakeholders | Strategies |
|---|---|
| School Counselor(s) | • |
| Administrator(s) | • |
| Teachers | • |
| Students | • |
| Student Organizations (clubs, teams, etc.) | • |
| Parents | • |
| Parent Teacher Associations | • |
| School Psychologists | • |
| Social Workers | • |
| Community Agency Members | • |
| Faith-Based Organizations | • |
| Youth and Community Associations | • |
| Colleges and Universities | • |
| Classroom Teacher Assistants | • |
| Other Support Staff (front office, custodial, cafeteria, playground) | • |
| School Improvement Team | • |
| Resources (grants, technology, etc.) | • |
| | • |
| | • |
| | • |

## *Step Five:* Results

Results: Restate your baseline data. State where your data are now. Did you meet your goal?

Restate baseline data:     Results (data now):     Met Goal: Yes_____ No _____

### Questions to consider as you examine results and revise your MEASURE:

Which strategies had a positive impact on the data?

Which strategies should be replaced, changed, added?

Based on what you have learned, how will you revise Step Four, "Stakeholders-Unite"?

How did your MEASURE contribute to systemic change(s) in your school and/or in your community?

The Educate step in MEASURE has been adapted with permission from the Student Personnel Accountability Report Card (SPARC) sponsored by the California Department of Education and Los Angeles County Office of Education. SPARC is a continuous improvement document sponsored by the California Department of Education and Los Angeles County Office of Education. SPARC has been adapted with permission as a complement to MEASURE.

## *Step Six: Educate*

Educate others as to your efforts to move data. Develop a report card that shows how the work of the school counselor(s) is connected to the mission of the schools and to student success. Below is an example of a report card.

---

### (School Name) MEASURE OF SUCCESS

**Principal:**                                    School Counselor(s):

**Enrollment:**

---

Principal's Comment

School Counselor's(s') Comment                   Results

Critical Data Element(s)

Systemic Changes

Stakeholders Involved                            Faces behind the Data

**Counselor(s):**

**Administrator:**

**Teachers:**

**Parents:**

**Students:**

**Colleges and Universities:**

**Business Partners:**

### Remember, the Steps Will Rarely Be Nice and Neat

The six steps will not always follow the sequence as outlined. You may enter this accountability process at different points or you may follow a different sequence. For example, you may want to look at the issue raised by the school board by first bringing the stakeholders together as in Step 5.

Sharing accountability can be messy and difficult, and the results sometimes are disappointing. It is frustrating when in collaboration with other stakeholders your goal still remains elusive. Whole-school efforts in collaboration and teaming are critical toward moving data elements. Do we give up after one year? Systemic change takes time. Remember, change is a process, not an event (Fullan, 1993, 2002).

When you become a school counselor, if you are not readily comfortable with retrieving data, learn who can get the disaggregated data for you; this is more important sometimes than having the technological skills to retrieve data. Make noise about needing good data when you hit roadblocks to retrieving data. Knowing the power of data, what data elements you need, and who to ask for help to retrieve the information in a form you and the other members of the leadership team can use is an exceptional start toward creating an accountable school counseling program.

### Change Is Hard

In implementing a data-driven school counseling program you are often asking people to work in a different way than they have become used to working. This is especially true if you are part of a department that has counselors prepared in the traditional approach to training school counselors. Teachers and administrators may not view the school counselor as someone who can help affect the academic success of students because it has not been their experience that school counselors have worked in this way. Change is hard and the stakeholders you want to bring to the table to help you make a difference for students may be the stakeholders who do not agree with your approach. You will experience naysayers and road blockers. You will hear a litany of reasons why you should not work differently. The "Yes, buts" can be endless:

It's not reality.

It's pie in the sky.

It's impossible!

We don't have the money.

You are getting us into something that is not our job.

This is fiscally impossible.

I don't have the time.

No matter what we do, things will always be the same.

Parents want me to do one-on-one counseling.

We've always done it this way.

We have already tried that and it did not work.

The problem is too complex.

We don't have the personnel or resources.

I don't want to rock the boat.

What's wrong with the way things are?

They won't take anything off my plate. I am already doing way too much.

This too shall pass.

Letting those kids in will make our test scores look bad.

I am too close to retirement to change now.

(personal conversation with Nan Worsowicz, Joni Shook, and Sejal Parikh, December 17, 2010)

Data can help counselors garner support for their programs and, more importantly, support more students. Are our sights too high, our goals too lofty, the work impossible to implement? Not at all! The wonderful, amazing work you will be doing to change students' lives will be enhanced by adding the next step, accountability, demonstrating your value to the mission of your school. Don't let the data naysayers deter you. Failure to establish recognizable school counselor results for student achievement is tantamount to being counted out (Martin, 2004). In the world of schools today where "increased academic performance for all students" is the mandated goal, school counselors must take this critical step—become routine users of data to inform and sharpen their focus. Data, those cold hard numbers, actually move us closer to children because we speak with assurance now that the school counselor has made an impact on students' learning (Dahir & Stone, 2004).

# TECH TOOLS

The Tech Tools section offers suggestions for you when you become a practicing school counselor to maximize the goals of your program. However, when appropriate and possible, learn and implement these tech tools before you enter the field.

- Technology can help you retrieve data to get a clear picture of student achievement. Data will help you identify the areas of concern and the patterns of achievement inform you where your school counselor program is most needed. Accountability and a data-driven school counseling program depend on student information.
- Work for good data through your school's or district's student information management system. Ask questions of the managers of student information for the district. Continue to ask questions and gently push until you get reports in a form that is usable to you.
- Monitor student progress by querying databases to see which students are not progressing, need special attention, or are being successful.
- Make informed decisions about individual students and large groups of students by accessing data on students such as scheduling, attendance, discipline, test history, attendance, test scores, current grades, and past academic performance. For example, if you find that certain students are chronically absent, then this is information that can help you to investigate and make a difference.

# LOOKING BACK: SALIENT POINTS

### Accountable Data-Driven School Counseling Programs

In this age of accountability, it is essential that school counselors contribute to the school success agenda and clearly tie successful outcomes for students to their presence in school. Documenting the results of our efforts is key to assessing program effectiveness. Time-on-task and process data have sufficed in the past for accountability, but student impact data are the logical next step. The accountable school counseling program utilizes student data to create vision and targeted change. Accountability measures involve systematically collecting, analyzing, and using data to inform and guide the development and construction of a school counseling program. Accepting the challenge of accountability propels us to demonstrate by words and actions that we accept the responsibility of removing barriers to learning and achievement and promoting success for those students from whom little is expected.

### ASCA Standards and National Model and Accountability

The ASCA standards were critical in starting the conversations about measurable results. The ASCA National Model speaks to the importance of having an accountability system and an organizational framework that documents and demonstrates how students are different as a result of the school counseling program.

### Time-on-Tasks and Results Based

Counting services delivered and looking at post tests for learning gains are important aspects of program evaluation but are soft data. Couple these soft data with the school counseling program's impact on critical data elements and the program is aligned with the accountability agenda of the school and school district.

### Equity and Accountability

Closing the gap in student performance is a central component of educational reform. School counselors are ideally situated to influence low expectations and course enrollment patterns. School counselors as leaders and advocates purposely behave in a manner that promotes entitlement to quality education for all students. Counselors' penchant for collaboration and their belief in a social justice agenda can influence systemwide changes that result in greater opportunities for all students, especially low-socioeconomic students and students of color who have traditionally been underserved.

### Building a Data-Driven School Counseling Program

A school counseling program built around data means using numbers rather than relying just on assumptions or perceptions to determine where to focus the efforts of the school counseling program. Critical data elements are examined to see where students' gaps and needs are and then, in collaboration with other stakeholders, strategies are developed and applied. Enrollments in college-prep courses, graduation rate, retention rates, special education placements, attendance, grades, and standardized test scores are just a few of the critical data elements that may receive attention in a data-driven school counseling program. Data, a telling story of achievement patterns, equity issues, career and college connections, and overall effectiveness of the school, are central tools in the school counseling program.

### Disaggregated Data

Disaggregating data is looking beyond averages and percentages to separate out the data by categories, ethnicity, gender, socioeconomic status, and teacher assignment to reveal where the needs are the greatest or the successes to replicate the strongest.

### MEASURE: A Different Way of Focusing Our Work

MEASURE, an acronym for Mission, Elements, Analyze, Stakeholders-Unite, Reanalyze, Educate, is a six-step accountability process that helps school counselors develop a data-driven school counseling program. MEASURE shows school counselors how to take baseline data, develop strategies with other stakeholders to move the data in a positive direction, and then report the results in hard data.

## KEY TERMS

Critical data elements p. 213

American School Counseling Association
  (ASCA) National Model p. 214

Results-based accountability p. 217

Performance data p. 219

Environmental barriers p. 220

MEASURE p. 221

Demographic data p. 228

Disaggregating data p. 229

Interventions and strategies p. 238

External stakeholders p. 239

---

## *School Counselor Casebook: Voices From the Field*

### Impacting Academic Achievement

### Here's How a Practicing College Counselor Responded to the School Scenario

Serving on our school's accountability committee uses all of my transformed school counseling roles as a leader, collaborator, student advocate, team member, and data-informed practitioner. There are other key people on this committee including our social worker who works with students and their families and representatives from each grade level and department. Once the committee is in place, our work begins with a focus on attendance, our main school improvement goal this year.

Since I have access to data that teachers might not easily access, I must come to the first meeting loaded with all the information that will help us to develop a plan of action. This includes attendance data for each 20-day cycle, which is how we monitor average daily attendance, the number of absences by grade level, and students who have missed over five days in the semester. I will bring a copy of the board policy for our school district, so we can make sure it is aligned with our action plan.

In my collaborator's role, everyone's opinion is important. After presenting the data, I will encourage a brainstorming session with all members to formulate a plan. Each person needs to be respected in her or his point of view. It is important my colleagues see me as a team player. Attendance is a schoolwide issue and it is everyone's problem. It is impossible for one person to shoulder the entire responsibility of getting every student to school and on time. All school personnel must be involved for the plan to be successful.

Each of us has a particular role to play and strategies could be put in place involving all stakeholders. For example, teachers will be asked to call students who are absent. Our attendance clerk will also play a key role in communicating with parents and providing us with data. It is my job as a counselor to find out what the problem is and to do my best to help resolve it. Using a report in my database I obtain information about individual students. I will meet with each student to ascertain the problem and create an individual plan as well as look at groups of students and grade levels to see where the problems are reoccurring.

We also brainstormed an incentive program, which rewards students for coming to school every day as well as target students whose attendance is poor. The rewards include a "jeans day" each Friday for students who have perfect attendance for the week, a monthly reward celebration for students with perfect attendance for the month, and a recognition ceremony for students who have perfect attendance for the nine weeks. Also, students who do not respond to the rewards system will be identified using data from our computer system.

We set a realistic goal for us to increase our current attendance percentage from 90 percent to 92 percent. This is an important step in the plan. Future committee meetings are scheduled. Responsibilities are divided and the action begins.

As a leader, consultant, and facilitator, I will prepare a presentation to share at the next faculty meeting and facilitate a discussion after the presentation. It is important all staff are aware of the plan and what their role will be. The plan must include all stakeholders so I will also present to the Parent and Teachers Association and to the students. Letters are sent home with each student and included in the enrollment packets for new students. With parental support enlisted, our plan is now in place.

Our committee is looking forward to sharing our plan with the faculty, getting their input, monitoring our data, and looking forward to helping students improve their attendance. We will have a MEASURE plan to share with our school board at the end of the year.

Sharon Eaves has been a middle school counselor for 20 years and the lead middle school counselor for Hamilton County for the past 15 years. Sharon serves on various committees within her district, is a member of the local university's advisory board, and is a frequenter presenter at the annual Tennessee School Counselors' Institute.

## LEARNING EXTENSIONS/MAKING CONNECTIONS

Read the five scenarios that follow. Chose two of the cases to practice the steps of MEASURE. Develop a MEASURE for your two cases by filling out all six steps as if you had met with stakeholders and everyone developed strategies (see the completed example in this chapter).

Visit a school counselor and retrieve a real piece of data that is troublesome for the school counselor (follow confidentiality rules). Sit down with the counselor and explain MEASURE and help her or his think through how she or he could implement a MEASURE. A MEASURE template can be found on the text's website. Finish the first three steps of the MEASURE.

1. Your state issues a grade to schools based largely on test scores. Like most report cards the grades range from an A to an F. Your school has been on the F list for two years and is now under threat of being taken over by the state if test scores do not improve during the current school year. What role will your school counseling program play in helping this school make a difference in the school's test scores?

2. In your school, Hispanics comprise 30 percent of the ninth graders but only 7 percent of the students enrolled in the college-preparatory science track. Yet, when you ask these students about their plans after high school, over 90 percent say they are planning to attend college. How can your data-driven guidance program help the Hispanics and all other students in your school whose curriculum choices are not matching their hopes and dreams?

3. The school district in which you work has mandated that Algebra 1 and Geometry are required for graduation beginning with the current ninth graders. After the first semester of implementation of this policy, 37 percent of the ninth graders were failing. In disaggregating the failure rates by teachers, it is apparent that some teachers are much more successful than others and some teachers have dismal failure rates. What other data will need to be gathered to illuminate this problem? What role will your school counseling program play in trying to support the ninth graders to meet their mathematics graduation requirements?

4. It is an unwritten policy by the teachers and administration of your school that all students who are in danger of being retained for the second time be screened and tested for possible placement into special education (SE) classes. SE students can have testing accommodations if they have identified disabilities and are offered different promotion and graduation policies. You believe that in your particular school there is an overreliance on SE as an intervention without aggressive searches for other effective means to support students before they get to their second retention. There are a disproportionate number of minorities placed into SE programs. What will be the role of your school counseling program in curbing the trend for SE placement as an intervention?

5. The school improvement plan for the year calls for an improvement in the orderliness and safety of the school's learning environment. It is believed that the disruptions in the environment and bullying behavior are contributing to the decline in test scores and grade point averages. What are some strategies you can use to enhance the school learning community? Discuss how you will gather baseline data and then how you will demonstrate that your strategies have been a success.

# Diversity Matters

## CHAPTER OBJECTIVES

*By the time you have completed this chapter, you should be able to*

- explore your personal beliefs, attitudes, and knowledge about working with diverse student populations;

- ensure that each student has access to a comprehensive school counseling program that advocates for all students in diverse cultural groups including affirmation of all ages, ethnic/racial identities, social classes, disability statuses, languages, immigration statuses, sexual orientations, genders, gender identities/expression, family types, religious/spiritual identities, and appearances (ASCA, 2010);

- understand the impact of poverty and social class on student achievement;

- discuss the impact of culture and ethnicity on student performance;

- use data to close the gap among diverse student populations;

- identify resources and methods of support for English Language Learners and students engaged in bilingual support;

- acquire knowledge of strategies and skills for promoting student success through culturally sensitive advising and counseling;

- develop consultation strategies to raise the consciousness level of faculty, administration, and staff to better serve students from an increasingly diverse population.

---

## School Counselor Casebook: Getting Started

### The Scenario

A classroom teacher asks you to come to his classroom and observe the following students: Manuela Perez, a Brazilian American child whose parents have lived in the United States for the past eight years; Tamika Washington, an African American student whose mother works in a finance office and whose dad is a professional, but not living at home; Shawn Brown's parents who are divorced with his mother working as a custodian while his father moved back to Barbados and Roberto Suero of Puerto-Rican descent, whose dad is a teacher and his mother is an interpreter. The teacher expressed concern about these students and suggested that they have poor peer relations and limited interactions, and erratic behavior in class. He also believes that all four are not working up to potential and will not achieve grade-level scores on the upcoming state exam. You agreed to observe the students and will sit down with the teacher and review the findings. You also talked about presenting your findings to the Child Study Team as needed.

### Thinking about Solutions

As you read this chapter, imagine yourself in the role of leader and advocate for these students. What factors will you look for that might be contributing to the students' lack of success? What diversity influences may be contributing to the teacher's concern about these four students? How will you address your findings with the classroom teacher? When you come to the end of the chapter, you will have the opportunity to see how your ideas compare with a practicing school counselor's approach.

---

## PROMOTING A SOCIAL JUSTICE AGENDA

[T]oo many children who enter school with equal yearning soon falter under the harsh light of adult assumptions and American cultural history. Our lowered sights precede their own (Roberts, 1997, p. 23).

Today's schools mirror the changing demographics of the neighborhoods and communities that reflect the diversity of America. Historically, public schools are the place where children can learn to get along with others and continue to be the primary institutions that create cohesion among diverse groups (Center on Education Policy, 1998). Not all public schools bring together children from various racial and ethnic backgrounds, or those who are rich with those who are poor. Some public schools today are racially and economically isolated, but this does not diminish the importance of teaching children to be accepting of differences, to understand and appreciate each other's culture, and to respect other peoples' points of view (Spradlin & Parsons, 2008). School counselors have a responsibility to observe, monitor, and modify adult and student behaviors that can foster learning community in which every student, regardless of color or wealth or ability, can flourish.

In the mid-19th-century wave of immigration, public schools were responsible for building a common culture and teaching democratic principles and ideals (McDevitt & Ormond, 2007). As large waves of new immigrants landed on our shores, they were encouraged to quickly assimilate. The cultural standard for immigrant children was to quickly master English, accept the normative culture, and become "mainstreamed" into American society; newly arrived children were labeled "culturally deprived" or "culturally disadvantaged" (Sadker & Sadker, 2005). The debates between **assimilation** and acculturation resulted in an acceptance of the beliefs that "native culture" was inappropriate or perhaps inferior (Woolfolk, 2009). Students developed internal self-doubts, creating conflict among students (Goldstein & Kodluboy, 1998).

In the 1960s and 1970s some ethnic groups did not want to assimilate completely into the mainstream and desired to maintain their unique pride, culture, and heritage (McDevitt & Ormond, 2007). The focus of attention was no longer only on color and race; ethnicity, culture, and tradition assumed a new prominence. The appreciation for diversity and the **integration** of multiculturalism in the schools became a goal (Woolfolk, 2009).

Today, in the tens of thousands of schools across our country, educators in classrooms and in school counseling offices respond to the complex influences of diversity. By the year 2050, it is predicted that there will be no majority race or ethnicity in the United States; every American will be a member of a minority group (Banks, 2002; Halford, 1999; National Center for Educational Statistics, 2010; Payne & Biddle, 1999).

Of the 49.3 million students enrolled in public schools and in private elementary and secondary schools during 2009, almost 45 percent represented groups designated as racial minorities (National Center for Educational Statistics, 2009). As the population demographics continue to shift (see Figure 9.1), school counselors are ethically obligated (ASCA, 2010a) to deliver a comprehensive school counseling program to every student from culturally diverse backgrounds and need the requisite awareness, knowledge, and skills to do so (ASCA, 2010).

Differences are not limited to race, ethnicity, or language; school counselors also must address identity, generation, cultural customs, geographical origin,

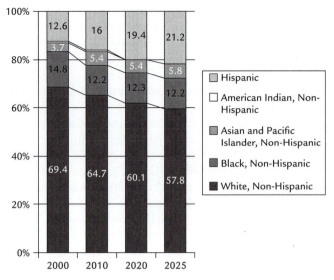

FIGURE **9.1** Projected Shifts in Population

Source: U.S. Bureau of Census, Population Projections (2009)

community, and family traditions (Capuzzi & Gross, 2003). Blending ethnicities, culture, and heritage can place educators in a cultural "minefield" where they must navigate a caring and respectful path that addresses the needs of many groups (Franklin, 2001; Holcomb-McCoy, 2004; Lee, 2007b). A child's worldview of harmony or discord will be influenced in great measure by her or his educational experience (Center on Education Policy, 1998). More recently, public schools have promoted an affirmation of human rights by focusing on social harmony, **tolerance,** and respect. By seeking ways of bringing together children from all races and ethnicities, prejudices and biases are reduced or eliminated (Teaching Tolerance, 2010).

According to the National Center for Educational Statistics (2009):

- Twenty-three percent of the children in school are immigrants or have parents who are immigrants. Most new arrivals to our nation come from Central and Latin America.
- In 2007, about 14 percent of the U.S. population was born outside of the United States; this included the approximately 69 percent of Asians and 44 percent of Hispanics who were foreign born.
- Thirty-five percent of children under the age of 18 were from minority groups. By the year 2020, this proportion is expected to increase to 45 percent.
- The United States is becoming more religiously diverse with Islam becoming the fastest growing religion in the nation.
- One in five children under the age of 18 was born poor and one in six is poor now.
- One in 5 children has a foreign-born mother.

- Nearly 34 percent of all African American children and 27 percent of Hispanic children are poor.
- By the year 2020, approximately 46 percent of all students in the United States will be students of color, many the children of new immigrants.

The data tells the story. As the lines continue to blur between what had been perceived as majority and minority populations, school counselors, as social justice advocates, should encourage students and faculty to be knowledgeable, open minded, and respectful of all cultures and all aspects of **diversity**. School counselors explore, understand, and work with the multiplicity of variables that comprise diversity and have a responsibility to value culture, race, ethnicity, gender, socioeconomic status and social class, sexual orientation, and promote awareness and **acceptance** among all student groups. These variables have a profound influence in students' lives and will continue to do so as they approach adulthood.

School counselors are in an influential position to challenge the status quo and assist those who have been victims or are potential victims of social and educational problems (Kiselica & Robinson, 2001; National Office for School Counselor Advocacy, 2010). Embracing a social justice agenda requires school counselors to acquire the awareness, knowledge, and skills to intervene at the individual level and at the systemwide level (Lee, 2007b). Working from a social justice mindset requires school counselors to give special care to those who historically have not received adequate educational opportunities or services including students of color, students from low socioeconomic backgrounds, students with disabilities, and students with nondominant language backgrounds (ASCA, 2010b).

## THE INFLUENCE OF CULTURE ON COUNSELING

Culture may be broadly defined as encompassing a group's common beliefs, including shared traditions, languages, styles, values, and agreement about norms for living. Culture, however, also intersects individuals' race, social class, gender, age, ability status, sexual orientation, and family traditions (Laird, 1998). Cultural intelligence is composed of those important competencies that allow us to effectively interact with people from diverse cultures in all kinds of settings (Bucher, 2008).

Culturally competent schools value diversity in both theory and practice in all aspects of teaching and learning as part of the overall school climate (Klotz and Canter, 2006). Schools considered *culturally responsive* forge a community out of cultural diversity, have the same high academic expectations for every student, deliver a curriculum that reflects many cultures, provide ways for students and staff to deal with racial/cultural tensions, actively hire a diverse and committed staff of educators, promote continuous staff development, involve parents in the educational process and are sensitive to their cultural needs, and define diversity in broad terms to include sexual orientation, ability and disability in addition to traditional concepts of race, religion, and ethnicity (Lee, 2001).

Holcomb-McCoy (2007) identified nine categories of cultural competence for school counselors: (a) multicultural counseling, (b) multicultural consultation, (c) understanding racism and student resistance, (d) multicultural assessment, (e) understanding racial identity development, (f) multicultural family counseling, (g) social advocacy, (h) developing school-family-community partnerships, and (i) understanding cross-cultural interpersonal interactions. Holcomb-McCoy suggested that continuous self-evaluation is the key to being more effective in counseling diverse populations.

School counselors recognize and acknowledge personal biases and **prejudices** that can influence their approach to counseling, guiding, advising, and encouraging students. Personal sensitivity to diversity also helps school counselors to determine how culture influences a student's perception of the problem and the choice of intervention. School counselors have an ethical obligation to be mindful of the influences of bias and prejudice (ASCA, 2010) and are responsible to act as "path finders," not "gatekeepers" (Hart & Jacobi, 1992) for students from all walks of life and backgrounds.

As counselors heighten their awareness as to how one's personal membership with regard to race, ethnicity, and culture can influence attitudes and beliefs, they have an obligation to participate in activities that allow them to explore their own identity (Bucher, 2008; Constantine & Gainor, 2001; Nelson, Bustamante, Wilson, & Onwuegbuzie, 2008).

## BOX 9.1

### *Exploring My Identity*
Considerations in Counseling and Cultural Competence

#### Cultural Identity
My racial identity is important to who I am.
My ethnic identity influences my interactions with others.
My gender is an important influence in the way I identify myself.
Social class influences how I relate to others.

#### Cultural Viewpoint
I am able to discuss the influence of racial and ethnic identity on student-adult relationships.
I seek to expand my knowledge about other cultures, especially those of the students and colleagues I work with.
I realize that people from the same culture may have divergent views, values, beliefs, and customs.

#### Intercultural Communication
I can use culturally competent communication skills with all parents, teachers, and school administrators.

I am aware of culturally insensitive topics, gestures, and body language.

I am aware when the race, culture or ethnicity of a student is a challenge for a colleague.

### Challenging Biases and Beliefs (Social Justice)

I can advocate for school policies, programs, and services that enhance a positive school climate and are equitable and responsive to diverse student populations.

I am willing to speak up when confronted with biases or prejudices about an individual or groups of students.

I am able to reduce social/institutional barriers that keep students from achieving their potential.

### Cultural Intelligence in Counseling

I can demonstrate sensitivity to others and skillfulness in relating to diverse individuals, groups, and classrooms.

I can recognize when my beliefs and values are interfering with providing the best services to my students.

I am aware as to how culture affects the help-seeking behaviors of students.

An individual's development is the totality of experiences and is greatly influenced by variables such as when one was born as well as the color of one's skin. Examining one's personal identity is a first step before one can explore the cultural norms and the diversity that represent others. Generational location strongly shapes how you see and live your life. Generations are influenced by the times and traditions that prevailed in any given period. The 1970s were about "breaking rules," the 1980s about "clouding conventions," and the 1990s about "getting by" in an era in which traditional rules no longer applied; these generational perspectives shape decisions, choices, and values (Howe & Strauss, 2000).

School counselors who embrace diversity understand the importance of crossing generational and cultural lines. "They make active attempts to learn about other cultures and interact with culturally different people (e.g., friends, colleagues); ... live and work effectively among different groups and types of people; understand the biases inherent in her or his own worldview and actively learns about alternative worldviews ... and are social activists, empowered to speak out against all forms of social injustice (e.g., racism, homophobia, sexism, ageism, domestic violence, religious stereotyping)" (Ponterotto, Utsey, & Pedersen, 2006, p. 130).

## DIVERSITY AND MULTICULTURALISM

When educators and community members refer to diversity in conversations in faculty rooms and classrooms, oftentimes race and ethnicity are what first come to mind. These terms are not interchangeable. Woolfolk (2001) defined *race* as "a group of people who share common biological traits (such as skin

# BOX 9.2

## *Reflections*

Self-reflection is an important component of professional identity (Council for Accreditation of Counseling and Related Educational Programs, 2009). Here are some questions that will guide you in reflecting on your own cultural identity and beliefs. Stop and reflect on them before continuing on.

1. What were the prevailing issues (social, historical, cultural, etc.) of your "developmental years" that helped to shape your thinking, belief system, and attitudes?
2. How did these issues influence or affect you, your family, and your relationships with your family?
3. How did the sum of all of these components create the person that you have become today?
4. How does your worldview affect how you work with or will work with students?

color, hair texture, etc.) that are seen as self defining by the people of the group" while *ethnicity* is presented as "**a cultural heritage shared by a group of people**" (p. 165).

In a broad context, diversity refers to the range of cultures and subcultures that represent attitudes, beliefs, values, rituals, symbols, norms and conventions, customs, behaviors, and ideologies (McDevitt & Ormond, 2007). School counselors recognize that diversity affects and influences the dynamics of learning, personal and social development, and school climate. The term *diversity-sensitive counseling* has been coined to reflect this wider range of variables (Baker, 2000). School counselors who seek further specific skill development acquire and develop intervention techniques that are appropriate to particular individuals or groups (Holcomb-McCoy, 2004).

The school experience can be supportive or disabling to our student populations. Regardless of the level of the work setting, school counselors must make a commitment to create a climate of caring and respect. Whether it is a racial slur or a comment about a student's ability to learn, school personnel are all too familiar with the tales told about some aspect of insensitivity in the school setting that has had a profound impact on student performance.

After race and ethnicity, culture is oftentimes the next thing that comes to mind when considering diversity. Culture is the sum total of ways of living including core beliefs, societal values, esthetics, patterns of thinking and communication, and behavioral norms that a group of people has developed to assure the group's position in a particular environment (Cooper, 1998). Culture is the response of a group of human beings to the valid and particular needs of its members and includes knowledge, values, traditions, and attitudes that guide the behavior of a group of people (Pedersen, 1991). Banks (2001) reminds us, "membership in a particular group does not determine behavior but makes certain types of behavior more probable" (pp. 13–14). We can gain insight about an individual's behavior, but we cannot assume to predict behavior. Most of us hold membership or have an identity with more than one group.

Traditionally, *race* and *ethnicity* are the terms that educators tend to consider when discussing the concept of **multiculturalism**. However, school counselors can take on a broader worldview that requires a look at multiculturalism as a "serious scholarship that includes all American peoples" (Halford, 1999, p. 9). "When we look around us, we realize that not all of us came from Europe. Many immigrated from Africa and Latin America, and others were already here in North America" (p. 9). School counselors must be most cognizant of norms that stem from the majority culture when working with students and their families (Holcomb-McCoy, 2007).

Multiculturalism is an awakening to our global interdependence. When working with children and youth, school counselors promote the ability to understand and appreciate differences and focus on the potential rather than on the prejudice. School counselors could approach all counseling as multicultural because each individual presents her or his unique blending of culture, heritage, and ability at the counselor's door. Pedersen (1991). suggested that multicultural counseling is a situation in which two or more persons, with different ways of perceiving their social environment, are brought together in a helping relationship; thus, cultural norms and expectations may vary between the counselor and the client (student).

Chisholm and Trumbull (2001) proposed a model that addresses a framework of individualism and collectivism that helps counselors better understand some of the large differences between the dominant Euro-American culture and new immigrants. For example, Hispanic students usually want to share what they have even at the expense of giving away a pen or pencil that leaves them without one to use in class, and they tend to want to work together to problem solve or help each other with an assignment or directions (Chisholm & Trumbull 2001). Asian students often present dress and religious affiliations that may stand out in a school setting (Axelson, 1999), while their cultural emphasis on restraint, respect for authority, and discretion may result in Asian American students choosing not to ask for help when needed (Spradlin & Parsons, 2008).

Counselors and teachers who understand that these cultural differences affect classroom behavior will clearly delineate the difference between students working together and working alone. "Singling out an individual's achievement can be seen as a negative in collectivistic groups because of its implicit slighting of other's abilities" (Chisholm & Trumbull, 2001, pp. 3, 4). This depth of understanding comes from taking the time to get to know the children, their families, and their culture through continuous communication. With the prediction from the U.S. Bureau of the Census (2009) that as many as one in 10 children will be foreign born, the value of understanding cultural differences becomes even more important to ensure student success in schools.

Cultural differences in our schools are often addressed by multicultural education, which teaches the value of cultural diversity (Sadker & Sadker, 2005). This is only one response to the increasingly racial, ethnic, and cultural diversity of our schools. Schools, as centers of learning, are in the best position to foster multicultural awareness in children and youth to encourage them to accept and appreciate cultural differences. Students and faculty need opportunities to acquire the experience, skills, awareness, and understanding to transcend the perceived barriers of differences (Johnson, 1995). Banks (2002) promotes multicultural education from a holistic perspective and emphasizes that it is much more than classroom instruction. One also faces challenges associated with acculturation in which the student identifies with the attitudes, behaviors, and values of the dominant culture (Lee, 2007a) while simultaneously relinquishing the traditions and customs associated with one's culture of origin (Spradlin & Parsons, 2008). Many young people seek to adapt to the dress, style, and lifestyle of the "American youth culture" and master the task of balancing an ethnic identity with one that will provide access to the mainstream culture. Students frequently find themselves caught between the two cultures (Lee, 2007a) and the expectations of family and peers.

What responsibility does the school counselor have in fostering a climate that is respectful of cultural diversity? School counselors should assume a critical position in social justice issues, advocate for marginalized youth, and be activists in schools and communities made up of predominantly poor and traditionally underserved families (Constantine, Hage, Kindaichi, & Bryant, 2007; Hipolito-Delgado & Lee, 2007). "Current perspectives on school counseling place advocacy at the core of the new vision of the profession" (Brown & Trusty, 2005a, p. 270). "Advocacy is the act of empowering individuals or groups through actions that increase self-efficacy, remove barriers to needed services, and promote systemic change" (McAuliffe, Grothaus, Pare, & Wininger, 2008, p. 613). Professional school counselors act as advocates for those who are marginalized by working with systems to address inequities in schools (Holcomb-McCoy, 2007).

School counselors are expected to "specifically address the needs of every student, particularly students of culturally diverse, low social-economic status, and other underserved or underperforming populations" (ASCA, 2005, p. 77). We do this by providing culturally competent counseling and consultation and through collaboration with all stakeholders to create a school climate that welcomes and appreciates the strengths and gifts of culturally diverse students (ASCA, 2009a).

One of the dilemmas that school counselors can help focus attention on is the overall impact of creating an empowering school climate that fosters an atmosphere of participation and acceptance. By identifying practices that may be inhibiting equity and access, it is necessary to seek ways to motivate staff and student interaction that transcends ethnic, cultural, and racial lines (Banks, 2002). These go far beyond moment-in-time interventions such as "Human Rights Days" and multicultural events. If an impact is to be made to create an environment that is empowering, accepting, and respectful, the process and planning must be

- multifaceted (varied in activity and services);
- inclusionary (engaging all school personnel, all students, and involve the community);
- developmental (proactive, not reactive in nature);
- continuous (ongoing); and
- supported throughout the school system (Johnson, 1995).

## BOX 9.3

### *Listen to Their Voices*

Student Perspective

My parents really care about my education. It is so hard for them to come to school as they are afraid of the language. I am not always a good translator.

We ran from country to country seeking a place to live and be free. Until that point I was always in school and did so well. Now I feel like I had to start all over.

I know I really need to learn English. I want to speak well. It is hard since I am the only one in my family that can speak English and Spanish.

My parents did not tell me we were moving forever. It was so hard to leave my home. I never had a chance to say good-bye to my friends. We just left. My parents said we had to leave to be safe.

In my country, if my brother and I didn't behave in school, we were slapped with a stick for things such as dropping books and forgetting homework. Here kids don't listen sometimes and no one does anything. I don't know why they do that. Our parents tell us to respect our teachers.

In this school, I know my teachers such as Miss Ann really care about me. That's why I came to talk to you today. I want you to care about me and what I want to become too.

Adult Perspective

These kids work harder than anyone else. School makes them happy. They make friends but we also make a second family for them. Many don't want to leave at the end of the school day ... they just like to hang out!

My students love interacting with each other—meeting others who are different from themselves but have similar stories to tell.

I use theater as the bond to get them to speak English. Imagine *A Midsummer Night's Dream* performed by ninth graders with 25 different accents representing their native languages. You have to love it and them. They want to learn to speak English and speak well.

They are hungry to learn. So many of our students had their education interrupted—war, famine, poverty, religious persecution. Their parents were looking for a safe and free world to raise them in.

I had a dialogue with a student about the negative implication of the word gay as he used it in a derogatory way. He stated, "I get it! It would be like if someone said that was so 'Mexican' if they were trying to say something is bad about me." He didn't really understand. This cultural inter-communication allowed my student to understand himself better and how his language could be viewed as hurtful by another person.

We listen, we hear. We have to go the extra mile. Each and every one deserves a chance for a bright and happy future.

Source: New York Institute of Technology: Listen to Their Voices: Newly Immigrated Students Speak Up! 2010.

In New York City alone, there are more than 20,000 designated students with interrupted formal schooling (New York City Department of Education, 2008). In large urban areas such as Los Angeles or New York City, 176 different languages are found, each representing a group of children whose heritage and ethnicity are far from the norm of what is considered traditional American culture (Roberts, 2010). Many immigrant students face the challenge of language acquisition. Custred (2002) makes the point that failure to ensure mastery of *theory to practice* of the "standard" language of American society will "deprive minorities of the tools necessary for productive entry into the economy and thus into society as a whole" (p. 237). For all of our newly immigrated students and for those whose first language at home is not English, this is an important reminder of the importance of blending academic progress with caring, understanding, and support. School counselors and teachers can help to foster resiliency by modeling empathy and ensuring that their school environment is conducive to making them feel that they belong, are competent, can learn, have opportunities to develop autonomy, and are safe. Changing the life trajectories of our newly immigrated youth from at-risk to resilient starts with changing the beliefs of adults in schools and communities.

## The Profile of a Culturally Competent School

Cultural competence is an integral component of school climate and the administration, faculty, and staff "promote inclusiveness and appropriate responses to difference as reflected by its policies, programs, and practices" (Nelson, Bustamante, Wilson, & Onwuegbuzie, 2008, p. 208). A school that has a broad view of cultural diversity includes not only differences in race and ethnic backgrounds but also "diverse sexual orientation, religious traditions, age groups and learning differences" and "typically invites everyone to learn and change" (p. 208). A school that is culturally competent

- recognizes the diversity of its students and promotes a sense of community around it;
- has high academic standards for all students;
- has a curriculum that reflects many cultures;
- has a mechanism for resolution of racial/cultural conflict;
- is committed to diversity among its staff; and
- provides staff development on culturally related issues.

You can assess your school's cultural competence in the following ways:

- Conducting a culture audit, which is a comprehensive means for assessing schoolwide cultural competence by identifying strengths and need areas to guide strategic planning.
- Collecting data from multiple sources regarding organizational policies, programs, practices, rituals, and artifacts that reflect the perspectives of diverse groups.
- Conducting surveys, interviews, and field observations (adapted from Nelson et al., 2008, pp. 208–10).

As a school counselor, your cultural lens will have a tremendous impact on your initial perception of others. Throughout your formative years, you were conditioned to see through the lenses provided by your family and environment. Cultural lenses filter our perception of others (Lehrer & Sloan, 2003). We view each other through the filters of our heritage, upbringing, race, religion, community, gender, and ethnicity (Bucher, 2008). Due to this perception, students form cliques and gangs within their own culture and oftentimes conflicts occur. Understanding our own culture and the culture of others gives us a better picture of ourselves and others. As our history constitutes an important part of our culture, listening to the stories that pass from generation to generation in our families helps us to develop a personal orientation. Inner curiosity motivates us to know our roots, where we come from, or where our families emigrated from. As we listen to the stories of others, we develop social awareness. How much do we know about the other students and families, especially those who have recently immigrated and whose cultural experiences differ dramatically from our own?

Self-awareness is only the beginning of multicultural awareness and cultural competence. Being aware of yourself as a cultural being has been described as a prerequisite for competent multicultural counseling. In fact, the first multicultural competency discussed by Sue, Arredondo, and McDavis (1992) stated, "Culturally skilled examiners have moved from being culturally unaware to being aware and sensitive to their own cultural heritage and to valuing and respecting differences" (p. 482).

When students are using inappropriate cultural lenses, school morale and students' grades will most likely be negatively affected. It is the job of the school counselor with the help of the teachers and the parents to sensitize the students to another way of viewing their peers through a different set of lenses. By wearing a different set of lenses, the students will have the opportunity to experience the world from the eyes of their peers who are a different culture, and they most likely will view school as a safe and harmonious environment where diverse student populations can peacefully coexist.

## Stereotyping

Intentional and unintentional **discrimination** affects both the equality and access to educational opportunities. The terms used for underrepresented students such as *at risk* and *culturally deprived* connote a bias. Thus, it is extremely important that all educators become self-reflective to identify stereotypes and biases. Limited knowledge regarding culturally diverse student populations creates challenges in the education of students considered minorities and not a part of the dominant culture. Biases and ethnocentrism, that is, the viewpoint that one's own group is the center of everything, can result in prejudice.

Students are frequently stereotyped by race and ethnicity. This **stereotyping** can become a self-fulfilling prophecy when students begin to see themselves through the expectations of their teachers and others. Stereotypes and discrimination can be internalized as "we become who others stereotype us to be instead of who we perceive ourselves to be" (Bucher, 2008, p. 45). For other students, they suffer from stereotype vulnerability and are afraid to even try for fear of perpetuating a stereotype. If some students have lost self-esteem and confidence and have succumbed to stereotypes and are no longer reaching for their potential, this will definitely impede achieving equity and access for all students. High expectations must be held and conveyed to all students.

> Recently, scientific research has shown that we can be fully committed to fairness and equality, yet still possess negative prejudices and hold on to stereotypes (Bucher, 2008). To continue to build cultural intelligence and become more culturally competent in working with children and their families, we have to maintain

self-motivation to make a long-term commitment to learn, change, and adapt. That motivation is based on understanding the value of cultural intelligence. However, social psychologists have found that "changing one's attitude does not necessarily lead to a change in behavior ... our behavior drives our attitudes." (Bucher, 2008, p. 212)

School counselors can model the continuous cycle of learning, acting, and reflecting. By placing ourselves in circumstances where we work with culturally diverse individuals, we'll find our biases to be unfounded and grow in cultural competence as we learn to understand ourselves and others as well. "Bias can be reduced significantly when members of racially and culturally mixed groups work together to accomplish common goals" (Bucher, 2008, p. 223). Awareness and skill development are essential to build cultural intelligence and become more culturally competent when working with children and families. Bucher presents "Nine megaskills," which are vital to cultural understanding (2008). The first megaskill is understanding one's own cultural identity and reflecting on the "cultural silo," experiences that restrict or limit our thinking and cultural understanding (Bucher, 2008, p. 39). This helps to develop one's sense of uniqueness so that in turn, others will be respected. Next, it is important to be aware and "check our culture lens" and recognize that each person possesses her or his own unique cultural lens. Third, becoming globally conscious will assist one in crossing cultural boundaries so that she or he will be able "to appreciate the talents and contributions of all people and cultures" (2008, p. 98). Another important megaskill is to shift perspectives. This means showing that we are trying to understand, listening with empathy, and "taking the role of the other" (2008, p. 105). The fifth megaskill is promoting intercultural communication, which involves being conscious of how we exclude people when we communicate, recognizing cultural miscommunications and learning to listen (2008). Another megaskill that is vital to cultural understanding is managing cross-cultural conflict. Conflict is viewed as a way "to learn more about ourselves and others" (2008, p. 173). Multicultural teaming, recognizing bias of ourselves and others, and understanding the dynamics of power when related to our position as school counselors are the last three megaskills essential in attempting to achieve cultural competence and intelligence. School counselors are professionally obligated to seek to enhance their own cultural competence and facilitate the cultural awareness, knowledge, and skills of all school personnel (ASCA, 2009a).

# DIVERSITY BEYOND CULTURE

## Social Class Distinctions and Poverty

There was a time when social class identification was synonymous with wealth, power, stature, and prestige. Children are acutely aware of upper-class, middle-class, and lower-class economic and social characteristics (Sadker & Sadker, 2005). Power and prestige are not always synonymous with wealth. Politicians and professors may have influence but often do not have the economic baseline to access upper-class social circles. Social class is influenced by perception. Values have begun to transcend what had been previously perceived as racial and ethnic barriers to demographic change

TABLE **9.1**

Percentage of Public School Fourth Graders Eligible for Free or Reduced-Price Lunch, by School Locale and Race/Ethnicity, 2009

| Race/Ethnicity | Total | City | Suburban | Town | Rural |
|---|---|---|---|---|---|
| Total[1] | 48 | 62 | 39 | 52 | 42 |
| White | 29 | 31 | 21 | 39 | 34 |
| Black | 74 | 80 | 65 | 83 | 72 |
| Hispanic | 77 | 82 | 70 | 84 | 72 |
| Asian/Pacific Islander | 34 | 45 | 25 | 41 | 23 |
| American Indian/Alaska Native | 68 | 67 | 52 | 70 | 72 |

Source: U.S. Department of Education, National Center for Education Statistics, National Assessment of Educational Progress (NAEP), 2009 Mathematics Assessment, NAEP Data Explorer.

whether these reference child-rearing practices or manicured lawns. Neighbors find that they have more in common with those of similar wealth, who share similar values, and are more accepting of racial, ethnic, and cultural differences (Woolfolk, 2009).

Educational aspirations are reflective of communities and school systems and the gap continues to widen among the "haves" and the "have nots" (Haycock, 2001). Low-income youth and children from affluent communities should have the same access to educational opportunity (House & Martin, 1998). This may not always be the case. As depicted in Table 9.1, the economic downturn and recession significantly increased the numbers of students eligible for free and/or reduced-price lunch, creating a widening of the gap for children who already had limited access to resources.

Although there are exceptions, poor students who attend poverty-stricken school systems usually have less opportunity as they progress toward high school graduation and postsecondary access, and this is more apparent as we examine the college attendance rates as shown in Table 9.2.

The data on the low-socioeconomic status of students of color and their families are cause for alarm. The 2010 census data revealed that 13.2 percent of all families of all races had incomes below the poverty level. The percentage

TABLE **9.2**

Four-Year College Attendance Rates by Income

| Achievement Level in Quartiles | Low Income | High Income |
|---|---|---|
| First (low) | 8% | 25% |
| Second | 16% | 42% |
| Third | 31% | 70% |
| Fourth (high) | 58% | 86% |

Source: Aud, S., Fox, M., and Kewal-Ramani, A. (2010). National Center for Education Statistics.

of families in this category increased dramatically for minority families. Rothstein (2008) reminds us that African American and Hispanic children are more likely to experience persistent poverty and continue to live in areas of concentrated poverty. The rise in the numbers of children of color has also increased the proportion of those living below the poverty line. Children who live in high-poverty communities have different life exposures, which include lack of access to public services and quality health care, poorly equipped schools, street violence, homelessness, drug racketeering, etc. (Rothstein, 2008). Children of poverty often live in single-parent homes, and most often, the single parent is a woman. When the head of household is female with no husband present, the poverty level almost triples (U.S. Bureau of the Census, 2009). These factors significantly influence each child's quality of life, school achievement, high school graduation, and ability to have all options after high school, including college. Closing the achievement gap requires a close examination of the socioeconomic inequalities that affect many students from underserved and underrepresented populations. Without closing the opportunity and information gap, the achievement gap will persist indefinitely.

Studies show that high-SES students stay in school longer and have higher levels of achievement (Conger, Conger, & Elder, 1997; Education Trust, 2001b; McLoyd, 1998). Students who are caught in a cycle of poverty are also caught in a cycle of low expectations. These cycles are self-perpetuating unless there is direct intervention on the part of educators to focus their efforts on both the obvious and the underlying symptoms. Several other contributing factors to perpetuating the cycle include low expectations, learned helplessness, peer influences, and resistance (Amatea & West-Olatunji, 2007; Gordon, 2006). Each of these factors offers additional insight and opportunities for school counselors. For example, students from poverty may not wear the "trendy" clothes that other young adolescents and teens consider as essential to their wardrobes; they may have little or no experience with cultural icons such as museums, theaters, and public libraries. Equally important, they often come to school with less background knowledge and fewer family supports (Payne, 2008).

### Self-Confidence

Students of poverty may also believe that it is extremely difficult or next to impossible to be successful (Gordon, 2006; McLoyd, 1998; Payne, 2008). As you may recall from Chapter 1, income is directly related to educational attainment. Low **socioeconomic status** (SES) children, particularly students of color, may firmly believe that they do not have access to participate in mainstream America (Payne, 2008). For some students making it in school, being successful, and getting good grades is translated by their peers to mean that they sold out or are acting "White," acting "Black," or acting "middle class" (Johnson & Duffet, 2005). This perspective affects students' ability to maintain stature in their peer group and they must reject the behaviors that would make them successful. This can result in insecurities about jumping into classroom discussions or an inability to participate in field trips resulting from a lack of self-confidence and low self-esteem (Conger, Conger, & Elder,

1997). Yet many adolescents are high achievers, despite their economic situation or pressure from peers (O'Connor, 1997). Regardless of race or ethnic background, young Americans believe that attending college makes a significant difference in how they will fare in the world (Wadsworth & Remaley, 2007, p. 26). Regardless of each student's economic status, school counselors are in an ideal position to identify the issues that stratify opportunity and work collaboratively with faculty and staff to close the achievement gap. No significant learning can occur without building a significant and respectful relationship (Comer, 1995).

### Ability Grouping

The national debate around ability grouping, which is a more contemporary interpretation of "tracking," continues to place attention on gate keeping vs. door opening. Ability grouping sorts students based on capability and should offer more flexibility to students who excel in one subject but need more reinforcement in another. Tracking suggests more permanence and can divide students from each other (Sadker & Zittelman, 2006) as students are assigned to classes based on above-average, average, or below-average achievement. Many educators believe that it is simpler for students with similar skills, aptitude, and intellectual ability to learn together in a homogeneous class (Sadker & Sadker, 2005; Sadker & Zittelman, 2006). When educators follow this belief, they sort students into groups based on their abilities and as a result set them on an educational path that can predetermine their futures. Parents and peers also influence these academic choices as students of the same race, ethnicity, and/or social class may find themselves in the same school "track," which can also lead to unintended racial segregation. *Tracking* is the term given to this process.

Although there are many complex arguments that focus on tracking and detracting, for purposes of this text, two basic philosophies are presented. The first one is homogeneously grouping students of similar ability together for purposes of remediation and acceleration. The second emphatically asserts that tracking stands in the way of equal educational opportunity (Loveless, 1999; Sadker & Zittelman, 2006). What is the appropriately ethical way to proceed? Reflect on the role that school counselors have played in the past on this commonplace practice of tracking or ability grouping by class.

School counselors have been part of the system that sorts and selects students according to perceived ability and/or achievement (Hart & Jacobi, 1992). School counselors have supported tracking systems by failing to inform students appropriately about the outcome and consequences of course assignment and placement (Hart & Jacobi, 1992). Tracking students has been the modus operandi in American education for many years. Children learn at an early age that they are sorted, selected, ranked, re-grouped, and classified according to ability as they compete each day for teacher approval, stickers, rewards, grades, bumper stickers, and access to honors and upper-level courses. Tracking also adds a socialization dimension to education. Expectations of teachers and parents differ and are dependent on student placement. Oftentimes differentiated instructional materials are selected for use in class, and adjustments are made in the rate of learner response and the teacher's delivery of the curriculum. Students, even the youngest, are aware of where they are placed and what level of achievement is expected of them.

A study by Stone (1998) revealed that placement into ninth-grade algebra was largely dependent on a student's socioeconomic status and school assignment. The ninth-grade mathematics placements for 6,000 students in this urban school district were examined. Low-SES students in the upper quartile on eighth-grade mathematics were not uniformly placed into algebra, despite their ability. Instead, they were placed into the general mathematics courses. Placement also was directly related to the attendance boundaries that defined which middle school a student attended. These also reflected the socioeconomic environment of the local community. Schools in the affluent areas of the city placed upper-quartile mathematics students into algebra at much higher rates while the low SES schools largely ignored algebra as an option for their students.

Critics of tracking suggest that it can be eliminated and students who arrive to school with diverse backgrounds can learn from each other and together (Sadker & Sadker, 2005). Detracked schools can become learning communities but teachers need time and support so that all can succeed—student and teacher. Although ability grouping should be more flexible and focus on closing the opportunity and information gaps, school counselors must be mindful that students are not isolated along cultural, racial, or economic lines and perpetuate in-school segregation (Spradlin & Parsons, 2008). School counselors have a moral and ethical responsibility to examine practices and policies that affect any student's right to a quality education. Predetermining a student's future is an action that speaks louder than words. School counselors can either support or challenge the philosophies and procedures that stratify opportunities for students.

## Gender Equity and Inequity

There is a tradition of thinking that suggests:

- girls do better in some subjects than boys do;
- some careers are for men and some careers are better suited for women;
- science and math are difficult for girls;
- girls and boys use computers for different purposes; and
- men and women receive unequal pay for equal work in certain job titles (Sadker & Sadker, 2005).

The question is not whether boys and girls are different in their learning, behaviors, personality traits, and interests, but rather, in what ways are boys and girls different? (Spradlin & Parsons, 2008). Figure 9.2 highlights researched-based differences.

The challenges of becoming a diversity-sensitive school counselor require an examination of the impact of gender differences on student success in school. For many, this may not be as obvious as race, ethnicity, and cultural differences when we work with students. Gender differences can influence what is expected as the "norm" and can contribute to some of the fundamental differences in

| Boys | Girls |
|------|-------|
| problems with homework | organized |
| distracted and restless | focused |
| low organization | higher grades |
| low preparation | good study habits |
| do not think school is important | care about education |
| lack of concern about education | cool to be smart |
| discipline problems | behavior well suited for classrooms |
| get over problems quickly | drag out problems |

FIGURE **9.2** Perceived Gender Differences in School

Source: Clark, Yacco, & Rant (2007)

---

personality development for boys and girls in the traditions of some cultures (Lee, 1998). Erickson's identity and intimacy stages influence male and female development differently and influence relationship building (Gilligan, 1993). However, like other forms of discrimination, messages of sexism may be subtle (Sadker & Sadker, 2005). Counselors and teachers may not always be aware of the messages that are communicated and how these affect student behavior and student choices.

**Gender** refers to the judgments that are made about femininity and masculinity, and often these are influenced by culture and context. Gender is a learned psychological, social, and cultural aspect of a person that describes expected and sanctioned male and female behavior that results from socialization (Spradlin & Parsons, 2008). This differs from sex, which refers specifically to biological conditions of maleness or femaleness (Woolfolk, 2009): the possession of the XY chromosomal configuration for males and the possession of the XX pattern for females (Spradlin & Parsons, p. 15). Gender identities form at an early age when girls and boys take on social and cognitive roles that are associated with a specific orientation of masculine or feminine. As their concept of their world develops, young children receive clues about distinctions between what is considered male and female. This is evidenced in that girls play with dolls and boys play with trucks; girls wear pink and boys wear blue. As children grow older they become more attuned to role models of their own gender. Their awareness of gender differences takes on a greater level of sophistication and this has implications for their self-concept and behaviors. As students move into adolescence their ideas about gender help them determine how they measure up to gender roles. Children and adolescents form mental images of what girls are supposed to do and what boys are supposed to do. Parents contribute to stereotypical expectations by setting different boundaries for girls and boys when it comes to personal safety. Societal influences and those of family, peers, and the larger community can reinforce the need to stay within boundaries (Ruble & Martin, 1998; Ward, 2002).

Traditional gender-role orientation can influence how we view students, raise children, and our personal worldview. Sometimes this appears as a bias in behavior that is translated into verbal phrases such as "boys will be boys" when classroom or playground behavior becomes unruly. Researchers also have discovered that teachers tend to interact more with boys than girls (Bailey, 1993; Gurian, 2001; Sadker & Sadker, 2005). Oftentimes teachers, parents, and even school counselors reinforce stereotypical expectations by not insisting that both male and female high school students continue their studies in math and in the sciences. Exceptions are made for female students more frequently than male students, thus reinforcing expectations around achievement related to gender (Sadker & Sadker, 2005).

Gender expectations can also affect students' career decision making, course-taking patterns, desire for "good grades," involvement in after-school activities, sports, and hobbies (Clark, Lee, Goodman, & Yacco, 2008). Recently, educational aspirations and postsecondary education completion have become female dominated. Data (NCES, 2008) have revealed that women earned the majority of associate's, bachelor's, and master's degrees. Educators' opinions of students can drastically affect student motivation and achievement. If a student believes that a counselor or teacher does not care about her or his contributions in class because of gender, or because of any other individual characteristic, a student can unconsciously and permanently lose interest and the willingness to work harder and to pursue her or his dream.

What can school counselors do? Here are some areas that are worthy of attention that school counselors can address:

- Becoming cognizant of any unintentional biases that may exist in delivering group or classroom activities. This bias could involve grouping students by gender or favoring one gender over another in the delivery or processing of the activity.
- Consciously and intentionally call on boys and girls equally.
- Utilizing current data and analyzing the trends that affect the aspirations and motivation of the student population in their care.
- Encouraging all students to explore their interests and realize their dreams. We need to pay close attention to the stereotyping of career paths and to what are considered traditional and nontraditional occupations from both our perspective and that of others (Graham & Taylor, 2002; Turner, Conkel, Starkey, Landgraf, Lapan, Stewart, & Huang, 2008). Career decision making is closely aligned with educational planning.
- Becoming "gate openers," not "gatekeepers." We can play an influential role in every student's course selection to ensure that talent and interest are nurtured. Upper-level math, science, and technology courses must become part of every student's academic portfolio to ensure later success and access to quality postsecondary opportunities.
- Addressing the influence of bias in language. Using words such as *department chairperson* instead of *chairman* are more in tune with an equal opportunity environment. Tendencies to use terms such as *OK, guys* can also reinforce a gender bias. Additionally, language should be inclusive and affirming and not discriminate in its intent.

School counselors can put aside personal gender prejudices and biases to encourage student initiative and motivate colleagues to do the same. Working with teachers to foster cooperative learning and teamwork in the classroom will help students feel that contributions of their own gender are important and noteworthy.

## Sexual Identity

Human sexuality is complex and refers to the degree to which we identify with the social and biological aspects of being a man or a woman (Spradlin & Parsons, 2008). Sexual orientation is part of sexual identity and is defined by who we are emotionally and/or to whom we are physically attracted (p. 18). Questioning is also an important consideration for educators to address as students may be "questioning" their sexual orientation at any point over the lifespan of the school year.

Sexual minority youth, as they progress through elementary, middle, and secondary schools in the United States, are confronted every day with taunts, epithets, and a host of other, negative, insulting, and derogatory words from their peers that are intended to bring them into conformity with the dominant majority culture's view of "normal" sexuality (i.e., a heterosexual or opposite-sex sexual orientation; Pope, 2004, p. 31). Peer-to-peer interactions can at times be cruel, especially during these formative years. A student who is questioning her or his sexual identity is often subject to stereotypical taunting or ridicule and fear being shunned as a classmate, friend, team member, and/or club participant (Chen-Hayes, 2000; McFarland & Dupuis, 2001). In public schools, 97 percent of students regularly hear homophobic comments from their peers (Parker, 2001). All students regardless of their sexual identity or sexual orientation are entitled to learn, grow, and develop in a bias-free environment.

What can school counselors do? School counselors have an ethical responsibility to be proactive in their attitudes and behaviors with students and colleagues around bias, sexual discrimination, sexual harassment, and sexual orientation and promote a school climate that permits students to study and socialize without fear of repercussion or stigma.

Additionally, we can

- help students become aware of their use of heterosexist or homophobic language in the classroom and in the hallways;
- intercede immediately when overhearing a hurtful remark;
- avoid heterosexist language that stereotypes male and female relationships; and
- use appropriate terminology and language when talking about Lesbian, Gay, Bisexual, Transgendered, and Questioning (LGBTQ) youth issues with colleagues and with students.

Support your students by withholding assumptions about sexuality and not assuming a particular student is "straight"; this assumption suggests that gay and lesbian students are invisible. Make sure you communicate to your students that you are a safe person to speak with and you can use a "safe zone" symbol such as a rainbow button or sticker to identify yourself as a safe person. Create a list of resources for students and families needing information and work collaboratively with colleagues to create guidelines for classroom discussions that include alternative family configurations and provide the perspectives and voices of the LGBTQ community.

Research suggests that sexual minority youth will first disclose that they are gay, lesbian, or questioning to a school counselor rather than other school personnel (Harris & Bliss, 1997). Professional school counselors must be prepared to work with sexual minority students when they present themselves for counseling (Pope, 2004).

As advocates and leaders, school counselors can develop and implement policies that eradicate the verbal and physical harassment of all students, including sexual minority students (Pope, 2004). All students are entitled to learn in an environment that is bias- and harassment-free.

# CREATING A CULTURALLY COMPATIBLE CLIMATE

Demographics and conceptual changes are reshaping America's schools. Given all of the variables that comprise diversity, school counselors and educators are challenged on a daily basis to respond to the needs of every student. Culturally compatible schools ensure that an atmosphere of respect, understanding, and caring for students is at the heart of the learning community. School counselors play an important role in fostering this environment.

ASCA reminds us that school counselors can use a variety of strategies to heighten the awareness and sensitivity of students and parents to culturally diverse persons and thus enhance the school environment (ASCA, 1999a). Counselors have the ability to consult with school personnel to identify the alienating factors in attitudes and beliefs impeding the learning ability of culturally diverse students and to ensure that students' rights are respected (ASCA, 1999a).

The Association for Multicultural Counseling and Development (AMCD) developed competencies (Arredondo et al., 1996; Sue, Arredondo, & Davis, 1992) around three domains: counselor awareness of own values and biases, counselor awareness of client's worldview, and culturally appropriate intervention strategies. Within each domain are competency areas: beliefs and attitudes; knowledge; and skills. Currently, AMCD has established 117 behavioral, outcome-based explanatory statements (1996) that can serve school counselors as well as learning goals (Arredondo & Arciniega, 2001).

Although one can acquire knowledge from a textbook, nothing can replace the awareness gained and the skills acquired from getting to know the students, their families, and the community in which they live. As you observe students' interactions, be sensitive to their beliefs, and try to understand the cultural sway that influence their way of thinking and responding.

ASCA's National Standards (Campbell & Dahir, 1997) specifically encourage school counselors to ensure that students will acquire the skills to understand and respect self and others. This serves as a reminder for school counselors to look beyond self-esteem and to focus attention on students' knowledge of self and acquiring how to extend respect to relationships with others. School counselors can powerfully influence colleagues to move beyond the traditional cultural exchange and focus the conversation on all aspects of diversity. Thus, all members of the school community can better understand the influence of culture on learning and life styles and consider class, race, ethnicity, gender, socioeconomic status, sexual orientation, and language. Cultural norms and expectations can also influence developmental benchmarks, sexual behavior, and educational choices.

In a culturally compatible climate the concept of respect for self and others is woven throughout the fabric of our schools and becomes part of the teaching and learning environment. The institution itself is oriented toward social harmony and cooperation. School counselors can provide the initiative and leadership to ensure that developmentally appropriate activities are an integral part of the school-counseling program and are directly linked to fostering a climate built on respect and caring.

School counselors can reinforce and extend awareness from the school to home and community and promote the need for effective school communication between home and school. Parents and/or caretakers need to feel welcome to ask questions, understand expectations, and learn strategies to help their children succeed. School counselors have a moral responsibility and ethical obligation to bridge the gap between school and home. For newly immigrated parents, guardians or caretakers, for those who are culturally or ethnically different from the majority in your community, for those who are uncomfortable with situations that are intimidating because of their personal educational attainment or experience, school counselors accept and embrace an advocacy role. Student success relies heavily on parental support and parental involvement.

## CHALLENGING BELIEFS AND CHANGING BEHAVIORS

Educational expectations continue to evolve and all educators must become open and sensitive to the preconceived attitudes and biases that may exist about students. Twenty-first-century schools are social arenas in which students that represent truly diverse behavioral styles, attitudes and orientations, and different value systems are brought together with one goal in mind, which is to maximize their potential as human beings (Lee, 1998).

Have school counselors "become the academic conscience of the school, insuring that the school remains focused on student achievement and accepts responsibility for student outcomes" (Hart & Jacobi, 1992, p. 49) as suggested many years ago? When school counselors embrace the ethical and moral obligation to reduce and eliminate the institutional and/or social barriers that may stand in the way of every student's academic, career, or personal-social development (Dahir & Stone, 2009; Lee, 2007a; Lee & Walz, 1998), they advance the moral dimensions of school to include a strong social justice agenda to "close the gap," especially for diverse populations of students who have been traditionally underserved or underrepresented.

School counselors now face the challenge of working with diverse student populations. Unique in its diversity, this is a generation that has aspirations for financial success, high expectations for educational achievement, and significant social pressures. It is also the first generation that has experienced emotional trauma as a result of a declaration of war by terrorists here on home soil and a decade of turmoil abroad. Youthful uniqueness and the many aspects of diversity that exist in schools is a positive force not to be shunned or ignored. School counselors are in a unique position to do the following:

- Examine policies and practices that address student placement in ability groups or individual courses to ensure equity and access among all student populations.
- Provide professional development on key diversity issues at faculty meetings including ethnicity, culture, gender, social class, and sexual orientation to create a bias-free and respectful school climate.
- Encourage faculty to explore issues of culture and diversity in the context of the curriculum and to use teachable moments to extend learning.
- Work with school leadership teams to promote sensitivity and bias-free language.
- Seek awareness, knowledge, and skill to work with cultural diversity of the student population that comprises your school.
- Support students who have declared their sexual orientation as gay, lesbian, transgender, questioning, or bisexual.
- Sponsor family group meetings to help new immigrants understand and address meaningful issues such as negotiating the school system, especially for those whose first language is not English.
- Seek to identify resources that will help to close the opportunity gap between privileged and less-privileged students.
- Make yourself known as a "safe person" to whom all students can talk.
- Advocate for a fair student code of conduct, equitable course taking options, and high educational attainment.
- Act as a visible and vocal social justice advocate for all students regardless of gender, race, ethnicity, culture, religion, sexual orientation, ability, or disability.

Changing attitudes and beliefs is no easy task; school counselors will face denial and resistance from colleagues. "If I wait long enough this will go away, or they will go away." Many will say, "We don't do that; we are not prejudiced." "We treat all students equally." Educators as a rule are good people with good intentions. Colleagues sometimes need support to examine their belief system and not focus on what was. Without sincere reflection on current practices, schools cannot move forward and create systemic change (Stone & Dahir, 2011). Resistance will be the modus operandi and is often accompanied by self-doubt, blame, anger, discord, and withdrawal. Similarly, it is important to also help students and colleagues eliminate pervasive stereotyping that can impair their ability to assess others appropriately (Ramirez & Smith, 2007). School personnel can explore biases and prejudices that result in stereotyping and search for alternative practices and seek solutions in eliminating practices that do not foster equality, harmony, and respect. School counselors must take action to ensure that strategies are in place to celebrate, value, and appreciate diversity within the school environment and beyond.

## BOX 9.4

### *Self-Assessment for Counseling Diverse Students*

Consider where you are on the continuum of acquiring knowledge and honing skills. Answer each question, then develop a plan for professional and personal growth.

1.  Am I familiar with strategies that promote equity when working with diverse student populations (e.g., utilizing culturally/gender relevant counseling practices, empathizing with and understanding the students' worldview)?
    Yes _____ Need to know more _____ No _____
    Action planned:_____
    _____

2.  Am I familiar with verbal and nonverbal language patterns of different ethnic/cultural groups in my school?
    Yes _____ Need to know more _____ No _____
    Action planned:_____
    _____

3.  Do I have high expectations for all students and assist students to acquire resources and opportunities necessary for success?
    Yes _____ Need to know more _____ No _____
    Action planned:_____
    _____

4.  In working with diverse student populations, do I consider the interaction of gender differences, class differences, language differences, and cultural differences?
    Yes _____ Need to know more _____ No _____
    Action planned:_____
    _____

5.  Do I provide career counseling on the basis of the students' abilities, interests, and skills rather than according to traditional roles based on gender, race, disability, or ethnicity?
    Yes _____ Need to know more _____ No _____
    Action planned:_____
    _____

6.  Do I encourage students to take courses nontraditional to their gender, race, disability, or ethnicity if the student shows an interest in one of those areas (e.g., mathematics, science, computer technology for girls and early childhood education for boys)?
    Yes _____ Need to know more _____ No _____
    Action planned:_____
    _____

7.  Do I assess and reflect on my values, attitudes, and beliefs and have the ability to refrain from imposing them on the student?
    Yes _____ Need to know more _____ No _____
    Action planned:_____
    _____

*(continues)*

## Box **9.4**

8. Do I participate in inservice programs or special skill sessions for counselors dealing with culturally diverse students?
Yes _____ Need to know more _____ No _____
Action planned:_____
_____

9. Do I meet with students outside of the office to show an interest in their needs beyond the classroom?
Yes _____ Need to know more _____ No _____
Action planned:_____

10. Do I use a multidimensional approach to identify the level and scope of a student's ability to succeed before recommending course selection, placement, and future schooling/career opportunities?
Yes _____ Need to know more _____ No _____
Action planned:_____
_____

Our effectiveness will rely on our ability and our ability to engage others to

- listen to students and hear their voices and their stories;
- take the necessary risk to make sure no student is left out of the success picture;
- ask questions and eliminate the excuses and "yea buts" from others' responses;
- challenge yourself and your assumptions and don't be afraid to bring others along; and
- seek multiple ways to help every student find success.

The 50th anniversary of the *Brown v. Board of Education* Supreme Court decision (1954) reminded us that without public education children would likely be segregated into school settings that reflected their racial, ethnic, cultural, or religious background. Without the common denominator of public school, perhaps people in general would be more divided and more fearful of those different from themselves. Schools as important learning and social communities are significant conduits in promoting understanding, acceptance, respect, and harmony.

School counselors must seek ways of collaboration that address diversity in our schools in a meaningful way. This is not only a challenge but also a moral and ethical responsibility. Acting as advocates and leaders, school counselors ensure that the diverse needs of our students are reflected in the teaching and learning environment of the place called school. It is through changing attitudes and behaviors that positive and constructive change occurs. Part of this responsibility is the reflection and introspection that is essential for school counselors to grow personally as well as professionally

(Holcomb-McCoy, 2007). Whether counselors are able to provide comprehensive counseling programs and services that are unbiased and culturally appropriate for students and their families can make a huge difference in student achievement, particularly with traditionally underserved and underrepresented students (Holcomb-McCoy, 2005). Accountability and responsiveness to the obvious and subtle needs of our diverse student populations presents a challenge that reflects the nature of participating in a democratic society and investing in the future.

## TECH TOOLS

- Explore the National Center of Education Statistics website to follow trends and shifts in population demographics nationally. Compare your findings to your state and local demographics: http://nces.ed.gov/pubs2010/2010015/tables/table_1a.asp.
- Want to know more about your own heritage? Genealogical websites provide insight about your family's background. You can use these tools with colleagues to better understand your ethnic and cultural heritage.
- Keeping up with federal and state laws to ensure compliance with the needs of special/exceptional student education is a challenge. Go to the Office of Special Education Programs (OSEP) at http://www2.ed.gov/about/offices/list/osers/osep/index.html?src=mr.
- Stay abreast of current initiatives and legislative changes in IDEA. Check out your state department of education's website that is devoted to exceptional/special education. Also go to the Council for Exception Children page at www.cec.sped.org for information and resources.
- Consider the ethical and legal implications of technology, including issues of equity and access. Take a look at the ASCA Ethical Standards at www.schoolcounselor.org and consider the implications.
- You have learned that socioeconomic status influences school success. Review the Children's Defense Fund website at www.childrensdefense.org/ to find out more about what you can do to advocate for the needs of every child.
- Use the test locator published by Buros Institute of Mental Measurement to research various instruments that are used in your local school district at www.unl.edu/buros/.
- Polish your presentation skills by looking at websites such as www.ncjrs.org/pdffiles1/ojjdp/178997.pdf. You will need to download Adobe Acrobat to read PDFs such as this one. Then use presentation software as a tool to educate, guide, and inform students, faculty, colleagues, and parents about the diverse needs of students in our schools.
- The National Center for Education Statistics (http://nces.ed.gov/nceskids/) has a KIDS ZONE on its homepage. Check out the easy-to-use *How to Make a Graph* section to present data you have on your students.
- The National Center for Education Statistics has data tables for you to examine the different patterns of changing demographics: http://nces.ed.gov/programs/projections/projections2018/tables.asp#Group1.

- *Teaching Tolerance* has many resources to support your work with diverse student populations: www.tolerance.org/.
- The Center on Education Policy provides research, papers, and information on school improvement: www.cep-dc.org/.
- The Education Trust: www.edtrust.org/issues/higher-education.

---

# School Counselor Casebook: Voices from the Field

## The Scenario Reviewed

At the end of the first quarter, a classroom teacher asks you to come to observe four students who he believes are not working up to their ability. The students are not getting along with others in the class and not completing assignments in a timely manner. He does not believe that they are keeping up with the expectations for the fourth-grade class and not sure if they are appropriately placed in a regular education classroom. You agreed to observe the students and review the findings with him. You are also aware that these four students represent various racial and ethnic backgrounds.

## A Practitioner's Approach

Here's how a practicing school counselor responded to the school counselor casebook challenge:

On visiting the classroom, I notice that these four students are the only culturally diverse students in the class. That is the only difference visually. As this is a middle-class school, all of the children are well dressed and all have the necessary school supplies required.

What I do notice rather quickly is how the teacher manages his classroom. Questions are directed to the other students in the class. Those students are encouraged to answer the questions. I observe the four students in question. Manuela begins to talk to the student next to him. Tamika and Shawn are taking notes. Roberto is distracted and talking to the students around him, with them asking him to stop. This continues for the remainder of the period. After class, I ask the teacher if this is typical. He replies that it is, though it has escalated recently. We discuss parent contact. The teacher shows me his parent contact log, which shows he has contacted all the parents. The parents promised to help their children with homework and discuss proper behavior with them. I told the teacher I would meet with each of the four students and re-confer with him.

When I spend time with each student individually, I see a different side to each child. Each child is engaging and verbal. Tamika expresses her frustration that she feels invisible in the classroom. She goes on to tell me that no matter how hard she tries to participate, the teacher never calls on her. Tamika feels that this is why the children in her class ignore her; she feels she is not one of the "teacher's pets."

Shawn spoke with me about missing his dad. He said that sometimes that distracts him. Shawn also says that he feels bad when he knows the answer, but is not called on when he raises his hand. He goes on to say that he feels embarrassed when he is not paying attention and gets called on and does not know the answer. Shawn sometimes feels that his classmates think he's "dumb" because of this.

Manuela and Roberto both expressed that they like working together or with other students in the class, but they always seem to get into trouble because they are "talking" in class. They both feel their classmates perceive them as troublemakers and avoid them.

As I review my notes on each session, the situation begins to make sense to me. As school counselors we have a responsibility to shift the focus of attention to create an overall school climate of full participation and acceptance. With that responsibility, we need to focus on student potential rather than stereotypical expectations.

I spoke with the teacher about my observations. He admitted he wasn't aware of how much the absence of Shawn's father in his daily life had an effect on him. I explained to the teacher that I would be setting up a meeting with Shawn's mom to discuss this issue with her. I also said that I would be seeing Shawn on a regular basis individually to work with him on the issues that are affecting him academically and social-emotionally.

I discussed with the teacher the idea of using the workshop model, which will group the students in clusters for instruction and for learning activities. This will help not only the four students he is concerned about but motivate all of the students to interact with each other in group activities. Students would experience learning, acquire social skills, and practice the strategies in small groups. Every student would be engaged in collaborative learning through participation in individual and group activities.

As an aside, I did have a private conversation with the teacher. I asked him in a friendly and honest discussion to explore his personal beliefs and attitudes about culturally diverse populations. Sometimes we all have stereotypes that we don't even realize we are bringing into the classroom or a counseling session. Sometimes we do work with cultures that we are unfamiliar with. School counselors have an ethical responsibility to teach awareness and sensitivity to all stakeholders. Self-reflection is sometimes the first step.

Marjorie Miller has been a middle school counselor in the New York City public schools for 12 years, and prior to that she worked on the college level as assistant director for student services for six years. Marjorie is an active member of the New York State School Counselor Association.

# LOOKING BACK: SALIENT POINTS

## Promoting a Social Justice Agenda

Today's schools mirror the changing demographics and diversity reflected in our communities. Census data show that minority population growth in the

United States is based on age distribution, birthrate, and immigration patterns. Public schools are a place where children can learn to get along with others in a diverse society. Schools must become the primary institutions to create cohesion among diverse groups. School counselors have a responsibility to value culture, race, ethnicity, gender, socioeconomic status and social class, sexual orientation, and promote awareness and acceptance among all student groups.

## The Influence of Culture on Counseling

School counselors recognize and acknowledge personal biases and prejudices that can influence their approach to counseling, guiding, advising, and encouraging students. Personal sensitivity to diversity also helps school counselors to determine how culture influences a student's perception of the problem and the choice of intervention.

## Diversity and Multiculturalism

In a broad worldview, diversity refers to the range of cultures and subcultures that represent attitudes, beliefs, values, rituals, symbols, norms and conventions, customs, behaviors, and ideologies.

When we think of diversity, culture is what usually first comes to mind. Culture is the sum total of ways of living including core beliefs, societal values, patterns of thinking and communication, and behavioral norms that a group of people have developed to assure their position in a particular environment. Culture is also the response of a group of human beings to the valid and particular needs of its members and includes knowledge, values, traditions, and attitudes that guide the behavior of a group of people.

## Profile of a Culturally Competent School

Cultural competence is an integral component of school climate and the administration, faculty, and staff promote inclusiveness and appropriate responses to difference as reflected by its policies, programs, and practices. A school that has a broad view of cultural diversity that includes not only differences in race and ethnic backgrounds but also "diverse sexual orientation, religious traditions, age groups and learning differences and typically invites everyone to learn and change" (Nelson, Bustamante, Wilson, & Onwuegbuzie, 2008, p. 208).

## Stereotyping

Students are frequently stereotyped by race and ethnicity. This stereotyping can become a self-fulfilling prophecy when students begin to see themselves through the expectations of their teachers and others. Stereotypes and discrimination can be internalized as we become who others stereotype us to be instead of who we perceive ourselves to be.

## Self-Confidence

Students of poverty may also believe that it is extremely difficult or next to impossible to be successful. Low-SES children, particularly students of color, may firmly believe that they do not have access to participate in mainstream America.

## Ability Grouping

Ability grouping sorts students based on capability and should offer more flexibility to students who excel in one subject but need more reinforcement in another. Many educators believe that it is simpler for students with similar skills, aptitude, and intellectual ability to learn together in a homogeneous class. When educators follow this belief, they sort students into groups based on their abilities and as a result set them on an educational path that can predetermine their futures.

## Social Class Distinctions and Poverty

Social class affects culture and has begun to transcend what had been previously perceived as racial and ethnic barriers to demographic change. Although educational aspirations are reflective of communities and school systems, the gap continues to widen among the haves and the have-nots. Poor students in our middle and more affluent communities should have the same access to educational opportunity as do their classmates, but this is not always the case. School counselors can either support or challenge the philosophy and procedures that stratify opportunities for students.

## Gender Equity and Inequity

Examining the impact of gender differences on student success in school may not be as obvious as race, ethnicity, and cultural differences when we work with students. Gender differences can influence what is expected as the "norm" and can contribute to some of the fundamental differences in personality development for boys and girls in the traditions of some cultures. However, like other forms of discrimination, messages of sexism may be subtle. Counselors and teachers may not always be aware of the messages that are communicated and how these messages affect student behavior and student choices.

## Sexual Identity

Students who are questioning their sexual identity are often subject to stereotypical taunting or ridicule and fear being shunned as a classmate, friend, team member, and/or club participant; however, students are entitled to learn, grow, and develop in a bias-free environment. School counselors have a responsibility to be sensitive to gender bias, sexual discrimination, sexual harassment, and sexual orientation and promote a school climate that permits students to study and socialize without fear of repercussion or stigma.

## Creating a Culturally Compatible Climate

The primary goal for creating culturally compatible schools is to ensure that an atmosphere of respect, understanding, and caring is at the heart of the learning community. Colleagues can move beyond the traditional cultural exchange and focus the conversation on all aspects of diversity and thus better understand the influence of culture on learning and lifestyles, which include class, race, ethnicity, gender, socioeconomic status, sexual orientation, and language.

## Challenging Beliefs and Changing Behaviors

Each individual develops as the result of the totality of life experiences and is greatly influenced by variables that include the era in which one was born as well as the color of one's skin. Generational location strongly shapes how life is viewed and valued. Students too are influenced by similar variables that can have a profound influence on their lives and will continue to do so as they approach adulthood.

Education has changed; we need to change attitudes about students, too. Schools have become the social arena in which students who represent truly diverse behavioral styles, attitudes and orientations, and different value systems are brought together with one goal in mind, which is to maximize their potentials as human beings. School counselors have a moral and ethical responsibility to act as advocates and leaders ensuring that the diverse needs of students are reflected in the teaching and learning environment of the place called school.

## KEY TERMS

Assimilation p. 253

Integration p. 253

Tolerance p. 254

Diversity p. 255

Acceptance p. 255

Prejudice p. 256

Ethnicity p. 258

Multiculturalism p. 259

Discrimination p. 263

Stereotyping p. 263

Socioeconomic status (SES) p. 266

Gender p. 269

## LEARNING EXTENSIONS/MAKING CONNECTIONS

1. Get in touch with your personal beliefs and attitudes by completing the following statements:

   a. When I meet a new Hispanic student I think
   b. African American youth are
   c. When I meet an Islamic family I think
   d. Our Asian students
   e. The gay and lesbian students in our school

   Write down your responses. Share them with a classmate or peer. Did you note any patterns? How are your perceptions similar, different?

2. What do you think about when you hear about "changing demographics"? How has your community changed over the past 10 years? Which ethnic groups have shown the greatest increase in population?

3. American society used to be referred to as a "melting pot." How does this differ from the model of multiculturalism that we use today?

4. Explore the impact that your name, first and last, had on your personal identity. Share this with a classmate. Consider how your name relates to your growth and development from a variety of diverse perspectives including race, ethnicity, and culture.

5. How does your school system respond to the diverse needs of students in your community? What aspects of diversity are the most important to address?

6. What can school counselors do to foster a multicultural atmosphere in their schools?

7. What traditional biases are you aware of that affect a student decision about her or his future goals?

8. Download your school district report card information; select one school to analyze in your community. What does it tell you about achievement of the diverse groups of students that comprise your community?

9. What resources exist in your school and community that support diversity in its fullest meaning?

10. Reflect on the scenario presented at the beginning of the chapter. What intervention strategies did you implement as an alternative to initiating the referral process for special/exceptional student education?

CHAPTER **10**

# Working with Special Needs Students

## CHAPTER OBJECTIVES

*By the time you have completed this chapter, you should be able to*

- describe the three tiers of Response to Intervention and the school counselor's involvement;

- explain the alignment of the ASCA National Model to Response to Intervention (RtI) and Positive Behavior Intervention Supports (PBIS);

- discuss the laws and regulations that guide the programs and services for students with special needs, including 504 and IDEA;

- describe the characteristics of the IDEA classifications categories of students with disabilities;

- detail the specific steps involved in the special education referral process and IEP development;

- identify contemporary issues that may affect the delivery of services to students with disabilities, including consideration of over identification of some student populations.

---

## *School Counselor Casebook: Getting Started*

### The Scenario

Gavin is in eighth grade and seems to have more difficulty with word problems in math and other abstract thinking areas than many of his peers. Although he is highly motivated, he still struggles. To succeed, he needs a lot of practice, and his approach is somewhat more mechanical than that of his peers. He comments, "I need to be able to 'see it' to understand it. Some of these ideas are just too abstract for me. I can get it, though, if I get enough practice."

When he gets frustrated with homework, he retreats to his room where he plays his guitar, and he is accomplished enough to compose his own arrangements. Gavin is skilled at working with people, and some of his peers turn to him as an arbitrator when clashes occur in club and other organizational meetings.

Gavin's team of teachers has asked for a conference. He is doing poorly this year in middle school and they are concerned that he may not move on to high school.

### Thinking about Solutions

As you read this chapter, think about possible solutions. Where would you begin in identifying the issues and seeking solutions? When you come to the end of the chapter, you will have the opportunity to see how your ideas compare with a practicing school counselor's approach.

# PROVIDING FOR THE INSTRUCTIONAL NEEDS OF ALL STUDENTS

Schools across the United States focus great resources to provide every child with a quality education and to accommodate learners who struggle to succeed. To determine how many students we are talking about is complex. But we do know that 68 percent of eighth graders read below grade level (NAEP, 2009) and approximately 1.3 million students don't graduate from high school on time (Education Week, 2010). Equally important, the graduation rate of students with identified special needs is only 57 percent, and 50 percent of the U.S. prison population was identified as students with special needs (National Center on Secondary Education and Transition, 2006).

School counselors and most educators ascribe to the belief that all children can learn and all children can achieve. All school personnel should be sensitive to the time needed to learn, especially for students who struggle to achieve a level of minimum proficiency. Learning ability is distinct to the individual; each child has unique talents, skills, and limitations (McDivitt & Ormond, 2007). So many factors can limit or extend the learning process.

Some theorists describe the individual's ability to learn and demonstrate success in the context of intelligence. Gardner's theory of multiple intelligences (1999), Sternberg's diarchic theory of intelligence (1985), and Goldman's theory on emotional intelligence (1995) provide insight into how children, adolescents, and adults gather and apply information to solve problems and behave appropriately. These theorists view learning as multidimensional and offer alternative explanations and rationales to traditional measure of intelligences that are often used to "label" students. When intelligence and learning are viewed in the context of a process, there is a greater array of options available to advocate for appropriate student services and supports (Goldman, 1995). Individual learning styles and preferences also influence how a student accepts, processes, understands, and applies knowledge (Gardner, 1999). When teachers utilize a variety of interventions and strategies, it helps to determine where the learning gap is as well as what will work best to help students learn.

Master teachers know that each student acquires and applies information differently. Traditional classroom settings and instructional plans often teach to the majority of students and even the best teachers acknowledge that annually a few students would be left behind and not meet grade-level standards. Successful classroom and school settings are committed to identifying all of the possible resources for those students who are slow learners, hyperactive, artistic, English language learners, from low-income families, newly immigrated, or technically inclined (Sadker & Sadker, 2005). Effective educators challenge all students to focus on their strengths and overcome the obstacles that are inhibiting their ability to learn. This goes far beyond those labeled as **special education** students and extends to meeting the individual and diverse instructional needs of every student in our schools and classrooms.

## A Social Justice Agenda

*Learning ability* is a student's capacity or aptitude to master a skill, task, or concept while the term *disability* describes a student's incapability to accomplish or acquire the same skills, task, or concept in certain situations

(Woolfolk, 2009). The current (traditional) system for identifying children as learning disabled, also known as the discrepancy model, limits the opportunity to provide targeted interventions early on and makes it almost impossible to focus on early intervention (Walser, 2007). Students are moved from general education classrooms to special education settings based on the discrepancy between students' IQs and standardized tests, particularly in reading and mathematics. Students who performed poorly on IQ tests and were labeled as slow learners were not entitled to additional help and were doomed to a school experience of low expectations, low achievement, and poor performance.

Special education students and/or students with 504 plans are sometimes viewed as second-class citizens in our schools (Sadker & Sadker, 2005). This perception is frequently held by some mainstreamed students as well as by some teachers and parents. Students with disabilities, like newly immigrated students, students from low-income families, and others who don't fit neatly into the "norm," need to be treated equitably and respectfully (Quigney & Studer, 1998). All students deserve a quality, challenging, and successful educational experience and school counselors have an ethical responsibility to protect the rights of every student and their families (ASCA, 2010b). School counselors, serving as social justice advocates, can ensure that students with learning and instructional differences are treated with the same respect and are given the same opportunities as all of the students who are considered part of the mainstream.

## RESPONSE TO INTERVENTION

> RtI is not a specific curriculum or program; rather, it is a framework for promoting access to high-quality core instruction and providing increasingly intensive educational interventions in a timely manner for students who struggle in core instruction. (National High School Center, National Center on Response to Intervention, and Center on Instruction, 2010, p. 1)

**Response to Intervention** (RtI) is a potentially powerful framework for organizing, allocating, and evaluating educational resources to meet the instructional needs of all students and to prevent long-term school failure. It is the practice of providing high-quality instruction with evidence-based core instruction and interventions that are matched to student need, monitored frequently to make decisions about changes in instruction or goals and using the student's "response" to determine effectiveness or changes in the instructional and learning plan (National Association of State Directors of Special Education [NASDSE], 2006). The purpose of RtI is to ensure that good instruction and teaching take place.

When President Bush signed into law the Individuals with Disabilities Education Improvement Act (IDEIA, 2004), one significant difference from the previous reauthorizations addressed the past practice of using IQ-achievement discrepancy to identify children with **learning disabilities** (LD). More commonly referred to as IDEA, the law permits practitioners to use RtI as both the means of providing early intervention to all children at risk for school failure as well as identifying students who may need more individualized instruction than the traditional classroom can provide

(Fuchs & Fuchs, 2006). IDEA regulations fall short of mandating RtI as a method for identifying children with learning disabilities. However, IDEA modified this requirement and changed, in part, the way in which struggling students can be diagnosed as learning disabled through the use of Response to Intervention.

> In determining whether a child has a specific learning disability, a local educational agency may use a process that determines if the child responds to scientific, research-based intervention as a part of the evaluation procedures. (IDEA, 2004, Sec. 614.b.6.B)

Thus, state departments of education cannot exclusively require the use of IQ tests to diagnose learning disabilities and are permitted to use "alternative methods" such as RtI for diagnosis (Walser, 2007).

RtI definitions may slightly vary, but in all situations, RtI integrates assessment and intervention within a multilevel prevention system to maximize student achievement and to reduce behavior problems (National Center on Response to Intervention, 2010). According to NASDE (2006), implementation requires an understanding of the core principles that guide practice as well as the components that define practice. The core principles of RtI are the following:

- Effectively teach all children.
- Intervene early.
- Provide a multitier model of service delivery.
- Use a problem-solving method to make decisions within a multitier model.
- Use research based, scientifically validated interventions/instruction to the extent possible.
- Monitor student progress to inform instruction.
- Use data to make decisions.
- Use assessments for screening, diagnosing, and monitoring progress (NASDE, 2006, pp. 19–20).

As instructional needs can vary from student to student, each requires targeted instruction, that is, teaching practices designed to meet the individual's particular learning needs (Buffum, Mattos, & Weber, 2010). All students do not learn at the same rate; some need extended time. As a multitiered approach to help struggling learners, RtI targets instruction with the appropriate levels of time and support, which is the purpose of RtI. Most importantly, RtI is for all students and helps to blur the lines between general and special education. Students' progress is closely monitored at each stage of intervention to determine the need for further research-based instruction and/or intervention in general education, in special education, or both.

The most essential barometer of student success is the use of data-driven practice. RtI shifts the emphasis from undocumented benefits to evidence-based student outcomes. Teachers and school counselors use outcome data to:

- determine the effectiveness of both general and remedial instruction and interventions;
- early identify students with academic or behavioral problems;

- prevent unnecessary or over identification of students for special education;
- decide which students need special programs, including special education; and
- assess the effectiveness of "interventions," individual education programs, and special education services (NASDSE, 2006).

Teachers, school counselors, and specialists monitor the instructional progress of students, identify those with poor learning outcomes, provide evidence-based interventions, adjust the focus and intensity of those interventions as determined by a student's responsiveness, and identify students with special needs who are not succeeding in the classroom or may have a disability. These activities are part of the scope of practice of effective educators in their day-to-day work with students. RtI is not a new concept or way of work; it is new terminology. Prior to IDEA (2004), researchers (Bergan, 1977; Heller, Holtzman, & Messick, 1982; Marsten, Muyskens, Lau, & Canter, 2003; Vaughn & Fuchs, 2003) proposed models that explored the quality of instruction in general education, debated whether a special education program is appropriate and of value in improving student outcomes, and examined progress monitored through the use of curriculum-based assessment tools.

Then, what makes RtI different? Evidence and data drive the decision to determine what the student needs to succeed, which targeted supports are necessary, and at which tier level of intervention is assigned. This must be done with fidelity. RtI forces us to examine all available resources and to reorganize or regroup instruction to create a time for intervention based on a team approach. Utilizing a problem-solving model, team members explore and annotate what is working and what has not been effective to address the learning issue. The intervention team seeks to work with students in a variety of different ways and goes beyond the traditional pull-out system of remediation. RtI systems use people resources where and when they are needed.

## RtI and Special Education

**Eligibility for special education** can occur when a student's response to both the core instruction and supplemental interventions does not result in achieving grade-level objectives such as academic benchmarks or expected peer performance levels (NASDE, 2006). There will be students who are *not* succeeding with tiered RtI interventions but also may *not* qualify for special education. When the RtI approach is used to identify students who need special education services, specific interventions at the Tier 1, 2, and 3 levels are closely monitored and student progress is closely scrutinized using student outcome data (NASDE, 2006). Students no longer move in a horizontal line from regular to special education without taking the steps to move vertically through a multitiered series of interventions.

We will further discuss the special education selection and classification process later in this chapter.

## A Multitiered Approach

Figure 10.1 provides a visual representation of the different levels of RtI interventions. Tier 1 reflects the school personnel's approach to providing a

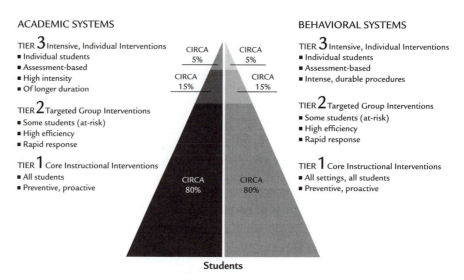

ACADEMIC SYSTEMS

TIER **3** Intensive, Individual Interventions
- Individual students
- Assessment-based
- High intensity
- Of longer duration

TIER **2** Targeted Group Interventions
- Some students (at-risk)
- High efficiency
- Rapid response

TIER **1** Core Instructional Interventions
- All students
- Preventive, proactive

BEHAVIORAL SYSTEMS

TIER **3** Intensive, Individual Interventions
- Individual students
- Assessment-based
- Intense, durable procedures

TIER **2** Targeted Group Interventions
- Some students (at-risk)
- High efficiency
- Rapid response

TIER **1** Core Instructional Interventions
- All settings, all students
- Preventive, proactive

CIRCA 5%   CIRCA 5%

CIRCA 15%   CIRCA 15%

CIRCA 80%   CIRCA 80%

Students

FIGURE **10.1** Response to Intervention Tiers

Source: National Association of State Directors of Special Education (2006). Reprinted with permission.

quality grade-level curriculum, with effective teaching to every student. Teachers operate from the principle that all children can learn and differentiate instruction accordingly. Teachers scaffold content and address the process on the basis of student needs while also making the time to meet with small groups of students to address gaps in learning (Buffum, Mattos, & Weber, 2010).

Tier 2 targets students in need of additional support and focuses on identified learning needs. Interventions are delivered through small-group instruction using specific strategies that directly target a skill deficit (D'Agostino & Murphy, 2004). Interventions are most effective when they are focused on the cause of a student's struggles rather than the symptoms such as a failing grade (Buffum, Mattos, & Weber, 2010).

Tier 3 is intensive support and ensures that every student who needs it receives it in addition to the core curriculum instruction. In other words, the core curriculum is not replaced with a remedial program. Intensive help must be individualized and the focus is on the specific needs that were not met by Tier 2 interventions and a plan is created for how to meet them. Each tier is additional time spent on targeted instruction above and beyond the time spent in that instructional area for all students.

When all students have guaranteed access to rigorous curriculum and effective initial teaching, targeted and timely supplemental support, and personalized support from highly trained educators, far fewer will experience failure (Sornson, Frost, & Burns, 2005). When RtI is diligently applied, the vast majority of students will never need to be referred for special education testing (Buffum, Mattos, & Weber, 2010).

## The School Counselor's Role in RtI

The core principles of Response to Intervention are grounded in equity, access, and social justice, and they promote the beliefs that we can effectively teach all children. School counselors recognize the critical importance of early intervention for struggling students as they assist teachers with differentiated instructional service delivery, closely monitor student progress to inform instruction, and use data to make informed decisions.

> Counselors need to have an understanding of how to recognize discrimination and other barriers to equal educational opportunity before he/she can take the appropriate steps to address barriers enabling all students to develop to their fullest. (U.S. Department of Education, 2005)

As a member of the RtI team, school counselors participate in the identification process of students who are struggling in the core academic areas and especially in the middle and high schools. They are frequently among the first of the professionals to become aware of the student who is struggling in several classes. School counselors are in a pivotal position to consult and collaborate with teachers around the challenges of creating a classroom environment that is conducive to every student learning and succeeding. Teachers are experts in differentiating instruction, organizing learning groups, and classroom-based assessment of an individual student's progress. School counselors are well-versed in the use and interpretation of assessments and collaborate with teachers for the purposes of screening, diagnosing, and monitoring progress. By bringing these specialized skills together through the problem-solving process, RtI teams determine which intervention(s) the classroom teachers should use to support the needs of the student. Problem solving identifies interventions as needed, to address both the learning and behavior problems that prevent students from acquiring and applying the academic skills needed for success (Clements & Sabella, 2010). School counselors and teachers *together* can determine to what degree the interventions are working and what needs to be done to best support the student for the greatest impact. From a strengths-based approach, the school counselor can identify when and how an individual student is succeeding and then shares these successes with the classroom teachers.

### MEET ARLENE CRANDALL: ENGAGING SCHOOL COUNSELORS IN THE PROBLEM-SOLVING MODEL

School counselors are essential to the successful implementation of RtI and have an important role to play in the Problem Solving Model (PSM). The problem-solving model has four parts to it: (1) What is the problem? (2) Why is it happening? (3) What should be done? (4) Did it work? These elements reflect the essence of scientific method. Many schools may not have implemented the use of specific curriculum-based measures at the secondary level, but the PSM can be used to frame the work of any building team to help discover the underlying needs of the struggling student rather than repeating courses or being placed in

*(continues)*

remedial services. The practice of using the PSM can help an entire faculty become more diagnostic in reviewing the needs of students rather than referring the student for more services.

School counselors look for the underlying learning need (What is the problem? Why is it happening?) by carefully reviewing the student's cumulative file and academic history. Does the record give us evidence of where learning started to become difficult? Did the student have a consistent program in her or his early elementary years (K–3)? This is especially critical for students who have had disrupted education, moved multiple times, or who are homeless. Perhaps this eighth-grade student may never have learned the basic elements of reading or math. Without a level of automaticity, students are distracted from problem solving, comprehension, and higher-order thinking by the energy they need to put into basic phonics or mathematical calculation.

School counselors can help school personnel by looking at these patterns and then providing the supportive information that administrators may need to make the case for the use of curriculum-based measures or new styles of scheduling that allow for regular intervention classes in the day. These are great challenges for any secondary school. But the most successful RtI interventions are regularly scheduled and consistent in implementation. Such advocacy and support of the school community can have a broad impact on increasing the learning ability of numerous students.

This impact is the real gem of RtI. It is systematic change that in the long run affects many more students than would previously be noticed or supported before they experience failure. It gives us the hope that we can prevent students from defining themselves as stupid or unable to learn. Imagine a school where all students believe they can learn!

*Arlene Crandall has worked in education for more than 30 years as a teacher, school psychologist, special education director, and staff developer for the New York State Education Department. Currently, she is an adjunct at New York Institute of Technology, is the president of ABCD Consulting, Inc., and provides staff development on implementation of the Response to Intervention framework.*

School counselors also serve as advocates for parents and/or families to best understand what RtI services are and how to maximize the instruction given in school with additional support at home. School counselors can be an important conduit and provide the information about RtI that is specifically written for parents. For example, school counselors, together with classroom teachers, can encourage parents to become partners to reinforce activities at home and follow up with the use of RtI interventions, particularly in the elementary level, especially in the areas of reading and math. Parents can learn to look for the evidence that the instructional interventions are making a difference and better understand how the resources from the home, school, and community can contribute to a student's ability to succeed.

## RtI and the ASCA National Model

Once you get to know the RTI process, you will realize that it is highly consistent with all the components of comprehensive school counseling programs as espoused by the **ASCA National Model** (Clements & Sabella, 2010). Here's how RtI and the ASCA National Model complement each other.

### *Foundation*

The foundation of the comprehensive program is built on the premise that "all means all." The mission and vision statements reflect the school counseling program's contribution to student development (academic, career, and personal-social). The faculty, administration, and perhaps the students themselves collaborate with the school counselor to identify which standards and competencies are needed by the students as the program is delivered, managed, and assessed for impact.

### *Delivery*

In Chapter 3, we discussed how to differentiate interventions to utilize the law of parsimony and ensure that every student benefited from the school counseling program. To achieve equity, some students need more than others to achieve the same goal.

Through the delivery system, individual student planning, responsive services, and the school counseling curriculum can be differentiated to reach every child in your building and provide knowledge and skills around important topics. Figure 10.2 shows the alignment of an "all student" instructional RtI model, with the delivery system of the ASCA National Model. In classroom

|  | From Classroom Teacher | From School Counselor |
|---|---|---|
| All Students Receive ⟶ | Subject Classroom Lesson | School Counseling/Student Development Curriculum |
| Some Students Receive ⟶ | Small-Group Remediation | Group Counseling |
| A Few Students Receive ⟶ | Individual Extra Help | Individual Counseling, Crisis Counseling, External Referral |

FIGURE **10.2** Differentiated Delivery

instruction teachers often deliver a lesson through whole-group instruction. Some students might need a small-group follow-up lesson; a few may need one-on-one tutoring. Similar to the classroom model, others will need additional "reinforcement" or group counseling, while a few students may require support through individual counseling.

Thus, the tiered interventions in RtI can be likened to the differentiated model of school counseling services delivery shown in Figure 10.2.

**System Support**   Participation on the RtI team is a clear example of system support. Using the collaborative consultation process with teachers and extending it to the parent/family members utilizes everyone's expertise. As part of the RtI team, a school counselor is often the only professional in the school building who is well-versed in group process and group dynamics, and additionally can utilize these skills as needed in a problem-solving, facilitative manner during the team meetings. School counselors also provide inservice sessions or PTA presentations with other members of the RtI team to provide information or to further illustrate services to teachers and families learning more about RtI interventions.

### Management System

The organizational structure and meticulousness of maintaining documentation is a management task that is organized by the RtI team and in particular by the classroom teacher and intervention specialist. A student's record can often reveal trails of evidence leading to the understanding of where the learning began to fall apart in a student's history, particularly if a student has been in a number of school systems. RtI also requires the use of multiple points of data. Managing data, developing action plans, and organizing the delivery of strategies through the use of calendars and counseling logs are some examples of school counselor-led activities that complement Tier 1, 2, and 3 interventions.

### Accountability System

Accountability and the evaluation of the school counseling program are absolute necessities (ASCA, 2005, p. 9). As with RtI, a quick look at the data alone does not tell the whole story about a student or groups of students. In Chapter 8, we learned how important it is to disaggregate all the critical data elements and examine them to shed light on areas of student success or areas in need of more attention. MEASURE (Mission, Elements, Analyze, Stakeholders-Unite, Results, Educate) showed us how to identify an important issue, gather the appropriate data, deliver strategies, monitor progress, modify strategies, and assess results. You can develop a MEASURE to monitor the effectiveness of activities provided to all students and Tier 2 and/or 3 interventions.

When RtI is aligned with the ASCA National Model and MEASURE, school counselors demonstrate their commitment to an effective, efficient,

## Lets's start with Step Two: Element

### Element
What critical data *element* are you trying to impact? (Examples include grades; test scores; attendance; promotion rates; graduation rates; postsecondary-going rate; enrollment into honors or AP courses, special education; discipline referral data; etc.).

What is the *baseline* for the data element? Where is the *goal*?

Element: standardized test score
Baseline: 50% of the eighth-grade students are not reading at grade level
Goal: Increase the percentage of students reading at grade level to from 50% to 75% before the students transition to high school.

## Step Three: Analyze

Analyze the data element. You can use percentages, averages, raw scores, quartiles, or stanines. You can aggregate or disaggregate the data to better understand which students are meeting success. You can disaggregate by gender, race, ethnicity, socioeconomic status, or in a multitude of ways to look at student groupings.

The baseline data revealed that 50% of the eighth graders are reading below grade level; 85% of the students targeted are boys. All have been reading below grade level for at least two years.

## Step Four: Stakeholders-Unite

Stakeholders-Unite to develop strategies to affect the data element
Beginning Date: September 1
Ending Date: June 1

| Stakeholders | Strategies |
|---|---|
| School Counselor(s) | • Develop a mentoring program for the boys utilizing local male university students |
| Administrator(s) | • Fund a breakfast and dinner program for the mentors with a focus on literacy<br>• Gather classroom observations of learning to see if there is a common pattern of need such as vocabulary work<br>• Work with RtI team to choose research-based model of vocabulary instruction for all teachers to implement at Tier 1 |

*(continues)*

| | |
|---|---|
| Teachers | • Pool Tier 1 strategies to motivate all eighth graders to read |
| Students | • Submit lists of books and magazines that they enjoy reading |
| Parents | • Encourage parents to participate in the monthly eighth-grade book club |
| Parent Teacher Associations | • Donate extra copies of the book club selection to parents |
| RtI Team | • Monitor the impact of grade-wide adjustment of vocabulary instruction—Tier 1 (grade-level interventions) <br> • Identify students for more targeted Tier 2 and 3 interventions using curriculum-based measures <br> • Identify interventions and how they will be implemented |
| Business Community | • Donate books, awards, certificates, wireless reading devices for reading motivation <br> • Fund computer-based reading intervention programs that can be used for increased practice of targeted instruction |
| Eighth-grade Faculty and Staff | • Participate in an eighth-grade monthly book club <br> • Work collaboratively to implement Tier 2 and 3 interventions |
| School Improvement Team | • Add eighth-grade literacy to this year's goals |
| Resources (grants, technology, etc.) | • Use wireless reading devices (e.g., Kindle, iPad) on a loan basis as motivators for the students to use to read the book of the month |
| Other | |

## It is now June! Let's look at Step Five: *Results*

Results: Restate your baseline data. State where your data are now. Did you meet your goal?

Restate baseline data: 50% below grade level
Results (data now): 70%
Met Goal: Yes _____ No _____ X _____ ALMOST!

Take your *Questions to Consider to your RtI Team* as you examine results and revise your MEASURE:

Which strategies had a positive impact on the data?

*The eighth-grade book club, which motivated students to want to read the next month's selection on the iPad or Kindle. Student submitted book selections. Grade-wide use of vocabulary instruction model supported all students in learning new vocabulary. Teachers noted more frequent recognition and use of new vocabulary in student work.*

Which strategies should be replaced, changed, added?

*Include seventh graders; explore how to get more donations for Kindles, iPads, reading software. Investigate the use of common vocabulary instruction at this grade level.*

Based on what you have learned, how will you revise Step Four, "Stakeholders-Unite"?

*We need to consider adding a mentoring program for the eighth-grade girls also. Get help from the librarian to screen student book selections.*

How did your MEASURE contribute to systemic change(s) in your school and/or in your community?

*We made huge strides in improving our eighth-grade test scores and in helping our eighth graders get ready for high school.*

## *Step Six:* **Educate**

Educate others as to your efforts to move data. Develop a report card that shows how the work of the school counselor(s) is connected to the mission of the schools and to student success. Below is an example of a report card.

*We published our Report Card on our school's website and wrote an article about our eighth-grade literacy project for the district bulletin and local weekly newspaper!*

data-driven, and highly collaborative process. These systems complement each other and take advantage of the collective expertise and experiences of the parents, the RTI team, and the students. When school counselors actively participate on the RtI team, the result will be a win-win process for all involved.

## POSITIVE BEHAVIOR INTERVENTION SUPPORTS (PBIS)

**Positive behavioral intervention supports** (PBIS) is the application of the RtI framework for the prevention of behavior difficulties. Like RtI, PBIS requires the use of continuous monitoring, data-based decision making, and an intervention continuum (Horner, Sugai, Smolkowski, Eber, Nakasato, Todd, & Esperenza, 2009). When PBIS is effectively implemented, the majority of students demonstrate appropriate behavior within the general education classroom without additional supports, thus saving the more intensive interventions (e.g., social skills classes, individualized behavior interventions) for the students who require these interventions (PBIS, 2010). PBIS is based on a problem-solving model and aims to prevent inappropriate behavior through teaching and reinforcing appropriate behaviors (OSEP Technical Assistance Center on Positive Behavioral Interventions & Supports, 2007), and the process is consistent with the core principles of RTI.

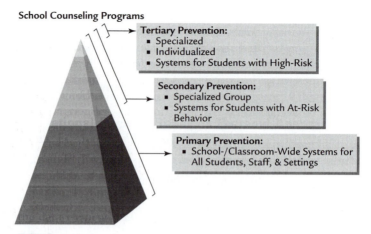

**School Counseling Programs**

**Tertiary Prevention:**
- Specialized
- Individualized
- Systems for Students with High-Risk

**Secondary Prevention:**
- Specialized Group
- Systems for Students with At-Risk Behavior

**Primary Prevention:**
- School-/Classroom-Wide Systems for All Students, Staff, & Settings

FIGURE **10.3** Multilevel Systems of Support

Source: Office of Special Education Programs, Positive Behavioral Intervention Supports (2010). Reprinted with permission.

PBIS offers a range of interventions that are systematically applied to students based on their demonstrated level of need. Both RTI and PBIS are grounded in differentiated instruction. Each approach identifies the components in place at the universal (Tier 1), targeted group (Tier 2), and individual (Tier 3) levels (OSEP, 2007) to meet the needs of children experiencing academic and social difficulties in school (Sandomierski, Kincaid, & Algozzine, 2007) as shown in Figure 10.3.

**Primary Prevention Tier 1**   Most students. This tier encompasses approximately 80 percent of students. Most students will find success under a schoolwide behavioral plan that creates and maintains a positive and respectful school culture and environment. In this type of culture, behavior expectations are common in every location in the building and students are taught what the behaviors look like and sound like, e.g., a clear example and definition is given for treating each other with respect in the cafeteria.

**Secondary Prevention Tier 2**   At-risk students. This tier comprises about 15 percent of the student body. Within this group are students for whom the schoolwide interventions won't work all of the time. Specific efforts can reduce the number of problem behaviors by working with targeted students on specific behaviors.

**Tertiary Prevention Tier 1**   High-risk students. These students make up about 5 percent of the school population. The schoolwide and classroom interventions have not made an impact on this group of students. At this level there is a need for specific, individual interventions for each student, and this tiered approach rewards positive behavior as well as teaches students appropriate behaviors to challenging situations.

Primary prevention is one of the significant factors that distinguishes the school counseling profession from other helping professions (American School Counselor Association, 2005), and the need for comprehensive prevention efforts is acutely felt in schools today where behavioral problems are prevalent (Curtis, Van Horne, Robertson, & Karvonen, 2010). The work of school counselors is closely aligned with the philosophy of PBIS and in particular with the delivery of prevention activities through the student development curriculum and "preventative" responsive services. School counselors are an invaluable resource in helping their administrators and colleagues find research-based programs to support good behavior in school. If the student has greater needs, she or he is involved in Tier 2 or 3 interventions and school counselors often provide both group and individual interventions.

In essence, PBIS can be construed as the prevention component of the ASCA National Model, which has as one of its goals to provide all students with the knowledge and skills to achieve success in school and develop into contributing members of our society. School counselors, utilizing the personal-social development standards, help students acquire the ability to respect self and others; make decisions, set goals, and take necessary action to achieve goals; and acquire coping and resiliency skills (ASCA, 1997b). When the school counselor serves in a consultation capacity, the counselor can:

- Help develop a systems approach for positive behavior for the entire school.
- Promote a team approach to working with students.
- Encourage teachers to look at the "whole child" when identifying issues.
- Design and monitor specific plans for schoolwide, classroom, non-classroom, and individual students to create a positive school culture.

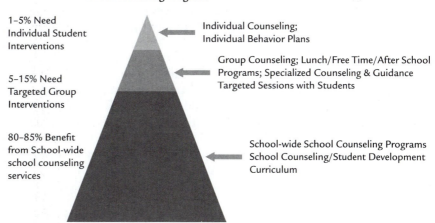

FIGURE **10.4** Comprehensive School Counseling and PBIS

Adapted from Office of Special Education Programs Technical Assistance Center on Positive Behavior Interventions and Supports, USDOE (2010).

School counselors are in a unique position to collaborate with faculty and to identify the essential resources and support systems that each student needs to achieve success in academic accomplishments and in personal-social relationships (Stone & Dahir, 2011). Some students need additional tools, time, and specialized instruction to achieve at a minimum proficiency. The next section of this chapter addresses federal legislation that offers additional help to students who need more intensive support than is provided by traditional academic supports and/or through Response to Intervention and Positive Behavior Intervention Supports.

# SPECIAL EDUCATION

Professional school counselors encourage and support all students' academic, personal/social, and career development through comprehensive school counseling programs. Professional school counselors are committed to helping all students realize their potential, and make adequate yearly progress regardless of challenges resulting from disabilities and other special needs (ASCA, 2010b).

Special education or, as it is sometimes known, exceptional student education began after a dark time in our history in which people with significant disabling conditions were often isolated or persecuted. The first organized initiatives for special education began with institutions for the deaf, blind, and "Idiotic and Feeble-minded Youth" (Osgood, 2008, p. 41). As these institutions grew, it became the "task of public school to identify, segregate, instruct, and control children whose disabilities were seen as difficult, dangerous, or un-treatable" (Osgood, 2008, p. 41).

Additional protection of children with disabilities began in earnest between the 1960s to the 1980s with the disability rights movement. The federal government increased the amount of resources given to disability and court decisions led to new expectations from agencies and schools serving people with disabilities Laws passed during this time include Section 504 of the Rehabilitation Act of 1973, Education for All Handicapped Children Act of 1975, and the 1986 Amendments to the Education for All Handicapped Children Act. These laws focused on protection against discrimination, parental rights, and increasing resources.

In 1990, the Education for All Handicapped Children Act was revised and renamed the Individuals with Disabilities Education Act (IDEA). In 2004, the act was revised and renamed the Individuals with Disabilities Education Improvement Act (IDEIA) to reflect a focus on improving educational outcomes. IDEIA greatly expanded the list of guaranteed services to disabled children (Osgood, 2008; Ysseldyke & Algozzine, 2006).

## Education for All Handicapped Children Act of 1975

The **Education for all Handicapped Children Act** (1975) commonly known as Public Law 94-142 protected the rights of all children and required states to provide a "free and appropriate education" for all children between the ages of 3 and 21, regardless of the handicapping condition or disability. PL 94-142 is the basis for *special education*, the term commonly known across the 50 states. Special education encompasses the entire range of learning, emotional, and physical disabilities, and in some states also includes students who have special abilities, gifts, or talents. Reauthorized in 1991 as the Individuals with Disabilities Education Act (IDEA), the word *handicapped* was eliminated and *disabled* was used in its place. IDEA requires that every disabled child have access to the program of study that will most effectively approximate a normal child's educational program. This is accomplished through the **Individualized Education Plan (IEP)**, which is the written record of the needs of each student and the procedures to provide services. The IEP must include education goals and the instructional services designed to meet the stated goals, as well as information on how progress will be monitored.

## SPECIAL EDUCATION AND SCHOOL IMPROVEMENT AGENDAS

IDEA and No Child Left Behind (NCLB) both addressed the needs of students with disabilities by focusing on student achievement and outcomes; emphasizing parental participation; and requiring the regular evaluation or assessment of students and staffs (Osborne & Russo, 2006). "The most important difference between the two statutes is that IDEA focuses on the performances of individual students in an array of areas, while the NCLB is more interested in system-wide outcomes" (Osborne & Russo, 2006, p. 18). One of IDEA's additions is a definition of "highly qualified" teachers, which also applies to related services personnel and paraprofessionals. This parallels the language of NCLB. To be classified as "highly qualified," a standard that is based on state rather than federal law, subject area teachers in public schools will not only have to be certified fully in special education or pass state-designed special education licensure examination, but they will also have to possess bachelor's degrees and demonstrate knowledge of each subject for which they are the primary instructors (Osborne & Russo, 2006). The standard is based on state rather than federal law as is all certification or teacher credentialing.

The issue of which standards to apply to students with disabilities and the consequences of failing to meet a given standard are questions that require professional judgment in each individual case as required by law (Hallahan, Kauffman, & Pullen, 2009). Requiring all students with disabilities, and those for whom the tests are inappropriate for other reasons, to take state exams is considered by some to be unfair. However, testing to determine outcomes is necessary to determine whether programs for students with disabilities are working.

> When it comes to special education, it's wrong to compare outcomes for students with disabilities to outcomes for students without disabilities. The right comparisons are contrasting students with disabilities who receive special education (or any given treatment) to those who don't receive it, or comparing students with disabilities before and after they receive special education. (Hallahan et al., 2009, p. 68)

The No Child Left Behind Act (Public Law 107-110) pushed for evidence-based interventions and extensive programs to support literacy instruction in the early grades and accountability (Ysseldyke & Algozzine, 2006). Under both the No Child Left Behind Act (NCLB) and the Individuals with Disabilities Education Act (IDEA), a school can now be identified as in need of improvement when it fails to meet standards for students with disabilities. This accountability imperative is suggested as a way of leading "to interventions that will produce enhanced outcomes for students with disabilities" (Ysseldyke & Algozzine, 2006, p. 38). Huerta (2008) expressed concern when special education programs are coupled with mandates such as No Child Left Behind due to unintended consequences from these expectations. "Some teachers and administrators may erroneously equate rigor with exclusive exposure to grade-level standards and curriculum at the expense of addressing individual student needs" (Huerta, 2008, p. 31).

### Blueprint for Reform

With the current reauthorization of the Elementary and Secondary Education Act, more than ever before, America's schools are responsible for meeting the educational needs of an increasingly diverse student population. The Blueprint for Reform requires school personnel to provide a wide range of resources and support to ensure that all students have the opportunity to succeed in college and in a career, regardless of ability or disability. Although the primary funding for programs specifically focused on supporting students with disabilities is through IDEA, the Blueprint proposes to increase support for the **inclusion** and improved outcomes of students with disabilities.

The Blueprint also encourages the use of assessments that more accurately and appropriately measure the performance of students with disabilities and to provide the curricula and instructional supports to meet all students' needs. All educators, including school counselors, should be well prepared through their preparation programs and professional development to meet the needs of diverse learners. As participant in the RtI and IEP teams, school counselors are the voice to ensure equity and access to the appropriate services and supports to educate every child. A thorough understanding of working with special needs populations is essential to ethically and responsibly consider every student's educational expectations.

## THE OVER IDENTIFICATION DEBATE

There is a growing concern about the over identification of children for special education.

> According to U.S. government figures, public schools have identified as learning disabled between 5 and 6 percent of students between six and seventeen years of age. Learning disabilities is by far the largest category of special education. About half of all students identified by the public schools as needing special education are learning disabled. (Hallahan et al., 2009, p. 191)

Some of the criticism has been leveled against the teacher: "teachers are too quick to label students with the slightest learning problem as 'learning disabled' rather than entertain the possibility that their own teaching practices are at fault" (Hallahan, Kauffman, & Pullen, 2009, p. 192). Others argue that the increase is due to "social and cultural changes that have raised children's vulnerability to develop learning disabilities (Hallahan, 1992). For example, the number of children living in poverty doubled between 1975 and 1993" (Hallahan, Kauffman, & Pullen, 2009, p. 192).

There is a growing concern about the over identification of children for special education. According to U.S. government figures, public schools have identified as learning disabled between 5 and 6 percent of students between 6 and 17 years of age. The overrepresentation of students of color means that they have limited access to general education experiences and the opportunities those experiences provide. Disproportionality refers to "the extent to which membership in a given ... group affects the probability of being placed in a specific disability category" (Oswald, Coutinho, Best, & Singh, 1999, p. 198).

> Nationally, Black students, particularly those identified as mentally retarded or emotionally disabled, have been consistently overrepresented for more than 3 decades. Native American students are also persistently overrepresented in special education nationally, and while the same is not true for Latino students, they are often overrepresented at the state and district levels where their enrollment is highest. (Sullivan et al., 2005, p. 1)

It has been well documented that Black students are often overrepresented in special education classrooms (Zehr, 2004). "Seventy-five percent of the national school enrollment is white, but white students make up only 71 percent of the special education enrollment. In comparison, students who are black make up 16 percent of public school enrollment but 21 percent of the enrollment in special education programs" (Algozzine & Ysseldyke, 2006, p. 30). "The overrepresentation of students of color means that they have limited access to general education experiences and the opportunities those experiences provide" (Rueda, Klingner, Sager, & Velasco, 2008, pp. 131–32).

The U.S. Department of Education (2004) recently concluded that LEP students are underrepresented with only 9.2 percent of English Language Learners receiving special education services as compared to 13.4 percent (NCES, 2010) of the 3- to 21-year-olds in public schools receiving services under the Individuals with Disabilities Education Act. A higher percentage of males are identified as learning disabled.

> Boys outnumber girls by about three to one in the learning disabilities category. Some researchers have suggested that the prevalence of learning disabilities among males is due to greater biological vulnerability. The infant mortality rate for males is higher than that for females, and males are at greater risk than females for a variety of biological abnormalities. (Hallahan et al., 2009, p. 192).

A body of critics suggests males are more vulnerable to referral bias. They suggest that academic difficulties are no more prevalent among boys than among girls but that boys are more likely to be referred for special education when they do have academic problems because of other behaviors (Hallahan, Kauffman, & Pullen, 2009).

## Procedural Steps in Special Education Placement

The complex process of special education eligibility and placement requires many stakeholders to include parent(s), guardian(s), or caretaker(s). The National Dissemination Center for Children with Disabilities (NICHCY) is an organization that offers resources and information on disabilities in youth and research-based information on effective educational practices (NICHCY, 2010). NICHCY also offers the following information on the procedural steps to special education placement:

1. Giving Parents Notice. It is important to know that IDEA requires the school system to notify parents in writing that it would like to evaluate their child. Before the school may proceed with the evaluation, parents must give their *informed written permission* (in a form the general public can understand and in the parents' native language).

2. Evaluation. A full and individual initial evaluation of the student must be conducted to see if the student has a disability and is eligible for special education. *Informed parent consent* must be obtained before this evaluation can be conducted. The purpose of conducting this evaluation is to see if the student is a "child with a disability," as defined by IDEA. Information is gathered that will help determine the student's educational needs and to guide decision making about appropriate educational programming for the student.

   IDEA, in section §300.8, lists different disability categories under which a student may be found eligible for special education. These are the following:

   (1) *Autism* means a developmental disability significantly affecting verbal and nonverbal communication and social interaction, generally evident before age three, that adversely affects a child's educational performance. Other characteristics often associated with autism are engagement in repetitive activities and stereotyped movements, resistance to environmental change or change in daily routines, and unusual responses to sensory experiences. Autism does not apply if a child's educational performance is adversely affected primarily because the child has an emotional disturbance, as defined in (4) of this section.

   (2) *Deaf-blindness* means concomitant hearing and visual impairments, the combination of which causes such severe communication and other developmental and educational needs that they cannot be accommodated in special education programs solely for children with deafness or children with blindness.

   (3) *Deafness* means a hearing impairment so severe that the child is impaired in processing linguistic information through hearing, with or without amplification that adversely affects a child's educational performance.

   (4) *Emotional disturbance* means a condition exhibiting one or more of the following characteristics over a long period of time and to a marked degree that adversely affects a child's educational performance: (a) An inability to learn that cannot be explained by intellectual, sensory, or

health factors. (b) An inability to build or maintain satisfactory inter-personal relationships. (c) Inappropriate types of behavior or feelings under normal circumstances. (d) A general pervasive mood of unhappiness or depression. (e) A tendency to develop physical symptoms or fears associated with personal or school problems.

(5) *Hearing impairment* means an impairment in hearing, whether permanent or fluctuating, that adversely affects a child's educational performance but that is not included under the definition of deafness in this section.

(6) *Mental retardation* means significantly subaverage general intellectual functioning, existing concurrently with deficits in adaptive behavior and manifested during the developmental period, that adversely affects a child's educational performance.

(7) *Multiple disabilities* means concomitant impairments (such as mental retardation-blindness or mental retardation-orthopedic impairment), the combination of which causes such severe educational needs that they cannot be accommodated in special education programs solely for one of the impairments. Multiple disabilities does not include deaf-blindness.

(8) *Orthopedic impairment* means a severe orthopedic impairment that adversely affects a child's educational performance. The term includes impairments caused by a congenital anomaly, impairments caused by disease (e.g., poliomyelitis, bone tuberculosis), and impairments from other causes (e.g., cerebral palsy, amputations, and fractures or burns that cause contractures).

(9) *Other health impairment* means having limited strength, vitality, or alertness, including a heightened alertness to environmental stimuli, that results in limited alertness with respect to the educational environment, that—(i) is due to chronic or acute health problems such as asthma, attention deficit disorder or attention deficit hyperactivity disorder, diabetes, epilepsy, a heart condition, hemophilia, lead poisoning, leukemia, nephritis, rheumatic fever, sickle cell anemia, and Tourette syndrome; and (ii) adversely affects a child's educational performance.

(10) *Specific learning disability*—(i) *General.* Specific learning disability means a disorder in one or more of the basic psychological processes involved in understanding or in using language, spoken or written, that may manifest itself in the imperfect ability to listen, think, speak, read, write, spell, or to do mathematical calculations, including conditions such as perceptual disabilities, brain injury, minimal brain dysfunction, dyslexia, and developmental aphasia.

(11) *Speech or language impairment* means a communication disorder, such as stuttering, impaired articulation, a language impairment, or a voice impairment, that adversely affects a child's educational performance.

(12) *Traumatic brain injury* means an acquired injury to the brain caused by an external physical force, resulting in total or partial functional

disability or psychosocial impairment, or both, that adversely affects a child's educational performance. Traumatic brain injury applies to open or closed head injuries resulting in impairments in one or more areas, such as cognition; language; memory; attention; reasoning; abstract thinking; judgment; problem-solving; sensory, perceptual, and motor abilities; psychosocial behavior; physical functions; information processing; and speech. Traumatic brain injury does not apply to brain injuries that are congenital or degenerative, or to brain injuries induced by birth trauma.

(13)  *Visual impairment including blindness* means an impairment to vision that, even with correction, adversely affects a child's educational performance. The term includes both partial sight and blindness (National Dissemination Center for Children with Disabilities, 2010b).

3.  What the Notice Must Contain. In the case of initial evaluation, the written notice the school system must provide includes notice of procedural safeguards that includes why it wants to conduct the evaluation (or why it refuses) and a description of the evaluation procedures and assessments. The purpose is to ensure that *parents are fully informed of all procedures* should they agree to go forward and also to understand their right to refuse consent for evaluation.

4.  Timeframe for Initial Evaluation. The evaluation must be conducted within 60 days of receiving parental consent or the state can establish its own timeframe and it takes precedence over the 60-day timeline required by IDEA.

5.  The Scope of Evaluation. A student's initial evaluation must focus on that student only. Large-scale tests or group-administered instruments are not enough to diagnose a disability. The evaluation must use a variety of assessment tools and strategies to gather relevant functional, developmental, and academic information about the student, including information provided by the parents about the student's health.

6.  Review Existing Data. Evaluation includes a *review of existing evaluation data* on the student such as classroom work or state or district assessments.

7.  Determine Eligibility. Parents are to be part of the group that determines their child's eligibility and are also to be provided a copy of the evaluation report. Some school systems will *hold a meeting* where they consider the eligibility of the student for special education and related services. At this meeting, assessment results are explained. If the evaluation results indicate that the student meets the definition of one or more of the disabilities listed under IDEA and needs special education and related services, the results will form the basis for developing the Individualized Education Plan (IEP).

8.  Triennial Evaluations. After the initial evaluation, *evaluations must be conducted at least every three years* (generally called a triennial evaluation) after the student has been placed in special education.

## Inclusion

Many schools across the United States are establishing inclusive environments in which students with disabilities, including those with severe disabilities, are integrated into the traditional mainstream classroom setting. This movement, based on the principle of normalization (Wolfensberger, 1972), was first championed in Scandinavia and then in the United States in the early 1970s. The goal was to make life for those with disabilities as culturally normative as possible. The resulting trend was one of gradual enlightenment, moving slowly from ignorance and fear of the disabled to increasing acceptance and understanding (Menzies & Falvey, 2008). Central to such discussions was the issue of integrating ("mainstreaming," in the then-current terminology) students with disabilities into regular school and classrooms.

> This topic had received significant attention for decades as a "should we or shouldn't we" question. With PL 94-142, it became a "how much and in what ways" question: the law required it but was not specific or clear on exactly how far school districts were expected to proceed in terms of accommodating all students with all kinds of disabilities and levels of intervention needs. (Osgood, 2008, p. 118)

In conclusion, the special education teacher and the regular classroom teacher work together to serve the needs of all of the children assigned to the classroom. Although some students appear to be in need of special education or exceptional student services, school counselors have a responsibility to seek not only the least restrictive environment but also provide to every student the most challenging educational opportunity possible. School counselors, by virtue of their training in human relations, group dynamics, and interpersonal skills, can play a vital role in inclusive education (Quigney & Studer, 1998). Although school counselors will also encounter situations in which teachers, parents, and administrators seek the placement of all children into special education as the only prognosis for success, they can help encourage interventions that do not include special education.

## The Dominant Classification: Learning Disabilities

There are two pervasive and widely accepted definitions of learning disabilities. The first of these was constructed by the federal government in 1975 and readopted and reauthorized in 1997 and 2004 in the Individuals with Disabilities Education Act (IDEA). The federal government describes specific learning disability as a disorder in one or more of the basic psychological processes involved in understanding or using language, spoken or written, which may manifest itself in an imperfect ability to listen, think, speak, read, write, spell, or do mathematical calculations. The federal definition includes the following disorders: perceptual disabilities, brain injury, minimal brain dysfunction, dyslexia, and developmental aphasia. Disorders excluded are learning problems that are primarily the result of visual, hearing, or motor disabilities (Hallahan, Kauffman, & Pullen, 2009).

Due to large advancements in neuroimaging techniques, researchers have found evidence that leads them to believe that learning disabilities stem from a dysfunction in the central nervous system (Hallahan et al., 2009). Possible explanations for this dysfunction fall into three categories: genetic, teratogenic, and medical factors. Research has found that there is a strong genetic link in many cases of learning disabilities, and researchers are now trying to pinpoint the exact genes involved in learning disabilities. In the case of teratogens, external agents can cause malformations or defects while the fetus is developing. Examples of this are fetal alcohol spectrum disorders. Finally, medical factors, such as premature birth, can put children at risk of developing a learning disability (Hallahan et al., 2009).

Learning disabilities have long been identified by looking for an IQ-achievement discrepancy. Critical objections to this method are based on the test's statistically flawed formulas, false sense of precision, and its weakness in predicting reading ability. Recently, a growing number of professionals have moved toward using a response to the intervention (RtI) approach as discussed earlier in this chapter (Hallahan et al., 2009), which is permitted under IDEA for special education evaluation.

Learning disabilities are manifested most in reading ability, specifically decoding, fluency, and comprehension problems. Reading disabilities are often coupled with attention problems as evidenced by 10 to 25 percent of those with a learning disability also having attention deficit hyperactivity disorder (ADHD). Social-emotional problems result as children with learning disabilities are at a higher risk for experiencing peer rejection, poor self-concept, and poor social cognition (Hallahan et al., 2009).

## THE SCHOOL COUNSELOR'S ROLE IN THE SPECIAL EDUCATION IDENTIFICATION PROCESS

School counselors are key collaborators in the special education process. "School counselors already possess the knowledge skills and training that can be beneficial to guiding all stakeholders in the special education process" (Geltner & Leibforth, 2008, p. 162). The school counselor's role varies by school assignment. It is especially helpful when the school counselor provides the support of the referral process, but does not have the dominant responsibility. School counselors want to be master consultants and this role fits nicely into the special education referral process. Many of the consulting roles associated with special education are discussed in the chapter on consultation, collaboration, and teaming. Additional areas of the special education process previously not discussed are as follows:

1. Individual Educational Plan Development. Often, IEP meetings are problem focused, and school counselors are well suited to shift this train of thought into a more strength-based approach (Geltner & Leibforth, 2008). ASCA recommends that school counselors engage in indirect services, such as participating on multidisciplinary teams (MDTs), to advocate for students with disabilities (Milsom, Goodnough, & Akos, 2007). IEP teams should include individuals who can share knowledge of the student, availability of resources, and curriculum options (Clark, 2000b). "School counselors may be the only school personnel who have formal training in group work. This group work training includes analysis of group dynamics and development to determine what is necessary from leaders and members for groups to function effectively, something that is critical for an IEP meeting" (Milsom, Goodnough, & Akos, 2007, p. 20).

2. Parent Involvement. School counselors can model appropriate IEP meeting flow for faculty and staff to ensure that proper consideration is taken to involve the parents in this process. School counselors can also provide training to IEP coordinators as to how to effectively communicate with the student's parents in a positive manner. They can also advocate for the use of evidence-based interventions and collect data to ensure the interventions are benefiting the students (Geltner & Leibforth, 2008).

3. Student Observations. School counselors can play a critical role in helping to bring focus to students' nonacademic needs as well. "School counselors should be prepared to assist students in academic, career, and transition planning and personal and social areas. With knowledge and training in interventions addressing these three domains, school counselors can assist IEP teams in developing relevant goals and identifying realistic individual or group counseling interventions to assist students in meeting those goals" (Milsom, Goodnough, & Akos, 2007, p. 21).

## Section 504 of the Rehabilitation Act of 1973

**Section 504** of the Rehabilitation Act of 1973 was the first congressional action to mandate that individuals with disabilities could not be discriminated against or denied benefit by any program (or activity) receiving federal funding solely based on being disabled (Jiménez & Graf, 2008). Part of the Rehabilitation Act of 1973 also applies to the provision of services for students whose disabilities are not severe enough to warrant classification but could benefit from supportive services and classroom modification (Pierangelo & Giuliani, 2007). The regulations with Section 504 provide equal opportunity for individuals to achieve the same results, earn the same benefits, or attain the same levels of achievement in the most integrated settings that fit the individual's needs (Jiménez & Graf, 2008). Section 504 explains that no otherwise qualified individual with a disability be excluded from participation in, be denied the benefits of, or be subjected to discrimination under any program or activity receiving federal financial assistance.

Section 504 defines an individual with a disability as one "who (i) has a physical or mental impairment which substantially limits one or more of such person's major life activities, (ii) has a record of such an impairment, or (iii) is regarded as having such an impairment (Osborne & Russo, 2006, p. 18). Under Section 504 physical or mental impairments include (A) any physiological disorder or condition, cosmetic disfigurement, or anatomical loss affecting one or more of the following body systems: neurological; musculoskeletal; special sense organs; respiratory, including speech organs; cardiovascular; reproductive, digestive, genitor-urinary; hemic and lymphatic; skin; and endocrine; or (B) any mental or psychological disorder, such as mental retardation, organic brain syndrome, emotional or mental illness, and specific learning disorders." Osborne and Russo note that this list is not meant to be exhaustive and that it provides examples of types of impairments that are covered by Section 504" (Osborne & Russo, 2006, p. 18).

For an individual to have a record of impairment, there must be documented history, or identification of having a mental or physical impairment that has substantially limited one or more major life activities. "An individual is defined as having an impairment if they have (a) a physical or mental impairment that does not substantially limit major life activities but that is treated by a recipient as constituting such a limitation; (b) a physical or mental impairment that substantially limits major life activities only as a result of the attitudes of others toward such impairment; or (c) none of the impairments ... but is treated by a recipient as having such an impairment." Section 504 defines "major life activities" as functions such as "caring for one's self, performing manual tasks, walking, seeing, hearing, speaking, breathing, learning, and work" (Osborne & Russo, 2006, p. 18).

There are three defenses school officials can rely on to avoid being issued a charge of noncompliance. They involve the following: (1) "officials can be excused from making accommodations that result in 'a fundamental alteration in the nature of [a] program'," (2) "to avoid compliance if a modification imposes an 'undue financial burden'," and (3) "and otherwise qualified student with disability can be excluded from a program if her or his presence creates a substantial risk of injury to himself, herself, or others" (Osborne & Russo, 2006, p. 19).

### Eligibility

First, a student must be identified as having a disability under the definition established by Section 504. Once this has been done, the student must be determined to be "otherwise qualified." "In order to be 'otherwise qualified,' as the term is applied to students, a child must be '(i) of an age during which non-handicapped persons are provided such services, (ii) of any age during which it is mandatory under state law to provide such services to handicapped persons, or (iii) [a student] to whom a state is required to provide a free appropriate public education [under the IDEA]'" (Osborne & Russo, 2006).

The provisions in Section 504 regulate four areas: pre-placement evaluation, evaluation, placement, and revaluation. Pre-placement evaluations call for school officials to evaluate all children who are believed to need special education or related services. This action is to be taken before the school officials make any decisions in regards to the children's initial placements in regular or special education.

The evaluation provisions call for school officials to do the following: validate tests and other evaluation materials for the specific purposes for which they are used, and the tests must be administered by trained personnel in conformance with the instructions provided by their producer. As educators apply placement procedures to students under Section 504, their interpretations of data must consider information from a variety of sources, including aptitude and achievement tests, teacher's recommendations, physical condition, social and cultural background, and adaptive behaviors that have been documented and carefully considered. In addition, not only must any decisions be made by a group of persons, including individuals who are knowledgeable, but each child must be periodically reevaluated in a manner consistent with the dictates of IDEA (Osborne & Russo, 2006).

This section offers a brief overview of a complex area of support for special needs students. School districts usually have someone on staff who is the Section 504 coordinator and who helps educators determine if a student is eligible for accommodations and, if so, what would be the appropriate modification(s). Once employed as a school counselor you will learn much more about how your district addresses Section 504.

# SUPPORTING EVERY STUDENT'S RIGHT TO A QUALITY EDUCATION

School counselors can assume stronger leadership roles in school improvement by advocating for and providing high-quality services to students with disabilities, creating a healthy climate in the schools, and serving as an essential resource for students, teachers, parents, and administrators (Bemak, 2000; House & Martin, 1998).

School counselors support and provide services to all students and staff in special education class settings as well as in the general education setting. RtI, as aligned with the ASCA National Model, is truly Myrick's "law of parsimony," i.e., do all you can for the most you can (2004). The RtI, PBIS, and special education processes provide both opportunities and challenges to all school counselors to use their advocacy and leadership skills to work with all special needs students, their families, and the professional school staff. ASCA's position statement on The Professional School Counselor and Students with Special Needs (2010) reminds us that school counselor responsibilities may include but are not limited to the following:

- Providing classroom guidance, individual and/or group counseling to students with special needs within the scope of the comprehensive school counseling program.
- Consulting and collaborating with staff and parents to understand the special needs of a student.
- Advocating for students with special needs in the school and in the community.
- Contributing to the school's multidisciplinary team, which identifies students who may need to be assessed to determine special education eligibility within the scope and practice of the comprehensive school counseling program.
- Collaborating with related student support professionals (e.g., physical therapists, occupational therapists, special education, speech and language pathologists) in the delivery of services.
- Providing assistance with developing academic and transition plans for students in the Individual Education Program (IEP) as appropriate (ASCA, 2010b).

School counselors also have an ethical responsibility to not stray beyond the bounds of their training to take on or be assigned inappropriate administrative or supervisory responsibilities that involve but are not limited to the following:

- Making singular decisions regarding placement or retention.
- Serving in any supervisory capacity related to the implementation of the Individuals with Disabilities Education Act (IDEA).
- Serving as the school district representative for the team writing the IEP.

- Coordinating, writing, or supervising a specific plan under Section 504 of Public Law 93-112.
- Coordinating, writing, or supervising the implementation of the IEP (ASCA, 2010b).

Ultimately, the goal is not to have school counselors facilitate or even attend every IEP meeting; the goal is to improve the IEP meeting process for all participants (Leibforth, 2008). School counselors often have training in group dynamics and group management skills that are useful for facilitating the work of the IEP team. Group facilitation skills that can be adapted for use during IEP meetings include (a) interpreting information and explanations during team discussions, (b) identifying and establishing goals, (c) assessing the interactivity and group dynamics, (d) providing alternative perspectives and/or solutions, (e) modeling appropriate communication skills, and (f) building group cohesion through common goals (Leibforth, 2008).

School counselors play a tremendous role advocating for students and families during the IEP meeting process, as well as helping students develop self-advocacy skills and encouraging parents to become advocates for their children (Rai & Amatea, 2009). As social justice advocates, school counselors are in the perfect position to talk with parents and students about how they are coping with the information they have received including the implementation of the IEP.

The majority of school counselors have within their caseload students who require special services, interventions, and support. While the specifics of the school counselor role in working with the processes of RtI, PBIS, 504, and special education may vary from state to state, the mandate for school counselors remains to assist *all* students to achieve in the areas of academic, personal/social, and career development (Trolley, 2008) and to improve the outcomes for all students, regardless of their ability or disability (Blueprint for Reform, 2010). It is essential that all school counselors, both preservice and those in practice, acquire the knowledge and skills to work with special needs populations and continuously stay abreast of the laws and trends pertaining to special needs students and their rights to a quality education.

## TECH TOOLS

Use the power of technology to learn more about resources available for special needs students.

- *U.S. Department of Education*

  This website provides a guide to educators, parents, and schools to implement IDEA in regards to IEPs for students who have disabilities: www.ed.gov/parents/needs/speced/iepguide/index.html

  U.S. Department of Education. (2005). The Guidance Counselor's Role in Ensuring Equal Educational Opportunity: www.ed.gov/about/offices/list/ocr/docs/hq43ef.html

  Counselors need to have an understanding of how to recognize discrimination and other barriers to equal educational opportunity before they can take the appropriate steps to address barriers enabling all students to develop to their fullest.

- *Council for Exceptional Children (CEC)*

  This international professional organization provides information to improve education for students with exceptionalities, students with disabilities, and/or the gifted. The CEC is an active advocate for all individuals involved. They provide news, policies, advocacy information, publications, and professional development opportunities: www.cec.sped.org

- *National Center for Learning Disabilities*

  A great site for counselors, educators, and parents. Everything you need to know about LDs: www.ncld.org/

- *National Dissemination Center for Children with Disabilities*

  Provides information on disabilities from infants to school-age children and adolescents about IDEA, No Child Left Behind, and research-based educational practices: www.nichcy.org

- *National Center on Response to Intervention*

  The National Center on Response to Intervention's mission is to provide technical assistance and dissemination about proven and promising models for Response to Intervention (RtI) and Early Intervening Services (EIS) to state and local educators, families, and other stakeholders. The center works in four areas: (a) knowledge production; (b) implementation supports; (c) information dissemination; and (d) formative evaluation, which involves an assessment of the quality, implementation, impact, and cost effectiveness of the services offered: www.rti4success.org

- *National High School Center*

  The National High School Center serves as the central source of information and expertise on high school improvement. Millions of high school students —particularly those with disabilities, with limited proficiency in English, or from low-income backgrounds—need additional support to succeed. To address this challenge, the National High School Center promotes the use of research-supported approaches that help all students learn and become adequately prepared for college, work, and life. The National High School Center identifies research-supported improvement programs and tools, offers user-friendly products, and provides technical assistance services to improve secondary education: www.betterhighschools.org

- *IDEA Partnership*

  The IDEA Partnership is dedicated to improving outcomes for students and youth with disabilities by joining state agencies and stakeholders through shared work and learning: www.ideapartnership.org

- *Center on Positive Behavioral Interventions and Supports*

  The Center on Positive Behavioral Interventions and Supports (PBIS), funded by the Office of Special Education Programs (OSEP), was established to address the behavioral and discipline systems needed for the successful learning and social development of students. The center provides capacity-building information and technical support about behavioral systems to assist states and districts in the design of effective schools: www.pbis.org

- *LearningPort National Professional Development Library*

  A national professional development library of learning modules, tool kits, archived webinars, and video resources conceived by the U.S. Department of Education's Office of Special Education Programs (OSEP) to support the use of ARRA funds. It was developed through supplemental funds made available to NASDSE's IDEA Partnership grant. To access LearningPort, go to www.learningport.us or www.learningport.info.

- *RtI Action Network*

  The RtI Action Network is dedicated to the effective implementation of RtI in school districts nationwide. Its goal is to guide educators and families in the large-scale implementation of RtI, so that each child has access to quality instruction and that struggling students—including those with learning disabilities—are identified early and receive the necessary supports to be successful: www.rtinetwork.org

---

## School Counselor Casebook: Voices From the Field

### The Scenario Reviewed

Gavin is in eighth grade and seems to have more difficulty with word problems in math and other abstract thinking areas than many of his peers. Although he is highly motivated, he still struggles. To succeed, he needs a lot of practice, and his approach is somewhat more mechanical than that of his peers. He comments, "I need to be able to 'see it' to understand it. Some of these ideas are just too abstract for me. I can get it though, if I get enough practice."

When he gets frustrated with homework, he retreats to his room where he plays his guitar, and he is accomplished enough to compose his own arrangements. Gavin is skilled at working with people, and some of his peers turn to him as an arbitrator when clashes occur in club and other organizational meetings.

Gavin's team of teachers has asked for a conference. He is doing poorly this year in middle school and they are concerned that he may not be able to move on to high school.

### A Practitioner's Approach

Here's how a practicing school counselor approached this challenge.

In advocating for Gavin, I would assess his current situation and gather as complete a history as possible from Gavin, his parents, and his teachers. A complete file review will show whether Gavin has been previously referred for any kind of special assistance. If so, I would note the findings, paying special attention to whether Gavin had previously been assessed for a learning disability. If interventions had been tried, I would review what Gavin's response to those interventions was, what seemed to help him improve, and what did not. In the file, comments from teachers on elementary and middle level report cards are often most revealing, as is attendance history and the number of school moves.

Gavin's statewide test scores will show his history with word problems in math, his ability to develop interpretations in reading, and any other areas of testing that require abstract reasoning abilities. If he has had previous intellectual assessments, I would look at any test scores that measure perceptual reasoning.

Gavin's comment, "I need to see it to understand," seems to point to a possible visual learning style, but I want to know what the experience of his teachers is with him in the classroom. Does he do better when given visual prompts? What has been tried (more visual prompts, extra time, minimal distraction)? Asking seventh- and sixth-grade teachers about their successes with Gavin will be helpful.

It is important to note Gavin's age and assess his relative development. Is he still somewhat concrete, and the ability to abstract will come with time? Can he abstract in other subject areas with an obvious difficulty when it comes to math only? His difficulty with abstract thinking may be a symptom of a learning disability. It might also be that he is behind developmentally, and still a concrete thinker, which will change with developmental maturity.

All along, I have been using a strength-based approach to build my relationship with Gavin. Although he is well liked and creative, Gavin, like many eighth-grade boys who are not doing well in their academics, may tend to give up more easily. While counseling with Gavin, I would draw as many connections to his music and composing skills as possible to help him see himself as capable and successful. I would also ask him to be his own arbitrator and use his arbitrating strengths in assessing his needs, helping him to look at his personal "clash" with learning. I would advocate for him with his teachers, prompting them also to build on his strengths.

When we all meet together, I would want to know how Gavin is doing in all of his subjects. Are his reading and writing skills strong? Is his statement, "I can get it if I get enough practice," borne out in the classroom? How does the curriculum suit Gavin? Does he get enough practice on a math skill before moving on, since he feels that success for him comes with plenty of practice? With parents, I would want to know at what point Gavin gets frustrated and what, if any, support gets him back on track.

*(continues)*

We would then develop a plan, tracking his successes with our interventions and assessing every couple of weeks. If he is doing well, we will monitor him for continued success. If not, we will continue to refine the plan, using Gavin's strengths to support him in his areas of difficulty. If our interventions have continued to prove ineffective, we would refer to our special services team for testing. The team would consider whether there is a discrepancy between Gavin's potential and his achievement, pointing to a learning disability. It is important to note, however, that the process of looking for successful classroom interventions continues, whether a learning disability is discovered or not. With high school approaching, our team needs to collaborate with high school staff for maximum transitional support. As Gavin's advocate, it is most important at this critical time in his life that he has a plan in place that will support his academic needs and help him move successfully from grade level to grade level with the necessary supports in place.

Linda Eby has been a middle school counselor for 26 years. She has presented at state and national school counselor conferences, and to educators and social workers internationally. She is a past president of the Oregon School Counselor Association, and a past middle level vice president for the American School Counselor Association.

# LOOKING BACK: SALIENT POINTS

## Providing for the Instructional Needs of All Students

School counselors and most educators ascribe to the belief that all children can learn and all children can achieve. All school personnel should be sensitive to the time needed to learn, especially for students who struggle to achieve a level of minimum proficiency.

## A Social Justice Agenda

School counselors, serving as social justice advocates, can ensure that students with learning and instructional differences are treated with the same respect and are given the same opportunities as all of the students who are considered part of the mainstream.

## Response to Intervention (RtI)

RtI is a highly organized three-tier approach to providing targeted supports as needed and as documented by data. Evidence and data will drive the decision to determine what the student needs to succeed and this must be done with fidelity.

RtI utilizes three tiers: Tier 1 reflects the school's approach to providing a quality grade-level curriculum, with effective teaching to every student. Tier 2 targets students in need of additional support and focuses on identified learning needs. Tier 3 is intensive support and every student who needs it receives it in addition to the core curriculum instruction.

## RtI and Special Education

There will be students who are *not* succeeding with tiered RtI interventions but also may *not* qualify for special education. The use of RtI to identify students who need special education services is similar to the traditional approach for identifying student access to special education service.

## The School Counselor's Role in RtI

School counselors recognize the critical importance of early intervention for struggling students as they assist teachers with differentiated instructional service delivery, closely monitor student progress to inform instruction, and use data to make informed decisions. School counselors are in a pivotal position to consult and collaborate with teachers around the challenges of creating a classroom environment that is conducive to every student learning and succeeding.

## RtI and the ASCA National Model

The RtI process is highly consistent with all the components of comprehensive school counseling programs. Each of the four quadrants—Foundation, Delivery, Management, and Accountability—can be aligned with the Tier 1 strategies, and Tier 2 and 3 interventions.

## Positive Behavior Intervention Supports (PBIS)

PBIS requires the use of continuous monitoring, data-based decision making, and an intervention continuum. When PBIS is effectively implemented, the majority of students demonstrate appropriate behavior within the general education classroom without additional supports, thus saving the more intensive interventions (e.g., social skills classes, individualized behavior interventions) for students who require these interventions.

## Special Education

Special education encompasses the entire range of learning, emotional, and physical disabilities, and in some states also includes students who have special abilities, gifts, or talents. In the Individuals with Disabilities Education Act (IDEA) the word *handicapped* was eliminated and *disabled* was used in its place. IDEA requires that every child with disabilities has access to the program of study that will most effectively approximate a normal child's educational program.

## Special Education and School Improvement Agendas

IDEA and the No Child Left Behind Act (NCLB) both address the needs of students with disabilities by focusing on student achievement and outcomes; emphasizing parental participation; and requiring the regular evaluation or assessment of students and staffs. Additionally, the Blueprint for Reform requires school personnel to provide a wide range of resources and support to ensure that all students have the opportunity to succeed in college and in a career, regardless of ability or disability.

## The Over Identification Debate

There is a growing concern about the over identification of children for special education. African American students have been consistently overrepresented in special education for more than three decades. Native Americans have also been consistently overrepresented, whereas the same is not true for Latino students. However, Latino students are often overrepresented at the state and district levels where their enrollment is highest (Sullivan, A'Vant, Baker, Chandler, Graves, McKinney, & Sayles, p. 1). The overrepresentation of students of color means that they have limited access to general education experiences and the opportunities those experiences provide.

## Inclusion

Many schools across our nation are establishing inclusive environments in which students with disabilities, including those with severe disabilities, are integrated into the traditional mainstream classroom setting. Based on the principle of normalization the goal was to make life for those with disabilities as culturally normative as possible.

## Procedural Steps in Special Education Placement

The complex process of special education eligibility and placement requires many stakeholders to include parent(s), guardian(s), or caretaker(s). The steps involved are many and require careful attention to both the process and the identification of the disabling condition(s) that are specified in the federal guidelines that determine a student's eligibility.

## The Dominant Classification: Learning Disabilities

The term *specific learning disability* means a disorder in one or more of the basic psychological processes involved in understanding or in using language, spoken or written, which disorder may manifest itself in an imperfect ability to listen, think, speak, read, write, spell, or do mathematical calculations.

## The School Counselor's Role in Special Education Identification Process

The role of the school counselor as a consultant fits nicely into the special education referral process. School counselors are actively involved in the development of the Individual Education Plan (IEP), involving parents, observing students, and providing recommendations.

## Section 504 of the Rehabilitation Act of 1973

"An individual is defined as having an impairment under 504 if they have (a) a physical or mental impairment that does not substantially limit major life activities but that is treated by a recipient as constituting such a limitation; (b) a physical or mental impairment that substantially limits major life activities only as a result of the attitudes of others toward such impairment" (Osborne & Russo, 2006, p. 18).

### Supporting Every Student's Right to a Quality Education

School counselors support and provide services to all students and staff in special education class settings as well as in the general education setting. The RtI, PBIS, and the special education processes provide both opportunities and challenges to all school counselors to use their advocacy and leadership skills to work with all special needs students, their families, and the professional school staff.

## KEY TERMS

Special education p. 286

Learning disabilities p. 287

Response to Intervention p. 287

RtI and special education p. 289

School counselor's role in RtI p. 291

RtI and the ASCA National Model p. 293

Positive behavior intervention supports p. 297

Education for All Handicapped Children Act of 1975 p. 300

Individualized Education Plan (IEP) p. 301

Inclusion p. 302

Section 504 of the Rehabilitation Act of 1973 p. 309

## LEARNING EXTENSIONS/MAKING CONNECTIONS

1. Discuss parental involvement in the special education process under IDEA. What are parents' rights? How are parents to be involved in the process? Discuss whether or not you believe a parent should have the final say as to whether or not their child gets special education.

2. Some students received special education services through a pull out program in which students would go to a resource room for a set time each day to receive special education services. Other students received special education services in a full-time self-contained special education program. First, discuss the opportunities and challenges using the inclusion model versus the traditional model of special education pull out resource room and self-contained classrooms.

3. How does Response to Intervention (RtI) support student achievement in your school system—either the one you live in or one that you may be seeking employment in?

4. Discuss the over identification of special education students through a social justice lens. In other words, who was being identified for special education and is there an equity issue? How can you as a school counselor help address this issue? Research at least two resources not cited in this chapter. Form your response and provide your two resources in APA style.

5. Discuss your understanding of learning disabilities as defined by the federal government.

6. You have been given permission to write the script as to how school counselors will be involved in the special education process. In a one-page, double-spaced paper, describe the school counselor's role.

7. Describe eligibility under Section 504 of the Rehabilitation Act of 1973.

8. A listing of Internet resources appears in the Tech Tools section at the end of the chapter. Familiarize yourself with three major organizations related to student disabilities and use the websites to summarize what a school counselor needs to know to work with students with these disabling conditions.

9. As a social justice advocate how do we best serve the following?

   a. The "Inherited" Special Education Student who has always been in special education, therefore always will be in special education.
   b. The Student in Academic Crisis who is in the middle to early high school years and struggling.
   c. The Student Not Performing Up to High Expectations who is in the early to late high school years.

## CHAPTER 11

# Creating a Safe, Supportive, and Respectful School Culture and Environment

## CHAPTER OBJECTIVES

*By the time you have completed this chapter, you should be able to*

- understand safe school concerns facing educators today;

- discuss techniques for preventing or deescalating violent situation in schools;

- discuss behaviors within a developmental and social context that are early warning signs of potential violence or other troubling behaviors in children;

- understand the value of conflict mediation and resolution programs for students;

- discuss strategies to prevent or deescalate bullying in the school environment;

- become familiar with the legal issues that affect school safety and a school climate;

- explore ways of integrating character education;

- develop strategies to create a safe and respectful school environment.

## School Counselor Casebook: Getting Started

### The Scenario

For the past two weeks several students in your caseload have complained to you about certain students who have been bullying them. Although students often complain about "being picked on," something about this situation just doesn't seem right. The students will not tell you who is involved but insist that you "tell" the teachers to do something about it. As you think this through, there are several courses of action available. You decide to discuss this with the other school counselors in your building, the teachers who are involved with these students, and your building principal. In your planning, consider how the American School Counselor Association National Model can help with a whole-school approach for prevention and intervention.

### Thinking about Solutions

As you read this chapter, imagine yourself as the school counselor in this situation and think about how you might answer this question. Keep the following questions in mind: How will you investigate the students' concerns about bullying especially because they will not "tell" who is involved? How will you get the teachers involved? What kinds of prevention and intervention activities might you suggest to address the bullying problem?

When you come to the end of the chapter, you will have the opportunity to see how your ideas compare with a practicing school counselor's approach.

# SAFE AND SUPPORTIVE LEARNING ENVIRONMENTS

> Every child deserves to be safe, respected, valued and able to focus on learning. (Jennings, U.S. Department of Education, 2010)

Since 1992, there have been 592 acts of **school violence nationwide** resulting in homicide (National Center for Educational Statistics, 2010). Schools are intertwined with their communities, where gangs, guns, and neighborhood volatility can cross the threshold of the schoolhouse door (Meyer & Furlong, 2010). Violence in America's schools cuts across all neighborhoods and although media attention on school violence often portrays violence as the reflection of inner-city norms, this is Hollywood's interpretation. Of the 28 reported cases of school shootings between 1982 and 2001, all but one occurred in a rural or suburban school setting (Kimmel, 2003). Schools nationwide seek assurances that targeted incidents will not occur in their community whether urban, rural, or suburban; however, research has shown that school personnel must take positive steps to develop a series of approaches that address safety, order, and an interpersonally supportive climate in the school (Borum, Cornell, Modzeleski, & Jimerson, 2010).

Although public perception is that schools are not safe havens and the media often present a picture that would indicate violence is on the rise, targeted acts of violence are the exception to the rule and have been decreasing (Modzeleski, Feucht, Rand, Hall, Simon, & Butler, 2008). The 2009 Indicators of School Crime and Safety gather the overall acts of serious acts of school violence nationwide and despite what appears to be a large number of occurrences, the incidents of violence in schools are declining. During the 2007–08 school year,

- there were 21 homicides and 5 suicides of school-age youth (ages 5–18) at school;
- there were 1,748 homicides of school-age youth at school;
- there were 1,296 suicides of school-age youth;
- the rate of violent incidents, 2 per 1,000 students, was higher in middle schools (41 incidents) than in primary schools (26 incidents) or in high schools (22 incidents);
- while 48 percent of schools reported at least one student threat of physical attack without a weapon, only 9 percent of schools reported such a threat with a weapon;
- the rate of the distribution, possession, or use of illegal drugs was higher in schools with 1,000 or more students (5 incidents per 1,000 students) than in schools with lower enrollments (1 to 2 incidents per 1,000 students); and
- approximately 13 percent of city schools reported at least one gang crime, a higher percentage than that reported by suburban (5%), town (5%), or rural schools (3%) (National Center for Educational Statistics, 2009).

Although homicides and serious acts of violence may be declining and U.S. schools remain relatively safe, any amount of violence is unacceptable.

TABLE **11.1**

Percentage of Schools Reporting Select Discipline Problems by School Level, 2007–08

|  | Racial Tension | Bullying | Sexual Harassment | Verbal Abuse | Gang Activities |
|---|---|---|---|---|---|
| Primary | 2.6% | 20.5% | 1% | 4% | 10% |
| Middle | 5.6% | 43.5% | 6% | 10% | 35.4% |
| High School | 5.4% | 21.7% | 6% | 12% | 43.1% |

Parents, teachers, and administrators expect schools to be safe havens of learning. Acts of violence disrupt the learning process and have a negative effect on students, the school itself, and the broader community (Centers for Disease Control, 2010). As Table 11.1 shows, discipline incidents that may lead to serious violent acts exist at all school levels.

The first step in preventing school violence is to understand the extent and nature of the problem. The Centers for Disease Control and Prevention, the U.S. Department of Education, and the U.S. Department of Justice gather and analyze data from a variety of sources to gain a more complete understanding of school violence as public policymakers, police officials, school administrators, and parents continue to search for explanations about violence in schools. The locations in which high-profile school shootings have occurred are generally perceived as those in which young people are given inadequate support in finding their own way in a difficult world (Lenhardt, Farrell, & Graham, 2010; U.S. Secret Service and the U.S. Department of Education, 2002a). Schools do not always present themselves as compassionate institutions. When parents become less stringent about discipline at home and in the school, the standards bar is lowered on "acceptable" moral and social behavior; this results in attitudinal and behavioral differences in children and youth (Shafii & Shafii, 2001; Swick, 2004).

## The Challenge for Educators

The Challenge: All children need a safe environment in which to learn and achieve, one free of fear and intimidation for teachers as well as children.

The Solution: Ensure a safe and orderly school by implementing programs that protect students and teachers, encourage discipline and personal responsibility, and combat illegal drugs. (Centers for Disease Control, 2010; Center for Mental Health in Schools at UCLA, 2007; Jennings, 2010)

Goal 4 of the No Child Left Behind Act (U.S. Department of Education, 2001) charged educators to ensure that every school needs to be safe and drug free. The act encouraged laws to be aggressively enforced and states that the first job of government is to protect its citizens. It further required states' departments of education and public schools to report on school safety to the public; provide protection to teachers and educators so they can teach and maintain order; and anticipate the potential for violence (NCLB, 2001). As part of the ESEA Reauthorization, six core areas are proposed in the Blueprint for Reform: accelerating achievement and ensuring equity; excellent instructional teams; educating diverse learners, effective teaching and learning; fostering innovation and success; and supporting student success (Jennings, 2010).

The principles of supporting student success intend to ensure that students are safe and healthy and have access to adults who care about their success. This is accomplished through fostering student engagement through relationships, school participation, and respect for diversity; emotional and physical safety; and creating school environments that address the physical surrounding, academic environment, wellness, and fairness in disciplinary enforcement (Office of Safe and Drug Free Schools, 2009).

Educators and communities have been working diligently to ensure that their schools are an emotionally and physically safe haven for students. A growing interest in character education is an acknowledgment that schools also believe principles such as responsibility, integrity, trustworthiness, care, kindness, and respect are foundational to creating a positive school climate and reducing incidents of aggression (Likona, 2004; Lockwood, 2008). The ASCA personal-social development standards complement character education efforts and emphasize respect for self and others, taking responsibility, acquiring resiliency, and personal safety.

Devine and Cohen (2008) state, "inculcating social and emotional skills both within classrooms and within the whole school context is the surest way to attain both academic excellence and social and emotional safety" (p. 5). They believe that if educators do whatever it takes to teach students how to be emotionally and socially aware, how to behave and handle situations in a nonviolent manner, and work together with parents and the community to create a safer learning environment for the students, it will improve student academic success as well. It is too easy for teachers to focus solely on the academic aspect of school and forget how important the outside factors are that affect learning. When students do not feel safe in their learning environment, they will not learn. When students acquire the skills, knowledge, and beliefs including reflective and empathic abilities; problem-solving and decision-making abilities; communicative capacities; impulse control and anger management abilities; cooperative capacities; ability to form friendships; ability to recognize and appreciate diversity; and altruistic capacities (p. 53), it increases their core social and emotional competence, which contributes to safer and more caring schools. School counselors are leaders and contributors to this collaborative effort and play a vital role in creating a climate that is both emotionally safe and supports student success.

## School Violence Defined

School violence can be defined as encompassing a wide range of activities, including assaults with or without weapons, physical fights, threats or destructive acts other than physical fights, robbery, harassment, dating violence, molestation, rape, bullying, hostile or threatening remarks between groups of students, and gang violence (Centers for Disease Control, 2010; Fischer & Kettl, 2001).

Educators and school counselors have a responsibility to understand youth behavior and establish a context that separates the healthy, normal, growing-up behaviors from those that are deviant, defy school policies or the law, and can result in a threatening situation. Educators and parents are often challenged to differentiate between youth experimentation and the attempt to establish a personal identity and risky behavior that can lead to antisocial and violent action. For example, do adults respond differently to the student who has a "short fuse" and "hangs out" with known substance users, then they do to the student who is academically on track and active in school events but has tattooed his neck and pierced his tongue?

Experimentation is a natural part of growing up and seeking independence is a normal developmental stage for adolescents. When a teen's interests and styles reflect popular peer-group standards, it is usually not a cause for alarm. When combined with falling grades, truancy, alcohol consumption or other aberrant behaviors, tattoos, body piercing, and bizarre clothing can be a call for help. Teachers, administrators, parents, and school counselors address inappropriate behavior every day. As with every preceding generation, behavior and appearances that vary from the norm can be seen as incongruous and often the typical response is to punish and exclude students (Skiba & Peterson, 1999).

### Student Behaviors: Violent or Disruptive?

It is equally important to differentiate between student behaviors that are seen as disruptive or violent. A disruptive student is one who interferes with the educational process or a teacher's authority over the students in the classroom (U.S. Department of Education & U.S. Department of Justice, 2003). Behaviors can range from more innocent disruptions, such as frequently strolling into class late, arguing with the teacher, or constantly shouting out, to a student who is violent and commits an intentional act of aggression on a teacher, other school employee, or another student. The violent student may possess or threaten to use a gun, knife, or a dangerous weapon; or damage or destroy school district or personal property (U.S. Department of Education & U.S. Department of Justice, 2003). Both situations require the intervention of school personnel, including school counselors—the first to maintain the school as a peaceful learning environment and the second to keep students out of harm's way (Dwyer, Osher, & Warger, 1998; Snell, 2005).

### Bullying

School **bullying** was once considered a childhood ritual or a normal part of development and was therefore often overlooked or ignored by school personnel. However, research has found that bullying is not a harmless phenomenon; rather, it is a widespread and serious problem that must be addressed. According to Olweus (1993), for a behavior to be considered bullying, it must have three elements: It must be intended to harm; it must be repetitive; and a difference of power, i.e., physical, social, age, size, etc., must exist between the bully and the victim. Bullying at school in the traditional manner is done by someone who harms individuals or groups intentionally and repeatedly by using physical strength, age, and power (Quiroz, Arnette, & Stephens, 2006).

Bullying has become the most common form of school violence and is on the rise (Dinkes, Kemp, & Baum, 2009), with 43 percent of all middle school children either victims or perpetrators (sometimes both) of chronic bullying that includes threatening, name-calling, punching, slapping, sneering, and jeering (Wang, Iannotti, & Nansel, 2009b). Experts in aggressive behavior believe there is no easy way to stamp out bullying (Beale & Scott, 2001; Carney, 2008; Swearer, Espelage, Vaillancourt, & Hymel, 2010). Traditional bullying behaviors can be categorized as direct, which tends to be more physical in nature than indirect bullying behavior, which can include behaviors such as hitting, tripping, shoving, threatening verbally, or stabbing. Boys who bully tend to engage in direct bullying (Farmer, Farmer, Estell & Hutchins, 2007) while female bullies tend to engage in indirect bullying including spreading rumors, blackmailing or imposing social isolation (Willard, 2006). Bullying is based on how power, control, privilege, and respect is defined in contemporary culture by adults and students alike (Wang, Iannotti, & Nansel, 2009a; Wiseman, 2002).

Research shows that when peers intervened, 57 percent of the interventions were effective (i.e., the bullying stopped within 10 seconds); however, peers intervened in only 11 to 19 percent of all bullying incidents (Hawkins, Pepler, & Craig, 2001). Students may feel ashamed or embarrassed to report bullying or fear that telling an adult will exacerbate the bullying problem. When students fail to ask for help in the case of relational bullying, it is difficult for school counselors or teachers to know that a student is having problems because of the covert nature of relational bullying (Singh, Lancioni, Singhjoy, Winton, Sabaawi, Wahler, & Singh, 2007). By collaborating with teachers, school counselors can teach guidance lessons about relational bullying and how to ask adults for help when being bullied. This establishes the school counselor as a concerned and knowledgeable professional who will work with and help students who are involved in bullying (Jacobsen & Bauman, 2007).

Since 1999, forty-five states have passed anti-bullying legislation (Simmons, 2010) to address the growing concern that bullying continues to increase dramatically among school-aged children and youth. Additionally, new guidance from the U.S. Department of Education's Office of Civil Rights is aimed at putting school districts on notice about their responsibilities to address bullying. Certain types of harassment rooted in sex-role stereotyping or religious differences may be considered a federal civil rights violation (Samuels, 2010).

### Cyberbullying

Teens live highly digital and media-rich lives with more communication choices than ever before, and this influences youth behavior in ways never imagined (OSDFS, 2009). Students today often are better prepared than adults in communicating technologically (Blair, 2003). **Cyberbullying**, a term not in existence a decade ago, is now a pervasive and growing problem that can have devastating effects on young lives and those around such affected youths. While definitions vary, most experts consider cyberbullying as electronic aggression involving the use of cell phones, computers, or other electronic devices to humiliate or harass someone, and possibly even threaten physical violence. Like traditional bullying, cyberbullying includes a wide range of behavior (Centers for Disease Control, 2010).

Technology and its misuse by students create challenges for school counselors, teachers, administrators, and parents (Kennedy, 2009). In a traditional sense, identification of the bully is typically easy. Research revealed that about half of middle school students who had been cyberbullied did not know who had bullied them (Limar, 2009). Cyberbullies frequently hide behind anonymity, which makes the identification of bullies so much more difficult (Strom & Strom, 2005). Limar (2009) identified five key factors that separate cyberbullying from traditional bullying:

1. *Anonymity.* A student who bullies through traditional means can be easily identified and potentially avoided. Someone who cyberbullies is often anonymous and her or his target is often left wondering who the perpetrator is, which can cause a good deal of stress.
2. *Disinhibition.* The anonymity afforded by the Internet can lead children to engage in behaviors online in which they might not engage in face-to-face contact.
3. *Accessibility.* Most children who use traditional ways of bullying terrorize their victims at school, on the school bus, or walking to and from school. However, children who cyberbully can wreak havoc any time of the day or night, including during the school day.
4. *Punitive fears.* Victims of cyberbullying often do not report their experiences to adults because of fear of retribution from their tormentors and fear that their computer or phone privileges will be taken away.
5. *Ambiguous bystander roles.* Most episodes of traditional bullying occur in the presence of other people who assume the role of bystanders and witnesses. The phenomenon of being a bystander in the cyber world may be quite different from witnessing bullying firsthand because bystanders may see the harmful material on a website or in a message but not witness face-to-face confrontation (The Challenge, 2009, p. 2).

Willard (2006) described school students who most often engage in cyberbullying as social climber bullies who are upper-social-class students who bully within the context of the interrelationships of groups labeled the "in crowd," the "wannabees," and the "losers." As leaders in the school, these bullies are often looked on favorably by administrators, teachers, and counselors. Students classified as "wannabes" and "losers" typically do not want to report cyberbullying to adults in the school for fear of exclusion or of retaliation. Victims of cyberbullies are often fearful of telling adults because they fear the bullying will become more harmful and intense.

Students can't learn if they don't feel safe. Period. (Jennings, 2010)

Cyberbullying can happen at any time and when least expected as the student who is cyberbullied often does not know the identity of her or his tormentor. She or he may be extremely anxious and distracted at school, concerned if the perpetrator is in homeroom, on the bus, or in gym class (Limar, 2009). Anxiety and stress is the result of wondering or worrying about embarrassing messages being spread. All of this can be extremely distracting to the entire student body.

To help reduce and prevent bullying and cyberbullying, school counselors can assume a leadership role in creating a climate that is safe and respectful (Chibbaro, 2007; Young, Hardy, Hamilton, Biernesser, Sun, & Niebergall, 2009).

School counselors are not the only people in the school who are responsible for the safety of students, but they may be the primary contact person for parents and students seeking information or help. Because many students are more tech-savvy than adults, school counselors can help to leverage that expertise to better understand how students are using technology and involve students to be a part of the solution to online bullying. School counselors can:

- provide leadership to advocate for policies that keep children safe;
- involve students in identifying bullying and cyberbullying problems at the school;
- integrate anti-bullying and cyberbullying lessons into the guidance curriculum;
- work with administrators, teachers, students, and parents to create a bully-free environment including respecting self and others, alternate ways of resolving differences, and acceptable use of technology;
- provide educational materials or training for parents and students on bullying issues and cyberbullying;
- develop a mentoring program for high school students to teach younger students about protecting themselves from bullies and Internet safety; and most importantly,
- empower students to speak up (adapted from Kennedy, 2009).

### Sexual Harassment

Sexual harassment has become an issue of national attention as a result of survey research conducted in the early 1990s that revealed 81 percent of the students, both girls and boys, had been the recipient of unwanted sexual attention in school (American Association of University Women, 1993). The updated Hostile Hallways Study (American Association of University Women, 2001) concurred that the problem continues to be pervasive with 83 percent of the girls and 79 percent of the boys reporting being victims of sexual harassment. In 1986, the Equal Employment Opportunity Commission extended the definition of sexual harassment from Title IX legislation (1972) to include sexual advances, request for sexual favors, verbal or physical conduct of a sexual nature when submission to such conduct is a term or condition of an individual's academic advancement, or the creating an environment that is intimidating, hostile, or offensive affecting the academic environment. This definition has been extended by the Office of Civil Rights (2001) to include a hostile environment that is severe or pervasive enough to interfere with a student's education.

The implications of sexual harassment provide school counselors with the legal muscle to bring the problem to the forefront of a school's attention. The Supreme Court Decision on *Davis v. Monroe County Board of Education* (526 U.S. 629, 1999) found the school district liable for severe, persistent, and pervasive incidences of sexual harassment if there is deliberate indifference. The Office of Civil Rights (OCR) requires that each school district, as part of Title IX compliance, have in place specific policies and procedure to address sexual harassment (Office of Civil Rights, 2001).

## The Etiology of School Violence

School violence may range on a continuum from subtle behaviors (e.g., teasing, name calling, bullying, and other forms of intimidation and harassment) to severe actions, such as physical fights and shootings (Center for Mental Health in Schools, 2007; Smith & Sandhu, 2004). With the help of counselors, schools can successfully identify students at risk of violent behaviors when effective prevention measures are put in place, including early assessment of students at risk (Canfield, Ballard, Osmon, & McCune, 2004; Cunningham & Sandhu, 2000; D'Andrea, 2004; Hernández & Seem, 2004; U.S. Department of Education & U.S. Department of Justice, 2003). Research has shown that the first steps toward preventing violence are to identify and understand the factors that place youth at risk for violent victimization and perpetration (Cunningham & Sandhu, 2000; D'Andrea, 2004). These factors are presented in Table 11.2.

The greater the number of risk factors to which an individual is exposed, the greater the probability that the individual will engage in violent behavior (Hawkins, Herrenkohl, Farrington et al., 2000). These contributing factors are translated into the attitudes and behaviors of

TABLE **11.2**
Factors Contributing to Youths at Risk of Violent Behavior

| Individual | Family | Peer/School | Neighborhood |
|---|---|---|---|
| History of early aggression; | Poor monitoring or supervision of children; | Associate with peers engaged in high-risk or problem behavior; | Poverty and diminished economic opportunity; |
| Beliefs supportive of violence; | Exposure to violence; | Low commitment to school; | High levels of transiency and family disruption; |
| Social-cognitive deficits; | Parental drug/alcohol abuse; | Academic failure; | Exposure to violence; |
| Hyperactivity, restlessness, risk taking; | Poor emotional attachment to parents or caregivers; | Frequent school transitions; | Availability of drugs and firearms. |
| Beliefs and attitudes favorable to deviant or antisocial behavior. | Child maltreatment; | Truancy and/or dropping out; | |
| | Parent criminality. | Gang membership. | |

Source: National Center for Injury Prevention and Control (2002).

students that are considered antisocial and impact school climate. Risk factors include the following:

Alienation: students who feel alienated usually perceive a lack of genuine love from significant others in their lives (Glasser, 2000a; Pollack, 1998). Alienated students may turn to gang involvement to provide an environment of "belonging" (Goldstein & Kodluboy, 1998).

Depression and Anxiety: Children who are consistently sad, anxious, moody, or negative may be experiencing the symptoms of an emotional problem (Shafii & Shafii, 1992). Suicide is one of the leading causes of death among adolescents (Hazler, 2000; U.S. Preventive Services Task Force, 2004).

Destructive Behavior: When a child hurts himself or others, it's a red flag that she or he needs help. This includes violent temper tantrums, fighting, threats, hurting animals, vandalism, setting fires, and being fascinated with weapons (Lowry, Powell, Kann, Collins, & Kolbe, 1998).

Gang Involvement: Adolescents and teens seek gang membership for affiliation and a sense of belonging. However, the community views gangs as engaging in activities that are intolerable, illegitimate, criminal, or a combination thereof (Goldstein & Kodluboy, 1998).

Manipulative: Children who have the ability to manipulate a situation know what to say, when, and where. Respect is selective and although students may appear to be obedient to authority figures, they are poised to intimidate the weak and powerless (Sandhu, 2000; Smith & Sandhu, 2004).

Peer Problems: Normal teens focus on their friends. In fact, their peer group often becomes more important than their family. When a teenager is a loner, it may be a sign that something is seriously amiss (Bluestein, 2001).

Bias and Prejudice: Attitudes of bias or prejudice may lead to involvement in hateful behaviors. Hate-induced activities can lead to violence that threatens and intimidates all students. Hate can be directed at ethnic minorities, surface in religious discrimination or gender-based bias, or target sexual minorities who are gay or lesbian, or at people with disabilities (Teaching Tolerance, 2003).

Use of Drugs: Over the past two decades, researchers have tried to identify the factors that differentiate those who use drugs from those who do not. Prevention of drug use, which is related to violent behavior, is based on identifying and reducing risk factors and the strengthening of **protective factors**. Risk factors are associated with greater inclination toward drug use while protective factors are associated with lessened inclination for drug use. Protective factors include bonding, healthy beliefs, and clear standards (Benard, 2004). The individual will be more resilient, prevent problems, and promote a healthy lifestyle (Hawkins, Herrenkohl, Farrington, et al., 2000).

Educators are better prepared to act with purpose to create a safer environment when they have a better sense of the warning signs that can place students at risk for potentially engaging in violent victimization and perpetration. Research confirms that most children who are troubled show multiple **early warning signs** (Hawkins, Farrington, & Catalano, 1998). Factors such as low educational achievement, low interest in education, dropping out of school, and truancy are potential contributors to criminal and violent behavior (Centers for Disease Control, 2010).

TABLE **11.3**
Early and Imminent Warning Signs of Violent Behavior

| Early Warning Signs | Imminent Warning Signs |
| --- | --- |
| Social withdrawal | Serious physical fighting with peers or family members |
| Excessive feelings of isolation and being alone | Severe destruction of property |
| Excessive feelings of rejection | Severe rage for seemingly minor reasons |
| Being a victim of violence | Detailed threats of lethal violence |
| Feelings of being picked on and persecuted | Possession and/of use of firearms and other weapons |
| Low school interest and poor academic performance | Other self-injurious behaviors or threats of suicide |
| Expression of violence in writings and drawings | Has a detailed plan to harm others |
| Uncontrolled anger | |
| Patterns of impulsive and chronic hitting, intimidating, and bullying behavior | |
| History of discipline problems | |
| Past history of violent and aggressive behavior | |
| Intolerance for differences and prejudicial attitudes | |
| Drug use and alcohol use | |
| Affiliation with gangs | |
| Inappropriate access to, possession of, and use of firearms | |
| Serious threats of violence | |

Source: Early Warning, Timely Response: A Guide to Safe Schools (USDOE, 1998).

Early Warning, Timely Response: A Guide to Safe Schools (U.S. Department of Education, 1998) heightens the awareness of educators to the behaviors and attitudes that students at risk of violent behavior present. The early and **imminent warning signs**, listed in Table 11.3, are research based and offer guidance to educators and stakeholders to identify the factors that can negatively affect individual and/or groups of students and school climate.

# SCHOOL COUNSELORS: COMMITTED TO SAFE AND SUPPORTIVE SCHOOLS

Educators and communities need to work diligently to ensure that their schools are an emotionally and physically safe haven for students. A growing interest in character education is an acknowledgment that schools also believe principles such as responsibility, integrity, trustworthiness, care, kindness, and respect are foundational to creating a positive school climate and reducing incidents of aggression (Likona, 2004). The personal-social development standards complement character education efforts and emphasize respect for self and others, taking responsibility, and personal safety. School counselors, as part of this collaborative effort, play a vital role in both prevention and intervention efforts.

School counselors as leaders and advocates who can motivate and collaborate are called on to join their fellow educators in creating and maintaining a safe and respectful school environment. Sandhu (2000) offered school counselors suggestions within their realm of influence to contribute to developing and maintaining a safe and respectful environment. These include the following:

- Proactively reach out to all students for primary prevention and to maximize every student's development.
- Collaborate and team with teachers to develop sensitivities about students who appear alienated or disaffected.
- Consult with teachers on the characteristics of the warning signs of troubled students and lend support to teachers to help them cope with difficult students in their classrooms.
- Engage all stakeholders in the process to comprehensively address the problem.
- Develop strong relationships with students who have been victims of violence themselves or who inflicted violence on others.

Glasser (2000b) reminds us that students who are alienated can be disruptive or violent. Sandhu's (2000) suggestions are designed to reduce this alienation. Unhappy individuals carry within them the potential to do harm, to themselves or to others, as do those who can motivate others to strike out in self-defense or as a result of peer pressure. School counselors are often the first personnel in a school building to be aware of individual student issues, interactions among groups of students, and climate and environmental changes. This positions counselors to play a vital role in bringing issues to the forefront of the faculty's attention (Capuzzi & Gross, 2000). Faculty can be advised to

- Establish a caring and supportive relationship with children and youth.
- Get to know needs, feelings, attitudes, and behavior patterns of students.
- Review school records with the school counselors to identify patterns of behaviors or sudden changes in behavior.
- "Do no harm" by making sure that the early warning signs are not used as a rationale to isolate, exclude, or punish a child.
- Understand violence and aggression within a context that realizes many factors can contribute to aggressive behavior. Some children may act out if stress becomes too great, if they lack positive coping skills, and if they have learned to react with aggression.
- Avoid stereotyping and be aware of false cues including race, socioeconomic status, cognitive or academic ability, or physical appearance. In fact, such stereotypes can unfairly harm children, especially when the school community acts on them.
- View warning signs within a developmental context due to children's different levels of social and emotional capabilities.

Understand that children typically exhibit multiple warning signs (U.S. Department of Education, 1998b).

As leaders and advocates, school counselors can publicly acknowledge the issues, be catalysts to seek solutions, and collaborate with colleagues to set in motion proactive prevention programs such as **peer mediation** and character education to address climate and relational issues.

School violence prevention is a challenging problem that requires a multifaceted response and utilizes services that link schools to the community. Research has shown that harsh measures and a repressive environment have not proven sufficient to create a school climate immune from disruption or acts of violence (U.S. Department of Education & U.S. Secret Service, 2002b). Zero-tolerance policies have become the norm, punishing minor and major infractions and sending a message that certain behaviors will not be tolerated (Skiba & Peterson, 1999). Student codes of conduct can more clearly delineate students' rights and responsibilities while additionally assuring consistency in the administration of consequences (New York State Center for School Safety, 2010).

Subtle or overt signs of aggression in parks, playing fields, the mall, and street corners continue to spill into the school's hallways and affect the school's climate. The basis for the hostility or confrontational acts has as much to do with communities and families as it does with schools (Leinhardt & Willert, 2002). Sports rage, for example, is a common way in which parents model unacceptable behavior to their children. Parents must be mindful of the example they set and the expectations that they hold for their children. Playing fields are not the place for directed frustration, anger, or violence in the name of competition. Children watch their parents and react accordingly (Heinzmann, 2002).

## Characteristics and Actions of Successful Programs

The Office of Safe and Drug Free Schools (2010) has identified common *characteristics* and *actions* of programs that have been successful in creating a positive climate and reducing acts of violence. Successful schools share the following characteristics:

1. An early start and long-term commitment that focuses on young children and sustains interventions K–12.
2. Strong administrative leadership that ensures consistent, clear disciplinary policies; staff development training to help teachers and staff appropriately work with **disruptive students**, mediate conflict, and proactively incorporate prevention strategies.
3. Parental involvement and training about the early warning signs of violence prevention and to engage them to serve as volunteers in school programs.
4. Interagency partnerships and community linkages to develop collaborative agreements for school personnel, local businesses, law enforcement officers, and social service agencies to work together to address the multiple causes of violence in schools and in the community.

Schools that are successful in creating a positive climate and reducing acts of violence employ actions that include the following:

1. Build a solid foundation for all children by supporting positive discipline, academic success, and mental and emotional wellness by creating a caring

school environment; teaching students appropriate behaviors and problem solving skills; positive behavioral support; and appropriate academic instruction with engaging curricula and effective teaching practices.

2. Identify students at risk for severe academic or behavioral difficulties early on and create services and supports that address risk factors and build protective factors for them. Approximately 10 to 15 percent of students exhibit problem behaviors indicating a need for such early intervention. It is important that staff be trained to recognize early warning signs and make appropriate referrals.

3. Provide intensive interventions for children who are experiencing significant emotional and behavioral problems. This involves providing coordinated, comprehensive, intensive, sustained, culturally appropriate, child- and family-focused services and supports. Such interventions might include day treatment programs that provide students and families with intensive mental health and special education services; multi-systemic therapy, focusing on the individual youth and her or his family, the peer context, school/vocational performance, and neighborhood/community supports; or treatment foster care, an intensive, family-focused intervention for youth whose delinquency or emotional problems are so serious and so chronic that they are no longer permitted to live at home.

4. Pull together with the community and determine and implement strategies essential to creating a safe-schools environment. Effectiveness generally requires the collaboration of schools, social services, mental health providers, and law enforcement and juvenile justice authorities. Because school violence mirrors the culture, norms, and behaviors of our communities and neighborhoods, schools are most successful in confronting school violence when the community around them is proactively involved.

5. Consider integrating the principles of character education across the content areas (Character Education Partnership, 2010; Likona, 2004; Likona, Schaps, & Lewis, 2000). Character education can address anger management, empathy, perspective taking, social problem solving, communication, general social skills, and peace building. Students develop empathy and learn acceptable ways to express thoughts and feelings.

> Conflict is a natural, vital part of life. When conflict is understood, it can become an opportunity to learn and create. The challenge for people in conflict is to apply the principles of creative cooperation in their human relationships. (Bodine, Crawford, & Schrumpf, 1996, p. iv)

## Conflict Resolution and Peer Mediation: Reducing Acts of Violence

Managing conflict is a life skill and everyone faces conflict in their daily lives. Students are no different than adults and are challenged by the many conflicts they experience with peers, teachers, and parents. Students are often quick to resort to violence to get what they want, which may be encouraged by what they observe in their community and depicted in the media.

Children may choose violence as a way to solve problems or to meet their needs because they lack adequate **conflict resolution** skills (Brinson,

Kottler, & Fisher, 2004). It is also important to identify and address the variety of pressures that students face that can influence their decision to resolve a conflict peacefully or resort to violence. Students become angry for a variety of reasons including being lied to; being blamed for something that they didn't do; being ignored; being put down; having their confidence broken; being made fun of in front of others; or through frustration with people or things including technology (Wolfe et al., 2009). The list, which is similar to adult prompts for anger, is endless.

Peer mediation is an approach to learn how to manage interpersonal conflict in elementary and secondary schools. These programs provide a unique opportunity for diverse students to use communication skills, human relations, and problem-solving skills in real-life settings. Effective programs can help to create a safe and welcoming school environment, improve interpersonal and intergroup relations, and assist in reducing school conflicts and violence, especially when part of a comprehensive violence prevention plan (Schellenberg, Parks-Savage, & Rehfuss, 2007). The qualities that mark an effective peer mediation program include youth empowerment, capable adult supervision, cultural competence, diversity, responsiveness to the specific needs of the population it serves, fair resolutions to mediated conflicts, and measurable outcomes (Association for Conflict Resolution, 2007).

### Defining Terms

School-based programs differ in their purpose and intent, and clarity in terminology is important to help you determine program goals and implement a prevention program.

*Conflict*—a struggle between two or more opposing forces (Cohen, 2005).

*Conflict resolution*—the process by which people resolve a dispute or a conflict so that their interests are adequately addressed, and they are satisfied with the outcome.

*Conflict resolution education*—educational practices that model and teach how to resolve conflict in culturally appropriate ways.

*Peer mediation*—a process in which students who have been trained in mediation skills and processes mediate the conflicts of other students.

*Peer mediation program*—an elementary or secondary school program that trains and supports student mediators to offer mediation as an option for resolving conflicts within the school community.

*Peer mediator*—an elementary or secondary student who has been trained in mediation and has the competence to facilitate the resolution of disputes between student peers using a mediation process.

*Mediation*—a process in which an impartial third party facilitates communication and negotiation and promotes voluntary decision-making by the parties to the dispute.

Peer mediation can be a powerful tool to assist in conflict resolution. The trained peer mediators bring both parties together with the goal of reaching a level of understanding, often taking the form of a written contract, which prevents friction between students from escalating to violence. Peer mediation programs, as with any school-based initiative, require thoughtfulness and careful planning to bring to fruition.

## Steps to Developing a Peer Mediation Program
### 1. Secure the Buy-in of Your Administrators and Colleagues
With any new program that will result in a change, colleagues must understand the rationale and momentum for change. Start with data and results of programs that have been successful. What difference will this make in my classroom or on the playground in my school? Secure input from all students, teachers, staff, parents, and the community.

### 2. Program Design and Planning
Solicit volunteers to form a steering committee and select a coordinator to plan meetings and outreach to the school community. Who will our program serve? What is mediate-able vs. what is a disciplinary infraction? How will the peer mediation program relate to other programs in our school?

As you establish program objectives, how will the mediation program influence policy and procedures? Also consider by what measures of progress to evaluate success; design a referral process and forms that can be used by students and teachers. Don't forget to designate a place where mediation can occur and the appropriate times for students to participate.

### 3. Training and Outreach
You cannot learn to mediate from a book; you cannot train others to mediate unless you are a mediator yourself (Cohen, 2005, p. 105). Take the time to find trainers in your community by contacting university personnel, agencies, and the court system. Use Noah's Rule to ensure that you include students representing all populations and subgroups in the trainings. Although you should start small, think big knowing that your program will grow and expand each year by including students and faculty in the trainings. Most importantly, outreach to the entire school community and involve students to "sell" the idea.

### 4. Mediating Cases
This is the basis of a credible and successful program. If you are not sure if a situation is appropriate for mediation, check with your principal or dean of students. After the session is scheduled, identify mediators based on the request of the referred parties, i.e., two students or perhaps one adult and one student. Know when not to take on a case if there is a potential conflict of interest or it presents an ethical dilemma. Make sure mediators have prompts/scripts to help them stay on task and to prepare a written agreement. Build in time to debrief with the mediators when the session is completed and decide the follow-up and when it needs to take place.

### 5. Program Maintenance and Evaluation

Successful programs require frequent attention on the part of the coordinator and steering committee. Meet frequently with student mediators and help them by reviewing scenarios to role play. Most importantly, keep the administration and faculty informed of the types of mediations, the frequencies, and the impact. Monitor your data so you can see the impact of the program on different types of discipline incidents and evaluate your progress.

School counselors can promote and help develop mediation programs that support clear and effective mechanisms for resolving conflict. By taking a leadership role, the school counselor can encourage staff to model behaviors that lend to resolving differences in a "win-win manner" and that also will spill over into the classroom. The mediation process differs from a counseling intervention and requires objectivity and addressing the facts at hand to bring the parties to an agreement that they can both live with and provide support, protection, and supervision to all students in an even-handed way.

## A Climate of RESPECT

RESPECT is an acronym that stands for the actions of Reflect, Educate, Secure, Prepare, Examine, Cooperate, and Transform. These verbs denote steps in a procedure for establishing a respectful school climate. RESPECT can act as a blueprint for the leadership team in developing an action plan but can also be applied to any number of situations to increase the potential for a safe and respectful school climate.

More fully, RESPECT represents

- reflect on the current climate;
- educate the faculty;
- secure a commitment;
- prepare for the unexpected;
- examine data;
- cooperate across all the content areas;
- transform the school culture and climate.

We will use the story of Main Street Middle School, a fictitious school that is representative of many suburban and rural middle schools, to illustrate RESPECT in action.

### Reflect on the Current Climate

Last year, the Main Street Middle School's leadership team was asked to develop an action plan to improve climate and help students acquire the attitudes, knowledge, and skills needed to resist violent acts, drugs, alcohol, and reduce other risky behaviors.

Using the resources from the U.S. Department of Education's Office of Safe and Drug Free Schools (OSDFS, 2010) as a guide, the school leadership team, which includes the school counselor, committed to the challenge of creating a school in which respect is the cornerstone. Everyone in the school community, both internal and external to the school, would be involved in the process. The leadership team surveyed faculty perceptions toward student behavior, discipline, drug and alcohol use, and related behaviors. Additionally a "town meeting" was held to discuss the concerns, needs, and problems of the school with the entire community.

Information gathered from the survey and the town meeting was used to develop a prevention plan to create a safe, respectful environment. Findings pointed to the controversy surrounding zero-tolerance policies. Although faculty believed well-defined discipline policies and school security were necessary to maintain order and a safe climate, students viewed the newly instituted "zero tolerance" as restrictive, unfair, and punitive; many more students had been suspended as a result of the policy's enforcement. The students asked for the discipline policy to be replaced by a code of conduct. The faculty acknowledged that a code of conduct could address students' rights and responsibilities and this could become the cornerstone for a character education program.

The survey and town meeting results helped the leadership team identify community stressors, discipline incidents, and places where bullying was occurring. It placed the team in a better position to reflect on the current situation and begin to consider measures to positively improve climate.

### Educate the Faculty

Creating a safe and respectful environment requires that educators ensure that no child will go unnoticed, unattended, or unconnected. Youth who have positive and caring role models in their lives are less prone to engage in risky behaviors. Educators who establish clear standards for acceptable behavior for themselves and others can be a powerful influence (New York State Center for School Safety, 2010). Students who feel "school connected" are less likely to engage in violent behavior, use substances, or experience emotional distress (McNeely & Blum, 2002). Implementing these protective factors will serve to reduce the potential of risk factors associated with acts of violence and aggressive behavior (U.S. Department of Education, 1998b). Classroom discussions and activities help raise students' awareness of what constitutes bullying and victimizing and in turn will help students develop appropriate actions that they can take when they witness or experience incidents of bullying (U.S. Department of Education, 2002a). To secure a safe environment, faculty can encourage students to

- seek immediate help from an adult when they are being victimized;
- privately support those being hurt with words of kindness or condolence;
- express disapproval of bullying behavior by not joining in the laughter, teasing, or spreading rumors or gossip;
- speak up and offer support to victims when they see them being bullied; and
- report bullying/victimization incidents to school personnel.

As its next step, the Main Street leadership team requested 20 minutes to deliver an inservice at the next faculty meeting to educate the staff and faculty. At the meeting, each member of the faculty received a copy of "Early Warning, Timely Response" (U.S. Department of Education, 1998b), which summarizes the early and imminent warning signs. Faculty were encouraged to become keenly aware of students who are at risk and consequently put others at risk. The inservice closed with faculty members sharing their personal concerns about what they have observed in student behavior. The process of educating the faculty as to early warning signs, the factors contributing to violence, and the ways to prevent problems were viewed by all concerned as a positive step toward establishing a safe environment.

### Secure a Commitment

To secure a safe environment, the leadership team at Main Street worked to obtain a commitment from every member of the school community from student to principal to pay close attention to what goes on among the student body. The team proposed that every member of the faculty establish a connection with a student who is isolated and troubled. Additionally, the leadership team suggested that the faculty establish clear standards for behavior, encourage character development, and motivate students to contribute to a safe and respectful learning environment.

The team believed that students and faculty could pull together with the common goal of creating an environment that is safe and respectful. By involving students in the process, the team offers the opportunity for them to assume responsibility and take ownership for contributing to the climate of their school where they spend as much time as they do in their homes. Students rise to the occasion when presented with opportunities to help create fair and respectful classrooms. School personnel organized programs that increased student confidence, knowledge, responsibility, and skills such as volunteering to be mentors to younger students, peer facilitators, and tutors.

### Prepare for the Unexpected

Understanding that crisis and tragedy can strike at any time, from within or from outside of the school setting, the Main Street team was determined to assess the school's preparedness. The Blueprint for Reform (U.S. Department of Education, 2010) urges schools to support student success by creating a safe school where every student feels like she or he belongs, is valued, and feels physically and emotionally safe.

No school is protected from tragic occurrences such as the death of a faculty member or student, car accidents, tornado destruction, kidnapping, suicide, or an event of terrorism such as 9/11. Crises can range in scope and severity from incidents that affect a single student to those who can wreak havoc on an entire community. Events such as 9/11 severely affected staff and students, leaving the nation feeling vulnerable and unprepared for tragedies of this magnitude (Dahir, 2001).

Tragedy leaves a permanent imprint on each one of us; grief and loss know no boundaries. Every school member, from student to counselor, needs to be aware of the protocols and procedures to follow for any crisis (U.S. Department of Education & U.S. Secret Service, 2002b). Crisis management plans have specific components mandated by state education regulations, legislation, and/or local school board policy. According to the U.S. Department of Education, the U.S. Department of Justice, and the American Institute of Research (2002a), these can include but are not limited to the following:

- The chain of command to implement procedures.
- Clearly defined roles and responsibilities for every staff member.
- Specific assignments for school personnel to monitor indoor or outdoor school areas and/or groups of students.
- Guidance for scheduled and unscheduled emergency preparedness drills.
- Internal and external communication guidelines.
- Collaborative procedures for working with police officers, firefighters, emergency trained personnel, bomb squads, parents, community agencies, and local officials.
- Guidelines for working with the media.
- Follow-up practices for the aftermath.

A crisis response plan addresses the personal and the human side of trauma, loss, injury, and grief. Key to providing immediate response is a well-trained crisis response team that meets periodically to update skills and retool each member's preparedness (Dorn, 2002; Vanderbilt Mental Health Center & Tennessee Department of Education, 2007). Crisis response teams often include school counselors, student services school personnel, and community-based mental health professionals. The work of the crisis response teams also is to attend to student and staff well-being so that they do not become overwhelmed or traumatized. Crisis response teams can offer support and structure for students, staff, and families to express their grief and sense of loss, while also identifying the interventions and resources necessary for those who may be in need of regularly scheduled counseling or therapy.

At Main Street Middle School, the leadership team desired to assure students that the adults of their environment will protect them. Routine evacuation drills were implemented with each school professional accepting the responsibilities and accountability for student safety. Police officers, firefighters, emergency medical technicians, and other community members partnered with school personnel to provide students with peace of mind that they will be protected (Office of Safe and Drug Free Schools, 2010).

Training was provided so that school personnel would know how to not only help their students through a crisis but also help them to return home safely. The leadership team used the suggestions from the U.S. Department of Education (2002a) to design plans in both crisis management and crisis response. Every detail was addressed from emergency exiting to updating classroom and office locations, and room assignments. Changes to any aspect of the plan would be communicated to all team and faculty members. A formal opportunity to review and evaluate the plan will be scheduled at least once a year.

Solid preparation for response and management of the critical incidents can save lives, affect the recovery and healing period, build bridges between school and community, and desensationalize media attention. In Box 11.1, we recount one school's readiness to respond to a tragic event that was beyond the scope of anyone's imagination.

## MEET ADA ROSARIO DOLCH AND THE STAFF OF THE HIGH SCHOOL OF LEADERSHIP AND POLICY STUDIES: NEIGHBORS TO THE WORLD TRADE CENTER

"How have we all become important in one day?" asked the social studies teacher of his colleagues at the High School of Leadership and Policy Studies, a high school two blocks from the World Trade Center. His purpose just three days after 9/11 was to help everyone gathered in the room put the World Trade Center tragedy in a different context so they in turn could help their students regain a sense of empowerment, purpose, and hope. It was a way to begin the healing process. The counselor and teachers wanted to help their students escape from the feelings of powerlessness and despair.

This, the first faculty gathering since 9/11 when they had to evacuate to Battery Park, was a time to tell the stories of that day. The heroism of these 70 adults in the midst of the crisis spoke to their preparedness to move students to safety for students and to set into motion a series of decisions that would protect and guard the students' emotional and physical safety to the extent possible.

Ada Rosario Dolch, the principal, related the chronology of events that took place that morning. Within seconds after the plane exploded into the World Trade Center, the security guards came rushing into her office and told her that they had to evacuate the building. It took only a second for the magnitude to sink in and she made an announcement directing everyone to go to the park. And they did. All of those drills and practices were now a reality. Student and faculty together were walking scared but moved quickly. In as orderly fashion as possible they made their way through the wave of anxious humanity that clogged the streets of lower Manhattan to Battery Park. Seven hundred students and their teachers protected and encouraged each other. They supported each other and helped the others who crossed their path, taking special care of those who were disabled, blind, and wheelchair-bound. Leaving behind their pocketbooks and keys, bankcards and credit cards, briefcases, lesson plans, backpacks and books—all of the ordinary trappings of an ordinary day in the life of high school teachers and high school students.

Seven hundred students were brought to safety and taken out of harm's way, protected by the compassion and caring of their school family. The staff protected their students as best they could as they stood in the park watching the horror intensify with a second explosion right before their eyes. Ada called it a tsunami wave that rolled over the lower part of Manhattan, descending on the crowds with debris, dust, paper, rubble. As students reached out to each other, they helped strangers also along the way. One rushed to rescue an older woman who was getting trampled and pushed up against the fence.

As the teachers shared their experiences they conveyed a spirit of hope and optimism about the future. They talked about how to bring from this crisis a message to their students that we are all important. With uncertainty about the future and with determination, they talked about how to help the students return to school and provide the structure of instruction and opportunities to talk.

"We will do our best," one teacher said. "We have all become important in one day. More so than any of us could have imagined on the first day of school. We will contribute to this effort to rebuild our lives, our families, our school, our neighborhood, our city, our hopes and dreams. We will make this world a better place. That's why we are here. We are survivors, not victims."

Reprinted with permission: Dahir, C. (October, 2001). We Have All Become Important, New York State School Counselor Association.

---

Schools are never emotionally prepared for violence, grief, and trauma. A structured crisis management plan helps all school personnel and students to better deal with the trauma and stress of the unexpected or unforeseen. The school counselor's ultimate goal, as part of the crisis response team, is to help the school community return to a semblance of normalcy as quickly as possible. ASCA reminds us that the professional school counselor's role is to respond to and advocate for the emotional needs of all persons affected by a crisis (ASCA, 2002). Putting structure back in place will help students and staff regains a sense of safety and security.

School counselors cannot easily separate their involvement on the crisis response or management team from the proactive commitment to ensure that every student will acquire safety and survival skills (ASCA, 1997a). School counselor initiative will help students function appropriately in an emergency situation; more importantly, students can acquire the coping and resiliency skills to successfully emerge from crisis, grief, loss, and tragedy.

### Examine Data

Student success data can be collected and analyzed systematically to inform and guide the development and implementation of a safe schools program. The use of demographic and performance data makes it possible for counselors to determine how policies and practices are affecting issues of equity and climate (Stone & Dahir, 2011). School report card data tell the story about attendance, suspension, and graduation rates, which have a significant impact on school climate. Collecting and disaggregating data is the critical first step in the school safety process (OSDFS, 2010) and provide a baseline for consistency in data-driven decision making.

At Main Street Middle School several sixth graders had reported "getting picked on" and "being pushed around," and the leadership team agreed that there were patterns of bullying that warranted investigating.

The leadership team agreed that data collection should be systematic, consistent, and unbiased to examine the disaggregated data in a variety of ways.

The data might provoke some new questions such as "Is there a relationship between attendance and bullying? What are the underlying contributors to suspensions or to hallway tussles?" A careful data analysis of discipline incidents could offer insight about the nature of the recent complaints of the sixth graders and help to identify the specific cause-and-effect relationships that contribute to both school safety and building a safe and respectful school environment.

The leadership team examined all of the variables that contributed to discipline referrals. The monthly data reports revealed the sixth-grade discipline referrals since September. The incident reports showed that 75 percent of the incidents involved verbal harassment and physical confrontation. Eighty-five percent of these incidents took place in the hallways, lunchroom, and/or on the bus. Almost 40 percent of the referrals involved the same 25 students, 17 of whom were boys. Would further data disaggregation reveal any connection of these to "bullying"? Has this physical and verbal harassment reduced the achievement of the students who have been victimized? The leadership team realized the value and importance of digging deep to uncover the roots of the problem and consider systemic implications.

Had this conversation and further investigation not taken place, the sixth graders' complaints may have been dismissed as isolated incidents. Data collection and analyses are necessary to transform the culture and create a positive climate by helping to identify the cause and effect of inappropriate behavior as well as develop proactive prevention and remediation strategies. If students do not feel safe in the school environment, they will not learn to the best of their ability (Bluestein, 2001). Student fear and concern for personal safety affect a classroom teacher's ability to engage students in successful achievement (McNeely & Blum, 2002). Specific strategies to eliminate this negative behavior would improve the school's climate and enhance the learning environment for the sixth grade.

### _Cooperate Across all the Content Areas_

Random events and assemblies or occasional thematic days on safety and respect are not enough to change the climate and culture of a school. Basic concerns of the faculty and stakeholders such as helping students cope with anger, resolve and mediate conflict, develop friendships, acquire a respect for self and others, and understand personal safety could be addressed in teachable moments across the academic areas (Dahir & Stone, 2004). This would require the cooperation among all school professionals.

When youth feel valued, are involved in positive relationships, and have external and internal guides, they perform better in school. Building character protects young people from many different "risky behaviors" and promotes positive attitudes (Search Institute, 2010). Students who demonstrate values and skills that make them less likely to engage in risky behavior tend to be more successful in school and in life (Benson et al., 1999; Scales & Taccogna, 2000).

The Search Institute (1997) promoted asset acquisition for students to help build youth of character, compassion, and commitment. The external assets are the relationships and supports that guide students to behave in healthy ways and make good choices, while the internal assets are the competencies, values, and self-perceptions that guide a young person's ability to self-regulate her or his behavior (Scales & Taccogna, 2000). Looking at student growth and development through an assets lens positively affects teaching, learning, relationships, and school climate as high-risk patterns of behavior diminished as students increased their acquisition of "assets" (Scales & Taccogna, 2000).

The **Developmental Assets** (Search Institute, 1997) and the three ASCA personal-social development standards offer guidance to develop competencies, the outcomes for what students should know and be able to do. Undertaking asset building across the content areas will aid in the design of a proactive safe schools action plan that has student needs at its core and affects the school climate in positive ways. Using the personal-social development standards will help students to acquire attitudes, knowledge, and skills to support both affective and academic development. The faculty's buy-in is revealed through beliefs and behaviors. Caring beyond the classroom and creating a positive moral culture in every school building are two of the many ways that a whole-school effort can focus on youth development.

The Main Street leadership team acknowledged the importance of securing the buy-in and the full cooperation of the faculty and staff. To start

## BOX **11.2**

### *Main Street Leadership Team Belief Statement #1*

To create a school climate of caring and respect, we, the faculty of Main Street Middle School, believe we can:

a.  Create a positive and collaborative classroom climate by looking at what we teach, how we teach, and what we ask students to do considering their point of view.
b.  Listen to students and give them opportunities to share their concerns, whether it's about why they failed a test, didn't do their homework, or reflect on what the particular lesson meant to them on personal basis.
c.  Give students choices and responsibilities in rule-making within the classroom and within the structure of the school environment.
d.  Look at each situation as a challenge for resolution rather than an action to be disciplined and think about how to problem solve rather than punish.
e.  Connect with the students and actively listen to their concerns.
f.  Use teachable moments to connect the curriculum with affective development. What novel exists that does not address conflict? Literature can become a venue for connecting academic content with character building.
g.  Make a commitment to use culturally sensitive and developmentally appropriate materials.
h.  Help students acquire coping and resiliency skills (Dorsey, 2000).

the process, several sample belief statements were developed to gain their support for the safe and respectful schoolwide action plan. These draft statements were the result of research, observations, and faculty-room and community conversations. At the next faculty meeting, the draft belief statements were presented and served as a basis for discussion.

Cooperation among faculty, staff, and administration will improve school climate and help students acquire the attitudes, knowledge, and skills needed to resist violent acts, drugs, alcohol, and reduce risky behaviors. School personnel who hold student needs at the core of their belief systems create safe and dynamic learning communities (Stein, Richin et al., 2001).

### Transform the School Culture and Climate

Ensuring a safe and respectful school environment requires close attention to students' social and emotional lives, the dynamics of relationships, and the environment in which students thrive and grow. Peer pressure, concerns for safety and well-being, harassment, and bullying are some of the challenges that students face every day in hallways that can be hostile or friendly. For some students, issues of personal safety and emotional balance are more important to them than meeting academic standards. Does the school faculty project an image of caring and concern? Or do students look elsewhere for support and personal, social, and emotional growth?

Schools and communities together have transformed the school culture and created climates of respect by developing comprehensive, integrated plans that embrace key sectors of the community—the schools, social services, mental health providers, and law enforcement and juvenile justice authorities (Departments of Education, Justice, & American Institute for Research, 2002).

When the Main Street Middle School prevention and intervention action plan was close to completion and ready for faculty review, the leadership team recognized that it was only part of the long journey ahead. To transform the climate and culture of the school would be a complex process that requires a commitment of time and a willingness to thoroughly examine policies, practices, and behaviors that stratify student opportunities. Transforming the school culture is a responsibility that resides not only with the adults; students too must assume responsibility for contributing to a system that is safe, secure, and respectful. The team acknowledged that although every act of hostility or aggression may not be eradicated, implementing the RESPECT strategies can make a difference with teachers, counselors, administrators, students, and community pulling together.

Planning for success was Main Street's first step in the journey. RESPECT, far from a perfect design, provided a starting point.

# PROGRAMS OF PROMISE

## Character Matters

According to the Character Education Partnership (2004), character education is an intentional effort to help students understand, care about, and act on core ethical values. The absence of the core values of respect, responsibility, trustworthiness, fairness, diligence, self-control, caring, and courage can lead to destructive youth behaviors. Thus schools that do not emphasize these core values are at greater risk of acts of violence or aggressive behaviors.

Connecting Character to Conduct (Stein et al., 2001) is a comprehensive methodology that promotes the core values of RICE:

Respect: Showing respect toward ourselves and others

Impulse Control: Doing the right things for the right reasons

Compassion: Showing concern and caring for others

Equity: Treating everyone with fairness

The Connecting Character to Conduct (CCC) method includes adult modeling of RICE behaviors and curriculum specific activities that are initiated anywhere there is an opportunity to learn, such as classrooms, hallways, or the cafeteria.

## MEET SUSAN SKLAR: A COMMITMENT TO CORE VALUES

Susan Sklar, chair of pupil personnel services, had the data to demonstrate that the students of Grand Avenue Middle School were well-behaved, academically successful, and involved in many extracurricular activities. It was a principal's dream. But Susan Sklar, along with the school leadership team, counseling staff, and faculty, believed that the students could do even better. They wanted their students to be kind and respectful, even if no one else was looking. Yet, everyone recognized that they could not force one more thing into the packed academic day. If they were to adopt an approach to character education, it had to be something everyone could do as a seamless, natural part of their role. The faculty chose Connecting Character to Conduct (CCC) to help them develop core values that everyone would abide by.

Through professional development and parent engagement practices, the Grand Middle School team adopted a shared vocabulary to clearly define their purpose, strengthen their sense of membership, and specifically articulate their roles and rules, or guiding principles. Today, everyone at Grand Avenue abides by the guiding principles/core values of RICE. Now every member of the school learning team, faculty, staff, and students alike are using their shared core values to achieve their individual goals while advancing the purpose of their school, which is to help all students learn well, stay safe, and graduate! Everyone has a specific role to play; roles clearly define areas of responsibility. Every Grand Avenue student has a dual role: to learn well, stay safe, and graduate, and to help other students do the same.

Grand Avenue Middle School is located in the Bellmore-Merrick School District on Long Island, New York.

# SCHOOL COUNSELORS TAKING THE NEXT STEPS

With almost every youth exposed to a barrage of visual violence in the media, and for some in their communities and homes, we must recognize that we live in potentially dangerous times (Garbarino, 1999). School violence can manifest itself in many different forms. Once remanded to the playground or streets, the definition of violence is far more than physical assaults in schools and can be displayed as hostility, aggressive language, threats, subtle and overt acts of peer pressure, put-downs, harassment, bullying, intimidation and extortion, and teasing (Leinhart & Willert, 2002). The stringent discipline policies and metal detectors may be important security measures but do not get at the source of the problem. High morale and strong leadership coupled with organizational and administrative support contribute highly to a school's prevention program (Gottfredson, 2001). Building a level of trust among and between all members of our school community can help to identify the shared values that all stakeholders embrace and support.

School counselors can help to put more extraordinary measures in place to help students navigate materialism, competitiveness, pressures, insensitivity, failure, and conflicting values. School counselors as responsible and caring adults play a key role in the lives of our youth (Daniels, 2002). The potential for healing lies not within a system of rules and punishments, but in a system that celebrates curiosity and caring, discovery and joy—and in the process, we will make it better and we will make it safe (Bluestein, 2001, p. 381).

To live in a world of hope one must put the fear aside. No longer can caring school personnel always protect children from hate, terrorism, and violence. The fear that some children experience when bullied on the playground is a similar fear used by terrorists for intimidation. Children can learn they cannot act out of hate, anger, and fear.

Alternative ways for children to learn to cope with emotions are possible. School counselors can assume a leadership role to help young children and adolescents build strong character, develop coping and resiliency skills, and set goals for the future. School counselors can help to transform the world of schools and through intentional efforts in our schools, create a more respectful and peaceful one in which we live in today.

# TECH TOOLS

When you become a school counselor, use the power of technology to maximize the efficiency and effectiveness of your contributions to create a safe and respectful learning environment. Use the Web to explore resources, programs, and data to create safe and respectful school settings.

- What Does the Data Tell Us? Indicators of School Crime and Safety is the U.S. Department of Education's annual report on school crime and student safety. This report provides the most recent data available from a variety of independent sources: http://nces.ed.gov/programs/crimeindicators
    - Centers for Disease Control and Prevention

Division of Adolescent and School Health
www.cdc.gov/healthyyouth
Division of Violence Prevention
www.cdc.gov/violenceprevention
http://www.cdc.gov/ncipc/factsheets/yvfacts.htm (use the Web to look at statistics for youth abuse of alcohol, or drugs, or tobacco)

Sourcebook for Community Action: This CDC sourcebook is the first of its kind to look at the effectiveness of specific violence prevention practices in four key areas: parents and families; home visiting; social and conflict resolution skills; and mentoring: www.cdc.gov/violenceprevention/pub/YV_bestpractices.html

The U.S. Department of Education's Office of Safe and Drug Free Schools has a wealth of activities, rigorous criteria to evaluate prevention programs, best practices, a newsletter, and information at www.ed.gov/offices/OESE/SDFS.

- Blueprints for Violence Prevention

The Blueprints for Violence Prevention identifies 11 model prevention programs that meet a strict scientific standard of program effectiveness. The 11 model programs, called "Blueprints," have been effective in reducing adolescent violent crime, aggression, delinquency, and substance abuse. To date, more than 800 programs have been reviewed: www.colorado.edu/cspv/blueprints

- Department of Education www.ed.gov
  National Youth Violence Prevention
  Resource Center www.safeyouth.org
  Stop Bullying Now Campaign www.stopbullyingnow.hrsa.gov
  Center for Substance Abuse Prevention: www.samhsa.gov
  Collaborative for Academic, Social and Emotional Learning (CASEL): www.casel.org

The National Institute on Drug Abuse. Preventing Drug Use among Children and Adolescents: A Research-Based Guide. Call 1-800-729-9989; www.nida.nih.gov/Prevention/Prevopen.html

## *School Counselor Casebook: Voices From the Field*

### The Scenario Reviewed

For the past two weeks several students in your caseload have complained to you about certain students who have been bullying them. Although students often complain about "being picked on," something about this situation just doesn't seem right. The students will not tell you who is involved but insist that you "tell" the teachers to do something about it. As you think this through, there are several courses of action are available for you to take. You decide to further discuss this with the other school counselors in your building, the teachers who are involved with these students, and

*(continues)*

your building principal. In your planning, consider how the ASCA Model can help with a whole-school approach.

### A Practitioner's Approach

Here's how a practicing school counselor responded to the school scenario:

Comprehensive counseling programs are data driven. With this in mind, I would begin by giving students, parents, and teachers surveys to collect baseline data. Post surveys could be used to assess whether interventions were effective at reducing bullying and improving the school climate. Using data in this way serves as part of a recommended management system under the ASCA National Model.

I would share the survey results at a faculty meeting, along with a brief presentation on bullying. Then I would meet with our school counseling advisory committee to brainstorm prevention and intervention activities. Including classroom guidance sessions on bullying as part of the prevention strategies would be important. Classroom guidance sessions are an important component of the Delivery System of the ASCA model and are useful in implementing the national standard for personal-social development.

Early in the school year, I would teach students how to recognize bully behaviors, bullying terms, provocative versus passive victims, relational aggression, reporting versus tattling, and the role of bystanders. This gives all students a common language and gives me a framework to use with students later when bullying situations surface.

Even with the best prevention activities you still need intervention strategies. I would have small-group sessions for victims and offer individual counseling for bullies to teach them positive strategies to gain the power and control they desire. Your advisory committee can help develop clear school procedures for bully reporting and consequences. Additionally, they can encourage the faculty to take on the bullying problem as a whole-school effort and encourage every teacher to do their part. As a final note, be sure to document and share your pre- and post data with your school community. It is important to demonstrate how the counseling program supports the overall mission of the school.

Joy Guss has been a school counselor for nine years at the elementary, middle, and high school levels. She has presented professional development sessions for school counselors and serves on her district's crisis response team. She was the first counselor in the Metropolitan Nashville Public Schools district to receive a MEASURE award for her work with students. Joy is currently a school counselor at Bellevue Middle School in Nashville, Tennessee.

## LOOKING BACK: SALIENT POINTS

### Seeking a Safer Learning Environment

Schools may look the same from the outside of the building as they did in the past; however, violent acts and the impact of trauma, tragedy, and terrorism have moved from the community into the schoolhouse. This constant barrage of violent images reinforced a false message: that violence is an appropriate choice of action. Our public schools must be reclaimed to once again become emotionally and physically safe havens for students.

## The Challenge for Educators

Many of our schools are unprepared to address the behaviors or the challenges that arise out of the ever-increasing complexity of societal trends and influences. School personnel struggle to strike a balance between holding all students accountable for their actions yet ensuring that all students receive the necessary resources and supports to achieve and succeed at the highest level. Developing safe and responsive schools is a comprehensive approach that includes acknowledging the risk factors, developing effective strategies, and involving all stakeholders.

## School Violence Defined

Although the factors and contributors to school violence may present a bleak picture, targeted acts of violence are the exception to the rule (U.S. Department of Education Office of Safe and Drug Free Schools, 2003; U.S. Departments of Education & the Secret Service, 2002a). Yet the public perceives that schools are no longer safe. The research both supports and contradicts this perception. Although it is clear that other kinds of problems in American schools are far more common than targeted violence, high-profile incidents in schools over the past decade have resulted in increased fear among students, educators, and parents (U.S. Department of Education & the Secret Service, 2002a).

Violence in schools (i.e., fighting, homicide, suicide, firearm injury, bullying) is usually the result of a series of factors that build up over a period of time. School violence is the result of an intentional action that leads to harm to oneself or another person. School personnel, including school counselors, work in a focused manner to help keep the school and students safe from harm's way (Dwyer, Osher, & Warger, 1998).

## The Etiology of School Violence

Schools can successfully identify students at risk of violent behaviors when effective prevention measures are put in place (U.S. Department of Education & U.S. Department of Justice, 2003). Research has shown that the first steps toward preventing violence are to identify and understand the factors that place youth at risk for violent victimization and perpetration (National Center for Injury Prevention and Control, 2002).

## Contributing to a Safe and Respectful School Environment

School counselors can proactively reach out to all students to maximize every student's development; collaborate and team with teachers to develop sensitivities about students who appear alienated or disaffected; consult with teachers on the characteristics of the warning signs of troubled students and lend support to teachers to help them cope with difficult students in their classrooms; and engage all stakeholders in the process to comprehensively address the problem.

### Implementing a Respectful Environment

RESPECT is an acronym for a series of steps that can help instill a safe and respectful environment in a school. It stands for Reflect on the current climate, Educate the faculty, Secure a commitment, Prepare for the unexpected, Examine data, Cooperate across all the content areas, and Transform the school culture and climate.

### Personalizing the School Experience: Advisory Programs

Secondary schools can be large and impersonal environments. Advisory programs can personalize the school experience and provide opportunities for students to establish an identity and a mechanism for self-expression and participate in school-based experience that emphasizes affective and life-skills instructional components.

### Character Matters

Character education is an intentional effort to help students understand, care about, and act on core ethical values. These core values of respect, responsibility, trustworthiness, fairness, diligence, self-control, caring, and courage promote school environments that are safe and respectful.

### School Counselors Taking the Next Steps

Building trust among and between all members of the school community can lead to a climate in which all stakeholders are involved, respected, and supported. The potential for healing lies not within a system of rules and punishments but in a system that celebrates curiosity and caring, discovery and joy. In the process, school counselors will make it better and make it safe. As school counselors build safe and respectful environments, it is time to make sure that no child will go unattended or unnoticed.

## KEY TERMS

School Violence p. 323

Bullying p. 326

Violent Students p. 326

Dyberbullying p. 327

Protective and risk factor p. 331

Early warning signs p. 331

Imminent warning signs p. 332

Peer mediation p. 334

Disruptive students p. 334

Conflict resolution p. 335

Developmental assets p. 345

## LEARNING EXTENSIONS/MAKING CONNECTIONS

1. Interview a school counselor or school administrator regarding her or his experiences with student violent/aggressive behavior and discuss effective solutions to these problems.

2. Research your state's department of education's policies and procedures regarding safe schools. What is expected of individual schools and systems? What documentation must be kept?

3. Develop one strategy for your school building to identify and intervene with those students who are at risk for aggressive or violent behavior. Consider involving all school personnel. Identify one national standard and one student competency that you will address. Also consider any building policy or procedures that must be considered to successfully implement your strategy.

4. Consider these five student incidents that you and your colleagues worked with this week:

   a. An angry girl who threatened others.
   b. Bullying in the bathroom.
   c. A student whose boyfriend started a fight in the cafeteria because she ate lunch with another boy.
   d. A student who is a victim of cyberbullying.
   e. A student who brought a box cutter to school.

   For each incident, discuss the feelings associated with the violent/disruptive student. Identify the behaviors manifested by the feelings and discuss which behaviors are early and/or imminent warning signs. Finally, identify the key issues and implications associated with each scenario.

5. Prepare a five-minute presentation on student engagement and fostering connectedness that you could share at a faculty meeting. Give a concrete example of how teachers and staff could utilize these strategies in the classroom to

   • Help students get to know each other's (and your) strengths.
   • Involve students in planning, problem solving, and identifying issues in the classroom.
   • Involve all students in classroom responsibilities.
   • Connect every student to one school club, sport, or community activity
   • Integrate the concepts of self-discipline, respect, and impulse control throughout your lessons.
   • Develop a mentoring program to support students who need a significant adult in their lives.

6. Analyze TV viewing for an hour during prime time. Log how many acts of violence children are exposed to, how many explicit sexual comments are made, how many ethical dilemmas are posed, Compare notes with your colleagues.

7. Pop culture is represented in many mediums. Watch the Grammy Awards show or an hour of MTV videos. What can we learn about youth culture from music?

8. Explore your local university, county, or community website for community-based organizations and governmental services that offer training in conflict resolution and peer mediation programs to reduce or eliminate youth violence.

# School Counselors as Consultants

## CHAPTER OBJECTIVES

*By the time you have completed this chapter, you should be able to*

- define consultation and apply models of consultation;

- explain the role of the school counselor as a consultant;

- understand the power of collaborative facilitation and how to use the model;

- define the relationship between the consultant and parent as consultee and teacher as consultee;

- describe effective parent conferences;

- describe the four Ds of the consultation process;

- develop a collaborative action plan.

---

### *School Counselor Casebook: Getting Started*

#### The Scenario

After the first nine weeks of middle school, Ms. Lawrence tells you that Susan has not completed any homework or in-class assignments since the school year began. The teacher tells you she has tried everything and is now requesting the paperwork to start the special education process with this student in hopes she can be placed before Christmas.

What should you do?

#### Thinking about Solutions

As you read this chapter, think about possible solutions. Describe the consultation role you might exercise in helping this student and other underachievers. When you come to the end of the chapter, you will have the opportunity to see how your ideas compare with a practicing school counselor's approach.

---

## THE EFFECTIVENESS OF CONSULTATION IN THE SCHOOLS

Research supports **consultation** as an effective method of service delivery in a school setting (Baker, Robichaud, Westforth, Wells, & Schreck, 2009; Brigman, Mullis, Webb, & White, 2005; Dinkmeyer & Carlson, 2006; Dougherty, 2009; Erchul & Sheridan, 2008; Parsons & Kahn, 2005). Consultation in schools is described by authors in many different ways but is commonly described as a problem-solving approach with the adults in the student's life that are in a position to affect positive change (Baker et al., 2009; Brigman et al., 2005; Erchul & Sheridan, 2008; Friend & Cook, 2009; Gibson, 2010; Kampwirth, 2006; Parsons & Kahn, 2005). The consultant brings expertise to another professional or parent in this triadic relationship to benefit the third party, the student, or the system (Crothers, Hughes, & Morine, 2008; DeBoer, 1995; Friend & Cook, 2009; Parsons & Kahn, 2005). Consultation is a specialized problem-solving process in which one professional who has particular expertise assists another professional (or parent) who needs the benefit of that expertise (DeBoer, 1995; Parsons & Kahn, 2005).

In the **triadic-dependent model**, the consultant is viewed as an expert in child behavior and advises as to the origins and causes of problems and makes recommendations as to how to alleviate the difficulties the student is facing (Brigman et al., 2005; Bergan & Kratochwill, 1990; Parsons & Kahn, 2005). In this model, the immediate goal of the consultant as expert is to increase the skills, knowledge, and objectivity of the consultee so that the consultee can more successfully help the consultant implement an intervention plan (Dougherty, 1990, as cited in Baker et al., 2009; Parsons & Kahn, 2005). Dinkmeyer and Carlson (2006) define consultation as a collaborative process in which the consultant and consultee share responsibility for designing and implementing interventions that are in the best educational interests of their students. "The emphasis is on equal relationships developed through collaboration and joint planning ... the consultant is not the problem-solving expert" (Dinkmeyer & Carlson, 2006, p. 12).

Dinkmeyer and Carlson (2006) provide a critical viewpoint for school counselors to consider when developing their role as a consultant. While others in the helping field speak of the differentiated responsibilities for decisions and accountability for outcomes (Friend & Cook, 2009), Dinkmeyer and Carlson (2006) discuss a shared responsibility with regard to decisions and outcomes:

> A superior-to-inferior relationship suggests that consultees seek advice that consultants dispense. Instead, we advocate an equal relationship. Equality means the consultant is not an expert dispensing advice on demand. The consultee has equal responsibility for changing the situation, which prompts the consultation relationship. (p. 13)

Dinkmeyer and Carlson's spirit of collaboration is an excellent fit for the school counselor/consultant as it maintains an equal partnership between all parties involved, including shared responsibility for outcomes and accountability.

In the past, collaboration and consultation were viewed as discreet skills, with consultation requiring an expert, which implied a differentiation of power. Collaboration had little to do with the consultation process but was considered a valued skill among educators in their role as team player and committee member. **Collaborative consultation** is now a consultation model for the school setting (Brigman et al., 2005; Crothers et al., 2008; Dougherty, 2009; Kampwirth, 2006). There is a consensus among many authors of consultation texts that in schools the expert model is far less effective than the collaborative model because in schools people are more likely to implement change if they are involved in discussing and creating the solutions (Brigman et al., 2005; Dougherty, 2009; Kampwirth, 2006).

"In essence, consultation has emerged as a primary service provided by helping professionals to assist a variety of other professionals (such as teachers) and caregivers (such as parents). Collaboration, as a direct service, has emerged as an alternative to consultation, particularly in settings where both the would-be consultant and consultee are employed in the same setting" (Dougherty, 2009, p. 3).

For example, teachers have a tough job and when they reach out for help it can be frustrating if the school counselor as "expert" comes in and without collaboration offers solutions that the teacher feels misses the mark because the counselor is unaware of the interpersonal dynamics, concerns, or issues involved in the teacher's daily struggles. In the collaborative approach, the synergy generated by an interchange of ideas will lead to relationship building and increases the potential for success. The remainder of this chapter will emphasize a collaborative consultation approach placing attention on relationship building, communication skills, problem-solving approaches, and accountability for results.

## Consultation as a Powerful Tool

Consultation is valued by school counselors as a powerful tool that allows them to have a far-reaching, lasting impact on the school's internal community members such as students, teachers, administrators, paraprofessionals, and external community members such as parents and counseling agencies (Baker et al., 2009; Brigman et al., 2005; Davis & Lambie, 2005; Dinkmeyer & Carlson, 2006; Gibson, 2010; Simcox, Nuijens, & Lee, 2006). The school counselor as consultant extends her or his reach to more students by working collaboratively with the adults in a student's life who can make a major impact on a student's academic, career, and social/emotional life (Baker et al., 2009; Brigman, 2005; Crothers, Hughes, & Morine, 2008; Davis & Lambie, 2005; Dinkmeyer & Carlson, 2006; Parsons & Kahn, 2005; Velsor, 2009). The American School Counselor Association recognizes the role school counselors play in students' academic, career, and social/emotional success and describes the process as "Counselors consult with parents or guardians, teachers, other educators, and community agencies regarding strategies to help students and families" (ASCA, 2005).

School counselors behaving as skilled consultants are key contributors in helping give students the gift of becoming successful in school (Dinkmeyer & Carlson, 2006; Gibson, 2010). There are so many **unalterable factors** that school counselors are powerless to affect, such as whether or not a student has at least one loving parent, comes to school fed, and is ready to learn (Hammond, 2010; Kenny, 2003; Stone & Dahir, 2011). However, there are alterable factors for which school counselors wield tremendous influence when as consultants they work with parents, teachers, and administrators to benefit a student or with a system that is impeding progress for a student. "Through consultation, partnering, collaborating and teaming, school counselors provide important contributions to the school system" (ASCA, 2005).

## Consultation as an Effective Use of Time

Parsimony is an efficient use of time by advocating that school counselors spend their time where they can impact the most students (Erford, 2011a; Myrick, 1997, 2003b). When working in partnership with an administrator or teacher to develop strategies to positively affect one student, the consultee can then apply those skills, knowledge bases, and resources to many more students. Even though counselor-to-student ratios are often too high, consultation helps meet the needs of many more students through the **rule of parsimony**. "Consulting with a teaching team about grade level concerns and helping to establish a framework for addressing individual student needs is one of the most efficient ways for school counselors to effect change. It is a time to clarify, explore, and create new strategies that will affect the classroom and school climate and ultimately student success in the classroom" (Brigman et al., 2005, p. 68). "By consulting (i.e., collaborating) with teachers, professional school counselors can assist teachers in improving their overall behavior management and instructional skills and increase their ability to more effectively deal with classroom problems as they occur" (Watson, Watson, & Weaver, 2010, p. 296).

The impact of consultation is exponential as the consultee and the school counselor together learn intervention strategies for future application. In a successful consultation, knowledge gained is transferred to new situations, ideas germinate into plans that benefit many more students, and highly skilled professionals emerge. Direct service delivery, such as individual counseling, reaches one student at a time while consultation indirectly affects the student by working with the other adults in the student's life (Brigman et al., 2005; Gysbers & Henderson, 2001; Myrick, 2003b).

"A primary rationale for providing consultation is that it is time-efficient. By working with teachers and parents, you can indirectly affect more students than you could by working directly with the students" (Brigman et al., 2005, p. 25).

Consulting is much more time efficient and therefore cost effective. The counselor who works with one client affects one person and her or his life. The consultant who works with one teacher indirectly affects the lives of 30 or more children. The consultant who works with one parent education group may affect the lives of 20 to 30 children (Dinkmeyer & Carlson, 2006).

There will always be a place for individual work with students; however, "consultation reaches the most students through the most effective use of the counselor's time" (Brigman et al., 2005, p. 5). "Counselors are able to help students function more effectively in their environment, while consultants are more likely to change the environment" (Dinkmeyer & Carlson, 2006, p. 11).

## The Consultant as Facilitator

The complex problems of children in schools often go beyond the expertise of even the most seasoned and skilled school counselor. Equal collaboration avoids placing on the shoulders of school counselors the unilateral onus to fix problems. The simple gesture of admitting that no one person has all the answers (no school counselor does) helps ease the burden to create magic and in many cases levels the playing field in promoting a partnership. Conveying that you don't have all the answers will at times encourage the consultee to voice her or his ideas and opinions and also communicates to the consultee that she or he is a valued player.

Consultation should focus on an equal partnership but there will be many occasions in which the school counselor will have greater knowledge and contribution to the problem solving required in the partnership. The point of an equal partnership in consultation is to focus on the facilitative role rather than placing the burden of acting as an "expert" in all the problems students and families face. School counselors, who understand the developmental issues and academic and personal social concerns, will often bring more expertise to the consultation partnership. Consultation is a process of problem solving; it is not an imbalance of power and having to possess all the answers. In school consultation, the power comes from the consultation partnership where equal problem solving is expected and helping others feel empowered is one of the goals (Dinkmeyer & Carlson, 2006; Friend & Cook, 2009; Kampwirth, 2006). Differentiation of power complicates the work and unduly burdens counselors to carry the load. A skilled consultant knows that an equal partnership better prepares consultees to handle their next crisis or obstacle. The school counselor's power comes not from being the child development expert, but rather from possessing strong interpersonal skills and a willingness to be engaged with the consultee.

We have observed that effective school counselors/consultants bring commitment, skill, resources, and knowledge to the consulting relationship. The counselor/consultant is resourceful; working to find answers, solutions, strategies, and resources; effective in interpersonal skills; and committed to collaboration. Textbook knowledge about causes and solutions to students' problems will not translate into an effective consultant.

Consultees may include **internal consultees**, such as a classroom teacher, an administrator, the media specialist, a special education teacher, and the school nurse. The **external consultee** may be a parent, agency personnel, mentor, tutor, community health care provider, or any other member of the larger community that has an interest in student success but who is not regularly housed in a school setting. School counselors as consultants will use both their internal and external resources to try and help their students.

Your primary consultees will be teachers, parents, and the system. The remainder of this chapter will be focusing on the consultation role with these three consultees.

## CONSULTING WITH TEACHERS

Teachers will seek you in the halls, the lounge, on email, through notes in your mailbox, and will appear at your office door. Teachers as consultees will be as varied as the myriad problems students face. In our experience, teachers as consultants generally fall into one of five categories: confident, questioning, dependent, absentee, or dominating.

1. *The confident teacher.* Highly skilled teachers who have sound ideas will collaborate with the school counselor to validate and confirm that the

approach they plan to use with a student is the right one. The Confident Consultee has a history of being successful with students and she or he reaches out to you to serve as a resource for agencies, tutors, mentors, materials, and as a sounding board. The Confident Consultee generally supports even your smallest effort and appreciates that you have listened and offered thoughtful comments and ideas.

2. *The questioning teacher.* These teachers come to the consultant because they have tried and failed to affect change in a student; they need a new voice and new strategies. These skilled teachers only ask for shared responsibility in trying to help their students. Questioning Consultees are rewarding to work with as they exercise a good-faith effort to follow through and to take responsibility for making the strategies work that were generated by your partnership.

3. *The dependent teacher.* Some teachers/consultees will demand immediate results. These teachers are often less skilled themselves at behavior and classroom management and are struggling or overwhelmed. These teachers have unrealistic expectations of you and maintain a "take this student and fix them and send them back cured by sixth period" approach. Rather than falling into the trap of unrealistic demands, the consultant has to spend time and energy reframing these teachers' request to be in the "fix it" business and skillfully coaxing a collaborative effort to examine the strategies that the teacher has tried in the past and to team in developing interventions and resources for the future. Dependency on the consultant may develop if the consultant is willing to act as the expert and own the problems as hers or his to solve.

4. *The absentee teacher.* Certain teachers will never call on you because they feel that they should be able to solve all problems in their class or they refuse to admit that any problems exist. For the Absentee Consultee there are ways to groom a collaborative relationship through other areas such as jointly planning classroom guidance lessons. Assisting in this way will place you in a positive light and help grow the teacher/counselor relationship.

5. *The dominating teacher.* The fifth type of teacher as consultee is the one who will try to monopolize your time. Unfettered, this teacher will deplete your energy. Setting boundaries is necessary to combat the teacher who behaves as if she or he is your only consultee, demanding your undivided attention. Setting and keeping specified appointment times, collaboratively developing action plans, and establishing one or two weekly check-in times for action plan evaluation may help to reduce the Dominator's dependence on you.

No one teacher/consultee falls neatly into these categories, but all display combinations or variations of these. With patience, flexibility, and interpersonal skills you are acquiring what West and Idol (1987) refer to as the art of consultation. Strong collaborative, communication, and negotiation skills will move teachers along the continuum to the Questioning or Confident Consultee.

### PREPARE for Effective Consultation with Teachers

To help you remember key concepts, best practices, and pitfalls to effective consultation consider using **PREPARE**, an acronym for Philosophy, Relationships, **Equity of power**, Professional development, Accessibility, Resources, Evaluate. The chart in Figure 12.1 is an advanced organizer to help you understand PREPARE at a glance. The chart is followed by an expanded version of each step.

### *PREPARE: Philosophy*

School counselors establish a philosophy of consultation that is in step with the philosophy of their school counseling program, which, hopefully, aligns with the mission of their school to support all students to be successful learners and productive citizens.

### *PREPARE: Relationships*

Relationship building is vital to each role you will perform as a school counselor, but never more so than in the consultation role where interpersonal skills can spell the difference between success and failure. Other chapters have addressed relationship building but this section focuses specifically on the consultation role. "One of the first steps in consulting with teachers occurs prior to the actual consultation. The most important step is establishing strong rapport and mutual understanding between counselor and teacher" (Gibson, 2010, p. 307). "A collaborative relationship with staff must precede all other efforts" (Dinkmeyer & Carlson, 2006, p. 89). Here are some guiding principles for building a reputation and interpersonal relationships with teachers:

Appreciate and understand how demanding and difficult it is to be a teacher. Avoid absolutes, blame, and judgment. It is not a function of the consultation relationship to assign guilt, blame, or categorize. Rarely are absolute statements true, such as, "her classroom is chaos," or "he could care less about teaching." Consultants usually cannot hide a judgmental attitude. Facial expressions, tone, and choice of words will convey true feelings. Consultees sense and react to a judgmental attitude by raising their defenses, which in turn lowers their willingness to cooperate (Parsons & Kahn, 2005).

- Follow through on commitments made to consultees. This is essential to achieve credibility.
- Identify teachers and parents who are open to working with you and start here with your consultation role to build your confidence before moving on to more challenging consultees.
- Recognize the irrevocable harm to your role if you are viewed as untrustworthy. For example, avoid reporting a colleague to the administration unless you are certain it will be handled skillfully. Once it is known that you deliver information to the administration, you have diminished your capacity to be effective. Work through other channels to help a teacher bring resolution to her or his problems before taking the drastic step of reporting. A good relationship with the administration will help you

| | |
|---|---|
| **P**hilosophy | • Establish a philosophy of consultation that aligns with the school's mission to support all students to be successful learners and productive citizens |
| **R**elationships | • Establish rapport and mutual understanding |
| | • Follow through on commitments made |
| | • Identify teachers who are open to working with you |
| | • Recognize the irrevocable harm to your role if you are viewed as untrustworthy |
| | • Provide a welcoming atmosphere and demeanor |
| | • Practice genuine respect and belief that the teacher can affect change |
| **E**quity of Power | • Help teacher feel empowered to be an equal partner |
| | • Reframe discussion when teacher wants to place burden on you to solve problem |
| | • Treat teacher with patience |
| | • Avoid condescending tone or behavior |
| | • Listen authentically |
| | • Solicit teacher's suggestions and show you value her or his input by incorporating ideas in plan |
| **P**rofessional Development | • Enhance your own skills: |
| |   ○ Join professional organizations |
| |   ○ Read current literature |
| |   ○ Attend conferences and inservices |
| |   ○ Observe effective counselors and teachers |
| | • Deliver staff development: |
| |   ○ Faculty meetings |
| |   ○ Grade level/Departmental meetings |
| |   ○ Newsletters |
| |   ○ PTA meetings |
| |   ○ Parent workshops |
| **A**ccessibility | • Be visible in the halls |
| | • Provide teachers with a note you are there to help them and/or a list of services you can deliver |
| | • Post your daily, weekly, monthly schedule on your door |
| | • Let it be known through various mediums you are an advocate for students, parents, and teachers |
| | • Be a part of the mainstream of the faculty (i.e., attending functions, socializing, and exchanging pleasantries) |
| | • Set up an electronic way for teachers to signal they need consultation services |
| **R**esources | • Broker and manage recourses, both human and material |
| | • Groom a relationship with community agencies |
| | • Develop a library of resources that address special needs students |
| | • Provide teachers with resources |
| **E**valuate | • Establish baseline data |
| | • Collaboratively implement strategies |
| | • Analyze impact data |

FIGURE **12.1** PREPARE at a Glance

forward the consultation role without risking being viewed by the faculty as being against them.

- Provide a welcoming atmosphere and demeanor. Personable individuals tend to be more successful in school consultation. "People are more willing to work with affable, outgoing, friendly people than with people who aren't" (Kampwirth, 2006, p. 108).
- Practice genuine respect and a belief that the consultee can affect change and contribute to the consultation process. Search your consciousness and truly believe in the inherent dignity and worth of each consultee (even those for whom you are offended by their actions). Beliefs determine actions (Hookway, 2005; Martin, 2004). **Positive self-talk** before each work session about the potential of the consultee to make progress will translate to positive interactions.

### PRE_PARE: _Equity of Power_

"One of the key concepts that underlies a collaborative approach to consultation is that of **egalitarianism**, or a non-hierarchical relationship between the consultant and the consultee" (Kampwirth, 2006, p. 110; bold treatment added). There is much wisdom in helping your consultee feel empowered to be an equal partner or dominant force in solving problems. Reframe discussions when the consultee wants to place the burden on you to solve the problem. A carefully worded request, "let's sit down and brainstorm some strategies," emphasizes the need for a partnership. Treating the consultee with patience, avoiding a condescending tone or behavior, listening authentically, soliciting her or his suggestions, and showing you value her or his input by incorporating all ideas into the plan promotes equity of power.

"Additionally, professional school counselors should remember that consultation is a partnership that is based on trust and respect. Therefore, teachers should be made to feel trusted and respected as they are asked for their own expertise in creating, implementing, and evaluating interventions that will help student" (Gibson, 2010, p. 308).

### PRE_PARE: _Professional Development_

Grow your body of knowledge and expertise while fostering the professional development of potential consultees. Professional development is two-pronged: enhancing your own skills and delivering staff development to support faculty members' and administrators' growth and development.

Professional organizations, literature, conferences, and inservices will contribute to your professional development. Observations of other counselors or teachers who are most effective in meeting the needs of difficult or troubled students can help you learn how to grow your skills.

Position yourself as a vital resource to teachers and raise your profile by making staff development a routine part of your work. A 10-minute staff development workshop at each faculty meeting where you convey information to help all faculty and staff places you in a favorable light as a willing respondent to teachers' and students' needs. Arrange speakers or present important topics in faculty meetings such as Response to Interventions, special education eligibility, eating disorders, attention deficit hyperactivity disorder (ADHD), suicidal ideation, or bullying. Other mediums for staff development would be grade-level/departmental meetings, a school newsletter, the PTA meetings, and parent workshops. Grant writing might help you bring in resources in the form of people and materials. Secure speakers by swapping places with another counselor who presents her or his forte to your faculty while you present a topic you are particularly competent in to her or his faculty. Without promoting unhealthy competition, find a way to focus on your teachers' best practices so as to replicate areas such as good classroom or behavior management.

### PREPARE: Accessibility

Being accessible, professionally available, and approachable will further your efforts to be taken seriously as a consultant and to be considered a partner in the educational process. Some guiding principles follow:

- Be visible in the halls, cafeteria, and classrooms consulting with teachers.
- Provide teachers and other potential consultees with a note that you are there to help them and/or a list of the different types of consultation services you can deliver.
- Post your daily, weekly, and monthly schedule on your door with time for consultation clearly marked. Be flexible and if at all possible accommodate people who come in unannounced for consultation.
- Let it be known through various medium that you are an advocate for students, parents, and teachers, publicizing consultation activities that extend beyond the traditional role of helping with troubled students to areas such as helping teachers with resources to support their classroom management or finding tutors and mentors for students.
- Be part of the mainstream of the faculty: attend functions, socialize, and exchange pleasantries. Avoid setting yourself apart as this will affect your ability to be an effective consultant to help the students in your school.
- Set up an electronic way in which teachers can signal you that they need your consultation services so that it is easier for both of you to make an agreed-on meeting time. A caution when using email is for both of you to avoid using identifying information about a particular student.

### PREPARE: Resources

Brokering and managing resources, both human and material, increases the effectiveness of the consultation role and allows you to widen your realm of influence. By becoming a manager of human resources, you extend your reach without overextending yourself. A consultant who brokers resources brings in as many agencies, business partners, parents, and other resources as possible to deliver strategies such as mentoring and tutoring. Just one eager, trustworthy volunteer under your direction can set the wheels in motion to garner support from a variety of sources to help you with specific needs. The chapters on coordination of resources and accountability offer extensive information on potential stakeholders and resources to bring into your program. Groom a relationship with community agencies so that you can have contact information when you need to refer parents and others to outside resources. Some agencies will reposition support personnel into your school if you provide them with facilities.

- Develop a library of resources that address the issues and special needs of your student population. Use other mediums for your consultation role besides face-to-face conversations. Have a newsletter with critical timely information. Make computers available with important websites earmarked for parents and educators to use in searches.
- Provide teachers with resource materials. When you find a valuable free resource, order one for everyone in the school and advocate for money when you need to purchase vital resources. For example, the U.S. Department of Education at www.ed.gov/index.jsp has online guides, programs, and the latest research to assist teachers and administrators (see the text's website for free publications you can order).

### PREPARE: Evaluate

Evaluate your effectiveness as a consultant by establishing baseline data, collaboratively implementing strategies, and then looking at the results in the form of impact data to see if the student improved in troublesome areas such as attendance, grade point average, promotion, etc. Refer to Chapter 9 to learn how to evaluate your work through MEASURE.

## CONSULTING WITH PARENTS

Now that we have discussed teachers, the first of our three primary consultees (teachers, parents, and the system), let us examine our work with an equally important partner: parents. Educational consultation is likely to be more successful when there is an effective parent-educator partnership (Delaney & Kaiser, 2001; Epstein, 2001; Epstein et al., 2009; Epstein & Sheldon, 2002; Sanders, 2000; Sheridan, Clarke, & Burt, 2008). Student success is not home or school, teacher or student, but the dynamic relationships between them; learning takes place where there are productive relationships among all participants in the educational process (Epstein, 2001; Epstein et al., 2009; Epstein & Sheldon, 2002; Sanders, 2000). It is a well-documented fact that student performance is enhanced by a strong relationship between parents and the school (Adams, Womack, Shatzer, & Caldarella, 2010; Bryan & Henry, 2008; Bryan & Holcomb-McCoy, 2007; Davis & Lambie, 2005; Griffin & Steen, 2010; Harris, Wierzalis, & Coy, 2010; Minke & Anderson, 2005; Sheridan, Clarke, & Burt, 2008).

Positive effects of parent involvement on student achievement are apparent across grade levels and for all socioeconomic status (SES) levels (Davis & Lambie, 2005; Epstein et al., 2009). When parents are involved, we know that students show improvement in grades, test scores, attitudes, and behavior; complete more homework; are more engaged in classroom learning activities; and have higher attendance rates and a reduction in suspension rates.

## PARTNER for Effective Conferences with Parents

PARTNER helps you remember a seven-step approach in facilitating the success of conferences with parents or guardians. PARTNER is an acronym for Planning, Acknowledging, Rapport building, Teaming, Negotiating, Ending, Regrouping. The school counselor as consultant can provide ongoing staff development to teachers and other educators about communicating effectively with parents and also facilitate the exchange of tips for conducting parent conferences and managing parent visits. Counselors acting as advocates can collaboratively create ground rules about how to conduct parent conferences. As a consultant, it is altogether appropriate that counselors help to establish a climate of acceptance, openness, and trust that will promote goodwill between the school and community (Gibson, 2010). It is dangerous to assume that everyone understands the basic dos and don'ts of communication. Be an advocate for all members of the school community by helping teachers understand the tenets of good written and verbal communication. By conducting staff development you can place the school in a better light, reduce the gossip and naysaying about the school, and minimize some of the problems teachers have with parents. When parents visit the school for a parent conference, school counselors and teachers have the opportunity to develop an ally or a foe (Gestwiki, 2010; Keys, 2000; Sheldon & Epstein, 2002). It is in everyone's best interest, but most importantly the best interest of the student, to try to maximize the school visit (Davis & Lambie, 2005). Figure 12.2 is an advance organizer to help you understand PARTNER at a glance. The chart is followed by an expanded version of each step.

### PARTNER: Planning for Success

School counselors can help teachers plan ahead and implement strategies before the parent conference to increase the likelihood of success. In advance of the conference, help the teacher:

- Recognize that she or he will be talking to a parent about their child, someone for whom parents would give their lives. Helping teachers keep this thought in the forefront of their minds will reduce the teachers' defensiveness and frustrations when the parent cannot be objective about their child's problems.
- Be prepared to hear angry words, accusations, and unfair statements with the realization that to respond in kind is not an option. Parents' defense mechanisms may mean that they will behave badly. Under these circumstances, the teacher can learn to react more kindly.
- Think positive thoughts about the student. Remember, beliefs and attitudes are conveyed in our faces, tone, words, and actions.
- Recognize that for parents to come to school is sometimes intimidating or embarrassing. Create a pleasant environment and interchange that helps parents feel welcome. Offering something to drink, walking them over to a bulletin board to see their child's displayed artwork, handing them a

| Planning for Success | • Recognize you are talking about *their* child<br>• Be prepared to hear angry words, accusations, and unfair statements<br>• Think positive thoughts about the student<br>• Recognize that parents may feel intimidated or embarrassed<br>• Help provide for an interpreter<br>• Keep the number of people in the room to a minimum<br>• Dress professionally |
|---|---|
| Acknowledging Parents as Equal Partners | • Understand that parents are doing the best they can or know how to do<br>• Convey confidence in having the parent as a partner<br>• Recognize and value the parents' rights |
| Rapport Building | • Use facilitation skills to defuse anger<br>• Begin with positives about the student<br>• Avoid absolute statements |
| Teaming to Identify the Problem | • Encourage parents to talk about how they see their child's progress<br>• Collaborate to recognize and acknowledge shared goals<br>• Avoid fixed problem-solving ideas<br>• Have resources material and agency referrals available |
| Negotiating a Plan of Action | • Search for congruence in defining the problem and the plan to be implemented |
| Ending Effectively | • Summarize the conference to check for understanding and willingness to work together<br>• End with affirmations |
| Regrouping | • Monitor interventions and adjust accordingly<br>• Be willing to try alternative interventions |

FIGURE **12.2** PARTNER at a Glance

folder with papers that have good grades on them, and showing them how neat their child keeps her or his desk are just a few ideas to start off on a positive note.

• Help provide for an interpreter and/or someone to be present from the family if the teacher believes it will put parents more at ease.

• Keep the number of people in the room to a minimum. It is sometimes intimidating when a parent has to come into a room full of people with titles such as school psychologist, social worker, and intervention specialist. If possible, spend some time with the parent(s) alone to discuss confidentiality, to work on relationship building, to increase parents' comfort level, to explain to them who will be in the meeting and why, and if necessary, to help them understand you are an ally before plunging parents into a room full of people.

• Dress professionally but in a way that helps parents identify with you. This approach may require professional dress that is more understated. Overdressing can intimidate parents and cause them to withdraw from the conversation.

### PARTNER: Acknowledging Parents as Equal Partners

School counselors can help teachers increase the likelihood of a successful conference if they can help the teacher validate and acknowledge parents as true partners in the problem-solving arena. Help teachers:

- Understand that parents are doing the best they can or know how to do. They love their children and just because they do not respond the way we believe they should, it does not mean that they should be dismissed.
- Convey confidence in having the parent as a partner. By having parents feel empowered to be a partner, teachers reduce the likelihood of one-upmanship that can drive a wedge between teachers and parents and places the burden on each party to solve the problem alone.
- Recognize and value the parents' rights to be the guiding voice in their children's lives and really listen to what they say in terms of their child's needs.

### PARTNER: Rapport Building

School counselors can help teachers build rapport with parents by helping the teacher:

- Use facilitation skills to defuse anger and to let the parents know that in the teacher resides a genuine listener. Ask genuine questions of the parents. Show an interest in their answers. Reflect and paraphrase. Avoid acronyms and education jargon that leaves parents confused. Check for clarity and understanding often.
- Begin with positives about the student. It may seem like a cliché, but get teachers to make positive comments, show successful work, praise behavior, or cite the child's skills before launching into a list of problems. You can build on the positives to affect problem areas.
- Avoid absolute statements such as "your child is out of his seat *all* the time," or "*never* does his work," or "*always* picks a fight on the playground." These statements usually give parents nowhere to go but on the defensive.

### PARTNER: Teaming to Identify the Problem

School counselors can help teachers build a team mentality with parents by helping the teacher:

- Encourage parents to talk about how they see their child's progress in school. This should come before a list of concerns from the teacher.
- Collaborate with the parent to recognize and acknowledge the shared goal of removing barriers so that the student can be a successful learner. Identifying common goals helps the teacher/parent/counselor partnership to pinpoint the problem (Henderson, Mapp, Johnson, & Davies, 2007). Accurate problem identification starts with common goals for the student's behavior and academic work (Parsons & Kahn, 2005). Discuss the parents' and teachers' perspectives of desired student performance early on in the meeting.

- Avoid fixed ideas about how the problem should be solved. Be open to the possibility that parents may really have the best ideas for addressing the issue or that a completely different approach may be needed. The agenda should be flexible and receptive to really hearing what a parent has to say with an urgency to accomplish preset goals.
- With parental input, prioritize concerns and settle on the area(s) of concern that warrant the greatest effort and attention (Parsons & Kahn, 2005). This hopefully will be an area that affects the child's ability to be a successful learner. Avoid trying to tackle all of the problems at once, with the hope that improvement in one area will affect others.
- Have resource material and agency referrals available to address the issues you plan to discuss.

### PARTNER: Negotiating a Plan of Action

Search for congruence with the parents in defining the problem to be addressed and the plan of action to be implemented. The plan of action should be in the form of goals, not in the form of problems. For example, "John will complete 75 percent of his work the first week." MEASURE is a good tool for framing a plan of action as illustrated in this chapter in the case of Susan that follows and in the chapter on accountability.

### PARTNER: Ending Effectively

Summarize the conference and check for understanding and the willingness for everyone to work together. If in doubt about the acceptability of the action plan, then speak up and raise the issue while processing what has been said. End with affirmations about the potential for making a difference and the 100 percent commitment that all parties plan to give in working together. Thank parents for their time, presence, and for demonstrating a commitment to be in partnership with the school for the greater good of their child's education.

### PARTNER: Regrouping

Monitor the interventions during the designated allotted time and adjust the interventions as needed. Be prepared for the possibility that all partners will need to return to the table and start anew on a plan. Accentuate and expand what worked. The plan of action may not be successful the first time around. Be willing to try alternative interventions without jumping to more restrictive classroom settings such as special education placement.

## THE FOUR Ds OF THE ACTION PLAN

The action plan is the heart and soul of the consultation process. The mechanics or steps in developing and delivering an action plan are presented as the Four Ds to serve as a memory aid: (1) Data gathering, (2) Devising the action plan, (3) Delivering the action plan, and (4) Debriefing. Figure 12.3 is an advance organizer to help you understand the action plan. Following is an expanded explanation of each step.

| Data Gathering | • Gather facts through a variety of methods |
| --- | --- |
| | 1. Educational record review |
| | 2. Interviewing the teacher |
| | 3. Interviewing the parent |
| | 4. Interviewing other educators |
| | 5. Interviewing the student(s) |
| | 6. Interviewing other helping professionals |
| | 7. Student observation |
| | 8. Systems observation |
| | 9. Educational Assessment |
| | 10. Psychological Assessment |
| Devising the Action Plan | • Use facts to accurately determine how student's needs will be met |
| | • The action plan is a partnership between all stakeholders |
| Delivering the Action Plan | • Set timelines for strategies to be implemented |
| | • Timelines ensure accountability |
| Debriefing | • Determine if the action plan was effective |

FIGURE **12.3** The Four Ds of the Action Plan

**Data gathering**    The first step, in collaboration with others, is to gather the facts through one or more of a variety of data-gathering methods. Rarely will you use every approach with each case but discussed are 10 frequently used approaches to gathering information:

1. Educational record review
2. Interviewing the teacher
3. Interviewing the parent
4. Interviewing other educators
5. Interviewing the student(s)
6. Interviewing other helping professionals
7. Student observation
8. Systems observation
9. Educational assessment
10. Psychological assessment

Data gathering helps participants in the consultation process make better decisions by accurately identifying the problem and narrowing the focus of the interventions so that the resources and energy brought to the table are addressing the critical issues.

**Devising the action plan**    After the facts have been collected by all parties involved to accurately determine the student's (or students') need, then the consultant and consultees will start devising an action plan. The action plan is a partnership using each person's skills and knowledge to help the student(s).

**Delivering the action plan**   Delivering the action plan will require all stakeholders to set timelines and strategies that they will be implementing. A timeline is important for interim accountability to see if the delivery of the plan is actually taking place.

**Debriefing**   The final step is the debriefing. This is the time to determine if the action plan was effective and what revisions, if any, are necessary.

# APPLICATION OF THE FOUR Ds IN THE CASE OF SUSAN

Application of the Four Ds will be presented here in the context of a most prevalent teacher complaint, underachievement. The case of Susan will serve as the context to learn how to develop an action plan. Imagine yourself as the school counselor in this case.

*Ms. Lawrence tells you that her student, Susan, "has not completed any work the entire year." Ms. Lawrence explains to you that she has "tried everything" and would like your help in trying to determine what to do next. Where will you start?*

## Data Gathering in the Case of Susan

Data gathering is the first step in the consultation process. What follows below are some data-gathering steps in this hypothetical case with some possible outcomes. You will usually not have the time, resources, or the need to complete all these steps for one student. The steps and the sequence will vary according to the specifics of the real situation and rarely would you attend to all these steps. However, as an introduction and to learn the application of the data-gathering methods, each data-gathering method will be applied to the case of Susan.

### Educational Record Review

A review of the student's educational record is usually a good place to start the data-gathering process. Critical information is kept in the educational record and differs by school district according to its policy. Typical information includes screening results for vision and hearing, cumulative grades and test records, attendance, as well as entry and withdrawal information. Cumulative information can determine patterns that may reveal the sudden onset of problems or chronic issues. Did the problem have roots in years earlier? Were there early or recent indicators that this student was going to have difficulty? Are there records of interventions already applied to the problem?

*Examination of Susan's educational record reveals a pattern of low marks and teacher comments regarding Susan's failure to complete work and her lack of motivation. Other discoveries added to the cause for concern. In the five years Susan has been in school, her grades and test scores were consistently just below the average range but her reading comprehension had never been above the 20th percentile. On the positive side, her attendance has always been good.*

### Interviewing the Teacher

Probably the most powerful tool in terms of information gathering for the school counselor as consultant is the interview, especially the interview with the teacher. Good teaching matters, and what happens between the student and teacher can spell the difference between a student who is academically successful and one who gets left behind. Using a face-to-face interview to question, gather, and probe, a school counselor can put together information that will get to the heart of the issue and help clarify, define, and focus the work of the consultant/consultee. The interview helps to set the stage so that the work of all stakeholders can be rendered more effective. In absence of good interviews, the alternative would be trial and error to get at the issues, unnecessary struggles, and false starts that an interview could curtail.

Interviews can yield anecdotal information. Allowing a teacher or parent just to talk about the student can provide information about areas that you as an interviewer may not even think to explore. Anecdotal information is an opportunity to learn about the strengths of a student and to discover some positive information from which to build, especially in terms of establishing rapport when you start to interview the student or parent. Anecdotal information gives you a stronger sense of the student as a person and begins to round out one's perspective of the student rather than compartmentalizing her or him as "the student who has a problem finishing work."

An interview can determine the scope of the problem and help to prioritize which issues should be the foci. Baseline data can be collected, goals set, and a timeline established (see Chapter 8 for information on establishing baseline and outcome data).

*In your interview with Ms. Lawrence, she says that Susan has not done any work all year. As is often the case with absolutes, you know that the word any is a blanket statement made out of frustration. So you gently focus on what is really meant by "all year" and you learn that Susan's work is uneven but not completely nonexistent.*

*You are able to get an accurate description of the problem with probing questions such as "Are there subjects in which Susan will complete work?" and "What percentage of Susan's math problems goes unsolved?" "Is there a difference in Susan's response if the problems are given all at once or a few at a time?" "Does Susan work better when collaborating on work with other students such as peer helpers?" "Does Susan participate in art, music, physical education?" "Does Susan respond better when she is isolated to do her work?"*

*Questioning and listening helps you to pinpoint that Susan's problem occurs most often when she is left alone to complete work. With carefully worded questions, you also learn what interventions have not been tried in the past. Together you and Ms. Lawrence generate ideas for interventions. Because it is a team effort, Ms. Lawrence is more willing to take ownership. For example, by asking about peer helpers, you have encouraged Ms. Lawrence to try this approach to keep Susan on task.*

The school counselor in this scenario was careful to avoid making the consultee feel like she was being subjected to the third degree. Interviewing is not just about questioning but effective listening as well. Skilled interviews can plant ideas that the consultee can implement.

### Interviewing the Parent

A partnership with parents is powerful. "A positive home-school partnership is almost always the basis for improvement in behavior and learning problems, and this is true from preschool through adolescence" (Kampwirth, 2006, p. 166). Parent interviews can provide rich information but these interviews are often fraught with landmines. "The idea that an outsider (an individual representing the school) is asking to get involved in a family's life may have threatening connotations, especially for families that traditionally handle problems within the family rather than seek outside resources. Many families are confused about how to deal with their child's school-related problems" (Kampwirth, 2006, p. 126). In his 1996 work, Maital (as cited in Kampwirth, 2006, p. 126) noted, "parents may seek, and at the same time build defenses against, information and advice that they find uncomfortable." Although professional school counselors can be resources for parents, many parents bring anxiety and anger to consultation. This anxiety and anger needs to be evaluated by the professional school counselor to determine the appropriate response to the parents. In many cases, anxiety appears as anger or aggression. The majority of parents are worried about their children, and this worry can prevent them from hearing or understanding the purpose of the consultation. Anger can be a natural response for parents who see their children as an extension of themselves and are asking, "What are they saying is wrong with my child (me)?" (Gibson, 2010, p. 206). Later in this chapter, we address partnerships with parents.

*In your interview with Mr. Kurtz, Susan's dad, he talked about his daughter's successes and challenges and described what he had tried in the past to help Susan such as rewarding good grades with money. Mr. Kurtz said he did not have the money to pay for a tutor and that he could not help with homework because his job required long hours. Because he is a single parent, Mr. Kurtz said he relied on Susan's older siblings to care for her, admittedly a poor plan as the older siblings had problems doing their own schoolwork. Mr. Kurtz said the house was often chaotic with teenagers everywhere and loud music. He expressed a determination to try to improve the situation so that Susan could study. Mr. Kurtz seemed genuinely interested in trying to help Susan be more successful academically. He was willing to cooperate on an action plan and to set a time to meet again to discuss progress.*

### Interviewing Other Educators

Often it is appropriate to interview other educators and support personnel. Examining how the student behaves with other teachers can lend insight. If the student displays acting out behavior, identify what the paraprofessionals observe while working with the student in the classroom or on cafeteria duty. Ask the administration about their opinions and observations regarding this student and her or his problems.

*Mr. Mott, Susan's teacher from the previous year, was willing to describe interventions that he had tried with Susan. Mr. Mott said he had his greatest success with Susan the three weeks before Christmas break. Susan's mother had promised to visit Susan and her brothers at Christmas. Mr. Mott said that Susan talked about the upcoming visit constantly and Mr. Mott would encourage her to write letters to her mother during English class, draw pictures for her mother, and receive free time in the art corner to make presents for her mother in exchange for completing her work. Mr. Mott said he was able to get Susan to work hard by putting her work in a portfolio in anticipation of showing Susan's mother her work. Susan's work was still below grade level but her efforts were yielding results. Mr. Mott said sadly, "I think Susan thought that if she could show her mother that she could be really good that her mother would come home." Mr. Mott says he never got the entire story but he believes the Christmas visit was not the happy occasion Susan had anticipated. Susan came back from Christmas break more erratic in her performance than ever and it was a constant struggle to find ways to motivate her. Mr. Mott said he occasionally had success by pairing Susan with an older student who would come and tutor Susan two times a week.*

Seek out other educators who have had success with students with similar problems. Gather ideas and interventions from these teachers and seek their input in developing an action plan. For example, an elementary counselor who enrolled a student with autism arranged to have a Special Education (SE) specialist come to his school to help the current ESE teacher as well as the rest of the school develop strategies for working with this student, as we all lacked experience with autistic students.

### Interviewing the Student

It is often appropriate to interview a student or conduct an individual counseling session to get the student's perspective about the problem. From the student's perspective, the school counselor can often learn what motivates the student and initiate strategies that will boost the student's success. Students of all ages can take part in problem solving, but the older the student, the more necessary her or his involvement becomes to ensure and increase the likelihood of success.

*You meet with Susan three times over the course of two weeks. She tells you that she feels she is dumb and that no matter how hard she tries, she will never be able to understand what the teacher is telling the class. Susan talks about her family but she paints a far better picture than what was described by her father and Mr. Mott. Susan talks about a family that does "great stuff together, like go out to eat." She describes brothers who take her places, a father who gives her things, and a mother who has a very important job.*

*Susan can't name anything that she likes about school but she does talk about Mr. Mott and how much she liked being in his class last year.*

### Interviewing Other Helping Professionals

Reaching out to other members of the helping profession can provide resources that the school would not otherwise be able to offer. Helping professionals internal to the school, such as a school psychologist or school social worker, or external to the school, such as agency or community mental health providers, may also offer experience or expertise to support internal school members.

*In Susan's case, you are becoming concerned about issues of abandonment. With the permission of Susan's father, you consult with an agency counselor to get some information that you can pass along to Susan's father. The discussion helps you understand that Susan may indeed be experiencing adverse effects from abandonment. Abandonment, or "withdrawal of support," involves rejection and/or being left behind by an important figure in one's life (Hyper Dictionary, n.d.). Susan's loss of her mother may mean she has abandonment issues (Auman, 2007; Wolchick, Ma, Tein, Sandler, & Ayers, 2008). Without a formal diagnosis yet with the observable behavior that Susan is struggling, you encourage Susan's father to seek counseling for her at an agency that offers a sliding fee scale and secures volunteers who will bring children to their counseling sessions when transportation is a problem.*

### Student Observation

Observations can be done by any qualified, certificated educator in the building and can take many forms. Sometimes a counselor will sit and work an educational game with a student to observe the student's thought and problem-solving processes, behavior, and social skills. An observation can take the form of recording what you see out of the direct line of vision of the student. Observations are best when they record overt information; those behaviors that are observed without interpretation such as "the student moves the chair from under the table, sits down, immediately leans over and whispers something to the student sitting next to him and then shares a laugh with the student." The observer then follows up the recording of overt behavior with the subjective part of the observation, in other words, putting an interpretation and opinion of what she or he believes is the meaning of the overt behaviors. Many observers skip the recording of overt behaviors and just report the meaning of what they observed. Observers will need to train themselves to record what the eye sees because it requires the observer to focus and not miss important messages while trying to prematurely interpret or bring meaning to the observations. The observation should not confirm preconceived ideas about what is believed to be the issue but to identify how the student functions in the school environment. Train yourself to record objective information and then connect the dots presented to form your opinions about the meaning of the information. Following is an observation of a reading lesson in which the teacher is checking for comprehension following a silent reading assignment.

*With the agreement of the teacher, you observe Susan in class. The students, including Susan, do not know why you are sitting in the back of the classroom and soon forget that you are there. Below is just the first 8 minutes of the 25 minutes of the observation and a partial interpretation.*

# *School Counselor Casebook: The Case of Susan: Student Observation*

Time: 8:52 to 9:17
Place: Room 224
Activity: Reading

Susan traces the pattern on the tile floor with her toe. She intently watches her toe as she carefully tries to remain within the lines of the pattern. She goes outside the line. She stops moving her foot, gets a distressed look on her face, and then she starts all over from where she began tracing. She repeats this pattern several times.

(The teacher asks a student next to Susan a question and the student responds.)

Susan appears startled at the sound of her neighbor's voice. She stops the movement of her foot and stares intently at the student answering the question. She raises the front legs of her desk off the ground and balances on the back two legs. She lifts her feet and the desk slams down. Susan twirls her hair into tight coils and pulls the hair straight out from her head and parallel to the floor. Susan continues to play intently with her hair for the next two minutes, bringing her hair around to cover her eyes, selecting strands to put in her mouth, and studying the ends by bringing them around close to her eyes.

(The teacher continues to ask closed questions so that all the students can respond in unison, e.g., "What was the name of Kindra's dog?")

The sound of her classmates responding in unison brings a puzzled look to Susan's face. She lays her head in her hands and gently rocks herself back and forth and back and forth. This movement continues for two minutes until the teacher switches from having the students respond in unison.

(The teacher asks the students to stand behind their desks and act out the part of the story where the main character had to crouch behind a table.)

Susan appears startled when she sees each of the students crouching behind their desks. She looks around as if to copy the other students but tentatively crouches and then stands and then crouches again. She smiles big and then laughs out loud.

(The teacher asks the students to sit and shifts into asking for individual responses again.)

Susan watches the other students take their seats and then after everyone is seated, she takes her seat too.

*Interpretation*: Throughout the lesson Susan was not engaged except to copy other students who crouched behind their desk, apparently unaware of the purpose of the crouch. Susan's affect led me to believe she felt sad, lonely, and disconnected from the rest of the class. Susan's face transformed when she was doing what all the other students were doing (crouching). It is as if Susan rarely is able to follow along and feels left behind most of the time. Being able to be part of the group seemed to be very important to Susan and brought a light to her face, animated movements, and laughter, the only sound I heard from Susan the entire 25 minutes.

### System Observation

Don't forget the system in which Susan is functioning. Observing and gathering information about how the system has added value or stratified Susan's opportunities is critical to help her and other student's progress.

*When looking at the educational institutional in which Susan is functioning several stratifiers are found. Susan has been missing school at least three days a month because the bus came early. Additionally, you find that Susan often is not allowed to eat breakfast on the days her bus is late, as the cafeteria has closed. Susan depends on the breakfast provided at school, as her home life does not include a morning ritual of breakfast. In addition to missing reading class when she is absent, Susan has been missing reading class when her bus is late. Not only has the late bus kept her from eating breakfast, but also she has had to wait in line at the office to get her re-admittance pass, and this cuts into the morning reading time. You have also learned that the special reading support is no longer being offered to Susan because a student must demonstrate progress to remain in the program. Last year Susan was not able to demonstrate progress, so this year she was not assigned to the program. Additionally the school has a special Saturday tutoring program for students who have a B average. You never paid attention to the requirements for the tutoring program or the special support reading program but it has become apparent to you that maybe students who need the most support in reading are really given the least, a systemic problem that you can advocate to have changed.*

### Educational Assessment

What assessment instruments do you have at your disposal to understand the reading problems and other academic problems Susan is suffering? An educational evaluation, such as the Woodcock-Johnson Psycho-educational Battery (Woodcock, McGrew, & Mather, 2001), can identify areas of strengths and weakness for Susan so that strategies can be brought to bear on those areas. For example, the Woodcock-Johnson provides information about general intellectual ability, specific cognitive ability, oral language, and academic achievement. This assessment then provides an extensive measure of achievement and ability (Woodcock, McGrew, & Mather, 2001). Data analyses of other test results that are part of the student's educational record can be used in lieu of or in addition to an individual educational assessment such as the Woodcock-Johnson.

*You have decided to give Susan the Woodcock-Johnson Psycho-educational Battery as a measure of her achievement. The results of her assessment reveal that her standard scores are close to the mean for her age in all areas with reading comprehension slightly lower than the other scores. The results of the test helped pinpoint where Susan's academic functioning is and can help provide guidance in how to address those deficits.*

### The Psychological Assessment

Sometimes a student may need to be referred for a battery of tests called a psychological assessment that includes an intellectual quotient (IQ), a personality assessment, or projective evaluations, to name a few possibilities. A school psychologist usually does this battery and in many school districts this step would be taken only if it were believed that the student might need special education placement (see Chapter 9 for more on psychological assessments).

*For Susan it was determined that classroom and home interventions were adequate at this time and that Susan would not be referred for special education nor for consideration for a full psychological assessment.*

The information gleaned from your data gathering provides the basic information for you and the consultees to start devising a plan of action for Susan. The data-gathering stage may include one or more data-gathering approaches listed under Step 1 and/or other data approaches not described. For example, it may be determined that a developmental history is needed, or a medical evaluation, or a visit by a social worker.

### *Devising the Action Plan in the Case of Susan*

Having finished the first step of the action plan, Data gathering, let us discuss Step 2 of the four steps, which is Devising the action plan. The second step of the consultation process is to organize the data and take them to the consultee(s) so that an action plan can be devised with strategies and stakeholders' responsibilities for implementing each strategy. This is also the time to establish your baseline data so that after the interventions are put into place, you can track Susan's progress on her reading comprehension scores. With data all participants can know if progress is being made and if certain interventions are more effective than others in addition to which interventions

TABLE **12.1**
Stakeholders-Unite to Carry Out Strategies

**Current critical data element:** Susan's reading comprehension scores

**Baseline:** Susan's reading comprehension: 14 percentile

**Goal:** Susan's reading comprehension: 20 percentile by the end of the year

**Beginning date:** Sept. 05

**Ending date:** May 06

| Stakeholders | Strategies |
|---|---|
| School counselor | • Assist in the preliminary data gathering and collaborate on developing strategies<br>• Administer or access a qualified educator to give the Woodcock-Johnson Educational Assessment<br>• Help Ms. Lawrence, the teacher, and Mr. Kurtz establish a behavior management program. For example, the program may look like the following: Just before school ends each day the counselor goes by for a report from Ms. Lawrence and brings Susan to the counseling office to chart her progress in completing her work. Each successful day gets a happy face sticker on the chart, with four per week resulting in a treat and five good days earning two movie passes, as movies are a favorite pastime for Susan. Her father agrees to take Susan to the movie when she earns this reward. Fewer than three happy faces a week means limited television. |

| | |
|---|---|
| Teachers | • Give work in small chunks rather than the complete assignment<br>• Assign a buddy student to help her stay on task<br>• Tape instructions and lessons and then allow Susan and her buddy to replay the tape as needed<br>• Provide older students to peer tutor with Susan<br>• Send home a daily assignment book to be signed by Mr. Kurtz<br>• Increase positive attention to Susan<br>• Advocate that Susan be allowed to participate in the reading recovery program |
| Previous teacher, Mr. Mott | • Serve as an adult mentor to regularly check in on Susan's progress and to give her support and encouragement |
| Susan's father | • Check and sign the daily assignment book<br>• Provide a quiet study environment<br>• Get the older siblings to work with Susan on her homework<br>• Take Susan to the movie when she completes her behavior management program and limit her television when she does not complete her program<br>• Contact Susan's mother and encourage her to become more involved in Susan's life. Ask her to come to school for a parent conference with the counselor and teacher. |
| Business Partner | • Provide movie passes for rewards for Susan<br>• Provide a desk and chair for Susan<br>• Set up a computer for Susan at home and at school<br>• Provide transportation to counseling sessions when Mr. Kurtz cannot |
| Big Brother Big Sister organization and Boys and Girls Club | • Help Susan develop confidence and academic skills by (1) involving her in sports; (2) giving her time and attention; (3) orchestrating opportunities for Susan to develop friendships; and (4) providing her with tutoring |
| Administration | • Change the breakfast policy so that food is always available for late arrivals<br>• Change the tardy policy so that student's re-admittance does not depend on waiting in lines<br>• Change the criteria for admissions into special programs and tutoring programs so that students who need the most help can get it |

should be replicated and which should be eliminated. Devising an action plan means that you and the consultees identify stakeholders to help you make progress with Susan's academic success, especially her reading comprehension skills.

### Delivering the Action Plan in the Case of Susan

Having finished the first two steps of the action plan, Data gathering and Devising the action plan, let us move to the third step: Delivering the action plan. The teacher, parent, and school counselor connect the other stakeholders to the effort of delivering the action plan. The Big Brother Big Sister organization and Boys and Girls Club are contacted. Stakeholders have agreed to deliver their component of the action plan, a timeline is established for completion or an interim check of progress, and a date is set for the next meeting.

### Debriefing

Having finished the first three steps of the action plan, Data gathering, Devising the action plan, and Delivering the action plan, let us move to the fourth and final step: Debriefing. At the close of the time period set for the action plan, the stakeholders meet to answer the following questions: Did Susan's reading comprehension scores increase, her behavior improve, and her completion of work increase? What part of the action plan worked and should be enlarged on or replicated? If no progress was made, what strategies of the action plan did not work and need to be adjusted slightly, altered significantly, or discarded? These are the questions that the consultees and all the stakeholders wrestle with during the debriefing stage. This is the time to look at the data (reading scores) to see if progress is being made and to reanalyze and refocus. A consultant who checks her or his progress by looking at the baseline data and impact data is a consultant who does not have to guess if the strategies she or he is suggesting and helping to implement have any value to the student. In the case of Susan, her reading scores have gone up 14 percentile points. She scored at the 28th percentile in reading comprehension by the end of the school year. All the hard work of the consultants is paying off! It is the savvy consultant who knows where they are (baseline data), where they are going (strategies), and if they ever got there (impact data) (MacGregor, 2004). Restate the baseline data. Where are the data after the action plan? Did the strategies have a positive impact on the data? Yes, Susan's baseline data was 14 percentile and her data after action plan was 28 percentile.

This consultation work also resulted in systemic changes in three policies:

1. Food is now available in the cafeteria for late arrivals.
2. The tardy policy changed so that students' re-admittance did not depend on waiting in lines.
3. The criteria for admissions into special programs and tutoring programs changed so that students who need the most help can get it.

## RESPONSE TO INTERVENTION AND SPECIAL EDUCATION (SE)

The work that has been happening with Susan is basically a detailed chronology of **Response to Intervention** (RtI). Response to Intervention is an "all" education initiative that requires educators use data to create behavioral interventions and academic instructional strategies. Essentially, educators must make data-driven decisions to provide high-quality instruction for all students. This concept is not new to the profession of school counseling as the ASCA National Model states school counselors maintain accountability for their work and make connections to student achievement. Another important aspect of RtI is that it moves away from "wait to fail" situations in which students do not receive services until they are unsuccessful either behaviorally or academically. RtI also shifts from the discrepancy model that historically looks at the child as having the problem. Instead, RtI frames student issues as the problem for educators to resolve by examining such factors as curriculum, instruction, and school environment and how they interact with the learner (S. Parikh, personal communication, August 12, 2010).

Clearly, RtI is a systemic and data-driven process that is collaborative in nature. All professionals in school settings such as administrators, curriculum specialists, school counselors, teachers, school psychologists, and social workers have a unique level of expertise. As such, these professionals must come together, build a consultative atmosphere, and use data to make decisions about learning and behavior in their school setting. These decisions include agreeing on strong core instruction, identifying and allocating appropriate resources, and identifying students who need additional instruction and support through Tier 2 and Tier 3 interventions (S. Parikh, personal communication, August 12, 2010).

What if RtI was not enough and Susan was in danger of repeating for the third time? It may be time to consider a special education placement under Public Law 94-142. In 1975 Public Law (PL) 94-142 was passed (renamed to Individual with Disabilities Education Act or IDEIA) and resulted in many students who had disabilities receiving educational support. Under the provisions of IDEIA, regular education teachers are responsible for teaching SE students mainstreamed into their classroom and are entitled to receive additional help (Alexander & Alexander, 2010). The school counselor as consultant can be one of the contributors to the support team for regular education teachers who have SE students.

There are some students whose behavior challenges the normal solutions to behavioral problems. In 1997, IDEA was amended to include the use of functional behavior assessments to develop intervention plans for the behavior problems that prevented students from learning. Functional behavior assessment is a problem-solving process that uses a variety of techniques and strategies to help the Individualized Education Plan team identify social, affective, cognitive, and environmental behavior and use the assessment results to develop an intervention plan. The intervention plan must address short-term prevention, teaching of alternative skills, responses to problem behaviors, and long-term prevention (Dettmer, Thurston, & Dyck, 2005; Truscott, Cohen, Sams, Sanborn, & Frank, 2005).

"Amendments to IDEA in 2004 rendered another name change, this time inserting 'Improvement' making the exact appellation, Individuals with Disabilities Education Improvement Act (IDEIA), signed into law by George W. Bush on December 3, 2004.... Overall the new statute refines the 1997 version, but leaves the body of law in place. The new law coordinates more closely with No Child Left Behind (NCLB), allocates funds to stimulate schools districts to provide special education services for eligible children in clerical and other private schools, changes eligibility definitions for children with learning disabilities, modifies dispute resolution procedures, and prescribes more refined, and possibly harsher, disciplinary rules for children with disabilities, but yet forecloses complete exclusion from public schools" (Alexander & Alexandar, 2009, p. 570). IDEIA has tremendously increased services for needy children; however, the downside is that large numbers of students are being placed in SE who with appropriate interventions could be successful in the regular education classroom. A benefit to effective collaboration is a reduction in referrals for SE. When effective consultation is in place to help teachers with appropriate interventions and strategies, then SE referrals can be reduced. Hopefully in all but the most severe cases, SE will be considered only after a serious action plan, such as the one described for Susan, has been put into place to try to help the student be successful in the regular education program. "It follows that ancillary personnel, such as those engaged in consultative responsibilities, should not search for intrachild deficits and treat them somewhere else but find ways of modifying and improving the regular program to enhance educational opportunities for these students" (Kampwirth, 2006, p. 28).

The consultation role in SE referrals has taken a giant step forward with the advent of the pre-referral team (Lane, Mahdavi, & Borthwick-Duffy, 2003; McEachern, 2003; Ormsbee, 2001; Truscott, Cohen, Sanborn, & Frank, 2005). Many states and school districts are now requiring Pre-referral Teams or Student Support Teams that provide consultation and collaboration regarding a student's problem for the purpose of eliminating over identification of students into SE and to ensure that when a student is referred for SE, the referral is an appropriate one (Leinbaugh, 2010). Pre-referral team members discuss a student's academic, personal, and social/emotional needs and pose strategies, deliver interventions, and establish timelines to try to address the problem in the regular education program, or if the problem is such that more intensive services are needed then a direct referral for SE testing may be made.

## PARENT EDUCATION

In addition to parent consultation, school counselors educate parents by providing training opportunities, programs, and materials. Parent education can take many forms such as workshops, trainings, written material, or one-on-one interactions via a phone call or meeting. Parent education, designed by a school counselor, has the purpose of helping parents achieve better parent-child communication, teach useful information that parents need to support and work with their child on academic issues, and/or to strengthen the home/school partnership. In a school setting, parent education is usually directed toward helping parents change specific behaviors in their child that are interfering with the educational process such as acting out behavior but can also include general information in how to help your child prepare for tests. Education can take a formal approach such as providing a predetermined number of sessions on specific topics, e.g., "Helping Your Child Prepare for Postsecondary Education" or newsletters or a more informal approach in working with parents as a topic emerges.

Parent education programs have been around for a number of years, and many have continued to exist. Parent Effectiveness Training (PET; Gordon, 1977) and Systematic Training for Effective Parenting (STEP; Dinkmeyer, McKay, & Dinkmeyer, 1997; Dinkmeyer & Carlson, 2006) are two popular programs that have longevity and attempt to help parents understand child development and behavior management. The intent of these programs is to help parents learn about motivation for behavior, reinforcers, and how to reward and extinguish certain behaviors. Other resources frequently used by school counselors are CICC—Center for the Improvement of Child Caring (www.ciccparenting.org) and Parent Project (www.parentproject.com).

Research results are mixed on the effectiveness of parent education programs, but research results on parent education and training programs that have a behavior modification component have received the greatest amount of attention and positive results (Fitch & Marshall, 2004; Friend & Cook, 2009; Kaiser & Hancock, 2003).

## TECH TOOLS

- Consider developing an electronic self-help library with links that will take parents and students to websites that inform them about specific issues.
- Using word processing (or a spreadsheet program if you are more technologically astute), develop a directory of all agencies, their phone numbers, and the services they offer for specific problems found in children and adolescents. Have this information printed and distributed in administrators' offices, the front office, etc. and through word processing you can easily update regularly.
- Find and publicize databases such as PubMed (www.ncbi.nlm.nih.gov/pubmed/) that can help parents with information on attention deficit hyperactivity disorder, school phobia, and other health issues.
- Technology can help parents link with other parents through focus groups, support groups, and/or learning teams. Provide information for parents in the form of websites and chat rooms.
- Use technology to help you improve communication. For example, send home the letters of concern, letters of praise, etc., more easily by developing a bank of letters that are appropriate for the different grade levels in your school. These letters can then be stored electronically, retrieved, and personalized.
- Provide teachers with a bank of letters and written approaches, such as templates for newsletters to keep parents informed. Paraprofessionals can tailor letters to the grade level or situation. For example, if you have letters congratulating the eighth graders on being on the honor roll, paraprofessionals can easily personalize the letters.
- Deliver PowerPoint presentations to teachers on effective consultation skills, parent-teacher conferences, and topics about special needs children.

---

## *School Counselor Casebook: Voices from the Field*

### The Scenario Reviewed

After the first nine weeks of middle school, Ms. Lawrence tells you that Susan has not completed any homework or in-class assignments since the school year began. The teacher tells you she has tried everything and is now requesting the paperwork to start the special education process with this student in hopes she can be placed before Christmas.

What should you do?

*(continues)*

### A Practitioner's Approach

Here's how a practicing school counselor responded to this school scenario:

We have been using RtI (Response to Intervention) for several years and the teachers know that documentation is required of one or more strategies that they have tried with a student before requesting forms to start the process that would lead to a special education referral. In my role as a consultant, I know how important it is for all of us to share our expertise and knowledge when working with Susan. I respect the expertise of teachers and parents to help guide the process. I would begin by scheduling a time when the teacher and I can sit uninterrupted for at least 30 minutes to share what she has observed and already tried to motivate Susan to complete assignments. I am especially interested in what if any parental involvement has taken place already and if there is any feedback from other teachers who have worked with Susan. If there has not been a teacher/parent conference I would offer to help such as organizing and/or attending the conference.

It is important during our discussion that the teacher feels confident that I am here to assist her and help her identify strategies, intervention, and support that Susan may need to help her with class assignments and homework. I would take notes and try to assist the teacher in focusing on one or two strategies to try. I would also offer to observe the student in one or more classroom settings.

As Susan's counselor, I need to meet with her to see if I can figure out the underlying issues that are related to her school work. In my consultation role, I may need to also meet with her parent(s) and Susan to talk about what is holding her back from completing class work and homework.

Once the teacher and parents and I have made a plan we will schedule a follow-up conference within two weeks to see if our efforts are making a difference. Then we can reevaluate our efforts and determine what we will need to do next, and that may involve consulting with the other professionals who work with Susan.

Lynn Haldaman
Counselor
Sweet Apple Elementary
Roswell, GA

## LOOKING BACK: SALIENT POINTS

### Consultation in the Schools

Consultation bring "experts" together, be they a teacher, parent, or community-based professional, to bring their collective knowledge to bear on resolving a situation for an individual child or group of children.

## The School Counselor as Consultant

Consultation extends the school counselor's reach by working collaboratively with the adults in a student's life who can make a major impact on a student's academic, career, and social/emotional life. The consultation role is becoming more and more important because consultation is effective and efficient in removing obstacles in implementing a standards-based educational system in challenging low expectations and in promoting access and success in rigorous academics.

Consultation follows the rule of parsimony because with each successful consultation you are helping a teacher, parent, or other adult gain the knowledge that they can use with other students in the years to come. In a successful consultation scenario, both the teacher and counselor are learning intervention strategies for application to future problems; ideas germinate into plans that spill over to benefit more people.

## Teachers, Parents, and the System as Consultees

Your consultees will include many people, agencies, and institutions but your primary consultees will include teachers, parents, and the system—meaning the school district and your individual school. Student outcomes of educational consultation are likely to be more successful when there is an effective parent-educator partnership. It is easier for counselors to concentrate on individual student needs and not to look at the system, but systemic consultation affects many more lives.

Consultation as a problem-solving process sometimes involving an expert helping give knowledge and skills to a consultee. The definition this textbook promotes is that of collaborative consultation or shared responsibility with regard to decisions and outcomes and relies on maintaining an equal partnership between all parties involved.

## Teachers as Consultees

Teachers as consultees vary widely in skills and confidence with some needing little support while others place unrealistic demands on the consultant to own the problem and fix it. Skillful consultants must be able to work with all teachers on the continuum and relationship building considerably facilitates the consultant's role. PREPARE is an acronym for Philosophy, Relationships, Equity of power, Professional development, Accessible, Resources, Evaluate—key elements of effective consultation with teachers.

## Parents as Consultees

Parental involvement yields positive effects on student achievement. When parents are involved, we know that students show improvement in all areas of academic and social achievement. PARTNER is an acronym for effective conferences with parents. PARTNER stands for Planning for success, Acknowledging parents, Rapport building, Teaming, Negotiate a plan of action, End effectively, and Regrouping. The school counselor as consultant has a wonderful opportunity to provide staff development to teachers and other educators about effective communication with parents and tips for conducting parent conferences and managing parent visits.

## The Four Ds of the Action Plan

Data Gathering, Devising an Action Plan, Delivering the Action Plan, and Debriefing are the four steps in the consultation process. After collecting the facts and beginning to get enough information to determine the student's need, then the consultant and consultees will start Devising an action plan. Delivering the action plan will require all stakeholders to set timelines and strategies that they will be implementing. The final step is the Debriefing. This is the time to determine if the action plan was effective and what revisions, if any, are necessary.

There are 11 basic approaches to gathering information: educational record review, interviewing the teacher, interviewing the parent, interviewing other educators, interviewing the student, interviewing other helping professionals, student observation, systems observation, educational assessment, medical information, and psychological assessment.

Data collection helps participants in the consultation process make better decisions by accurately identifying the problem and narrowing the focus of the interventions so that the resources and energy brought to the table are really addressing the critical issues.

## KEY TERMS

Consultation p. 355

Triadic-dependent model p. 356

Collaborative consultation p. 356

Unalterable factors p. 357

Rule of parsimony p. 358

Internal consultees p. 359

External consultee p. 359

PREPARE p. 361

Equity of power p. 361

Positive self-talk p. 363

Egalitarianism p. 363

PARTNER p. 366

Response to Intervention p. 380

## LEARNING EXTENSIONS/MAKING CONNECTIONS

1. Using the power types described in Chapter 4, i.e., (a) Position Power or Jurisdictional Power; (b) Referent Power or Relationship Power; (c) Caring Power; (d) Transformational Power or Developmental Power; (e) Connection Power; (f) Reward Power; and (g) Technical, Information, or Expert Power, apply each of these power types to ways they can be used in the consultation process and discuss the benefits of each.

2. Dinkmeyer and Carlson (2006) provide a unique standpoint describing the collaborative nature of consultation. While others speak of the expert role of a consultant, Dinkmeyer and Carlson discuss a shared responsibility to decisions and outcomes. Consider the continuum of consultation with *expertise* on one end of the continuum and Dinkmeyer and Carlson's *collaborative problem solving idea* at the other end. Where are you on the continuum? Do you

believe you tend toward needing to be an expert in behavioral issues or do you lean toward the collaborative problem-solving approach? Discuss the merits of your position on the continuum in relation to your role as an effective consultant.

3. The author's definition of *consultation* stresses a partnership. Consultation is a partnership that the school counselor enters into with other adults in the internal or external school community for the express purpose of collaborative problem solving and supporting the implementation of strategies designed to increase a student's opportunity to be a successful learner. Rewrite the definition in an attempt to add your own opinion about the definition of *consultation*. Defend the merits of your definition.

4. PARTNER is an acronym for **P**lanning, **A**cknowledging, **R**apport building, **T**eaming, **N**egotiating, **E**nding, **R**egrouping. Consider the last time you worked with another adult in any consultation capacity. This occasion could have been a consultation outside the realm of an educational setting such as problem solving with a friend about how to lose weight or it may have been a complicated consultation about a student in a school who was underachieving. Think back to your role as consultant and take one of the areas above and describe how you behaved in this real consultation and what you would do differently as a result of reading about the PARTNER process.

5. Debate with your classmates your opinion of the merits of the following recommendation: "Dress professionally but in a way that will help parents identify with you. This approach may require professional dress that is more understated. When practicing as an elementary school counselor, our Child Study Team meetings were fashion shows with each person wearing and commenting on everyone's designer clothes and tons of gold jewelry."

6. Revisit Data gathering and the 11 basic approaches to gathering information. Contact a school counselor and discuss with her or him your willingness to assist in gathering information regarding a student in need. In collaboration with the counselor, implement three of the nine data-gathering areas and deliver the information you glean to the teacher, parents, and/or counselor. Be certain to get written permission from the child's parents before you start gathering information.

7. Develop and deliver a PowerPoint presentation to the faculty on effective parent conferences. The presentation should be 8 to 10 minutes long. Create a written feedback form so that you can grow your presentation effectiveness.

## CHAPTER 13

# School Counselors as Coordinators, Collaborators, and Managers of Resources

## CHAPTER OBJECTIVES

*By the time you have completed this chapter, you should be able to*

- explain the role of the school counselor in coordinating a school counseling program;

- discuss the benefits, barriers, and limitations of collaborating and partnering for student success;

- describe the skills needed to collaborate and partner;

- describe the benefits, barriers, and limitations of managing resources to deliver services to students;

- take a problem that affects student academic success and delineate strategies you would use to bring support and resolution to the problem through coordination, collaboration, partnering, and managing resources;

- explain the power of technology to considerably enhance your school counseling program.

---

## *School Counselor Casebook: Getting Started*

### The Scenario

For the second consecutive year your school has been placed on the Critically Low Performing Schools list, which means that if test scores do not improve over the next two years, the state will take over the school. You believe that as a member of the leadership team, instructional success and student achievement are as much your job as that of the principal, teachers, and other critical stakeholders. Your principal does not assign you extraneous duties and you have a solid and meaningful comprehensive, developmental school counseling program that is already supporting the achievement of students, yet, like everyone else in the school, you feel pressure of a pending state takeover. You want to extend your reach to support more students' academic success, but your day is already packed with important tasks that you do not want to relinquish.

### Thinking about Solutions

As you read this chapter, think about how you might extend your reach to support more students' academic success without relinquishing the important functions you already perform. When you come to the end of the chapter, you will have the opportunity to see how your ideas compare with a practicing school counselor's approach.

# COORDINATION, COLLABORATION, AND MANAGEMENT OF RESOURCES

*Coordination of services*, *collaboration*, and **management of resources**—three terms that are used interchangeably—are the mechanics or the "how" in delivering a school counseling program. In practice these three terms have unique aspects. The distinctiveness of coordination, collaboration, and managing resources as well as their interlocking components all work to the advantage of the school counseling program. The common denominator of the three is the power they have to extend the influence of the school counseling program to enhance the personal and academic success of each student in their charge. Coordination of school counseling means prioritizing, organizing, and delivering the components of the program such as individual/group counseling, classroom guidance lessons, consultation services, career and academic advising, and systemic support. Collaboration is a process of partnering and teaming with other educators, individuals, and groups of the internal community (the school site) and the external community (outside the school site) to deliver the components of the school counseling program. Working collaboratively with the administration, teaching, community, and agency programs in overarching, interlocking commonalities strengthens the impact of the school counseling program by collectively focusing on common goals. Managing resources is extending the school counselor program beyond what just the counselor could do by bringing in human and material resources such as parents, students, teachers, administrators, community members, business partners, and technology. Resource management requires minimal or no additional funds to add support and redistribute some of the duties of the school counseling program.

> A teacher stood in front of his group of high-powered, overachieving students and said, "Okay, time for a quiz." He pulled out a one-gallon, wide-mouth jar and a dozen fist-sized rocks that he carefully placed into the jar. When no more rocks would fit inside, he asked, "Is this jar full?" Everyone in the class said, "Yes." He reached under the table and pulled out a bucket of gravel. Then he dumped some gravel in and shook the jar, causing pieces of gravel to work themselves down into the space between the big rocks. Then he asked the group once more, "Is the jar full?" By this time the students were on to him. "Probably not," one student answered. "Good!" he replied. He reached under the table and brought out a bucket of sand and poured it, filling up spaces left between the rocks and the gravel. Once more he asked the question, "Is this jar full?" "No!" the class shouted. Then he grabbed a pitcher of water and began to pour it until the jar was filled to the brim. Then he looked at the class and asked, "What is the point of this illustration?" One student replied, "The point is, no matter how full your schedule is, if you try really hard you can always fit more things in it!" "No," the speaker replied, "the point is if you don't put the big rocks in first, you'll never get them in at all." (adapted from Covey, 1990)

What are the "big rocks" in your school counseling program? The big rocks are the components of your school counseling program that need to be in place before everything else spills over into the school counseling office. Once these important rocks or components are firmly anchored, when the flood of "other duties as designated" comes your way, you have a solid framework in place and you can better protect your time and program. Your role as **coordinator** requires that you determine the components of your program or the big rocks and then collaborate with others to fulfill an optimum educational opportunity for students. Managing resources allows for an extended reach.

Through coordination, collaboration, and managing resources, school counselors are able to deliver a comprehensive program that reaches beyond the "top" 5 percent and the most "at-risk" 5 percent to 100 percent of the students or every student in the school. Now we have a high-profile, powerful school counseling program. The "jar" in your program is full and heavy. You can lug this jar around, losing water, sand, and gravel as contents spill, and you do damage control or you can be proactive by having a program with set components and collaborating and brokering resources to see the components fulfilled.

## Coordination

Coordination of services means prioritizing, organizing, and delivering the components of the school counseling program, e.g., individual/group counseling, classroom guidance lessons, consultation services, career and academic advising, and systemic support, so that you increase the likelihood that the program will successfully affect the personal/social, career, and academic outcomes of every student in the school (Galassi & Akos, 2007; Gysbers & Henderson, 2006; Kerr & Dahir, 2007; Martin & Robinson, 2011; Moore-Thomas, 2010). In the coordination role the school counselor sets short-term targets and long-term goals. The school counselor as coordinator determines the goals of the school counseling program and identifies the mechanisms and resources needed to carry out those goals. The coordinator role of school counseling requires putting into place a program that reaches each student through both direct service delivery and, more importantly, indirect service delivery through the brokering of resources. The coordination role has become one of the most important roles a school counselor can perfect (Bryan & Holcomb-McCoy, 2004; Galassi & Akos, 2007; Staley & Carey, 1997). "Inherent in the provision of a full range of counseling services is the understanding that professional school counselors are pivotal to but not the sole service providers of a school counseling program. Comprehensive developmental school counseling services are most effectively offered through a team approach. Professional school counselors work in consultation and collaboration with guidance advisory committees; school staff (including teachers, resource teachers, principals, school psychologists and social workers, pupil personnel workers, nurse, secretaries, building services workers, and instructional assistants); parents, grand-parents, and guardians; and community stakeholders" (Moore-Thomas, 2010, p. 201).

School counselors will more and more come to rely on the expertise and services of others to deliver optimum programs. You will become much more familiar with the four components of the comprehensive school counseling program in Chapter 8 that addresses the ASCA National Standards (1997b) and the ASCA National Model (2005).

a. Guidance Curriculum (e.g., structured groups, classroom guidance);
b. Individual Planning with Students (e.g., advising, assessment, placement, academic, career and personal-social goal setting, and follow-up);
c. Responsive Services (e.g., individual and group counseling, consultation, and referral); and
d. System Support (e.g., program management, coordination of services, community outreach, and public relations) (ASCA, 2005; Erford, 2011c; Gysbers & Henderson, 2006; Stone & Dahir, 2011).

This chapter focuses on one of the four components, System Support. Begin your systems support role by answering these questions.

"Are the goals of the school counseling program aligned with the mission of the school?"

"What will be the priorities of the school counseling program for the year?"

"What data set(s) (see Chapter 8) will the school counselor collaborate to move in a positive direction?"

"Who in the internal and external community is working toward the same goals as that of the school counseling program?"

"Which components of my school counseling program must I deliver and which can I broker resources so that others can help me?"

"How can the school counseling program intersect with the other programs and resources to collaborate and partner to meet these goals?"

## Setting Priorities

There will never be enough school counselors to meet all the needs of students; furthermore, counselors must work within the limits of time, resources, and their abilities (Gysbers & Henderson, 2006; Myrick, 2003b). With too many demands on their time, school counselors establish priorities by first identifying the guidance needs of the school. This can be accomplished by speaking with administrators and teachers to assess what they believe to be the pressing issues affecting students. Students and teachers can participate in establishing needs by responding to a questionnaire and giving their perspectives on schoolwide problems, areas of concern, their needs, etc. (Bartlett, 2010; Erford, 2011a; Myrick, 2003a; Schellenberg, 2008). The school counseling program advisory committee may also be helpful in setting priorities (Myrick, 2003a). "Advisory councils provide a mechanism for input, feedback, and evaluation of the school counseling program's activities for a wide range of individuals. The community advisory council, also known as the school counseling program advisory committee (SCPAC), serves as a sounding board and steering committee" (Erford, 2011c, p. 52). "The advisory committee, sometimes called the group advisory team or advisory board, is composed of representatives of the stakeholders in the school—individuals in the school and community who are committed to the success of the school and students" (Bartlett, 2010, p. 212).

The PTA can survey parents and report their findings back to the school counseling program advisory committee. State and community reports may also shed some light on issues being faced by students such as a rising drug problem or an increase in school violence (Fusco, 2009; Myrick, 2003a). However, critically important to determining the priorities of your program should be needs of your school as determined by the gaps and glaring problems revealed by the school report card data (Erford, 2011a; Stone & Dahir, 2011).

## Time Management

Time management is an important aspect of priority setting (Erford, 2011c; Myrick, 2003a). One way to prioritize time and energy is to decide how much time you will spend with different types of interventions. For example, you may decide that you will only do small groups for 10 sessions per week or two sessions per day. By scheduling time for each of your interventions, you are better able to achieve a balanced program. Develop a weekly schedule broken down into blocks of time and display the times that you are available and the times that you have interventions scheduled.

# GETTING ORGANIZED

In organizing the school counseling program, four phases are suggested: (1) planning, (2) designing, (3) implementing, and (4) evaluating (Gysbers & Henderson, 2006).

## Planning

In the planning phase, desired student outcomes have been identified and the current school program has been scrutinized to determine what can be kept and what needs to change. Program goals are set in the planning phase based on the needs identified under the preceding setting priorities section. School counseling programs in the past have rarely utilized student information data to try to establish their program's goals (Dimmitt, Carey, & Hatch, 2007; Erford & McCaskill, 2010; Stone & Dahir, 2011). It is the school counselor of the 21st century that starts setting program goals by looking at the academic data for her or his students and asking questions such as, "Where are students' deficits? Who is being left out of the academic success picture?" (Bartlett, 2010; Stone & Dahir, 2011). School counselors who start their program goals by looking at the identified needs of their students through hard data and not just **needs assessments** will avoid running down rabbit trails and implementing services that are not needed and do not make a difference in students' lives (Bartlett, 2010; Stone & Dahir, 2011). Data tell you where your students are, where you need to help them go, and if your program's strategies helped you realize your goals (Dimmitt, Carey, & Hatch, 2007; Erford, 2011a, 2011c; Erford & McCaskill, 2010; Lapan, 2001; MacGregor, 2004).

## Designing

Once planning and priorities have been set, the designing phase is the focus in which the strategies needed to achieve the goals of the school counseling program are identified (see Chapter 9 on accountability). Then the components of the program should be assigned and school personnel should be assessed for their abilities (Gysbers & Henderson, 2006). Erford (2011c) states that all school personnel should be included to accomplish program goals. "It is important to emphasize that the counselor is but one player in a team effort. Without collaborative partnerships with other school personnel and community agencies, it is quite likely that a professional school counselor trying to stand alone will fall flat on her or his face" (Erford, 2011c, p. 55). The final task in the designing phase is to provide staff development, to inform them of the changes and new goals of the school counseling program.

### Implement and Evaluate

The counselor starts to implement the program and then evaluate the program to see if the program is an accountable, data-driven school counseling program. The school counselor must collect data on the efficacy of program components (Dimmitt, Carey, & Hatch, 2007; Gysbers & Henderson, 2006; Johnson & Johnson, 2001; Stone & Dahir, 2011). The data must then be analyzed and a report should be prepared to have a better idea of how the program contributed to desired student outcomes. Chapter 8 provides considerable detail on evaluating the effectiveness of the school counseling program.

## COLLABORATION AND MANAGEMENT OF RESOURCES

You stand staring at a stack of 450 educational records, each representing a student in your case load who has career, academic, personal, and social needs. How do you get your arms literally and figuratively around all these students to close the gaps in their information, to support their social development, and to widen their opportunities to fully participate in the U.S. economy? Stiffer standards, shrinking education dollars, and increased social stresses demand that educators, especially school counselors who have always had demanding student/counselor ratios, collaborate with each other to optimally prepare students. Linkages in and among administrators, teachers, businesses, and community agencies, properly initiated and carefully nurtured, will improve school counseling programs and promote student success (Bartlett, 2010; Bryan & Henry, 2008; Griffin & Farris, 2010; Herr, 2001; Martin, 2004; Miller, 2006; Muller-Ackerman & Shelton, 2006; Schellenberg, 2008; Schmidt, 2007; Stone & Clark, 2001).

### Collaboration

"Schools and school counselors cannot function alone to meet the needs of all students, and student success depends on collaborating with other stakeholders" (Griffin & Farris, 2010, p. 253). Requirements for effective collaboration begin with a sincere need to make collaboration work, a commitment to the time and energy required to develop relationships, articulated common goals, and supportive key players who can smooth the way such as principals and assistant principals for curriculum. Effective collaboration requires a willingness to share credit, blame, rewards, and penalties. Fairly healthy organizations are invaluable.

In a climate for collaboration, the leadership provides mechanisms for collaboration such as site-based teams and shared decision-making teams (Doyle, 2004; Holcomb, 2009).

Communication and problem solving among individuals are critical as they are introduced to new ways of doing things (Doyle, 2004; Edwards, 1994; Schellenberg, 2008). School counselors usually have an advantage in collaboration as they generally have a facilitative leadership style, good communication skills, an understanding of the nature and function of schools, and the "sink or swim" imperative to make collaboration work!

Collaboration is not for the faint of heart; it involves risk, relationship building, personal interaction skills that are above the norm, a spirit of cooperation, leadership ability, mediation skills, a thorough understanding of the nature and function of schools, likability, the ability to think on your feet, flexibility, a willingness to compromise, confidence, and an attitude and sincere belief that you can and will make a difference regardless of the attestations of the naysayers.

## Management of Resources

Implementing outreach efforts to get human, monetary, and technological resources from the internal community and the external community is managing resources. Grabbing and utilizing internal and external community members allows the school counselor to better deliver strategies to enhance student success. "The school counseling program does not belong to the school counselor; it belongs to the stakeholders" (Schellenberg, 2008, p. 15).

School counselor service delivery is widening its impact from a direct service deliverer to a coordinator of resources, from individual focus to a systemic focus, from a small percentage of the population to a program focusing on all students (Karcher, 2009; Schellenberg, 2008; Stone & Hanson, 2002). "New vision school counseling programs meet the needs of the system vs. the needs of the selected few" (Schellenberg, 2008, p. 15). The dilemma that many school counselors face today is how to adequately perform the varied roles teachers, students, and parents demand of them without diluting their effectiveness (Butler & Constantine, 2005; Stone & Hanson, 2002; Wilkerson, 2009). Efficient use of time and resources is a major issue for schools to be able to address increasingly heavy caseloads for counselors. Student service personnel partnering with regular education teachers and parents to collaboratively solve problems can positively affect many more students than direct services allow (Anderson-Butcher & Ashton, 2004; Bryan & Henry, 2008; Dahir & Tyson, 2010; Griffin & Farris, 2010; Myrick, 2003b). "School counselors who feel overwhelmed by the numerous tasks that they already perform may see a partnership approach to school counseling as inapplicable or impossible. A partnership approach to school counseling requires a paradigm shift among school counselors. They must recognize that schools and school counselors cannot create the strengths and assets that children need alone, especially children who face numerous economic and societal struggles. Bridging connections with teachers, school staff, families, and community members allow school counselors to impact children's lives by creating supports and assets that empower them and their families long after they leave the school" (Bryan & Henry, 2008, p. 115).

Beyond reducing student/counselor ratios, what delivery system can meet the needs of so many students? A delivery system is needed that places the school counselor at the hub of managing different stakeholders and resources to help the efforts of the school counseling program. "All stakeholders in the community will have valuable information and opinions to share regarding the direction for the school counseling program" (Bartlett, 2010, p. 215).

This model requires that the school counselor must be comfortable being a leader and motivator to get others to be part of the school counseling program (Galassi & Akos, 2007; Lieberman, 2004). A school counseling program comprised of many resources besides the school counselor is critical if all students (with "all" being defined as every student in the school) are going to be supported by the school counseling program. "Collaboration and consultation with stakeholders, namely school administrators, parents and teachers, are essential to developing a customized school counseling program that meets the unique needs of diverse students and the total school environment" (Schellenberg, 2008, p. 15).

The comprehensive school counseling program that reaches beyond the school counseling office to bring in resources such as parents, students, teachers, technology, school-based administrators, central administration, the larger community, and the business community redistributes duties so that counselors not only provide direct services but also manage other resources and utilize other approaches to get the job done. When the school counselor is the direct deliverer, purveyor, and implementer of all activities, then it is impossible to provide a school counseling program that affects all students. "All" is not possible in an overburdened model where the school counselor protects the school counseling domain as a one-person operation. Educators and others already employed by the school system are primary resources to tap and can be assisted in many ways with minimal or no additional funds (Erford, 2011c; Stone & Hanson, 2002). Outside resources are especially welcome and can be an incredible boost to the school counseling program and student success (Anderson-Butcher & Ashton, 2004; Bryan & Holcomb-McCoy, 2007; Erford, 2011c; Galassi & Akos, 2007; Miller, 2006; Myrick, 2003b).

Resource brokering is an aspect of the school counselor's role that is only limited by the counselor's tenacity, creativity, and initiative. It is the school counselor who can determine the extent and variety of brokering efforts that can increase the resources of the school counseling program. It is impossible to adequately describe all the wonderful, available resources that are out there for the asking.

## CASTT A WIDER NET

*CASTT* is an acronym for community, administrators, students, teachers, and technology. School counselors who have built a high-profile, powerful, resource-rich school counseling program have *CASTT a wider net* by involving community members, administrators, students, teachers, and technology in the daily work of their school counseling programs.

Collaboration is capacity building so that the future work can be redistributed and the school counseling program will cast a wider net in a more efficient manner with minimum duplication of services. The payoff to collaboration and team building is a resource rich program with an increased commitment to the school counseling program.

## CASTT a Wider Net in the Community

External community members such as agencies, businesses, organizations, civic groups, and other community members are feeling the responsibility of helping educators deliver the daunting task of educating our citizenry (Anderson-Butcher & Ashton, 2004; Arriaza, 2004; Moore, 2003; Sanders, 2006). Increasingly, schools are receiving public support in meeting complex demands of an ever-increasing diverse student population. Educators are realizing that it is implausible to meet the needs in isolation of our larger communities (Griffin & Steen, 2010; National Dropout Prevention Center/ Network, 2009; Schellenberg, 2008; Shipman, Queen, & Peel, 2007). Collaboration and partnership building with the community bolsters public faith in our schools but more importantly supports the efforts of educators.

Community volunteers, the greatest untapped resource, can come from churches, postsecondary institutions, the military, businesses, or essentially from all walks of life. Community members can serve individually or collectively on school improvement teams, citizen advisory committees, and/or **neighborhood associations** to affect the likelihood that students will be successful. Discussed here are just a few community resources to partner with your school counseling program: (1) parents; (2) agency members; (3) neighborhood associations and groups; (4) businesses; (5) colleges, universities, and other postsecondary institutions; and (6) alumni.

### *Partnering with Parents*

Parent-teacher associations or individual parents can serve as partners in the school counseling program. A few of the many ways in which parents can volunteer are to sponsor field trips, get students involved in community service,

---

**MEET CINDY FUNKHOUSER: PARENT VOLUNTEER AND FULL PARTNER OF THE SCHOOL COUNSELING PROGRAM**

Cindy Funkhouser, PTA President, was a solid partner to MaryAnn Dyal, school counselor, in the following ways:

1. *Bully-Proofing Program.* Under Cindy's guidance, the PTA assisted mightily in implementing a schoolwide bully-proofing program. Through provision of resources, financial assistance, people power, time and energy, faculty trainings, school counseling lessons, and an essay/ poster contest, this program affected every student, faculty, and staff member.

*(continues)*

2. *Mentoring.* This program was developed for at-risk boys in the fourth grade. Here, Cindy and MaryAnn reached out to a helicopter squadron of the US Navy to provide role models for their at-risk students. The mentors had lunch one day per week with their student over a one-year period. The PTA, under Cindy's leadership, provided lunch for the participants and teachers were included to reinforce the program's goals. The PTA also provided events such as ice-cream sundae parties for the participants. This program partnered not only the PTA but with teachers, students, and business partners as well.

3. *Tutoring.* Cindy and the PTA helped recruit volunteers from the USS *Kennedy* aircraft carrier. This program provided a safety net for those students who were struggling academically.

4. *Parent Fair.* Parents were not attending functions so the PTA provided the financial backing to offer dinner for the whole family before the meeting began as well as entertainment for the children while the parents were attending sessions on parenting skills. Some examples of the entertainment were movies, science experiments, and PE activities. Cindy and the PTA helped the school counselor pull in community agencies to provide valuable information to the parents.

5. *Character Education.* With the urging of the PTA, a business partner purchased a character education program for the school (it was so successful that the company branched out to other schools to provide the program). The business partner provides all the materials each month for the program and Cindy helps coordinate the effort. For example, one month's character theme was "Respect," and the PTA placed a table card at each place in the cafeteria with the word *respect* for each student to take home and place on their own dining room table for a family discussion about respect (adapted from Stone, 2003).

---

serve as mentors and tutors, participate in advisory groups, participate in telephone trees for emergencies, and to advertise school events.

### Partnering with Human Services Agencies

Both public schools and human services are being challenged to rethink and redesign their efforts to educate, socialize, and intervene in the problems of children and their families (Atkins, Graczyk, Frazier, & Abdul-Adil, 2003; Brown, Dahlbeck, & Sparkman-Barns, 2006; Griffin & Steen, 2010; Peebles-Wilkins, 2003; Schellenberg, 2008). "The current state of our society and, thus, our schools compels us to continually improve the way we educate all students, particularly those who could benefit from additional support and resources to meet their needs and help them become academically successful" (Griffin & Steen, 2010, p. 218). School counselors and other members of the human service profession are searching for increased coordination and collaboration among disciplines to better serve students and their families (Brown, Dahlbeck, & Sparkman-Barns, 2006; Simcox, Nuijens, & Lee, 2006). "This is in contrast to the past when these professionals worked in isolation on compartmentalized functions that emphasized their respective expertise" (Simcox, Nuijens, & Lee, 2006, p. 273). Many proponents of these changes point out that schools are a natural place for human services activities because they provide maximum access to the majority of children and families (Allen-Meares et al. 2009).

School counselors can tap community agencies to work in the schools as part of an outreach effort. For example, full-service schools take the agencies that serve the school community and move those resources onto the school grounds. This approach helps more students through easy access but the biggest payoff is the collaboration between agencies and educators who are in a position to see the daily struggles of the student. Bringing agencies into the school facilitates the examination of the multiple and interrelated etiologies of children's problems and reduces isolated treatment of the family situation; medical concerns, academic achievement, and emotional health can be addressed in isolation. Even without full-service schools, counseling agencies can be repositioned onto the school campus. Seeking alternative ways of delivering family and individual counseling services is especially important given the counselor-to-student ratios, complex psychological issues, and the amount of contact hours needed by families. Agencies that can help provide counseling services to students will be a tremendous boost to the school counseling program as, out of necessity, this area usually catches a small percentage of the school population.

> A community school (also called full service schools) is both a place and a set of partnerships between the school and other community resources. Its integrated focus on academics, health and social services, youth and community development and community engagement leads to improved student learning, stronger families and healthier communities. Schools become centers of the community and are open to everyone—all day, every day, evenings and weekends. Using public schools as hubs, community schools or full service school bring together many partners to offer a range of supports and opportunities to children, youth, families and communities. (Coalition for Community Schools, 2010, para. 1–2)

School counselors, social workers, school nurses, and other student support service providers can provide the nucleus around which a collaborative service delivery system can be built to help children and their families. The complexities and relatedness of student issues reinforce the need for school counselors to partner with agencies in an interdisciplinary manner (Anderson-Butcher & Ashton, 2004; Griffin & Steen, 2010; Gysbers & Henderson, 2006).

### Partnering with Neighborhood Associations and Groups

Neighborhood associations are generally interested in education, housing, recreation, and community improvements. These groups offer another community resource as they have a vested interest in making certain the schools of the neighborhood survive and thrive (Langhout, Rappaport, & Simmons, 2002; Vigoda, 2002).

Community asset mapping consists of three levels: (1) gifts, skills, and capacities of individuals living within the community; (2) citizen associations through which local people come together to pursue common goals; and (3) institutions present in the community such as businesses, local government, hospitals, education, and human service agencies (University of Missouri, n.d.). Within these three levels, local people and organizations are encouraged to explore how problems might be interrelated, and to respond to pressing issues in a coordinated, collaborative fashion (Griffin & Farris, 2010, p. 249).

Often real estate prices are tied to the success rate of schools and here is a group just waiting for the asking to come in and help with student needs. Even informal neighborhood groups can be an asset. Recently administrators in El Paso, Texas, related a story about a principal who stopped the nightly graffiti spraying of his school walls. This smart principal started to talk to the gang members who came to the school in the evenings to play basketball. In working with the gang members he learned that they could and would protect the school if they were allowed to play basketball later into the night. Gangs do not usually have the distinction of being neighborhood associations but they can be more powerful than a formal group. The point is that that all neighborhood groups, including those we generally feel are disenfranchised, can bring support to the school (H. Lopez, personal communication, September 12, 2004).

### Partnering with Businesses

School counselors can usually cite numerous ways business partners have helped the school with person power and financial backing. Start tapping into this resource to support elements of your program that will lend themselves to business support such as having businesses provide mentors and tutors, securing funding for T-shirts for the most improved citizens, and getting restaurants to provide food for your parent fair. There are endless opportunities for businesses to be part of the school counseling program.

### Partnering with Colleges, Universities, and Other Postsecondary Institutions

Counselor educators, particularly those who teach the school counseling and career courses, can provide school counseling or mental health counseling candidates for brief experiences, practicum, or for full-time internships. Ask counselor educators to deliver professional development to programs for your school or for the school district. Counselor educators can be involved in your school counseling program in research projects such as measuring the impact that your program or particular service delivery has on student outcomes. Consider asking to be a professional development school or a place where counseling candidates are prepared.

### Partnering with Alumni

Universities have long courted alumni as a resource for economic support and status. Secondary education has not tapped this resource as a gold mine of potential volunteers. Many times alumni feel a sentimental attachment to the school and would like to be asked to contribute to their former institution. When you take a position as a school counselor, why not invite alumni to participate in a school counseling program event? For example, alumni probably represent many varied professions and you could invite them to present at your career fair. You may find allies who have talents and interests they want to lend to your program; former students who are mental health therapists, graphic artists, costume designers, writers, firefighters, professional athletes, politicians, or photographers. By grooming a relationship with alumni the possibilities of benefiting from their time and talents are endless. To get your alumni involved, take some lessons from higher education who feature graduates in their newsletters, name buildings after them, honor their achievements, and have annual alumni events. When you are trying to find people who will bring a real commitment and sense of responsibility to the school counseling program, look for alumni.

## CASTT a Wider Net with Administrators

Collaborating with administrators can strengthen the leadership team of the school. Counselors and administrators evolved from strikingly different origins but are practically indispensable to each other in a necessary partnership representing contiguous services for students (Connolly & Protheroe, 2009; Schellenberg, 2008). The relationship between counselor and administrator has long been recognized as a marriage needed to meet the needs of students (Connolly & Protheroe, 2009; Schellenberg, 2008). When school counselors view themselves as a partner on the leadership team, their credibility, visibility, and power to effect change is strengthened and the principal has another set of eyes and ears helping her or him affect student success.

Partnering with administrators is powerful. Counselors and administrators no longer think of administration as unconnected to the school counselors' work; rather, counselors and administrators are inseparable partners. "The relationship between counselor and administrator can enhance or exhaust a school's ability to meet the needs of its students. We are married in a tight, necessary partnership representing contiguous services for our students. As in a good marriage, we need to think of ourselves as both individuals and a single unit. Our positions may have evolved from strikingly different origins, but at present, we are practically indispensable to each other" (Wesley, 2001, p. 60). "School principals and school counselors have something in common: both want to see students succeed. And although their individual roles and responsibilities are very different, both principals and counselors face difficulties and challenges in their efforts to improve student outcomes within the school. When principals and counselors can work effectively together, their efforts stand a far better chance of making a difference and helping all students succeed" (Finkelstein, 2009, p. 2).

Counselor/Administrator partnership activities include the following:

- supporting the school counseling program in spirit and in funding and personnel support;
- keeping each other informed, e.g., forewarning about a phone call from an angry parent or consulting and debriefing on a change in policy;

- sharing critical data elements needed to develop a data-driven school counseling program and highlighting the successes of the school counseling program;
- providing input on evolving district policy;
- Supporting a school climate conducive to success;
- working together to support classroom management programs and alternatives to ineffective discipline;
- sharing the burden of crisis intervention so that the counselor can count on delivering a program that reaches beyond crisis intervention to program implementation;
- building confidence that comes from a commitment to one another.

## CASTT a Wider Net with Students

Students can be an extension of your school counseling program, serving as allies for students who are being bullied, sounding boards for students who need another peer to talk to about personal issues, and can bring talent and skills to serve as tutors, mentors, mediators, aides, speakers, and developers of materials. Students are accessible, willing, and can sometimes be instrumental in influencing their peers when adults cannot.

Peer helpers or **peer facilitators** are defined as students who assist other students in exploring ideas or feelings about a situation, look for alternatives, and make responsible decisions (Barton, 2009). The terms *peer helper*, *peer facilitator*, *peer mediator*, *peer tutor*, and *peer supporters* often are used interchangeably. Students can learn to be peer facilitators by learning basic skills to help others with academic and personal issues. Those who participate in comprehensive peer facilitator programs will be especially helpful in their interactions with others. Peers can have quite an impact on preventing social problems and can help other students gain positive experiences from school.

**Peer mediators** help resolve conflicts. Here they act as peacekeepers and work closely with administration to develop a set of procedures in handling student conflict. For example, two boys were found fighting in the cafeteria. After being escorted to the mediation conference room, the mediation process was explained to the boys. Once they agreed to participate, the mediators clarified the events that unfolded to cause the conflict, asked questions, and helped the boys discuss how they were feeling. Finally, they discussed how they might resolve this conflict and avoid any conflicts in the future. Peer mediation reduces discipline referrals and increases a positive attitude toward the school because students are no longer handed referrals or suspension without telling their side of the story (Barton, 2009).

Peer tutors are used in all subject areas. With training, peer tutors not only assist students who are struggling academically, they build a relationship with the students so they can identify what problems arise that affect their study habits and what other issues occur in class that may be distracting. Students often feel embarrassed to ask for extra help and may worry about what their friends might think; however, peer tutors are responsive to these feelings and increase the students' ability to access extra help (Gordon, 2005).

Peer facilitator training also has a positive impact on the work of student assistants (Gordon, 2005) and this role is one of indirect assistance to peers. Students as aides or student assistants provide teachers and counselors assistance by working in offices, helping with bulletin boards, distributing materials, or helping with planning activities.

## CASTT a Wider Net with Teachers and Other Staff Members

Teachers and other educators such as teacher assistants (a.k.a., paraprofessionals, guidance assistants, or teachers aides), special education teachers, school psychologists, and social workers are accessible and vital partners.

### *Partnering with Teachers*

School counselors team with teachers and can strengthen classroom management, bring attention to learning styles, provide safety nets for students, promote programs such as cooperative discipline, and deliver schoolwide programs such as character education to improve the school climate. Teachers can considerably promote and spread the influence of the school counseling program. Through teachers we get support for classroom guidance lessons, mentoring and tutoring programs, and interventions for special needs students. Teachers can instruct school counselors in how to disseminate effective instructional techniques to other teachers. Teachers can help develop schoolwide interventions such as behavior management programs, awards programs, and staff development.

Special education (SE) teachers must use many of the same skills in their jobs, albeit to differing degrees. Both professionals are prepared in separate programs to assess student needs, pose appropriate developmental interventions, and consult with parents and teachers to analyze situations and generate possible alternatives for resolving them. Both school counselors and SE teachers are required to collaborate on teams when developing Individualized Education Plans (IEPs). The SE teacher/school counselor partnerships are natural allies to perform the sophisticated, demanding function of consulting effectively (Erford, 2011c). "Connecting with special education teachers is one way to ensure that all students receive comprehensive school counseling services" (Erford, 2011c, p. 55). School counselors and SE teachers can greatly affect students when working together on teams to gather information and explore alternatives to help parents and teachers who control so much of the physical, affective, and cognitive environment in which the child lives (Tarver-Behring & Spagna, 2005). Helping parents and teachers with their immediate problems improves their future functioning (Whitbread, Bruder, Fleming, & Park, 2007). Teachers and counselors who serve as catalyst in the problem-solving conference can help further the goals of the school counseling program by

- assisting with remediation and prevention;
- developing strategies to assist many students with academic and social problems, not just special education students;
- offering consultation services to regular education teachers;
- closely monitoring a student's progress;

- enabling the prevention of some problems as well as the remediation of others, reducing special education placements and the time students will spend in an SE placement;
- consulting with parents, which can enhance problem-solving by learning the skills of reducing broad problems into measurable and observable terms (Dardig, 2008); and
- establishing, staffing, and supporting a prereferral team. This strategy has been adapted nationwide to provide more comprehensive consultation services before SE is considered.

Response to Intervention (RtI), sometimes known as **pre-referral**, assistance teams have emerged due to (1) excessive numbers of students inappropriately referred to and declared eligible for special education, (2) the need for greater levels of consultation and collaboration, and (3) the need to support teachers who have too many students and a struggle to accommodate special learning needs (Brownell, Sindelar, Kiely, & Danielson, 2010; Bursuck & Blanks, 2010; Klotz & Canter, 2007). SE teachers can serve as the backbone of pre-referral work, which will considerably reduce the work school counselors have to do to get children through the child study team process in preparation for SE.

### *Partnering with Other Educators/Staff Members*

Schools have tried to alleviate poverty and respond to student needs by providing lunch programs, health clinics, and a full range of services. In addition to regular classroom instruction, professionals such as social workers, nurses, and school psychologists provide information in areas such as personal health, safety, sex education, and serve as a critical link between the school, home, and community (Erford, 2011c). These same educators can be brought into the school counseling effort. For example, school psychologists or social workers can serve on SE pre-referral teams, can serve as a resource for interventions, and can help set up behavior management programs for teachers. Social workers can help set up a parent night or parent fair, and attendance teachers can help us identify the students who need intervention and attention. The attendance teacher can help identify absentees and help provide interventions to get these students back in school. For example, the attendance teacher can alert others and seek help if she or he learns a student has been absent due to bullying, a bus schedule that does not work, or is homeless. Occupational specialists can help with career programs. The point is that school counselors can creatively and assertively look to each employee of the school district as a potential partner in the school counseling program. The teacher assistants, the custodian, the cafeteria workers, the computer, music, art, and physical education teachers can all be extensions of the school counseling program.

## CASTT a Wider Net with Technology

Technology is an area proving to have great potential for school counselors in efficiency while encumbering a small outlay of resources. Computers have been considered the tool to expedite tedious repetitive tasks, but computer potential for the roles, responsibilities, and effectiveness of school counselors is being expanded (Hayden, Poynton, & Sabella, 2008; Schellenberg, 2008; Tyler & Sabella, 2004; Wilczenski & Coomey, 2006).

According to Sabella (2003, as cited in Hayden, Poynton, & Sabella, 2008), "Technology can help counselors in one or more of four areas:

1. *Information/Resource*: In the form of words, graphics, video, and even three-dimension virtual environments, the Web remains a dynamic and rapidly growing library of information and knowledge.
2. *Communication/Collaboration*: Chat rooms, bulletin boards, virtual classroom environments, video conferencing, online conferences, electronic meeting services, e-mail—the web is now a place where people connect, exchange information, and make shared decisions.
3. *Interactive/Productivity tools*: The maturing of software and web-based programming has launched a new level of available tools off the shelves and on the Net. These technology tools can help counselors build and create anything ranging from a personalized business card to a set of personalized website links. Interactive tools help counselors to process data and manipulate information such as calculating a GPA or the rate of inflation, convert text to speech, create a graph, or even determine the interactive effects of popular prescription drugs.
4. *Delivery of services*: Most controversial, yet growing in popularity, is how counselors use the web to meet with clients and deliver counseling services in an online or 'virtual' environment" (para. 3).

Chris Bryan, a Florida high school counselor, says it best: "I believe that in the not too distant future, technology itself will be the biggest advocate for our teachers, students, and parents. Technology is all about communication, information, and potentially, the truth. The types of experiences technology can provide are becoming more and more immediate with audio and visual Internet connections. These connections have the potential to make education a much more transparent process than it is today. Right now our classrooms are windowless rooms. Parents can't see in. Teachers can't see out. Some school districts already have systems in place where direct internet communication, including students' attendance, behavior, and grades, takes place among parents, school counselors, and teachers." The speed with which counselors are now able to get information ideally positions us to use technology to our advantage in our advocacy role.

School counselors who understand equity issues and have technological skills to aggregate and disaggregate student information have critical, powerful skills that can allow them to act as advocates to identify and eliminate school practices that deter equitable access and opportunities for student success in higher level academics (Stone & Dahir, 2011). In the Tech Tools feature in every chapter of this text, we have included specific ways to employ technology to achieve your goals as a school counselor.

## BARRIERS TO COLLABORATION AND MANAGEMENT OF RESOURCES

Barriers to partnerships usually occur in the form of time, space, and personnel, usually in short supply in schools. Other barriers such as weak interpersonal skills can prevent educators from establishing and maintaining collaborative efforts. An atmosphere of **collegiality** starts with an administration that encourages collaborative efforts. Without administrative support the collaboration can become an arduous chore. Collegiality models shared-decision-making, multifaceted/multidisciplinary efforts, and reacts with enthusiasm for new ideas.

External members are harder to manage as services are often fragmented; the logistics of managing resources can eat up large chunks of precious time (however, it is time well spent as you meet the needs of more students). Rules and regulations of agencies, businesses, and other civic organizations can severely limit the work that can be accomplished, and services cannot always be repositioned into the school and this means families may have to find transportation and finances for services.

Parental involvement for some schools seems impossible to obtain. It can be frustrating when parents do not respond even when it is a matter of importance to their child's future. Barbara Barry, Florida elementary counselor, was not to be denied in her high-needs, urban school. When the traditional efforts of bringing parents into PTSA meetings failed, she brought in a couple of digital cameras and color printers, a stack of paper, and volunteers, and they advertised family portrait night. They were rewarded with a huge response. Approximately 35 family members showed up and a year later five times the number came. While parents were waiting for their family portrait, Barbara and other educators were busy getting important messages across. Thinking outside the box is what Barbara does best when it comes to parental involvement.

Herculean efforts to secure parental involvement can sometimes go unrewarded. For example, the University of North Florida's (UNF) school counseling candidates do one of their three internships at a critical needs school. The school had low parental involvement, high dropout rates, low postsecondary going-rates, and was designated by the state as a failing school (students were offered waivers to go elsewhere). The school counseling interns made over 900 phone calls to the parents of 320 students over four months to get the parents to participate in a joint career and academic advising session with their child. Information about the sessions was also issued in visits to the local faith community, in written information disseminated to students and parents at school, sporting events, and through the mail. Parents were offered sessions at their convenience, i.e., Saturdays, daytime, nighttime. The results were that a disappointing 11 parents participated in a face-to-face advising session. However, the counselors did feel there was a payoff as during the 900 phone contacts, parents were given critical career and academic information; the evidence revealed that the seeds planted paid off (e.g., an increase in test scores for the 320 students that received career and academic advising). The school counseling interns regrouped and redoubled their efforts to give students assignments and information to take home to discuss with their parents and turned to the faith community as a vehicle to reach parents. Research clearly indicates that children perform better, both academically and socially, if their parents are involved in their children's education. The home-school connection is vital but sometimes impossible to realize in the traditional sense of parents coming to the school for PTA meetings or advising sessions. Rather than lament and sit on their hands, Barbara Barry and the UNF interns looked for alternate ways of reaching parents.

## COLLEGIALITY: TAKING COLLABORATION TO A HIGHER LEVEL

When schools have a climate of collegiality much is gained. The benefits must be substantial for educators to put aside other activities to work with colleagues, for principals to promote and organize such work, for super-intendents to endorse it, and for school boards to pay for this work (Barth, 2006; Roberts & Pruitt, 2009). "As colleagues find opportunities to interact with each other, they typically deepen their understanding of what each other can offer and develop scholarly connections" (Gappa, Austin, & Trice, 2007, p. 305).

School counselors can contribute mightily to an environment of collegiality. Collaboration is critical but collegiality is collaboration at a different, deeper, and more professionally satisfying level. You can collaborate with other educators and not feel you have been collegial with them. Collegiality means the educator grows as a professional intellectually, personally, and in statute and standing. Collegiality means greater job satisfaction and attracts able and talented candidates by affording them work that is stimulating, meaningful, economically rewarding, and well regarded in the larger community (Gappa, Austin, & Trice, 2007). Most importantly students benefit from collaborative climates. "The nature of relationships among the adults within a school has a greater influence on the character and quality of that school and on student accomplishment than anything else" (Barth, 2006, p. 9).

Collegiality results in a school that taps the collective talents, experience, and energy of their professional staff (Hord & Sommers, 2008). "Collegiality is hard to establish. A famous baseball manager Casey Stengel once muttered, 'Getting good players is easy. Getting 'em to play together is the hardest part'" (Barth, 2006, p. 11).

Most teachers can point to a treasured colleague, but few work in schools where cooperative work is a condition of employment. Many teachers are satisfied with their peer relationships, but few claim that those relationships make their way into the classroom (Roberts & Pruitt, 2009). Many schools offer congenial work environments, but few offer a professional environment that makes the school as educative for teachers as for students (Hord & Sommers, 2008; Lassonde & Israel, 2010; Roberts & Pruitt, 2009). Collegiality increases the social aspect of schools. Social interactions with other adults, especially one's peers, can increase job satisfaction and negate the loneliness and stress some educators feel (Gappa, Austin, & Trice, 2007). Congenial relationships are personal and friendly and can lead to strong collegial relationships. "The promise of a good congenial relationship is one that allows us to shut off the alarm each day and arise" (Barth, 2006, p. 11).

Teachers who have worked together closely over a period of years celebrate their accomplishments by pointing to gains in the achievement, behavior, and attitude of students (Phelps, 2008). What are the implications for school counselors? As we work on systemic change, as we collaborate and partner, and as we manage human resources, we will want to concentrate on collegiality as a central focus and not just a happenstance byproduct of good collaboration.

# APPLICATION OF CASTT IN BUILDING A SAFE AND RESPECTFUL SCHOOL CLIMATE

Using a typical example in our schools, let's look at how school counselors can broker resources to affect the No Child Left Behind Act (2000) goal of a safer, more respectful school climate for all students.

*The climate at your school is dangerous for gay, lesbian, bisexual, and transgender students. You want to try to promote a safer, more inclusive school climate for this at-risk minority. How will you and the other members of the school's leadership team coordinate, collaborate, partner, and manage resources to help create a safer, more respectful school climate for this vulnerable student population?*

1. *Community Resources.* Gay, lesbian, bisexual, and transgender students often are isolated from the normal family support that is vital for successful identity development. Parents who have already been through the revelation that their child is gay, lesbian, bisexual, or transgender can offer support to families of students who are in the throes of trying to learn how to support their child as they wrestle with sexual identity issues.

   Agency counselors who work often with gay, lesbian, bisexual, and transgender youth can provide information about the best way to support these students. The local chapter of Parents and Friends of Lesbians and Gays (PFLAG), an international support group, can serve as a resource for information about other local resources and support groups to assist students and their parents. Lambda Legal Defense and Education Fund (email lambda@lambdalegal.org) can deliver professional development on the *Davis v. Monroe County Board of Education* (1999) so that teachers will understand the implications of the Supreme Court's decision on school safety and management of harassment.

   Community groups can work to reduce hate crimes and heighten understanding among all citizens. For example, two weeks after Matthew Shepard was killed in a gay hate crime in Laramie, Wyoming, in 1998, 17 school and community groups comprised of straight and gay students, parents, teachers, and counselors came together in Rockland County, Massachusetts, to develop strategies aimed at reducing hate crimes. Supported by GLSEN–Hudson Valley, participants left with action plans to attack one area of prejudice in their school or community (GLSENTalk, 1998). The Matthew Shepard Law was signed into law by President Obama on October 28, 2009, in response to the problem of violent hate crimes committed against individuals based on actual or perceived sexual orientation, gender, gender identity, and disability (www.matthewshepard.org).

Faculty, staff, and students from postsecondary institutions can provide speakers, money, facilities, and materials to help school counselors and others forward a safe and respectful school climate for gay, lesbian, bisexual, and transgender youth.

2. *Administrative Resources.* Administrators can promote the implementation of a policy protecting all students against sexual harassment to include a clause that expressly mentions sexual orientation. Elements of an effective sexual harassment policy should include the applicable laws, a zero-tolerance statement, and due process procedures to address complaints.

   According to the 2007 National School Climate Survey, published by the Gay Lesbian Straight Educators Network (GLSEN), nearly three-fourths (73.6%) of students heard homophobic or antigay remarks used often or frequently at their school and 9 out of 10 (90.2%) students surveyed heard the term *gay* used in a negative way often or frequently at school (Kosciw, Diaz, & Greytak, 2008, p. xii).

   Additionally, more than half (60.8%) of students reported that they felt unsafe in school because of their sexual orientation, and more than one-third (38.4%) felt unsafe because of their gender expression. Nearly nine-tenths of students (86.2%) reported being verbally harassed (e.g., called names or threatened) at school because of their sexual orientation. And two-thirds (66.5%) of students were verbally harassed because of their gender expression.

   Almost half (44.1%) of students had been physically harassed (e.g., pushed or shoved) at school in the past year because of their sexual orientation and 3 in 10 students (30.4%) because of their gender expression. For some students, victimization was even more severe with 22.1 percent reporting being physically assaulted (e.g., punched, kicked, injured with a weapon) because of their sexual orientation and 14.2 percent because of their gender expression. The majority (60.8%) of students who were harassed or assaulted in school did not report the incident to school staff, believing little to no action would be taken or the situation could become worse if reported.

   Administrators can support an assembly on diversity and tolerance and allow written information on bulletin boards advertising support groups and community activities for all minority groups to include gay, lesbian, bisexual, and transgender students. It is less threatening to school officials to have a bulletin board that gives referral resources in the community for support groups for a number of minority groups, and gay, lesbian, bisexual, and transgender groups are one more minority group in the information exchange.

3. *Student Resources.* Students can establish the role of heterosexual allies and call for systemic reform. Students can promote bully-proofing efforts and serve as another set of eyes and ears to identify, intervene, and/or report bullying. Students across Colorado returned to school wearing tiny patches that had the single word *respect*. The patch was designed to promote harmony among the school cliques exposed in the Columbine High School shooting.

4. *Teachers and Other Staff as Resources.* Teachers can include in their curriculum and instruction diversity awareness and multicultural initiatives aimed at promoting tolerance. Teachers can use inclusive language whenever possible to talk about famous gay, lesbian, bisexual, or transgender historical figures in social studies, English, and science (Campos, 2005). Teachers can challenge antigay verbal or written remarks made in their presence.

   Other educators can provide support in the form of information, acceptance, staff development, counseling, etc. For example, the media specialist can influence the choice of library books so that gay, lesbian, bisexual, and transgender students can begin to see themselves in the curriculum. Nurses can educate teachers as to the prevalence of suicide and development issues for this at-risk group.

   The assistant can establish a packet of documents for teachers and other educators to raise awareness of this at-risk minority. A study examined the coverage of sexual-orientation topics within 77 public university secondary teacher preparation programs across seven U.S. states, and represented programs preparing 8,300 to 11,500 teachers annually. Findings indicated that 40 percent of programs did not address sexual orientation as a diversity topic. Further, even programs that did address sexual orientation tended to abandon the topic in practicum courses, perhaps limiting students' abilities to apply the information to practice (Sherwin & Jennings, 2006).

   The school counselor managing resources can direct the guidance assistant to provide information to close the gap in information and understanding.

5. *Technology Resources.* Through technology, teachers and other educators can gain access to legal information on creating a safe, respectful school climate such as http://web.lexis-nexis.com/universe/document?. Also, technology can help us track discipline referrals that involve hate crimes and tell us where the incidents are taking place and who the perpetrators are.

In addition to the coordination of CASTT, school counselors provide specific strategies to support individual students as well as offer activities and services that educate the wider community to promote a safe and respectful environment. You can develop strategies to help students ease into the discussion of sexuality. For example, have students respond to verbal or written questions in which sexuality is but one of a number of questions and given the same weight as other questions (Stone, 2003). Encourage students to involve their parents and offer to be available for a joint conference; persuade students to express the fears they hold in telling their parents. Help students anticipate their parents' reaction and assist the student in developing coping strategies (Campos, 2005). Display the pink triangle "safe place" stickers supplied by Gay Lesbian Straight Educators Network (GLSEN) or other support symbols to send a message to heterosexual and gay, lesbian, bisexual, and transgender students that the school counselor is an "ally" or "friend." Continue to enhance collaboration between families and school. Involving parents routinely helps facilitate communication in tougher times. Provide onsite workshops for faculty and staff.

## TECH TOOLS

CASTT a Wider Net by using technology in your coordination role.

- School counselors often develop patterns in their recommendation letters, repeating key phrases and expressions when describing different students' academic prowess, character, athletic performance, service, and leadership. By taking these standard phrases that are your own words and creating files by type, you can go to your file, choose the paragraph that most closely matches each student, and tailor the paragraph to accurately reflect the individual student.
- Develop electronic bank forms, handbooks, addresses, and other information for easy use. Teachers and others can personalize and send information much more efficiently if templates are provided for them and all they need to do is personalize them so that the information is specific to their class or student(s).
- Technology plays a critical role in having accurate, timely data from student-information-management systems. School counselors using these data increase their ability to be another set of eyes and ears for social justice and advocacy, monitoring patterns of course enrollment, student access and success in higher level academics, delivering career and academic advising, managing resources to extend the reach of the school counseling program.
- Make technology your partner in career and academic advising, helping you close the information gap in areas such as helping students understand that financing a higher education is possible.

## *School Counselor Casebook: Voices from the Field*

### The Scenario Reviewed

For the second consecutive year your school has been placed on the Critically Low Performing Schools list, which means that if test scores do not improve over the next two years, the state will take over the school. You believe that as a member of the leadership team, instructional success and student achievement are as much your job as that of the principal, teachers, and other critical stakeholders. Your principal does not assign you extraneous duties and you have a solid and meaningful comprehensive, developmental school counseling program that is already supporting the achievement of students; yet, like everyone else in the school, you feel pressure of a pending state takeover. You want to extend your reach to

*(continues)*

support more students' academic success, but your day is already packed with important tasks that you do not want to relinquish.

## A Practitioner's Approach

Here's how a practicing school counselor responded to this school scenario:

As a counselor I would examine my resources first to see what options I have at my disposal. For example, I would look at my time and at already scheduled activities on my calendar: How much time can I personally allocate to improving our school's performance on this year's test scores? What interventions am I already doing? What interventions would I like to implement and how much time will I need to implement them?

Next I would look at the faculty resources available: Are there other stakeholders who can assist with some of the interventions I have in mind? For example, would our school social worker, school psychologist, and other student service personnel be available to assist? Would I be able to utilize parent volunteers, students from the high school, and other community based persons to assist? And then I would look at my financial resources: What type of funding will be needed to implement the interventions and are those types of funds available to me through my local school budget? If not, what other types of system funds could be accessed, i.e., Drug-Free Schools, PTA mini-grants, etc.?

After examining my resources, the next step would be to meet with the School Leadership Team to present my ideas to them. If they are interested, then I can move forward with an action plan, but if they do not want to see a particular program implemented, I would need to explore other options. Without administrative support and the support of the School Leadership Team, little can be accomplished. The most significant aspect of reviewing my ideas with the School Leadership Team is to make sure that my suggestions fit with the school's overall strategic plan for school improvement. Our strategic plan drives our school focus and must be utilized as the overall force behind implementation of our school counseling plan.

Once the resources have been reviewed and the support from administration and Leadership Team has been gained, it is time to move ahead with implementation of strategies and ideas. I would utilize an action plan format to formulate the structure and timeline of any intervention I plan to implement. This would allow me to spell out what my goals and objectives are and what strategies I want to use to reach those objectives. It will also keep me on track in terms of who is responsible for what, what my timelines are, what benchmarks I can use to gauge my success by, which national standards we are meeting, and what the final evaluation component will be.

These are some more specific suggestions for strategies I might utilize: I would identify which students are performing below the proficient expected levels on the state or national test by examining test scores. I could also use student grades to help identify underperforming students. Once students are identified, I could assess what services these students are already receiving in terms of remediation, tutoring, and other forms of academic assistance. If there are students who are not receiving these types of services, I can find out how to get them involved in a tutorial program, after-school help sessions with teachers, etc. If it appears that students need assistance with study skills and school success skills, I can set up small-group counseling sessions with these students. If I have not had the opportunity to implement classroom guidance sessions on these topics, I could also set these up with teachers.

Another useful strategy to assist students in becoming responsible for improving their own areas of weakness is to utilize individual advisement sessions with each student to review their last year's test scores and areas of weaknesses and strengths. Helping the student come up with a plan for improvement is the focus of the advisement session. This is a strategy where it is important to enlist the time of other persons in the school system including central office personnel who are usually willing to come out and assist students on assigned dates. Each advisor is given a group of students to work with on a specific date and is scheduled with students every 15 minutes during that day.

Reaching out to parents of identified students in several areas such as interpretation of test scores, how to help your child be test-wise, and other related topics is another way to work on improving your school's test scores. Parents need to know how important the test dates are for their child and what the various things are that they can do to help their child do their best on test dates.

Finally I would review the resources I acquired from past conferences and counselor's meetings and talk with other counselors to see what ideas they are utilizing in their schools. I find other counselors to be the best resource in coming up with ideas that they are familiar with from their schools and adapting those ideas to fit my own school. Resources exist—but it is truly a matter of identifying and coordinating them if we are going to improve the situation in our school. Who better than the school counselor to take a leadership role in making this happen!

Susan McCarthy is currently working as a middle school counselor at Sandy Springs Middle School, Fulton County Schools, Georgia, and has extensive school counseling experience at the elementary and secondary levels. Susan has also served as the state guidance consultant for the Georgia Department of Education and as a supervisor of counseling for a large suburban/urban school system in Atlanta, Georgia. Susan is the editor of the GSCA Journal, president of the Georgia Association of Counselor Educators and Supervisors, and is an ASCA National Standards Trainer.

## LOOKING BACK: SALIENT POINTS

### Coordination of Services, Collaboration, and Management of Resources

Skillful coordination, collaboration, and brokering of resources will determine the success or failure of your school counseling program. Coordination, collaboration, and management of resources are the mechanics or "how to" that guide your school counseling program. "Of all the counseling services, Gerler (1992) argued that coordination needs to come first if counselors are to influence the educational and personal development of students, and that it is one of the most important skills for serving at-risk students" (Galassi & Akos, 2007).

Coordination of services means prioritizing and efficiently organizing and delivering the components of your school counseling program, e.g., individual/group counseling, classroom guidance lessons, consultation services, career and academic advising, and systemic support. Collaboration is entering into a partnership or liaison with other individuals, groups, or members of other institutions who share a common mission of student success and who work with you and other members of the educational community for the purpose of enhancing the personal/social, career, and academic outcomes of every student in the school. Managing resources extends school counselors' reach beyond the school counseling office to bring in resources such as parents, students, teachers, technology, administrators, community members, and business partners with minimal or no additional funds to garner support and redistribute duties.

## Coordinator of Services

The coordinator's role is to decide the goals of the school counseling program and to identify the mechanisms and resources needed to carry out those goals. The coordination role has become one of the most important roles of a school counselor as we must increasingly rely on the expertise and services of others to deliver optimum programs. School counselors' roles need to change from just direct service delivery to becoming staff developers, consultants, collaborators and team builders, brokers of resources, and supporters of instruction.

## Collaboration and Partnering

However do we meet the needs of all the students in our charge? A school counselor stands in her or his office staring at a stack of 450 educational records, each representing a student who has career, academic, personal, and social needs. How do we get our arms around all these students to close the gaps in their information, to support their social development, and to widen their opportunities to fully participate in the U.S. economy? School counselors take ownership of individual counseling, consultation, leadership, and advocacy that need specialized skills that their master's level preparation and job experience provide. There are many duties that school counselors want to see successfully completed but that do not need to be under their exclusive purview. Stiffer standards, shrinking education dollars, and increased social stresses demand that educators, especially school counselors who have always been outnumbered with demanding student/counselor ratios, collaborate with each other to deliver optimum services to students. Collaborative efforts among administrators, community members, teachers, and school counselors will promote student success.

### CASTT a Wider Net: The Benefits of Collaboration

School counselors can cast a wider net when they commit to collaborate. CASTT is an acronym that stands for Community members, Administrators, Students, Teachers, and Technology. These are the people who will benefit the most from a collaborative school counseling program and who will also be our partners in this collaborative program increasing our effectiveness and widening our reach. Technology is an efficient and effective way of disseminating information and analyzing results. The benefits of collaboration are to meet the needs of students with a high-profile, powerful school counseling program that will match student aspirations the opportunities needed to support the realization of dreams. Collaboration is capacity building so that the future work can be redistributed and the school counseling program will cast a wider net in a more efficient manner with minimum duplication of services.

### Barriers, Limitations, and Collegiality of Collaboration

Limitations exist that make partnerships in schools a challenge. External members are harder to manage. Lack of interpersonal skills prevents educators from establishing and maintaining collaborative efforts. Collegiality models shared-decision-making, multifaceted/multidisciplinary efforts, and reacts with enthusiasm for new ideas. School counselors usually have an advantage in collaboration as they generally have a facilitative leadership style, good communication skills, an understanding of the nature and function of schools, and the "sink or swim" need to make collaboration work! It helps immeasurably when there is a climate for collaboration where the leadership of the school district and school site encourages collaborative efforts with mechanisms such as site-based teams and shared decision-making teams.

### Management of Resources

School counselor service delivery has widened from a direct service deliverer to a coordinator of resources, from an individual focus to a systemic focus, from a small percentage of the population to a program focusing on all students. The dilemma is how to have efficient use of time and resources to be able to address increasingly heavy caseloads for counselors. A delivery model is needed based on having the school counselor at the hub of managing different stakeholders and resources to help the efforts of the school counseling program. This model requires that the school counselor must be comfortable being a leader and motivator to get others to be part of the school counseling program.

## KEY TERMS

## LEARNING EXTENSIONS/MAKING CONNECTIONS

1. Discuss the benefits and limitations of collaboration. Can you be collaborative without being collegial? Why or why not? What are the benefits of collegiality?

2. Briefly discuss how you plan to use each of these 11 potential resources in your school counseling program: (1) administrators; (2) regular education teachers; (3) exceptional student education teachers; (4) other educators; (5) parents; (6) students; (7) guidance assistants; (8) agency members; (9) community members; (10) colleges, universities, and other postsecondary institutions; (11) technology.

3. Besides the above 11 resources, identify and explain the role of two other resources to bring in to partner with your school counseling program.

4. Think about the makeup of a pre-referral team for your future school. Who would you want to see on the team? How will you go about organizing the team? What other educator could take ownership of the team besides you? Develop a plan for your future school.

# CHAPTER 14

# Preparing All Students to Become Career and College Ready

## CHAPTER OBJECTIVES

*By the time you have completed this chapter, you should be able to*

- understand the importance of college and career readiness to every student's future aspiration;

- help students connect student motivation, achievement, and future goals;

- understand the influence of parents, peers, and economic pressures on career success;

- identify the career planning elements in your comprehensive school counseling and career guidance program;

- assess your current college and career readiness practices based on nationally accepted criteria;

- develop appropriate K–12 strategies for addressing the career development needs of students based on knowledge of the National Career Development Guidelines and the career development component of the National Standards for School Counseling Programs in the ASCA National Model;

- demonstrate familiarity with college and career assessment and planning resources and other tools to support students' comprehensive dreams and aspirations;

- develop strategies to motivate colleagues, school administrators, parents, and members of the community to collaborate to create bright futures for every student.

---

## *School Counselor Casebook: Getting Started*

### The Scenario

Two ninth-grade students stop by your office. You know that both of these students are in the honors program and they have done well so far this school year. The students tell you that they no longer want to be in the more challenging program. They claim that the work is not too difficult and they are clueless as to why they are in this class and not taking regular grade-level courses. When they asked their homeroom teacher why they have to be in the honors program, he said that it will help them get into college. The students told you that other members of the class have asked the same question and were not able to get any additional reasons. After you speak to these two students you realize that they have no awareness of career opportunities, why students go to college, and what it will take to succeed in life. What would you do?

**Thinking about Solutions**

As you read this chapter, think about what you might do as a new high school counselor to help students become better informed about career options and increasing importance of postsecondary education to succeed in a competitive global environment. When you come to the end of the chapter, you will have the opportunity to see how your ideas compare with a practicing school counselor's approach.

# SUCCEEDING IN THE GLOBAL ENVIRONMENT

> Together, we must achieve a new goal, that by 2020, the United States will once again lead the world in college completion. We must raise the expectations for our students, for our schools, and for ourselves—this must be a national priority. We must ensure that every student graduates from high school well prepared for college and a career. (President Barak Obama in ESEA Blueprint for Reform, U.S. Department of Education, Office of Planning, Evaluation and Policy Development, 2010)

College and career ready is the "catchphrase du jour" (Paulson, 2010) and has become the mantra for this decade. The focus in the proposed Blueprint for Reform (U.S.D.O.E., 2010) is to ensure that all students are ready to successfully transition to postsecondary education and a career. This is a shift in thinking only about graduation rates to focusing on the readiness of high school graduates to enter a globally competitive world. U.S. public schools are charged with developing a curriculum that fosters critical thinking, problem solving, and the innovative use of knowledge to prepare students for college and career. Regardless of the educational path after high school, all Americans should be prepared to enroll in at least one year of higher education or job training to better prepare our workforce for a 21st-century economy (White House Issues Education, 2010).

> Overwhelmingly, Americans agree with the President and believe a college education is essential for success in today's world. In 1978, only 36% said it was very important; in 1983, that increased to 58%; and this year, 75% of Americans agreed a college education is necessary. Eighty-four percent of Americans agree that all high school students should be well-prepared for college and a career. That increases slightly to 91% when you substitute the word "college" with "more education beyond high school," suggesting that Americans are not "hung up" over the concept of preparing all high school students for college. Without question, Americans equate more education, including college, with greater readiness for the world of work. (Bunshaw & Lopez, 2010, p. 21)

The complexity of this situation has escalated the importance of career development and effective student planning has escalated (Feller, 2003).

Leaving the future of America's youth to happenstance places young people at risk in an increasingly competitive job marketplace. In recent decades, the advancement of technology and increasing demand for highly skilled workers has placed a strong emphasis on increased academic achievement and a renewed emphasis on the delivery of career development and career guidance programs in schools across the United States. Every student needs the motivation and support to complete high school with the academic preparation to have all options after graduation (Education Trust, 1997), which includes two- and four-year colleges, career and technical schools, and military opportunities. Preparing students to select a career pathway and guiding them to enroll in appropriate coursework that is essential to support their goals is critical to meeting the global and economic challenges of this century. The U.S. Council on Competitiveness (2007) claims that continuing prosperity will require greater investment in postsecondary education and training.

**College and career readiness** preparation have become synonymous. Business and industry recognized the need for workers to come to the corporate office or to the factory with the affective and academic competence that complement employability preparation skills. Responsibility, self-management, respect for diversity, initiative, diligence, punctuality and teamwork, and collaboration are needed in the workplace and on campus. Today's young people will need to be better educated and prepared as the United States continues to move to a knowledge/information economic model. College readiness goes far beyond the ability of students to file an application and is far more complex and multidimensional than eligibility. It means to be able to continue to learn and succeed in coursework beyond high school. With this in mind, the National Governors Association and the Council of Chief State School Officers have released the Common Core State Standards (2010), which include rigorous content and application of knowledge through high-order skills and are aligned with college and work expectations.

> These [Common Core Standards] standards, fully implemented, will provide all students with a K–12 education that will give high school graduates a full range of options and opportunities to choose their path after high school. High expectations for all students that reflect the demands of the real world will open more doors for all, rather than just a few. (Cohen, 2010)

Efforts to place and maintain the U.S. position as first in the world of education, as discussed in Chapter 1, have been part of the national agenda for years. The National Commission on Excellence in Education (1983) and the Carnegie Forum on Education and the Economy (1986) issued reports that our nation's economic future is dependent on providing students with access and success in higher-level educational opportunities, critical thinking and analysis skills, and the development of affective competence.

In 1991, a joint commission was formed comprised of representatives from business, industry, and education. The Secretary of Labor's Commission on Achieving Necessary Skills (SCANS) produced a report titled *What Work Requires of Schools*. The document emphasized the development of strong affective and academic competence and identified competencies, foundation skills, and personal qualities that are needed for solid performance in the workplace. The five SCANS' competencies included the ability to

1. Identify, organize, plan, and allocate resources such as time
2. Work with others
3. Acquire and use information
4. Understand complex interrelationships
5. Work with a variety of technologies

The SCANS report encouraged schools to teach higher-order thinking skills, while providing opportunities for students to apply selected personal qualities including responsibility, sociability, self-management, integrity, and honesty in a meaningful way. These competencies brought attention to the importance of employability skills and for the first time, educators were urged to integrate academic and affective education in the areas of basic skills, thinking skills, and personal qualities (see Table 14.1).

The School to Work Opportunities Act (STWOA, 1994) encouraged educators to integrate academic and technical knowledge and skills to better prepare graduates of our high schools to meet the needs of both employers and postsecondary institutions (Worthington & Juntunen, 1997). School to Work (1994) called for **career awareness**, exploration through mentoring, shadowing, internships, and school–business partnerships. STWOA also provided for a closer monitoring of at-risk students who would benefit from career and technical education with the expressed purpose of preventing dropouts who become entrenched in entry-level, low-wage jobs with little opportunity for advancement (Herr, 1997). When students develop a strong sense of self and understand the connection between their studies and future opportunities, they have an easier time learning academic subjects (Sciarra, 2004). Both STWOA and the Tech Prep initiative were significant federally funded initiatives that promoted high achievement and the acquisition of employability (SCANS) competencies. Both emphasized collaboration with business and industry with the ultimate goals to improve labor market preparation.

The Partnership for 21st Century Skills (2006), a consortium of major business industries and education organizations, identified a skill set of essential outcomes for personal, educational, and economic success for 21st-century students. Recommendations include the following: students need to obtain *Learning and Innovation Skills* (creativity and innovation, critical thinking and problem solving, etc.); *Information, Media and Technology Skills, Core Subjects and 21st Century Themes* (global awareness, financial literacy, etc.); and *Life and Career Skills* (initiative and self-direction, among others). Despite the significant pressures placed on educators to raise the bar of achievement and for students to acquire the core competencies, the partnership recognized that

TABLE **14.1**
SCANS Competencies

| Basic Skills | Thinking Skills | Personal Qualities |
|---|---|---|
| Reading | Creativeness | Self-Esteem |
| Writing | Decisiveness | Self-Management |
| Mathematics | Problem Solving | Integrity |
| Speaking | Reasoning | Sociability |
| Listening | | |

Source: SCANS, 1991.

"today's life and work environments require far more than thinking skills and content knowledge. The ability to navigate the complex life and work environments in the globally competitive information age requires students to pay rigorous attention to developing adequate life and career skills such as: flexibility and adaptability; initiative and self-direction; social and cross-cultural skills; productivity and accountability; and leadership and responsibility" (Partnership for 21st Century Skills, 2009). Thus, it is recognized that the themes from the SCANS competencies and the goals of the School to Work Opportunity Act persist, encouraging educators to produce workers and citizens who are academically competent and have the affective skills to succeed in a global environment.

Currently, the need for higher educated and skilled workers continues to increase faster than the supply of workers, especially with the dramatic fluctuations in the economic outlook. As the United States struggles to recover from the Great Recession with repressed hiring rates and high unemployment, the United States faces fundamental challenges about its role in the global workplace and economic order (Feller, 2009). Employed workers are experiencing more stress and less satisfaction as employers continue to downsize to reduce costs and produce even minimal profits. To achieve this, students and adults must face tough choices about how to invest in their future.

The American Dream, and until recently the American reality, was that "people could start at the bottom and, without much formal education, work their way to the top" (Carnevale & Desrochers, 2003a, p. 228). With continuous changes in the workplace and the shrinking availability of high-paying blue-collar jobs, students today realize their "approach to career planning [will be] quite different from that of their parents" (Niles & Harris-Bowlsbey, 2002, p. 230). The school-to-work/career efforts in the 1990s helped underperforming students engage in relevant skill-based learning, motivating them to stay in school and graduate by making education relevant (Brand, 2005). At-risk students were engaged in career development activities (Plank, 2001) and participated in face-to-face social networks through work experience (Kazie, 2005). With increased economic pressures, these opportunities for career employment without education beyond high school have been marginalized.

According to the Bureau of Labor Statistics (BLS) Occupational Employment statistical projections (see Figure 14.1), occupations in a category with some postsecondary education are expected to experience higher rates of growth than those in an on-the-job training category (Bureau of Labor Statistics, 2010). Occupations in the associate's degree category are projected to grow the fastest, at about 19 percent. In addition, occupations in the master's and first professional degree categories are anticipated to grow by about 18 percent each, and occupations in the bachelor's and doctoral degree categories are expected to grow by about 17 percent each. However, occupations in the on-the-job training categories are expected to grow by 8 percent each.

The data tell the story: The more you learn, the more you earn, and the less likely you are to be unemployed. Increasingly, income is determined by the level of educational attainment. More education leads to higher income, which in turn produces higher standards of living for families. As shown in

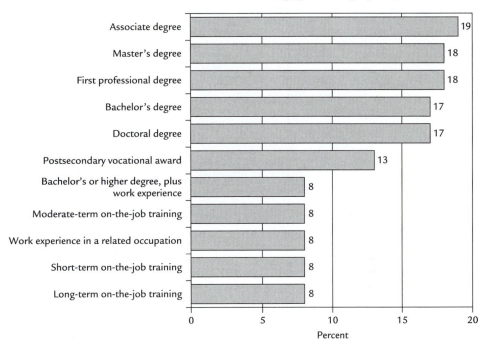

FIGURE **14.1** Employment Change by Education and Training Category
Source: Bureau of Labor Statistics Division of Occupational Outlook.

Figure 14.2, education continues to pay because employers believe that an educated worker can learn tasks more easily and are better organized, and this results in higher earnings and lower unemployment rates.

Job stability and a market outlook require a different workforce for the 21st century. As recently as the 1980s, it was fairly commonplace for a high school or college graduate to take a job with a company and stay with that company throughout her or his working life (U.S. Department of Labor, 2004). Statistics show that this is no longer a way of life; a person entering the workforce will change jobs an average of eight times before retirement (U.S. Department of Labor, 2004). What's more, the same person will change career paths three or more times (U.S. Department of Labor, 2004).

Although no one can predict with complete accuracy which jobs will exist in the future and which jobs will become obsolete, it is possible to assess a specific job's outlook (Occupational Outlook Handbook, 2010). Young people who drop out or seek entry-level jobs on graduation do not realize that employment at this level may not provide a living wage. Yet, the data tell the story. Over the course of a lifetime, a high school dropout in the United States earns $260,000 less than a high school graduate and $1 million less than a college graduate (Postsecondary.org, 2009).

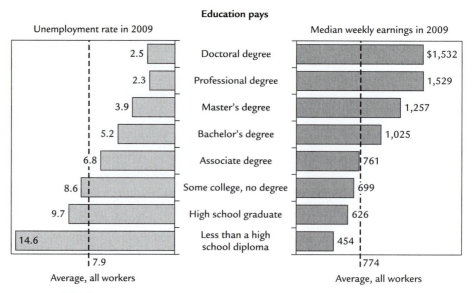

**Education pays**

FIGURE **14.2** Education Pays

Note: Data are 2009 annual averages for persons age 25 and over. Earnings are for full-time wage and salary workers.
Source: Bureau of Labor Statistics, Current Population Survey.

School counselors can guide students to examine opportunities that exist in the field now, including the average age of the employees in that job title, the number of people in training and preparation programs; developing technology, economic, and demographic trends do this. There is a wealth of information available on the Internet such as the *Occupational Outlook Handbook* (Department of Labor, 2010) and myriad websites devoted to **career guidance** (see Tech Tools at the end of this chapter). School counselors are key information brokers serving as the gateway to curricular connections to career opportunities as students develop career and educational plans. Career information support helps students better understand the connection between earning and learning.

As noted in Figure 14.2 there are substantial earnings differentials from the lowest to highest levels of educational attainment. When school counselors help students analyze the correlation between educational attainment and income it can have a powerful influence on young people who dream of lifestyles that offer financial independence, advancement, and success. Helping students realize their dreams is a critical and essential component of the work of school counselors. When students discover their passion and see the connection between their dreams and their education, it serves to motivate students to get higher grades, better attendance, and a stronger commitment to their education.

Demographics also provide key information in preparing the worker of the future. The millennial generation will surpass the size of Generation X and may become as large as the baby boom generation (Howe & Strauss, 2000).

Competition is strong and consumer demands continue to influence the need for goods and services. The high-tech industry is a prime example. When a product is in high demand, jobs in that industry are generally plentiful. However, unforeseen events such as 9/11 and financial market instabilities can cause changes in consumer confidence, affecting individual occupations or industries in this decade.

Emerging technologies create both obsolescence and opportunity. Company downsizing, due to technological innovations, significantly affects the workforce, causing many people to lose their jobs and seek new employment and careers (Bureau of Labor Statistics, 2010; Lawhorn, 2004). Technology innovations create shifts in the job market rapidly. Today's graduates will need to transition to the workplace with the ability to adapt to changing environments and to acquire new knowledge and skills to keep pace with innovation in the workforce.

## THEORETICAL UNDERPINNINGS

You will recall that school counseling's origins are in vocational counseling and Parsons (1909) believed there was "no part of life where the need for guidance is more emphatic than in the transition from school to work—the choice of a vocation, adequate preparation for it, and attainment of efficiency and success" (p. 4). Major theorists' writings and practice have strongly influenced career development. **Career counseling** is guided by theory that provides a point of reference from which the counselor develops a personal perspective of human growth, development, and behavior (Gladding, 2009). Developmental theory is a strong influence in career counseling as the life stages and changes affect career counseling. Career maturity is demonstrated by the successful accomplishment of age-appropriate and developmental learning across the lifespan (Super, 1980).

Super's (1980) **Life Span–Life Space** approach suggested that **career development** evolves along a continuum from birth throughout the lifespan. These early stages of growth in children addressed fantasy (4–10), interest (11–12), and capacity (13–14), and assisted children in developing an early awareness of the world of work and of their interests. In the exploration stage (15–24) youth and young adults acquire career awareness by discovering skills, talents, motivation, strengths, and weakness. They begin to understand that a strong commitment as well as acquiring coping and resiliency skills is essential to educational and career success. As young adults evaluate their strengths and weaknesses, career counseling can lead one to a better understanding of fear of failure, the influence of parents and guardians, and the individual's willingness to overcome obstacles to achieve her or his goals. This growth in self-concept informs decisions, choices, and eventually career selection. Because Super uses the concept of career maturity as a means of identifying which developmental tasks have been accomplished on the continuum of life development, career success therefore is the result of the congruence of abilities, personality, and aptitude with the choice of career environment. The concept of career maturity has been used to describe both the process by which individuals make career choices appropriate to their age and stage of development and their ability to successfully resolve and transition through the specific tasks of each of these stages (Brown & Lent, 2005, p. 358).

Using the perception that people are attracted to a given career by their personalities, Holland (1997) proposed that the environment could greatly influence a person's orientation to a career choice, personal satisfaction, and stability. Holland's typology approach to career development is based in self-knowledge and includes the following:

*Consistency:* Career choice is an expression or extension of one's personality into the world of work.

*Differentiation:* Individuals who match a personality type will demonstrate little resemblance to other types.

*Identity:* Individuals can acquire a clear and stable picture of their interests, goals, and talents.

*Congruence:* Individuals' personality type is in harmony with the choice of work environment.

Holland's **Self-Directed Search** (Holland, Fritzsche, & Powell, 1994a), an assessment tool, is based on the theory of career typology and is the basis for most of the career inventories in use today. The typology categorizes the relationship of personality to the work environments with respect to six types of personality orientations. Known as the "Holland Codes," these factors of influence on career choice are briefly described below.

*Realistic:* Individuals show an interest in working with objects such as tools and machines. Mechanical creativity and physical dexterity are important skills for this area. Individuals who score high on this theme prefer dealing with things rather than with ideas or people.

*Investigative:* Individuals display an interest in science, theories, ideas, and data. Analytical skills are important and a high score in this theme is indicative of someone who is creative, prefers to think through problems, and enjoys challenges.

*Artistic:* Individuals are concerned with self-expression and art appreciation. High scorers have artistically oriented interests and a greater need for individual expression, and they generally describe themselves as original, expressive, and unconventional.

*Social:* Individuals prefer to work with people in areas such as human welfare and community service. People skills such as listening and showing under-standing are important for this category. Someone who scores high in this category tends to be sociable, humanistic, and gets along well with others.

*Enterprising:* Individuals have an interest in business and leadership roles. Communicating with others and an ability to motivate and direct others are important skills for these occupations. Those who score high in this theme are often described as ambitious and enthusiastic. They tend to prefer social environments in which they can assume leadership and enjoy persuading others to their viewpoints.

*Conventional:* Individuals have an interest in organization, data, and finance. A high score in this theme indicates that an individual is most effective when dealing with well-defined tasks. In addition, these individuals prefer to know precisely what is expected of them and could be described as orderly and dependable.

According to Holland (1980) these personality descriptions can help one better understand how individual skills and interests relate to career choice and help find careers that best match interests and abilities.

Krumboltz (1976) approached career development theory from a cognitive-behavioral orientation. The theory stressed that each individual's learning experiences, such as generalization of self, sets of developed skills, and career entry behavior, influence an individual's career choice. The process of career development involves four factors: genetic endowments and career opportunities, environmental conditions and events, learning experiences, and task approach skills. Since the career decision-making model is a lifelong process, it is a critical skill to be taught.

More recently, Krumboltz (1998) has proposed that career success often results from "planned happenstance," that is, the individual creates and/or transforms an unplanned event into a life opportunity. Although individuals will admit that unplanned life events influenced their career paths, many see these as happenstance. Krumboltz suggests that the individual often overlooks the intent of their actions, which resulted in the action taken to get to know those who significantly influenced their lives or the purposeful actions that they took to change the event from serendipity to impactful.

The confidence and self-efficacy level of individuals can also influence career development. Bandura's concept of self-efficacy (1993) suggests that an individual's concept of confidence in performing tasks creates the balance between what an individual knows and the resulting action. An individual's beliefs about her or his ability to accomplish a task may be more influential than the actual ability to complete a given task. Turner and Lapan (2002) applied social cognitive career theory (Bandura, 1986) and examined the influence of perceived parental support to career self-efficacy. It was reported that parental support accounted for as much as one-third to almost one-half of their adolescent's career task-related confidence. Once again we are reminded of the influence of parents on youths' decisions about future career choices.

These four approaches—Super, Holland, Krumboltz, and Bandura—offer school counselors a philosophical and theoretical knowledge foundation to construct age-appropriate career-oriented systems that consider developmental life stages, personality influence, learning experiences, and self-confidence to best prepare today's youth for the careers of tomorrow.

## Using a Systemic Approach to Career Development

Career development is the sum of all of the processes and factors that influence and inform career choice and career success over one's lifetime. School counselors are committed to ensuring that each student is prepared to move forward to the next step of life, from grade level to grade level, and to life after high school. Career development provides the pathway.

Niles and Harris-Bowlsbey (2002) define career development as "the lifelong psychological and behavioral process as well as the contextual influences shaping one's career over the lifespan" (p. 7). According to Maddy-Bernstein (2000) career development is "the constellation of psychological, sociological education, physical, economic, and chance factors that combine to influence the nature and significance of work in the total lifespan of any given individual" (p. 2). Theorists have acknowledged that career development is intertwined with personal development (Niles & Goodnough, 1996; Super & Savickas, 1996).

The career development process crosses the lifespan and informs and influences various stages of a person's education and personal growth as she or he seeks career satisfaction. Preparing students to select a career goal and guiding them to enroll in the appropriate coursework that will lead them to achieve their career goals is essential to their success in a 21st-century global community. It should come as no surprise that associations including ASCA, The College Board, the National Career Development Association (NCDA), and the National Association of Secondary School Principals (NASSP) encourage school counselors to provide every student with the necessary help and direction to be successful in school and, ultimately, in life. The need for career development knows no boundaries.

## SCHOOL COUNSELORS: CRITICAL PLAYERS IN CAREER DEVELOPMENT

> Never before in the history of our nation have we had a greater need to prepare every student for the greatest range of opportunities after leaving high school. (National Office for School Counselor Advocacy, 2010, p. 6)

Career development is often the component of the school counseling program that receives the least attention. Every child dreams of success; school counselors are ethically obligated to focus our energies and help every child identify the path to success to realize her or his dreams (Schwallie-Giddis & Kobilaryz, 2000). Transformed school counselors use leadership, advocacy, teaming and collaboration, the use of data, and integrating technology in a meaningful context (Education Trust, 1997) and ensure that all students acquire the career awareness and **career planning** skills to make the connection between today's success in school and ensuring all options after high school.

Osborn and Baggerly (2004) surveyed Florida school counselors in which 79 percent of elementary counselors, 59 percent of middle school counselors, and 31 percent of high school counselors reported spending less time on career guidance than they preferred. They urged school counseling professionals to assist students in their career choices to help every student achieve her or his highest career potential. A national survey (Anctil, Schenk, Smith, & Dahir, 2009) of more than 1,000 practicing ASCA members revealed that career development is practiced at a significantly lower level than academic and personal/social development. Closing the information and opportunity gaps through improved career development activities for students is a prime example of social justice advocacy.

Recently 600 young adults were polled as to the reasons they were not able to complete their postsecondary degrees in a study conducted by Public Agenda (Johnson, J., Rochkind, J., Ott, A., & DuPont, S., 2010). High cost was a major contributing factor in causing them to drop out and these non-degree completers also revealed that their choice of the program of study was selected based on cost and convenience rather than on career choice and quality of program.

A subsequent report by the same organization, Can I Get a Little Advice Here?, concluded that the current high school career and college counseling system is weak in terms of helping to increase college access, attendance, and completion, which is considered a national educational and economic imperative in the Blueprint for Reform. Both degree completers and non-completers gave poor marks to high school counselors with regard to planning for future careers, deciding what postsecondary institution to attend, providing advice on how to pay for college, and working through the college application process. About 50 percent of the respondents indicated that their high school counselors make them feel like "just another face in the crowd." Further findings revealed that non-completers often came from families that had limited financial resources and/or that the student would be the first-generation college attendee, thus relying heavily on the college and career planning advice offered from the school counselor. These respondents assigned a low grade to their school counselors. Research shows that the high school students who are in most need of counseling about getting into and doing well in college are the least likely to get that assistance because of conflicting priorities of counselors (National Office for School Counselor Advocacy, 2010). Too many disadvantaged students are not aware of their career and educational options and they are not academically prepared for college completion despite earning a high school diploma.

The career development process "can be approached systematically and intentionally, or, it can be approached haphazardly and passively" (Niles & Harris-Bowlsbey, 2002, p. 261). At its best, career guidance and counseling offers a sequential, integrated, and coordinated system to connect education with future career opportunities.

# CAREER DECISION INFLUENCERS

Erikson (1968) noted that youth are particularly sensitive to the experiences and influences of those who surround and support them. Students' experiences and familiarity undeniably influence the actions they take about their future. Bandura's (1977) observations remain true today and remind us that social learning can greatly sway aspiration and motivation.

## Parents/Guardians

Parents or guardians have a profound effect on youth decision making. The 42nd Annual Phi Delta Kappa/Gallup Poll (Bunshaw & Lopez, 2010) asked parents if their child will go to college; 92 percent said yes, up from 82 percent in 1995 and 57 percent in 1982. Despite the economic climate, three of four parents believe they are very or somewhat likely to pay for their

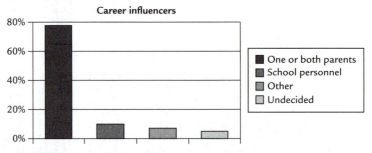

FIGURE **14.3** Career Influencers

Source: Adapted from *Decisions without Directions*, 2002.

child's college education. Parents also provided the reasons for wanting their child to attend college: (1) more job opportunities and better income; (2) have a better life; and (3) people need more education today. Interestingly, these are the same top three reasons parents gave when asked this question in 1982 (Bunshaw & Lopez, 2010, p. 21). However, at the same time, the Gallup poll respondents believed students today are less well-prepared for work or college than when the respondents themselves graduated from high school.

A prior national study of high school juniors and seniors, *Decisions without Directions* (Career Institute for Education and Workforce Development, 2002), concluded that the students surveyed received little or no career guidance outside of their home. Not surprisingly, Figure 14.3 reveals that parents are viewed by their children as the primary influence on career decision making.

Parents and students need to be well aware of the myriad options available to them that will result in satisfying career opportunities, especially with the understanding that parental influence plays a major role in college aspirations. The Phi Delta Kappa/Gallup Poll (Bunshaw & Lopez, 2010) reaffirms the beliefs of parents that college education will lead to a more rewarding career. Hoyt (2002) encouraged educators to inform both students and parents about postsecondary options, including the need to acquire high-tech skills, specialized programs, and facilitation in computer usage. With the job market undergoing rapid change, parents rely on school counselors and career guidance personnel to provide career information and guidance that is aligned with the educational choices that students seek after high school (Bardwell, 2010; Feller, 2003). School counselors can place themselves in the forefront of opening doors to opportunities and closing the information gap, by career guidance programs to support students to meet today's economic challenges (Feller, 2010).

## Educators

As shown in Figure 14.4, educators influence career choice. The study also revealed that teachers can have greater influence on student career decisions than school counselors.

Students also reported that teachers have provided advisement on career options or presented options to help further their education. Sixty-eight percent of the students who participated in *Decisions without Directions*

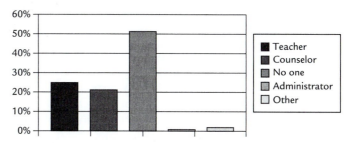

FIGURE **14.4** Educators' Influence on Career Choice
Source: *Decisions without Directions*, 2002.

(2002) believed that the best jobs and career required at a minimum a four-year degree. The prediction is that 90 percent of the fastest-growing jobs of the future will require more than a high school diploma and some postsecondary education (Alliance for Excellent Education, 2007b).

Many students attempt a two- or four-year college degree; however, a much smaller percentage prevail. Although 67.2 percent of high school graduates enroll in college each fall with the intent to complete a four-year bachelor's degree, only 78 percent of full-time students across the nation who enter a four-year institution with the intent to earn a degree are retained from the first year to sophomore year. Similarly, 59 percent of full-time students across the nation who enter a public two-year institution with the intent to earn a degree are retained from the first year to sophomore year. Almost one in four will drop out after the first year and approximately 56 percent will achieve a bachelor's degree in six years or fewer (National Center for Educational Statistics, The Condition of Education, 2009).

School counselors and teachers can help to bury the fallacy that a four-year degree is the only option to a rewarding career and thus help students best match their interests and abilities with their motivation and achievement. Teachers and school counselors are in critical positions to help high school graduates understand that those who do not receive any kind of postsecondary education or training are unlikely to obtain what most persons would describe as a "good" job and one with a "future" (Hoyt, 2001).

## Peers

The influence of the culture and of peers on youth's decision-making ability has been the subject of numerous publications (Howe & Strauss, 2000). Youth share interests and perspectives with their peers but this influence is greater on socialization issues than on career choice (Lesko, 2001). Peer-to-peer influence is focused predominantly on school achievement, substance abuse, and gang involvement, all of which can have a profound impact on students' ability to successfully complete high school (Janosz, Archambault, Morizot, & Pagani, 2008).

Knowing the significant influence that parents and peers play in the college and career planning process, students more than ever need accurate and timely information to help them choose wisely in school and plan for their transition after high school.

# CAREER PLANNING AND COLLEGE ACCESS

Students of privilege may envision themselves in a prestigious four-year college; whereas impoverished youth might see themselves thrust into the workplace as soon as they graduate from high school. Young people growing up in poverty perceive career options differently than more privileged youngsters (Education Trust, 2001a). The postsecondary educational attainment of low-SES students can be facilitated by greater internal locus of control and higher student academic expectations during early adolescence (Lee, Daniels, Puig, Newgent, & Nam, 2008).

Cultural norms and family expectations also can influence career goals. School counselors must be knowledgeable about the cultural traditions that could potentially limit a student's choice of options after high school or create a discord between the student and her or his parents or guardian. Every student, regardless of race, culture, socioeconomic status, or learning ability or disability, can benefit from a career guidance and counseling program. Educators, teachers, school counselors, and school administrators in partnership with parents or guardians have a responsibility to support students to ensure that they all have options after high school and find meaningful paths to careers. *Breaking Ranks* (NASSP, 1996, 2004) encouraged schools to provide every student with a transitional experience to prepare for life after high school and recognized the ultimate need for each student to become a contributing member of the community.

## The ASCA National Model and Career Development

Without the firm commitment and involvement of school counselors and other educators taking a proactive leadership role and assuming the responsibility for designing and implementing a sequential and integrated career development program, many students will receive little or no career guidance support. The American School Counselor Association strongly urges school counselors to provide a balance of academic, career, and personal/social development as the foundation of the comprehensive school counseling program (ASCA, 2005; Campbell & Dahir, 1997).

Career development is one of three student development domains in the comprehensive model (ASCA, 2005). Data present a strong case to provide career development for every student. The foundation of school counseling is strongly grounded in vocational guidance, which emerged in the late 1890s and has been a consistent focus of attention since the origins of the profession.

### *Defining Terms*

**Career counseling** assists students in acquiring a greater understanding that they have choices and the realization that their behaviors affect decisions. Counseling helps students connect their desire for self-efficacy, establish a sense of who they are, and initiate the necessary and essential changes to help them get where they are going.

According to Myrick (2003b) career guidance is the convergence of services that focus on personal and career growth and school adjustment, which assists individuals to choose, enter, and/or progress in an occupation. "Guidance is an

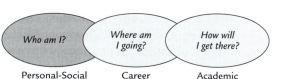

FIGURE **14.5** Connecting to Student Development

instructional process in which a student is given information and told how to move progressively toward a personal goal" (Myrick, 1997, pp. 2–3). In a school setting, we use career guidance strategies to involve students at developmentally appropriate stages in career development. These strategies include career awareness, exploration, assessment planning, and career counseling.

**Career awareness** helps students identify the world of options and opportunities that await them. For many students their familiarity with the world of work is limited to the experiences of parents and family members or what awareness they have acquired from TV and other media. Career awareness helps students connect self-knowledge and information gathering and helps them to see a world of opportunity as they begin to think about their personal and professional futures.

**Career exploration** offers students opportunities in the context of real-life and hands-on experiences to supplement traditional classroom instruction. Experiences such as connecting school learning with part-time work, project-based learning, career and technical education, mentoring and shadowing experiences, service learning, apprenticeships, internships, and co-op education are motivational and help students become more aware of the world of possibilities.

**Career assessment** helps students use the information they gain from appraisal of skills, abilities, achievement, and interests to better understand who they are, where they are going, and how they will get there as they acquire skills in personal-social, career, and academic development (see Figure 14.5).

### Career Assessment and Planning Tools

School counselors use a variety of achievement, interest, and ability assessments to consult with students, parents, and teachers and help all involved in understanding the outcomes of the results and how to use the information in meaningful ways. Assessments can be as simple as a one-page interest survey or as complex as the Armed Services Vocational Aptitude Battery (ASVAB), which involves several hours for a student to complete. Many interest inventories (Self Directed Search, the Strong Interest Inventory) and Computer Assisted Career Guidance Systems (Discover, Choices, SIGI-PLUS) are based on Holland's theory and help students identify the relationship between personality type and career preference.

The **Myers-Briggs Type Indicator** (MBTI) is a widely used personality assessment for high school students and provides feedback about an individual's patterns of behavior. Based on the theory of psychological types by Carl Jung, the MBTI can help students understand their preference in making decisions, organizing one's life, and acquiring information. The MBTI use four categories of behavior that address the focus of a person's orientation (extraversion or introversion); the way a person gathers information (sensing or by intuition); the way a person makes decisions (thinking or by feeling); and how a person deals with the outer world (judging or perceiving). The MBTI also helps students understand personal preferences in relationship to the outer world of people and things or to the inner world of ideas, and this understanding is articulated with career environments that may be best suited to their personality. After students gather information, participate in assessments, and engage in exploratory experiences, they are ready to create a career plan.

New and emerging technologies bring us Computer Assisted Career Guidance Systems (CACGS) to deliver career awareness, exploration, and career planning across a broad range of student activities and experiences. These Internet-based systems offer students and adults the ability to explore the world of work, gather information, participate in interest surveys and other career assessments, and help clients with career decision-making. CACGS assist individuals in making current career decisions as well as improving their capacity to make effective career decisions in the future and offer current information, immediate feedback, interactive simulations, and data storage (Gore & Leuwerke, 2000).

Similarly, College Information Systems are comprehensive search engines that help students to research interests, college majors, and work their way through the maze of information about the more than 3,000 institutions of higher education available in the United States. Additionally, 20 percent of the states have college- and career-ready assessment systems in place, while 45 percent are in the process of developing systems (Achieve, 2009). So much information is available that the challenge for students and parents is to have the assistance they need to understand and sort through available options and prioritize. A representative list of College and Career Resources can be found in Tech Tools and the end of this chapter.

Several states have developed "Career Plans," which align education goals with career goals. These systems recognize that students should begin the career planning process as early as elementary school and encourage all stakeholders to help students acquire the skills students needed to transition from grade level to grade level, and from high school to quality postsecondary and career opportunities. A career plan helps students establish a focus and a motivation for their achievement and can identify the strategies and tasks necessary to accomplish future goals. It guides students to make decisions about academic preparation, work experience, and the education and training necessary after high school to make successful transitions to the career path of their choice. The New York State Career Plan and Utah's Student Educational/Occupational Plan are examples of two statewide systems.

A career plan also documents the results of aptitudes, skills, interests, and personal preferences achieved by each student throughout their elementary, middle, and high school experiences. As part of an annual process to review educational and career goals, students can make necessary adjustments as knowledge and skills are attained and/or interests change. Career planning documents and demonstrates student acquisition of the competencies in the *National Standards for School Counseling Programs* (1997) and/or those in the *National Career Development Guidelines* (1989, rev. 2004). Students, teachers, and parents are now more aware of the knowledge and skills acquired as a result of participating in a school counseling program.

Practicing school counselors use the comprehensive school counseling program model to incorporate and integrate career guidance strategies into the academic, career, and personal-social development activities and services as part of the implementation of the Delivery System quadrant of the ASCA National Model: guidance curriculum; individual student planning; responsive services, and system support (ASCA, 2005).

## Career Development Is Everyone's Responsibility

Professional school counselors are faced with the daunting task of helping students develop the necessary skills, knowledge, and self-awareness needed to actively engage in effective educational planning as they progress from middle school to high school, to a postsecondary opportunity and to their future careers. The good news is that school counselors do not have to do this alone. Reaching out to teachers and college/university partners, school counselors can develop and implement a collaborative career and early college awareness program to help students identify their interests, skills, and aspirations, while helping them develop the decision-making and planning skills they will need to begin to implement short- and long-term goals.

---

### MEET LOURDES RIVERA, MARYBETH SCHAEFFER, ELIZABETH OPHALS, AND EBERTO (BOBBY) PINIERO

## The Career Institute: A Pathway to Decision Making

*"I liked that I was able to see what options I have available for me as a career. It is exciting to see how many career occupations I can have that match my interests."*

—a seventh-grade student

The Career Institute (CI) is a collaborative effort designed to integrate career development and early college awareness into the culture and mission of an urban city school that opened its doors five years ago to its first sixth-grade class. Developed by two university faculty members in collaboration with the school staff, the CI currently offers career-related interventions for sixth-, seventh-, eighth-, ninth-, and 10th-grade students. As the school continues to grow, interventions will be developed for the 11th and 12th grades, which will eventually be added to the school.

*(continues)*

The main activities of the CI take place over a three- to four-week period. During that time, students participate in a series of interventions specifically designed to engage them in the process of identifying and examining their interests, values, abilities, and skills and begin thinking about and planning for their post–high school educational and career goals. Ongoing collaboration among the school counselor, teachers, and college faculty assures that all stakeholders remain invested in the program. The lesson plans are delivered in the classroom setting by teachers during teacher-led advisory class periods with the support and assistance of the school counselor. Advisory lessons that require more in-depth career development theory or instruction (e.g., teaching students about the Holland types) are conducted by the school counselor and college faculty with assistance from the teachers.

As part of the college partnership, students participate in activities organized on the college campus. Last year all seventh-grade students attended a large lecture-type class during which they received information on Holland's theory. Students were excited to attend "class on campus" and participated in the lecture class as would be expected of college students. These types of on-campus events expose students to the college environment and help foster a sense of belonging that is expected to positively influence students' overall planning for the future.

Each year, the CI activities are followed up with a Career Day (CD). To make CD an integral part of the CI and the school's academic goals, speakers are asked to provide a brief career-oriented biography that students read in their advisory class prior to the visit. The advisory teachers use the biographies and the experiences students have had in the CI to help students develop interview questions for CD speakers. In follow-up advisory sessions, students discuss their experience with CD, process their thoughts, and reflect on their developing sense of self as it relates to career awareness and college readiness. Students then complete a reflective writing assignment focused on what they have learned through the CI and CD.

Developing and implementing a systemic career development and early college awareness program and getting the participation and commitment of the entire school staff can be a monumental endeavor for even the most enthusiastic and energetic school counselor. Here are strategies that can contribute to making the effort more manageable:

1. Establish an ongoing dialogue with the school principal that focuses on ways in which the school counseling program can contribute to achieving the school's mission. In developing the CI, the school principal was involved in every step of the process from the conceptual to the more pragmatic issues that needed to be addressed. These types of conversations not only help to educate the principal on what could be done but

also provide the school counselor with a broader understanding of the administrative issues that need to be attended to. Providing the principal with a vision of how school counseling can contribute to achieving the mission of the school is essential.

2. Gain the active participation of the teachers. With the principal's support, opportunities for discussions between the CI coordinators (i.e., school counselors, college staff) and teachers were organized. These discussions focused on how career development interventions throughout the students' education at the school might help teachers motivate and engage students in the classroom. Teachers participated in professional development workshops on career development, the importance of fostering self-awareness among students, and helping students make connections between school work and their future.

3. Provide ongoing opportunities for the school faculty to collaborate on the development of the CI activities and invite teachers to identify and develop activities they believe would contribute to meeting the goal of college and career readiness for all students. This may be accomplished informally, through hallway dialogues and shared lunch hours, and formally through surveys and professional development.

## Sample CI Activities by Grade Level
### Sixth Grade

- Complete a series of activity sheets to identify interests and skills (e.g., drawing, writing)
- Small-group discussions in which students share and discuss their interests and strengths
- Debriefing activities to encourage students to discuss what they have learned and relate this information to school achievement and the world of work

### Seventh Grade

- The Self-Directed Search-Career Explorer (SDS-CE)
- The Holland type theory (Holland, 1997)
- Use the type codes to organize information about themselves and the world of work
- Identify career options related to their type and unrelated to their type

### Eighth Grade

- Conduct online research on a particular occupation
- Investigate colleges that offer majors in their areas of interest
- Engage in class discussion with peers and adults about the information they have acquired
- Prepare a brief research report that becomes part of their school portfolio

*(continues)*

### Ninth Grade

- More in-depth research of occupations and college majors (e.g., what, where, and entry-level requirements)
- Research colleges (e.g., admission requirements)
- Draft initial personal statement/college application essay

### Tenth Grade

- Administration of the Strong Interest Inventory-College Profile
- In-depth exploration of interests, college majors, and college courses
- Decision-making and time management
- College visits

*Attending to the career development needs of students and providing appropriate interventions to facilitate students' career development has always been an essential role of the professional school counselor. Working with college/university partners and teachers, school counselors can ensure that students' career development needs are addressed and that they have ample opportunities to make connections between the learning that is taking place in their classes and their future educational and career goals.*

*Lourdes M. Rivera, PhD, is an associate professor in Counselor Education at Queens College. She previously worked as a counselor in a college setting providing academic, career, and personal counseling. MaryBeth Schaefer is an assistant professor in Curriculum and Teaching at St. John's University. Elizabeth Ophals is the school principal and Eberto (Bobby) Piniero is a school counselor at the School of Inquiry.*

## CONNECTING TO STANDARDS AND COMPETENCIES

Student attitudes, skills, and knowledge are the foundation for the comprehensive model (ASCA, 2005). The majority of career development and career guidance systems and programs use either the *National Career Development Guidelines* (2004) or the *National Standards for School Counseling Programs* (1997) to select the competencies that ascertain what students should know and be able to do.

### The National Career Development Guidelines

Recognizing the benefits of a systematic career guidance program across the lifespan, the National Occupational Information Coordinating Committee (NOICC) designed the **National Career Development Guidelines** (1989b, rev. 2004). These guidelines offered the counseling and career guidance community a framework to help students and adults acquire the skills necessary for success in the workplace. Through a developmental and organized process, adults and students could explore their interests, apply acquired skills and abilities, discover the many educational and occupational opportunities and options available, become aware of the education and training required for their career choice, and begin to develop and manage their career pathway. The National Career Development Guidelines help students and adults:

- Understand the relationship between educational achievement and career planning
- Understand the need for positive attitudes toward work and learning

- Acquire skills to locate, evaluate, and interpret career information
- Acquire skills to prepare to seek, obtain, maintain, and change jobs
- Understand how societal needs and functions influence the nature and structure of work

(NOICC, 1989b; rev. 2004)

The guidelines address three major competency areas: self-knowledge, educational and occupational exploration, and career planning.

*Self-knowledge* guides students to become competent in their knowledge and understanding of self-concept, acquire skills to interact with others, and to recognize and understand the importance of growth and change. As students transition into adulthood, they learn and apply these skills to maintain a positive self-concept and demonstrate behaviors that are effective at home and in the workplace.

*Educational and occupational exploration* assists students to acquire competency in making connections between educational achievement and career planning. Students acquire skills in locating information, evaluating and interpreting career information, and learn to apply this information to seeking, obtaining, maintaining, and changing jobs.

*Career planning* provides students with knowledge of the career planning process and support to make the decisions that align their educational goals with career goals. Students combine what they have learned about self-knowledge and the results of their educational and occupational exploration to develop a plan that will help them make informed decisions about their present and the future. Students begin to understand the influence of affective and academic skill development in the context of life-career choices.

The *National Career Development Guidelines* (1989, 2004) were carefully examined for their applicability and relationship during the development stages of the *National Standards for School Counseling Programs* (ASCA, 1997). The guidelines, summarized below, offered a strong foundation for the academic, career, and personal-social domains.

## The Career Development Domain and the ASCA National Model

The ASCA National Model (2005) emphasizes the use of the ASCA National Standards (1997b) to employ strategies to support student achievement and success, provide career awareness, open doors to opportunities, encourage self-awareness, foster interpersonal skills, and help all students acquire skills for life. "[T]he standards assist students in acquiring and using life-long skills through the development of academic, career, self awareness and interpersonal skills" (Campbell & Dahir, 1997, p. 9).

The national standards for career development guide school counselors to implement school counseling program strategies and activities that will help students acquire attitudes, knowledge, and skills to successfully transition from grade to grade, from school to postsecondary education, and ultimately to the world of work. Career development activities include the employment of strategies to achieve future career success and job satisfaction, as well as

## BOX 14.1

*National Career Development Guidelines: Career Development Competencies by Area and Level*

## Self-Knowledge

*Elementary*
- Knowledge of the importance of self-concept
- Skills to interact with others
- Awareness of the importance of growth and change

*Middle/Junior High School*
- Knowledge of the influence of a positive self-concept
- Skills to interact with others
- Knowledge of the importance of growth and change

*High School*
- Understanding the influence of a positive self-concept
- Skills to interact positively with others
- Understanding the impact of growth and development

*Adult*
- Skills to maintain a positive self-concept
- Skills to maintain effective behaviors
- Understanding developmental changes and transitions

## Educational and Occupational Exploration

*Elementary*
- Awareness of the benefits of educational achievement
- Awareness of the relationship between work and learning
- Skills to understand and use career information
- Awareness of the importance of personal responsibility and good work habits
- Awareness of how work relates to the needs and functions of society

*Middle/Junior High School*
- Knowledge of the benefits of educational achievement to career opportunities
- Understanding the relationship between work and learning
- Skills to locate, understand, and use career information
- Knowledge of skills necessary to seek and obtain jobs
- Understanding how work relates to the needs and functions of the economy and society

*High School*
- Understanding the relationship between educational achievement and career planning
- Understanding the need for positive attitudes toward work and learning
- Skills to locate, evaluate, and interpret career information

- Skills to prepare to seek, obtain, maintain, and change jobs
- Understanding how societal needs and functions influence the nature and structure of work

## Adult

- Skills to enter and participate in education and training
- Skills to participate in work and lifelong learning
- Skills to locate, evaluate, and interpret career information
- Skills to prepare to seek, obtain, maintain, and change jobs
- Understanding how the needs and functions of society influence the nature and structure of work

## Career Planning

### Elementary

- Understanding how to make decisions
- Awareness of the interrelationship of life roles
- Awareness of different occupations and changing male/female roles
- Awareness of the career planning process

### Middle/Junior High School

- Skills to make decisions
- Knowledge of the interrelationship of life roles
- Knowledge of different occupations and changing male/female roles
- Understanding the process of career planning

### High School

- Skills to make decisions
- Understanding the interrelationship of life roles
- Understanding the continuous changes in male/female roles
- Skills in career planning

### Adult

- Skills to make decisions
- Understanding the impact of work on individual and family life
- Understanding the continuing changes in male/female roles
- Skills to make career transitions

Source: National Occupational Information Coordinating Committee (NOICC), U.S. Department of Labor (1992, 2004).

fostering understanding of the relationship between personal qualities, education and training, and future career goals.

School counselors are encouraged to identify competencies for their students that will help them developmentally acquire the attitudes, knowledge, and skills that are integral to a career development program. The standards and competencies encourage students to participate in a series of structured activities that result in applying decision-making and planning skills in building their futures. The competencies selected should involve students in all aspects of a comprehensive career guidance system, which include career awareness, exploration, assessment, counseling, and planning.

Thus, by the time a student graduates from high school, she or he should formulate and bring into focus tentative career goals, select the appropriate academic and career/technical postsecondary options, and identify the levels of competence, certification, and/or achievement necessary to reach their goals.

# ALL STUDENTS: COLLEGE AND CAREER READY

The goal for America's educational system is clear: Every student should graduate from high school ready for college and a career. Every student should have meaningful opportunities to choose from upon graduation from high school. (President Barack Obama in ESEA Blueprint for Reform, in ESEA Blueprint for Reform, U.S. Department of Education, Office of Planning, Evaluation and Policy Development Blueprint for Reform, 2010, p. 7)

In today's global, knowledge-based economy, a college education is the gateway to social mobility and better lifelong opportunities. The vast majority of America's high school students (86%) expect to attend college, but many lack the support and guidance they need to prepare for enrollment and success in college (U.S. Department of Education, NCES 2010-170). Furthermore, as depicted in Table 14.2, college-going rates differ disproportionately by family income, parent education level, and other demographic characteristics. Too few students are graduating from high school ready for college. This education deficit is an urgent concern for the future of the nation as a whole and for our most underserved communities.

## TABLE **14.2**
Percentage of 25- to 29-Year-Olds Who Attained Selected Levels of Education in 2009.

| | African Americans | Asians | Latinos | Caucasian |
|---|---|---|---|---|
| Graduate from High School | 89% | 96% | 69% | 95% |
| Complete at Least Some College | 53% | 79% | 35% | 68% |
| Obtain at Least a Bachelor's Degree | 19% | 56% | 12% | 37% |

Source: Aud, S., Hussar, W., Planty, M., Snyder, T., Bianco, K., Fox, M., Frohlich, L., Kemp, J., & Drake, L. (2010). The Condition of Education 2010 (NCES 2010-028). National Center for Education Statistics, Institute of Education Sciences, U.S. Department of Education. Washington, DC.

## MEET ROBERT BARDWELL

### Comprehensive Counseling Changes the College and Career Culture

While the career and college culture in a school is influenced by the community in which the school is located, the school counseling program can inspire, cultivate, and motivate the college-going population.

At Monson High School, Massachusetts, the school counselors deliver a comprehensive and developmentally appropriate career and college program. Piggybacking on work begun in middle school, the two school counselors and career facilitator begin with ninth graders completing interviews within the first month of school during which future plans are discussed as well as finding out if the student is a first-generation college-going student. Students then complete a four-page career plan folder in ninth-grade health class that includes setting goals and strategies to accomplish those goals as well as a four-year plan, listing which classes would be taken in each year of high school.

Specific evening programs for students and parents are held in grades 10–12. In the early fall of grade 10 students and parents are encouraged to start thinking about college options, appropriate course selection, and extracurricular involvement with a presentation by a local college's director of admission. In collaboration with the English department, students write a research paper on a career linked to their previous career inventories and assessments. Junior year provides SAT prep classes at night both in the fall and the spring, college prep night with speakers from regional colleges, a field trip to the local national college fair, and an individual parent conference for each student during the school day in the spring. Senior year offers individual counselor appointments in early fall, an evening refresher program, and a financial aid night in November. Woven throughout each year are activities in our student advisory program held every other week for 27 minutes as well as activities during our annual Career & College Awareness Week each March, including the ever-popular door decorating contest, a competition between advisory groups where they choose a college and must decorate the door, which is then judged according to an established rubric.

Since implementing many of the above programs, the postsecondary rate increases from 78 percent in 2002 to a high of 93 percent in 2008 and dipping slightly to 88 percent in 2010. This could not be accomplished without the collaboration of administration, teachers, and counselors, as well as the vital role played by parents, community members, and business owners. The counseling staff ensure that every student can be successful in selecting a career commensurate with goal. Establishing a college-going culture takes a coordinated and consistent effort by all school staff. If done right, college-going success is not an accident but rather the result of a comprehensive school counseling and career guidance program.

*Robert Bardwell has been a school counselor for the past 17 years and serves as the director of guidance and student support services at Monson High School in addition to his student caseload. He is a past president of the New England Association for College Admission Counseling and secondary level vice president for the American School Counselor Association. Robert is an adjunct professor at several colleges, teaching both school counseling and college admission counseling courses for school counselors.*

## College and Career Readiness Counseling

Recently, the College Board National Office for School Counselor Advocacy released a comprehensive, systemic approach for school counselors' use to inspire all students to, and prepare them for, college success and opportunity intended especially for students from underrepresented populations. These eight components offer enriching activities, foster rigorous academic preparation, encourage early college planning, and guide students and families through the college admission and financial aid processes. By implementing these eight components, school counselors close the college and career planning information and opportunity gap and provide information, tools, and perspective to parents, students, schools, and their communities that build college and career readiness for all students.

*The Eight Components of College and Career Readiness Counseling*

A systemic approach for school counselors to implement, across grades K–12 and beyond, to build aspirations and social capital, and ensure equity both in process and results.

1. *College Aspirations*
   *Goal:* Build a college-going culture based on early college awareness by nurturing in students the confidence to aspire to college and the resilience to overcome challenges along the way. Maintain high expectations by providing adequate supports, building social capital and conveying the conviction that all students can succeed in college.
2. *Academic Planning for College and Career Readiness*
   *Goal:* Advance students' planning, preparation, participation and performance in a rigorous academic program that connects to their college and career aspirations and goals.
3. *Enrichment and Extracurricular Engagement*
   *Goal:* Ensure equitable exposure to a wide range of extracurricular and enrichment opportunities that build leadership, nurture talents and interests, and increase engagement with school.
4. *College and Career Exploration and Selection Processes*
   *Goal:* Provide early and ongoing exposure to experiences and information necessary to make informed decisions when selecting a college or career that connects to academic preparation and future aspirations.
5. *College and Career Assessments*
   *Goal:* Promote preparation, participation and performance in college and career assessments by all students.

6. *College Affordability Planning*
   *Goal:* Provide students and families with comprehensive information about college costs, options for paying for college, and the financial aid and scholarship processes and eligibility requirements, so they are able to plan for and afford a college education.
7. *College and Career Admission Processes*
   *Goal:* Ensure that students and families have an early and ongoing understanding of the college and career application and admission processes so they can find the postsecondary options that are the best fit with their aspirations and interests.
8. *Transition from High School Graduation to College Enrollment*
   *Goal:* Connect students to school and community resources to help the students overcome barriers and ensure the successful transition from high school to college.

Source: The College Board, 2010, reprinted with permission.

## Equity and Access

We can't really afford to sort people into those who have access to privileged knowledge and so find it relatively easy to go on to college and those who might be first-generation college students and don't have easy access to that knowledge. Those students are not being given the same opportunities. Whether we believe education is entirely for one's personal growth and development or whether we believe it's a means to an end, this country as a whole probably can't survive in the form we know if we don't ensure that postsecondary access and success are attainable now by students who would be the first in their families to attend college, and not something that takes those children and their families generations to achieve. (Conley, D., 2010, p. 34)

The National Center for Education Statistics (2008) reminds us that only 58 percent of low-income-family high school students are enrolling in college right after graduation. Low-income-family students dropped out of high school at rates twice as high as that of White students (National Center for Education Statistics, 2008). Only 10 percent of low-income students earned their bachelor's degrees by age 24 in 2006 (U.S. Census Bureau, 2008); conversely, 72 percent of high-income students earned their bachelor's degrees by age 24 in 2006.

As Table 14.3 indicates, even though college enrollment is increasing for low-income students, they still haven't reached the rate of high-income students in the mid-1970s.

The Education Trust (1997) expressed concern about the number of low-income and minority students who leave school prior to graduation not because of their inabilities to succeed, but because they are not being challenged academically; additionally, they are being placed disproportionately in special education and low-level or remedial classes. The Education Trust (2009) also reminded us that many of our high schools in the 21st century, especially those serving concentrations of low-income and minority students, don't prepare their college-bound students for postsecondary education.

TABLE **14.3**

Students' Family Income Level and College Enrollment

| Year | Low Income | Middle Income | High Income |
|------|-----------|---------------|-------------|
| 1978 | 39% | 41% | 63% |
| 1988 | 34% | 49% | 71% |
| 1998 | 49% | 63% | 78% |
| 2008 | 51% | 61% | 81% |

Source: U.S. Department of Education, NCES, the Condition of Education, 2010.

Table 14.4 additionally notes the disparities in college completion. The graduation rates reveal unequal success rates and also point to the need to improve all four-year college degree completion rates across all populations to reach the goal of all students "college and career ready."

> It is time to "own the turf." If not you, who? Who in the school is responsible for helping students nurture their dreams for bright futures and for helping them create successful pathways to those dreams? All of our students need school counselors to champion their cause. Each one of them is entitled to a rigorous education that prepares them to successfully attain their college and career goals. (National Office for School Counselor Advocacy, Patricia Martin, 2010, p. 6)

There is an endless array of career development and career guidance options and opportunities available to school counselors to motivate students to strive to reach their future goals. Often, it is hard for us to understand why some students just don't seem to "get it"! Why can't they see the connection between education and future success? The influence of parents, culture, and a child's self-confidence will always significantly influence one's decision about future career choices. Culture of origin can influence their life-career choices. Gender matters whether it's breaking down parental or community biases or working closely with a student needing support to choose a nontraditional career path.

Helping students make connections is the key to affecting future choice between and among students, their counselors, teachers, peers, family, and,

TABLE **14.4**

National Six-Year Graduation Rates of Bachelor's Degree-Seeking Students by Race/Ethnicity, 2007

| African Americans | Asians | Native Americans | Latinos | Caucasian |
|-------------------|--------|------------------|---------|-----------|
| 45% | 65.5% | 38.6% | 46.8% | 59.4% |

Source: U.S. Census Bureau, Current Population Survey, 2010. U.S. Census Bureau, American Community Survey, 2010. http://factfinder.census.gov.

most importantly, seeing the relevance of school to their dreams and aspirations. School is a place for youth to exert their influence and establish an identity. School is a place to explore, learn, apply, and acquire academic and affective attitudes, knowledge, and skills. School counselors face the challenge of helping students meet expectations of the higher academic standards and simultaneously assist students to successfully be prepared to become productive and contributing members of our society. Career motivation contributes strongly to a student's willingness to work a little harder, put forth a little more effort, and better understand the relevance of school to future opportunity. Comprehensive school counseling programs that include a strong career development and career guidance component will help our students to

- understand who they are, their interests, motivation, and ability;
- develop skills in the career planning process;
- establish career goals;
- become involved in career awareness and career exploration activities;
- visualize a positive future, close the information and opportunity gaps; and
- make connections between personal qualities, achievement, the motivation to get an education, and dreams of success.

Career development can no longer be put on the back burner. The ASCA National Standards remind us that is a full one-third of the work of school counselors with preK–12 students. Our Ethical Codes and our commitment to social justice require all school counselors to motivate students to discover their passions and work with them to develop goals and strategies, which invaluably contribute to helping students realize their dreams. The time is now for school counselors to step up to "own the turf."

## TECH TOOLS

When you become a school counselor use the power of technology to maximize the efficiency and effectiveness of career planning.

- Update your school counseling department website every week to highlight an occupation and include the skills, abilities, and education necessary to successfully perform that occupation. No website? Set one up. Try www.weebly.com.
- Collaborate with academic teachers to identify ways they can highlight the array of careers that require particular knowledge and skills in their subject areas. For example, social studies teachers can emphasize careers in fields such as journalism, communications, politics, travel and tourism etc., that require an understanding of history and geography as well as excellent writing skills.
- On giving an interest inventory, provide lists of occupations that fit that interest area. Try http://online.onetcenter.org for initial information. Have students identify the educational requirements of the occupations that seem most interesting to them at this point.

- Use search engines such as CollegeBoard.com to help students identify colleges that match their wish lists and collect and save data about each one.
- Record your parent workshops on career and college planning college applications, financial aid, time management, costs, and other important topics on web-based systems such as Elluminate.com or Voicethread.com so that parents/families who could not attend the face-to-face session have another opportunity to access the information. Use a translator to have the session available in languages spoken by the families in your student population.
- Track your students' two- and four-year college applicants to (a) see if they have been admitted and (b) if they finish their certificates or degrees. Interview non-completers to identify the obstacles.
- Create or search for YouTube videos on topics related to career development that are directed to students and parents.
- Update your professional knowledge by looking at career development resources from the American School Counselor Association (www.schoolcousnelor.org); National Career Development Association (www.ncda.org); and the Association of Career and Technical Education (www.acte.net).
- There are many free career exploration tools, such as the following:
  www.Careerzone.net
  www.careervoyages.org
  www.careerweb.com
  www.careeronestop.org
  www.MyeCareers101.com

These are most helpful in your work with students. Review your state department of labor's website as this is often a good place to find additional resources.

- If your school does not have the resources to build a career center consider a virtual career center and link this to the school counseling department website.
- Design an electronic newsletter for parents and students on career planning.
- The National Association of College Admissions Counseling (NACAC) can be found at www.nacac.net. Look on the NACAC website for resources to help you prepare and present a multimedia presentation on career or college planning to an audience of students, parents, or faculty.

## Internet Resources

Associations

National Association of College Admissions Counseling: www.nacac.net

National Career Development Association: http://ncda.org/

College Board: www.collegeboard.com

Career Information Resources

### America's Career InfoNet—Career Resource Library

Review a collection of links to local, state, and national career and labor market information sites: www.acinet.org/acinet/library-redirect.asp?category=1.6.

### America's Career Resource Network (ACRNA) Fact Sheets

ACRNA is excited to release three fact sheets outlining the critical role that teachers, counselors, and families play in assisting young people to make informed career and academic choices: www.acrna.net/.

### Junior Achievement (JA)

Check out these jointly produced materials designed to teach students about the world of work and engage them in the career planning process: www.ja.org/near/near_map.asp.

### National Career Development Guidelines (NCDG)

Use these guidelines to identify activities and strategies for developing high-quality career programs: http://associationdatabase.com/aws/NCDA/asset_manager/get_file/3384; http://cte.ed.gov/acrn/ncdg/ncdg_framework.aspx.

### Office of Vocational and Adult Education (OVAE)

Obtain information to help prepare young people and adults for postsecondary education and careers: http://www2.ed.gov/about/offices/list/ovae/index.html

ACT: www.act.org

Bureau of Labor Statistics: www.bls.gov

Discover: http://Act.org/discover

Into Careers: http://Intocareers.com

Focus: http://Focuscareer.com

Journal of Technology and Counseling: http://jtc.colstate.edu

My Future: http://Myfuture.com

Next Steps: www.nextsteps.org/

Occupational Outlook Handbook: www.bls.gov/oco/

Occupational Outlook Quarterly: www.bls.gov/opub/ooq/ooqhome.htm

U.S. Department of Labor: www.dol.gov

SIGI Plus: http://ETS.org

U.S. News and World Report: www.usnews.com/usnews/edu/eduhome.htm

Careers and Colleges

Blueprint for Reform: www2.ed.gov/policy/elsec/leg/blueprint
College Major Resource Kits: www.udel.edu/CSC/mrk.htm
University of Delaware Career Services Center's Major Resource Kits: Link academicmajors to career alternatives.

What do I do with a major in?

www.uncwil.edu/stuaff/career/majors.htm
Part of the University of North Carolina's website.

Researching Colleges

College View: www.collegeview.com
By combining a database of 3,300 two- and four-year colleges with multimedia "tours," College View gives students and parents a general overview of a college, plus a direct email option for requesting additional information.

College Board Online: www.collegeboard.org
A college search software online, free, to find colleges that match your goals and interests.

Embark: www.embark.com
A comprehensive site that can help you navigate the college research process.

Peterson's Education Center: www.petersons.com
Peterson's college database is available on this homepage, as is other educational and career information.

Maricopa Center: www.mcli.dist.maricopa.edu/cc
The Maricopa Center for Learning and Instruction (MCLI) site contains a searchable index to the websites for 773 community colleges in the United States, Canada, and elsewhere around the world.

RWM: www.rwm.org
RWM provides information on Private Post Secondary Vocational Schools in all 50 states.

The Princeton Review: www.review.com
You may search the Princeton Review's site by the school's name, region, state, size, and cost.

# School Counselor Casebook: Voices from the Field

## The Scenario Reviewed

Two ninth-grade students stop by your office. You know that both of these students are in the honors program and they have done well so far this school year. The students tell you that they no longer want to be in the more challenging program. They claim that it is not that the work is too difficult but that but they are clueless as to why they are in this class and not taking the regular grade-level courses. When they asked their homeroom teacher why they have to be in the honors program, he said that it will help them get into college. The students told you that other members of the class have asked the same question and were not able to get any additional reasons. After you speak to these two students you realize that they have no awareness of career opportunities, why students go to college, and what it will take to succeed in life.

What would you do?

## A Practitioner's Approach

Here's how a practicing school counselor responded to the school counselor casebook challenge:

I explained to the students that graduation requires successful completion of prescribed coursework. However, being a high school graduate is not the same as being prepared for college. *College readiness* implies rigorous coursework that challenges students to think beyond their levels of comfort and venture into unchartered territories. Demanding courses provide opportunities to develop global career-related skills and values applicable both in college and the workplace: problem-solving strategies, persistence, tolerance, perseverance, self-management, and strong work ethics. Most importantly, I want to make sure that they recognize the value of being in an honors program and how this path can lead to the opportunity to take Advanced Placement (AP) courses next year or enrolling in college-level (dual enrollment) courses as a senior. Although the students nodded in agreement, I was not convinced that they made the connection between today's program of study and their readiness for college-level work four years from now.

Ninth-grade students don't always understand the connection between their classes and their future. Although my colleagues and I visited the ninth-grade classes several times this year, and talked about goal setting and selecting the appropriate course work for future plans, we realized that we may need to do more to help them make the connections. Our comprehensive school counseling program aligns the career development standards with the academic development standards and our state's academic expectations. It would be appropriate to show the ninth graders how this all fits together.

Ninth graders are caught in the difficult time of transition and adjusting to a different level of rigor and expectations than in middle school. On a broader scale, a comprehensive approach to career preparation needs to be implemented where *all* students can readily understand the connections between school success and job success. When students explore the educational requirements for various careers they will be able to understand the need to take particular high school courses and how that coursework will support their future endeavors as they begin to explore postsecondary options.

*Dr. Kim H. Rodriguez has worked in the school counseling field since 1989 as both a school counselor and counselor educator. On the university level, Kim served as Coordinator of the School Counseling Program and Chair of the School Counseling Advisory Board and published her research on various counseling issues. An active member of the professional community, Kim Rodriguez has supervised numerous school counseling interns and is presently the lead school counselor in a large suburban high school.*

# LOOKING BACK: SALIENT POINTS

## Succeeding in the Global Environment

Increased academic expectations, pressures from the global economy, changing technology, and the continuous shifts in societal issues and values affect and influence today's schools. Preparing students to select career goals and guiding them to enroll in the appropriate coursework that will lead them to achieve their career goals is essential to their success in a 21st-century world.

Although no one can predict with complete accuracy which jobs will exist in the future and which will not, school counselors can communicate to students that jobs with a prediction of decline will need workers to replace those who leave the labor force through attrition and retirement. Data also strongly suggest that education pays.

## Theoretical Underpinnings

Career counseling is guided by theory, which provides a point of reference from which the counselor develops a personal perspective of human growth, development, and behavior. Career counselors also recognize and choose the appropriate orientations and strategies, theories and approaches according to the models applied and the assistance that a student needs.

## School Counselors: Critical Players in Career Development

School counselors can take a leadership role and assume the responsibility for designing and implementing a sequential and integrated career development program. The American School Counselor Association urges school counselors to provide a balance of academic, career, and personal/social development as the foundation of the comprehensive school counseling program.

## Career Decision Influencers

Youth are particularly sensitive to the experiences of those who surround and support them. The circumstances and influences that students face undeniably influence the actions they take about their future. Key influencers include parents, educators, and peers.

Many students struggle with weak academic preparation, little career guidance, and few workplace experiences. Without the commitment of school counselors and other educators who take seriously the responsibility to design and implement sequential and integrated career development programs, many students will receive little or no career guidance support.

## Career Planning and College Access

Educators, teachers, school counselors, and school administrators in partnership with parents or guardians have a responsibility to support students to ensure that they have all options after high schools and find meaningful paths to careers. Every student needs a transitional experience to prepare for life after high school.

## Career Development Is Everyone's Responsibility

All educators have a responsibility to support students to ensure that they have explored all options available after high school and identify meaningful paths to careers. Involving all stakeholders shows community commitment and support to prepare today's students for an ever-changing and complex world.

## Connecting to Standards and Competencies

The majority of school counseling programs use the National Career Development Guidelines or the National Standards for School Counseling Programs (1997) to identify specific competencies for student career awareness and development.

### All Students: College and Career Ready

Helping students make connections is the key to affecting future choice between and among students, their counselors, teachers, peers, family, and, most importantly, seeing the relevance of school to their dreams and aspirations. Ensuring equity and access is the school counselor's contribution to closing the information and achievement gaps and will assist students to become productive and contributing members of our society.

## KEY TERMS

College and career readiness
  steps p. 420

Career awareness p. 421

Career guidance p. 424

Career counseling p. 425

Life span–life space p. 425

Career development p. 425

Self-directed search p. 426

Career planning p. 428

Myers-Briggs type indicator p. 433

Computer assisted career guidance
  information systems p. 433

National career development
  guidelines p. 438

## LEARNING EXTENSIONS/MAKING CONNECTIONS

1. What career project might you engage your high school students in that would help them identify what they want to be doing two years from now, five years from now, and 10 years from now?

2. Take a close look at the Partnership for the 21st Century Skills. Ask your students to identify which skills they believe are most important to achieve their educational and career plans.

3. Your school is situated in a suburban community, in the shadow of a large metropolitan area. You ask your fourth graders what they know about the differences between working in the city and working in the suburbs. You find out that they know little except the fact that many of their parents work in the city. How can you use this information to help them understand the influence of lifestyle on career choice?

4. Your principal asked you to attend a local community partnership meeting. As you look around the table you begin to realize the diversity of professional and technical skill represented at the meeting. You are thinking about how your elementary students would benefit from exposure to the bigger picture of the world of work. What will you do?

5. Your school is located in a small town in a rural community. Main Street is only four blocks long, yet there is a good variety of shops and services represented there. How can you use your community resources to help your seventh graders become more aware of career opportunities?

6. Service learning can have a strong influence on building character. How can it also influence career choice?

7. Your district has asked the school counselors to develop an educational and career plan. You need to decide if you want to develop a plan that will work preK–12 or if you want to create a different plan for each grade level. What are the key elements that need to be included? There are many samples for you to look at on the World Wide Web! Investigate existing career plans and draft a career plan and present it to your colleagues.

8. Identify and write a descriptive paragraph for eight websites that can be used for college and career planning for the grade level you want to work with.

9. College and career ready can mean something different to the teachers in your school. Brainstorm with your colleagues what this means in your school.

CHAPTER **15**

# Transitioning into the Field of School Counseling

## CHAPTER OBJECTIVES

*By the time you have completed this chapter, you should be able to*

- explain how you will implement the elements of a comprehensive school counseling program;

- integrate the major themes of the textbook into a comprehensive school counseling program;

- identify practical suggestions you will use to strengthen your professional relationships and allies;

- define how your belief system will be demonstrated in delivering equitable and quality education for all students;

- explain how you will examine and enhance the physical, academic, and social climates in schools for optimum success;

- explain how to use a school's power base, your leadership style, and your own power base to enhance student learning;

- describe specific steps you will take to build your professionalism.

---

## *School Counselor Casebook: Getting Started*

### The Scenario
It is the last day of the school year and you have just finished your first year as a school counselor. You feel good about what you consider a successful first year. You believe you have made significant strides in grooming relationships and garnering support from administration and teachers for your program. You wonder if your perceptions of a successful year match others' evaluations of you and your program. You think about the things that surprised you most about the job. You also think about the things you wish someone had told you before you began your first day in the profession.

### Thinking about Solutions
As you read this chapter, imagine yourself as the school counselor in this scenario. When you come to the end of the chapter, you will see how four new counselors (2–4 years of experience) and two interns responded to these questions.

---

## ENVISIONING YOUR FUTURE

We hope you are excited about the great places this amazing profession is going to take you. Our sincere hope is that this textbook has served to inform and energize you about your journey ahead. As you move ahead you can be secure in the knowledge that the work you do along the way will improve the lives of hundreds of students. You will make a difference. How many professionals can say this with assurance?

For the past few months you have studied, reflected, and grappled with the traditional and the transformed practices of school counseling. Whether you are preparing for an immediate induction into the profession of school counseling or still have several courses ahead of you, it is our hope that you are developing a strong belief system and formulating in your mind how your beliefs will be demonstrated in your actions. At the core of this book's belief system is that:

- Every student can learn and achieve to high standards.
- Every child is entitled to an equitable and quality educational experience and an environment that is safe and respectful.
- All students can benefit from an effective school counseling program.
- School counseling programs are most successful when delivered in collaboration and in partnership with students, families, community members, educators, and administrators.

We also hope that you are developing strong beliefs about the role and responsibilities of a school counselor. The authors believe that:

- School counselors, as leaders and advocates, identify and rectify school-based practices that inhibit the success of individuals and groups of students.
- School counselors model behavior that contributes to a climate of caring and academic rigor and play a significant role in raising aspirations and motivating every student to succeed.
- School counselors help students develop effective interpersonal relationships and establish individual plans to achieve successful futures.
- School counselors, like every educator, are accountable for student success and have a responsibility to contribute significantly to systemic change (Hanson & Stone, 2002; Stone, 1996).

Your entrée into the profession can be facilitated by calculated moves on your part starting with the first day of school. Following are seven guiding principles from the American School Counseling Association for counselor education and school counseling programs.

- Act as a *counselor, advocate, leader, collaborator, and consultant* to maximize opportunities for students to succeed academically, emotionally, and socially.
- Strive to develop in all students *ambitious goals* and a *commitment to achievement* and to provide the positive environmental conditions that enable students to realize high aspirations.
- Become a **steward of equity**; be able to use data to recognize *institutional and environmental barriers* that impede students' ability to realize their full academic potential and be equipped to take the lead in remedying these inequalities
- Provide all students with *academic/career advising* to help them form values and attitudes about the significance of education to their future economic success and their quality of life.

- Become an effective *manager of resources* and partnership builder, enlisting the support of parents, agencies, and community members (Stone, 1996).

Green, Conley, and Barnett (2005) also developed guiding principles.

- Promote self-contextual awareness.
- Utilize an ecological framework for problem solving.
- Utilize indirect service models.
- Use collaboration to achieve comprehensive program objectives.
- Align school counseling goals with local reform and improvement strategies.
- Use evidence-based best practices.
- Use outcome-based evaluation strategies (Green, Conley, & Barnett, 2005).

## PLANNING FOR YOUR SUCCESS

Before you begin your new job spend as much time as you can learning about the physical, structural, academic, and social climate of the school, starting with the community in which it is situated.

### Learning about the Home and Community Environment

If possible drive, walk, or ride public transportation around the neighborhoods where your students live. Physically placing yourself in your students' neighborhood can be an eye-opening experience and will help you start to develop a solid understanding of your students' needs. Ask questions of other faculty and community members about the range of socioeconomic levels in the community, about incidents of child abuse, and about the degree of parental involvement with their children's education. The front office staff are a good source of valuable information, such as how many students are on free or reduced lunch, which student came in upset, attendance rate, etc. Letting them know that you consider them a valuable resource has a dual purpose: You learn a great deal and you start to groom a relationship with a group of people who can considerably smooth your induction into the school. Learn all you can about the stressors and support systems of your school's families so that you can be prepared for the students who walk through your door.

#### *Community Standards*

Become familiar with the prevailing community standards. Are you in an ultra-conservative part of the world, a bastion of liberalism, a solid middle-class suburb, or an urban setting? Remember that ethics are situational. You will need to know the community and institutional standards to discern how to behave ethically in this particular environment. Would your community be respectful of a poster on your door advertising a support group for gay, lesbian, bisexual, transgender, and questioning youth? Could you encourage a student to go to a neighborhood health clinic if she tells you she is pregnant? It is important to have a feel for the level of tolerance for school interference in value-laden issues. We have to be highly sensitive to the fact that parents have been given the legal right to be the guiding voice in their children's lives.

## Learning about the School Environment

Try to determine the nature of the school environment. What is the working climate like at this school? Is there a sense of camaraderie and cohesiveness among faculty or is the general atmosphere one of strife, tension, and unhealthy competition? Ask questions. Which departments or grade levels are functioning well? Are there pockets of problems or model areas?

### *Leadership and the Power Structure*

Leadership and power are important aspects of the **school climate**. Where is the power base for decision making on schoolwide issues? How are school counselors involved? Who are the formal leaders and what is the formal organizational structure of your school? Does the formal organizational structure match the power structure? Critically important is the informal power base. Who are the teachers who hold the power, have the principal's ear, or wield the greatest influence among the faculty? You will need these teachers and their influence even though some of them may have negative attitudes. Think back to the chapter on leadership. Identify those who have the referent power, connection power, and expert power. These are the people to know and court. Jim MacGregor, a high school counselor that you met in the chapter on advocacy, understood the power of buy-in and relationship building. He opened doors for his students to be enrolled in higher-level academics because he tenaciously tackled building a relationship with the external and internal community.

### *Culture and Beliefs of Administration and Faculty*

Learn about the administration and faculty culture and belief system. What is their belief about student learning? Almost all educators espouse the belief that given the right conditions all children can achieve to high levels. Do the educators in your school live this belief in programs and actions that support all students to be successful learners? How does the school use data to understand student achievement?

Ask questions about how students are disciplined in your school and look to see if there is a disciplinary plan in place. Read the disciplinary plan and see if you agree with it and discreetly check to see if the plan is carried out uniformly.

### MEET CAROL MCLEOD-ORSO: CHANGING THE CULTURE AND THE BELIEF SYSTEM

As a University of North Florida School Counseling student, Carol Orso interned at a rural high school that had a history of minimal course offerings in higher-level academics. Carol knew that course assignments in high school significantly differentiate students' opportunities beyond high school and their economic futures. Carol worked with the administrative team to use the school's database to provide her with information about students' mathematics scores on the state tests. Carol learned that a

*(continues)*

significant number of students taking the higher-level mathematics courses were scoring the highest on the state tests regardless of their grades or success rate in higher-level mathematics courses. In other words, she found a direct correlation between taking higher-level mathematics and doing better on statewide tests and no correlation between mathematics course grades and statewide test scores. Armed with this information, Carol looked further and found that failures in mathematics were largely due to factors such as not completing homework, excessive absences, and other variables that did not have to do with the students' ability to do higher-level mathematics. Carol started a critical dialogue with her administration about her findings. Using the school's database, she identified ninth graders who made a final grade of D or F in Algebra 1 in eighth grade and therefore were not recommended to take geometry, yet these students had demonstrated solid mathematics scores on their standardized tests. Understanding that knowledge can raise aspirations, she decided to ask the administrative team and chair of the mathematics department if she could help these students understand the interrelationship between higher-level mathematics and student future economic opportunities. Carol will follow this academic advising with student performance contracts and advance them to geometry in ninth grade and Algebra II in 10th grade—the year they take the state test to determine eligibility to graduate. Students at this school who have had poor grades in mathematics in the past—regardless of state test scores—have regularly been scheduled to take dead-end mathematics courses. Carol is a social justice advocate who used data to give her knowledge and power when advocating for greater opportunities for the students in her school.

---

Observe how teachers interact with students. Walk the hallways, listen, and keenly observe. You will be one of the few people in the school who has a finger on the pulse of the school and who understands which teachers have good classroom management, which rule by intimidation, or which employ cooperative discipline. Capitalize on this knowledge by helping other teachers to replicate the practices that result in a safer, more respectful school climate for all children.

### The Students

Student morale is an aspect of school climate. Are the students engaged, enthusiastic, positive, and motivated? Find out how school spirit is demonstrated. What percentage of the student body feels disenfranchised? To gain a better understanding of the student body, go into the cafeteria and sit down and talk with groups of students. By asking students what they think of their school and their school counseling program, you can open a dialogue, learn how the school counseling program is perceived, discover if the program has any public relations problems, and solicit ideas on areas to include in your program. Talking about bullying is a great introduction to learn about students' thoughts regarding their school climate. There is a discrepancy between bullied victims' experience and their parents' misunderstanding of the situation. Parents fail to notice their child's victimization. To provide support, the truth must be realized by the parent. The failure to see this victimization is a risk factor that can cause further harm or damage to the young student (Matsunaga, 2009). Engage a cross-section of the student body—this group is comprised of the ones who had been bullied, the ones who had bullied others, as well as those who feel they have been both the bullied and the bully (Frisén, Jonsson, & Persson, 2007). Students have different experiences and perceptions of bullying. They can tell us why children are being bullied, the idea behind why some bully others, and why the students feel it is important to stop bullying. Giving students the opportunity to talk about their school climate gives counselors great insight into what students are thinking (Frisén, Jonsson, & Persson, 2007).

### Curriculum/Instruction and Student Support

To the extent possible, learn as much as you can about the school's curriculum offerings, the special education program, and all support systems in place for struggling students. What is the philosophy and belief about what makes effective instruction? In elementary and middle school, getting advice about resource schedules such as physical education, music, and art can help you develop your classroom guidance schedule and further your understanding of the nature of this particular school.

# HEADING TOWARD SUCCESS

On or before your first day, begin heading toward success by organizing your space, your time, your resources, your data sources, and your support system.

## Organizing Your Physical Environment

You may have little or no control over the physical environment you are assigned. However, try to optimize your environment before the first day of school because as the year progresses you will have little time to fuss over making changes, moving furniture, and nailing pictures. Set yourself up early in a comfortable arrangement for the year. Vie for an office near equipment and people you most often need to access. You may have to scavenge if resources and furniture don't meet your needs. Find out what your school district has in the form of a surplus furniture warehouse. Place your furniture with attention to traffic patterns and have a space that allows you and students to be comfortable and in close proximity to each other without a desk or other barrier between you. A small table with chairs is ideal if you are lucky enough to have an office that will accommodate this.

## Organizing Your Time

A weekly, monthly, and yearly calendar can be a support. Establish a weekly calendar and place it on your door. Even if you have no idea as to what your month or year will actually look like, taking the step to have a semblance of organization and voice in your weekly schedule will help you establish a feeling of being in control of your time and job assignments. You can make adjustments and changes as you go along but getting started is an important first step.

## Organizing Your Resources

What technology resources are available? Hopefully your school has a wonderful infrastructure for high-speed Internet use, computers on every desk, technology labs, closed circuit television, and a computer teacher(s). Ideally your equipment will include computers for you and the students, a phone with multiple phone lines, a copy machine, and a fax machine. It is likely that you will not have the perfect situation. Be resourceful and seek support from business partners and others to help meet the equipment needs of your office. Often you will be hired into an already established program and things will be set up for you. You have to use your judgment about how much change you should ask for right away and what items you will want to table for a more opportune time. You are working to establish an inviting space for you and your students.

## Organizing Your Data Sources

Chapter 8 covered the rationale and mechanics of identifying and using critical data elements also known as report card data. As early as possible you will want to study your school's report card data. An easy way to start is to find the person in your school most familiar with the data and capture a few minutes of their time to discuss student performance and other critical data. The principal is usually a great resource for this information and will likely cooperate with vigor and appreciation. Improving student data elements is a "do or die" proposition for principals, so when you ask about the school's report card data, you are placing yourself in a positive light as someone who believes that the accountability imperative includes you (Stone & Dahir, 2011).

## Organizing Your Support System

Many school systems assign new counselors a buddy or mentor who is usually a talented, seasoned counselor who can assist new professionals in negotiating the first year and avoiding some of the pitfalls. If there is not a formal program in place in your district, reach out to someone and ask her or him if they will mentor you. As a new counselor, I did not have the benefit of a formal mentoring program but I was desperate for help. I called a veteran, master elementary counselor who most generously agreed to sit down and share with me all the knowledge that she could, and she continued to be my telephone mentor. When I moved to high school, Rosemary English, the assistant principal for curriculum, was my lifeline. If your school district does not have a formal mentoring program, find someone to support you in this way.

Find fellow colleagues in your own building who can support your efforts, such as your fellow counselors, a talented influential teacher, or a grade-level or department chairperson. Orchestrate success for yourself. For example, present your first classroom guidance lessons in teachers' rooms that have the best classroom management. Deliver a 5- or 10-minute staff development presentation early in the year on a topic that is sure to be of interest to all and that will place you in a positive, proactive light in the eyes of others. Find a sounding board, an ear, someone you can talk to with whom you can share all the frustrations that you don't want to air at school.

How else can you prepare to help your first day in the profession go smoothly? Attend to some public relations efforts that will help launch your program. Establish a bulletin board and give each teacher a newsletter or flyer to distribute to students that highlight components of your program. Contribute to an invitational environment for students by joining existing efforts or suggesting ways to welcome students. In addition to your bulletin board, flyer, or newsletter, greet students with a message over the public address system.

# ENSURING YOUR SUCCESS

As you launch into your first year as a transformed school counselor, put the mechanisms in place for developing your professional skills and knowledge, maintaining your energy, and resolve to meet the professional commitments you made as a graduate student and build the relationships that will support you in all your efforts at building a successful program.

## Professional Development

Professional organizations offer support and can help you increase your **professionalism** in the field. As a new counselor, I never missed an opportunity to go to the state conference. I would always return energized and excited about my profession in addition to bringing back armloads of ideas. I have continued this practice as I find my peers to be my best teachers and motivators. When looking back to the "Standard of Care" principle in Chapter 6, remember that you increase your commitment to professional growth and raise your Standard of Care when you are an active member of your professional organization. If you ever find yourself in legal hot water, your attorney is going to ask you what professional organizations you are a member of and how you demonstrated your commitment to the organization. Your lawyer's intent in this type of situation would be to show that you behaved as a reasonably competent professional in supporting your own professional growth.

Professional organizations such as the American School Counselor Association (ASCA) also provide informative publications and discussion lists as part of your membership. Every dollar spent on ASCA is returned to you in terms of the wonderful benefits you receive in professional development.

District level inservices, regional workshops, and summer institutes are but a few of the many ways you can continue to grow your professionalism. It is the responsibility of each of us to seek ways to continue to stay abreast of an ever-changing profession. It is time-consuming to read all the entries on a discussion list and you will probably have to pick and choose based on the subject. However, this forum benefits you when you need an answer.

## Management Agreement

Following the American School Counselor Association (ASCA) model, it is important to create a management agreement to keep your goals in line with what your co-counselors and administrators see you doing. This agreement is for each counselor at your school and it is signed within the first two months of the school year. In this agreement, information should be found regarding the percentage of time designated to each of the four areas of the delivery system. These percentages may vary with individual assignments, but the overall comprehensive program should be closely aligned with the recommended use of time as described by ASCA. You may use a sample management agreement provided in the Application Templates section of the RAMP website or create your own with more specific areas you want to see tackled (ASCA, 2008). As an end result of creating a management agreement for yourself, you will be able to use data to prove the positive light a counselor creates in promoting a healthy and positive school climate for all students.

## Practicing Wellness

What do you do for wellness? School counselors expend considerable energy. How do you sustain your energy? The more you give of yourself to support others, the more you need to take care of your own personal wellness. Every organization has its drawbacks and unfortunately in some cases unhealthy people, toxic environments, bureaucracy, and other drains on one's emotional well-being. The nature of most school counseling situations is one of satisfaction that we have made a positive impact on students, but it is also a demanding profession with too many students with unmet needs. While developing student resiliency, cultivate and guard your own. Find outlets that renew your spirit and seek opportunities to do them regularly. Does travel, exercise, or friends and family renew you? Does your serenity come from reading, spiritual pursuits, writing, or hobbies? Find allies among your colleagues to help buoy and support your resolve to do all you can for students. Orchestrate opportunities for tangible successes to help sustain the enthusiasm necessary for what you are doing.

## Professional Comportment

Behave in a professional manner at all times. But also be your own best advertisement. Positive self-talk is usually translated into a positive demeanor and hangs a welcome sign on your back that says, "I am approachable." Attitude is everything. Instead of being frustrated with barriers, develop a sense of humor about the absurdities of institutions, people, and bureaucracies. Your work is critically important, but give yourself permission not to be consumed by it. Set boundaries, develop coping skills, keep whatever comes your way in perspective because in the end your attitude will determine the beliefs and behaviors from which you operate and assist students.

Build and protect your relationships. A good portion of the coordination, consultation, and theories chapters focused on building relationships, but offered here are some cautions about protecting your relationships. Avoid behaving as a divisive element and be vigilant not to give the appearance of siding with one faction of the administration or faculty over another. Refuse to be a party to tearing down the administration, other faculty members, parents, or students. Build bridges.

Respect the experience of others and share your knowledge. Teachers and staff may look with suspicion on the new person who comes in eager with new ideas, ready to save the world. The climate and morale undertones may influence their receptivity to your ideas. Respect the traditions and established procedures of the school to the greatest extent possible and astutely make your changes so that you can be as effective as possible in the long run. Find the gems in current practices to celebrate and then with solid relationship building, you can start to make systemic changes.

## Maintaining Your Professional Commitments

Adhering to many of the ideals you learned in graduate school will be tougher than you think. Be prepared to fight the good fight.

### *Stay Passionate about Advocacy*

Advocacy is hard work. Expect at varying times support, praise, and ridicule. How do you stay invigorated when the response from others may be, at best, indifference and, at worst, resistance? One way to stay the course when you feel your resolve wavering is to walk into classrooms and look into the eyes of the students sitting there. Throughout this text you have been presented with the statistics of lost potential. When you feel your advocacy wavering, go into the kindergarten classes, look into the eyes of 100 students, and identify the 47 students who you are willing to sacrifice. By keeping the children's faces in your mind's eye, you will be spurred on to make the system work for all students. When teachers or others say to you, directly or indirectly, that certain students are "a lost cause," find a way to gently, politically, skillfully remind them that the hopes and dreams they want for their own children are the same as what you want for all students. If all of us in our communities and schools would do for each child what we would want done for our own children, then we would have a system committed to finding ways to widen students' opportunities. If as an advocate you can remember that the alternative to making waves is allowing some students to be left out of the success picture, then it will help fuel your passion to stay the course.

> There have been too many examples of academic success in the face of tremendous adversity to conclude that intelligence and ability are handed out sparingly or based on only genetic endowments, or that they cannot be affected by educational environments. These examples are powerful reminders that great potential exists in all students. What needs changing first is the expectations teachers hold for different students. Hold all students up to a high expectation. As a class and as a school, teachers and counselors need to approach the students universally and expect the best from all individuals. (Rubie-Davies, 2010)

## JIM MACGREGOR: CHANGING THE STATUS QUO

Like most school counselors Jim is outnumbered by a heavy counselor/student ratio. Not content to accept that he would only be able to be a career and academic advisor to a few students, Jim developed a computer-based four-year plan that interfaced with students identified career clusters. Using the career cluster as a guide, Jim's program informed students as

*(continues)*

to which mathematics and sciences they would need to match their career plans. Jim's efforts to help students see that they would have brighter futures if they would stretch and strive academically was made considerably easier when he tied course taking to a student's career goals and the four-year career plan became a living document, changing as the student's career cluster changed. Over six years, Jim's advocacy resulted in a 40 percent increase in African American students choosing higher-level mathematics and science courses. School counselors who act purposefully to connect students to their future opportunities affect the instructional program and change the status quo of who will reach graduation with a wide range of paths from which to choose.

### Support the Instructional Program

Good teaching matters! Throughout the text you have been given many techniques for supporting the instructional program. Constantly think of new ways to implement strategies to support teaching and learning, and send the message at every turn that you respect the tough job teachers have and that you are there to support the instructional program and the teachers' efforts. Be slow to judge. Teaching and school administration are hard jobs, indeed among the hardest jobs in America today with tough accountability, few resources, and minimal support. Be a cheerleader, never a thorn, for teachers and administrators.

### MEET MELISSA HIPPENSTEEL HOWELL: GOOD TEACHING MATTERS

Melissa was assigned to a school in which all previous teachers except the coach were removed and replaced by proven master teachers. This school was designated by the state for takeover at the end of the year if test scores did not improve. The PE teacher marveled at the change in the school: "In the past, all the teachers slept or took turns watching each other's class while they left campus. There was no education going on here." Melissa knew how to teach. It was said of Melissa that she could teach anyone to read and motivate even the most troubled child. She set her jaw with determination, rolled up her sleeves, won her third graders' hearts, and, oh, how they worked for her. Test results arrived and the principal called all staff together to inform them that the school had excelled and that they were now off the F list. Each teacher received her or his students' scores for sorting into two stacks to indicate which students fell "below basic." Melissa had no sorting to do;

none of her students scored "below basic." When Melissa returned her "one stack" this reserved, low-key principal let out a whoop, grabbed her, hugged her, and said, "Don't you realize what you have done?" Many students drop out in third grade but wait until they are 16 to leave school. In Melissa's class that year, no one dropped out. Good teaching matters!

---

# LAYING THE FOUNDATION FOR YOUR SCHOOL COUNSELING PROGRAM

Every chapter in this text has given you pieces of the puzzle to build a solid school counseling and program. The ASCA standards and model chapter laid out the components of a comprehensive school counseling program. Chapters on counseling, consultation, leadership, advocacy, theory, and counseling applications gave you the knowledge and skills to implement the components of your school counseling program. This chapter is about laying a solid foundation on which to build your program. Here are some suggestions for getting started on the major components of a successful program.

## Prepare a Mission Statement

Study the school's mission statement, then write the mission statement for your counseling program. Recall from Chapter 9 that the mission of the school counseling program should be closely aligned with the school's mission. For example, "The mission of the school counseling program is to provide all students, preK to 12th grade, professional school counseling expertise that will ensure that, regardless of their race, gender, religion, heritage, ability, or economic status, every student will be afforded the opportunity to achieve the skills needed to become lifelong learners and productive members of society." Printing out and displaying your mission statement will serve two purposes: (1) it will provide you with transparency, letting everyone—including students, teachers, and administrators—know what you stand for and what you hope to accomplish; and (2) it will keep you focused by reminding you every day what you stand for and what you hope to accomplish.

## Start Building a Belief System

As we discussed earlier in this chapter, beliefs shape how we view our world; behaviors reflect our belief system. What we believe, what we hold fast and true about students, families, teachers, and the educational process, drives our ability to support success for every student. Our beliefs are derived from our background and experiences. You had an opportunity to develop a personal belief statement. To develop a core belief system for your programs requires a dialogue among school counselors and their colleagues to explore the complexity of educational issues from all vantage points. A belief statement may read, "We believe that all students can learn and achieve to high levels. We believe that a comprehensive developmental school counseling program will help promote equity and access to educational opportunities. We believe as leaders in our schools, advocates for our students, and collaborators with students, teachers, parents and administrators we serve every student and provide equal access to school counseling programs." To launch the building of the school's formal belief system, draft a core belief statement and circulate it among your new colleagues, asking for their comments and contributions.

## Begin Building Your Team

The key to the development and implementation of a successful program is readiness. Before charging forward, identify a team who can help to implement your program. The core team members would include administrators, teachers, student service personnel, parents, students, and business and community representatives. Your team can start small and grow as needed. Table 15.1 shows the typical program implementation team and their responsibilities.

TABLE **15.1**

Program Implementation Team

| Implementation Team Members | Responsibilities in a Comprehensive School Counseling Program |
| --- | --- |
| School Counselors | Provide proactive leadership to ensure every student is served. Determine with the administration the management agreement for the comprehensive school counseling program and commit to the collaborative process of fulfilling the agreement. They manage the comprehensive program and coordinate strategies and activities with others (teachers, support staff, parents, community agencies, business representatives) to meet the stated goals and standards/competencies. |
| Teachers | Are partners with school counselors. They develop and infuse guidance activities into the instructional program that are integral to good learning, *not* extraneous, disconnected, added material. They may serve as advisors or mentors to students. |
| Pupil Personnel Services (school psychologist, social worker, school nurse-teacher, etc.) | Collaborate and team with the school counselors to ensure that school psychologists, school social workers, school nurses, student assistance counselors, and other support personnel are actively involved in supporting each student's academic, career, and personal-social development. They support students and families with information regarding outside agencies and assist students with mental health issues, physical health issues, or social issues. |
| Administrators | Determine with the school counselor(s) what the management agreement will entail and commit to the process of supporting how the management agreement will be fulfilled. Provide leadership in developing the program and in the ongoing program improvement. They provide continuous support and emphasize the importance of the program to others. They promote cooperation among counselors, faculty, and others. Additionally, they provide facilities and resources and allow time to facilitate the program process. |

| Parents | Work cooperatively with school personnel in delivering the program. They serve on committees and provide linkages to the community by communicating program goals to others. |
| Students | Actively participate and assume responsibility for meeting standards/competencies. They will be able to identify the skills, knowledge, and attitudes they have gained in structured guidance sessions. |
| Business/Community Representatives | Representatives from business and industry and others in the community serve on committees, talk with classes, act as mentors, provide financial support, and generally serve as partners in the education of youth. |

## Making the Shift to a Comprehensive, Transformed School Counseling Program

What do you do if you start a new job in a school that does not have a comprehensive, transformed school counseling program as prescribed by ASCA? Ideally you would negotiate the political landscape skillfully and move toward a collaborative effort in which key players will analyze existing practices (see Table 15.2). The purpose of the analysis would be determine to what degree comprehensive school counseling is in place and clearly identify aspects of a comprehensive model that need to be implemented.

TABLE **15.2**
Analyzing Existing Practices

| Current Practice | Analysis |
| --- | --- |
| Individual Counseling | How much time have school counselors been spending in individual counseling sessions? |
| | How many students per year receive individual counseling? |
| | What program initiatives can be instituted that help more students while lessening the need for individual counseling? |
| Group Counseling | How many group counseling sessions have counselors been hosting each month? How many students are involved with group counseling? |
| | How can group counseling be used to meet the needs of all students? |
| Collaboration | What are the resources available within the district and community to assist students and families and how do counselors currently collaborate with these services? |
| | In what ways can collaboration with district and community services be improved? |
| Consultation | How often do school counselors consult with other members of the school community? |
| | How could this consultation process be improved? |
| Leadership | In what manner do the school counselors currently demonstrate leadership? |
| | How might your leadership skills be better used to assist all students to reach their potential? |

| Advocacy | How does the school counseling program advocate for equity and support students who are at risk of failure? |
| | How can the advocacy component of the program be improved? |
| Teaming and Collaboration | How often and in what ways do counselors collaborate with members of the school community to assist students? |
| | How can teamwork and collaboration at this school be improved? |
| Data-driven Results | What type of data does the school district collect? |
| | How can those data be used to drive the comprehensive school counseling program? |
| Use of Technology | Take an inventory of the technology available at this school. |
| | Is the available technology sufficient to help you assist students and their families? |
| | What additional technology do you need and how will you justify its purchase? |

# ONE YEAR LATER: ENVISIONING YOUR TRANSFORMED SCHOOL COUNSELING PROGRAM

In an ideal world, what might your transformed school counseling program look like one year after it is launched? The ASCA national standards and ASCA school counseling program model form the foundation of your program, support the mission of your school, and provide the direction as to how every student will benefit from the school counseling program. The implementation team has determined a mission statement, philosophy, and guiding beliefs in line with the school, district, and ASCA mission. The team has identified an appropriate delivery system to include classroom teachers and support personnel. Parents, students, teachers, and support staff are aware of their roles within the delivery system. Newsletters, parents' nights, and presentations to faculty and community members promote the delivery system; career and business partners are included in the delivery model.

The implementation team meets regularly to discuss implementation at each level and acting as a support team, sharing the burden of change, and celebrating the victories achieved. Additionally, the members monitor whether one or more aspects of the preK–12th Comprehensive Counseling Program have *not* been addressed. If so, discussions take place to ensure that implementation progresses holistically and remains focused on improving student academic success.

Your comprehensive school counseling program is in a constant state of growth and change so that it will continue to address the specific needs of all students each year. A concerted effort is made to meet students in small and large groups. School counselors are now more visible to a greater number of students and faculty and viewed as leaders, advocates, and team players working toward school improvement and systemic change.

Your newly developed program supports the school's academic mission by promoting and enhancing the learning process for all students through an integration of academic, career, and personal/social development. The comprehensive school counseling program is an integral component to the total educational experience of all students. The program fosters student achievement and school improvement and is developmental and systematic in nature, sequential, clearly defined, and accountable. By addressing student needs in academic, career, and personal/social development throughout their preK–12 schooling, the comprehensive school counseling program promotes and enhances the learning process for all students.

Your school counseling program is now aligned with the broader goals of the primary mission of today's schools (Brown & Trusty, 2005b). The program promotes educational excellence through individual excellence, provides strategic interventions and academic achievement strategies such as tutoring, creates collaborations that span the boundaries of professions and agencies that integrates the expertise of school counselors, other pupil services personnel as well as business and community into the total program, and is current with the needs and expectations of education agenda and societal issues (Brown & Trusty, 2005b; Brown, Dahlbeck, & Sparkman-Barnes, 2006).

## A CLOSING WORD FROM THE AUTHORS

Traditionally, professional school counselors have been ancillary to the mission of schools. The National Standards, the ASCA Model, Transforming School Counseling, and now your program place professional school counselors at the forefront of school reform. With current data indicating achievement and opportunity gaps between underrepresented students and poor students and their peers, there is an ethical and moral imperative for professional school counselors to utilize all resources available to acquire the knowledge, skills, and attitudes to close the gaps.

You are preparing to be a professional school counselor, an educator, who like your colleagues will be at the heart and soul of the educational process, not a visitor whose job it was to be a clinician, but an educator who will bring unique counseling skills and specialized knowledge. You will have a major impact on your students through a repertoire of powerful roles: counselor, leader, advocate, collaborator, team builder, consultant, data analyzer/consumer, systemic change agent, steward of equity and access, manager of resources, career and academic advisor, and didactic counselor. This text has introduced you to school counselors who understand that they are uniquely positioned to touch all the students in their schools through their skills.

Emulate these role models and embrace your future as a leader, advocate, and systemic change agent; wielding influence and contributing to student success. Find your focus and implement your belief system. Being a counselor and an educator is an amazing privilege that allows us to use our skills to give young people the gift of access and success in learning—a gift that will carry them beyond the school walls. How exciting to be part of the most crucial profession that society has to offer—counselors/educators who touch the future through the lives of our students.

As a newly minted school counselor, build a support base so that you can attack barriers to student success and tackle the daunting task of changing attitudes and beliefs about students and their ability to learn. Make that mythical level playing field your sparring ground where you tackle institutional and environmental barriers that continue to adversely stratify students' opportunities. Embrace a social justice agenda and kick dirt in the proverbial eye of inequality.

## TECH TOOLS

The Tech Tools section offers suggestions for you when you become a practicing school counselor to maximize the goals of your program. However, when appropriate and possible, learn and implement these tech tools before you enter the field.

- Contact Educational Testing Services of the College Board and the ACT organization to learn what they have available in disaggregated student data and survey information that will help you better understand your students' test scores, and their survey responses.
- Use a search engine to look for grants to purchase equipment for your school counseling office and for other needs.
- Find the data wizard in your school, the person who can help you better understand which groups of students successfully mastered the annual achievement exams and other critical data.
- Read how school counselors could benefit from E-government Solutions: The Case of paperwork posted on the Indiana School Counselor association website to gain further insights into streamlining and automating cumbersome "paper pushing processes."
- Join a discussion list so that you have colleagues to readily consult with.
- Bookmark websites that will prove especially helpful to you by putting them in the "My favorites" category on your computer's desktop. Some examples are www.Schoolcounselor.com, E versions of Education Week websites, www.cyberguidance.net
- Develop an electronic newsletter for your students and parents.
- Learn to use the closed circuit television equipment or find someone who can help you so you can deliver daily messages to students.
- Attend to your professional development by taking advantage of American Counselor Association's courses that they have available on video. Many are excellent and can increase your knowledge on everything from brief therapy to legal and ethical issues.

## *School Counselor Casebook: Voices from the Field*

### The Scenario Reviewed

It is the last day of the school year and you have just finished your first year as a school counselor. You feel good about what you consider a successful first year. You believe you have made significant strides in grooming relationships and garnering support from administration and teachers for your program. You wonder if your perceptions of a successful year match others' evaluations of you and your program. You think about the things that surprised you most about the job. You also think about the things you wish someone had told you before you began your first day in the profession.

## A Practitioner's Approach

Here's how four new counselors (2–4 years of experience at the time of the interview) and two interns responded to this question.

> I never could have imagined the amount of serious family issues that elementary children must deal with (i.e., divorce, domestic violence, single parents, death, drugs and alcohol, sexual/physical abuse, neglect) in varying degrees, lack of parenting skills, and patterns of blame. Before becoming a school counselor I wish I had known the time spent (and very needed) as a sounding board (listener and problem solver) for parents, teachers, and administrators. I have found it so important to work with the parents and teachers to provide interventions and accommodations for children. It is because of the special needs of my students that classroom guidance, systemic changes, and grant writing are a big part of my life as a school counselor.

> *Laura Lee Kinard is a counselor at a rural elementary school in Bryceville, Florida. Lee graduated from the University of North Florida's School Counseling Program in 2003.*

Before becoming a counselor I never could have imagined how much I would worry about my students' future, especially my high school and continuing education students. I work with students who are all deaf or blind with additional special needs. As I work on their final Transition Individual Education Plans it is like a huge scavenger hunt to try to research resources for these students who are from all over the state of Florida. I want my students to experience the best opportunities out there as they deserve the best. I am constantly amazed at how much trust the parents put in the school counselor. Parents have a huge responsibility and they need all the support school counselors can offer them. In the preparation program we talked about the importance of working as part of the team and collaborating with others. I never would have imagined how huge this part of the job is. Learning how to relate with students, school staff, parents, community agencies, and local businesses in positive ways is so important. I've also been amazed by how valuable my relationships with the other students in my counselor preparation program have become. We are always there for each other and can offer support and feedback.

I never had a complete picture of how important it was going to be to be creative and to be able to take initiative. I've learned in this job that if you can dream it you can make it happen. If you have supportive administration, teachers, support staff, and parents, the sky is the limit. Sometimes it may be a balancing act, but always working on building positive relationships allows for me to attain these dreams.

I wish I had known just how important time management really is! Each year that I perform my job, my skills and techniques for time management grow and improve. I am able to do so much more this third year as compared to my first year. At the end of a year, I now sit down with my planner and pencil in the entire next year making sure I have time for Classroom Guidance Sessions, Transition Planning/Counseling Sessions, Career Fair, Red Ribbon Activities, Testing/Assessment Training/Consultation, Special Projects, and

*(continues)*

Team Meetings. I get so much more done if I plan out my year in advance rather than just taking each day as it comes. I have learned that it is so important to take care of myself and to nurture a wonderful support group (friendships) beyond school and get plenty of rest so that I can meet the demands of a job I truly love.

*Karen Kolkedy is a school counselor at The School for the Deaf and Blind in St. Augustine, Florida. Karen graduated from the University of North Florida's School Counseling Program in 2002.*

I would never have imagined the extent to which there are inequities in our public schools. The problem is compounded because so many educators are not trained to teach low socioeconomic, urban students. The resiliency of elementary students to survive and thrive under adverse conditions always surprises me and gives me hope. I wish I would have known before becoming a school counselor how better to work with fellow educators that are not invested in their school and their students. This daily struggle has been very taxing.

I never could have imagined how rewarding it is to work with students. Each day I learn something new from them. I'm always on my toes! As a counselor, we have more freedom to work with students without having the curriculum constraints that teachers have and can impact a student as a whole. I have been very surprised about how entrenched school counseling departments can be. Entering into an already established school counseling office makes it difficult to implement schoolwide comprehensive guidance programs; buy-in is difficult to obtain as a new counselor.

*Shirin Mitsis is an urban high school counselor in Jacksonville, Florida, and is in her first year as a school counselor. Shirin graduated from the University of North Florida's School Counseling Program in 2004.*

Making the transition from the graduate school classroom to the counseling department may leave you feeling a bit unprepared, but there is no time to hesitate. There is simply no substitute for being in the school environment and watching events unfold. I know I have a lot to learn, even though I feel well prepared. There never seems to be enough time. I learned fairly early that counseling, especially at the elementary level, is not a linear process. The truth is that as I grow as a school counselor, I will be more able to define where the book knowledge ends and the real-life knowledge begins. Every experience is a learning experience, even though it might not feel that way at the time. Internship has taught me the value of small steps. I can think of no better preparation for new counselors than spending time "on-the-job" as interns.

*Julie Van Nostrand interned at Southampton High School and Southampton Elementary School and graduated from the New York Institute of Technology School Counseling Program in 2004.*

Some counselors initially question the intern's abilities and she or he needs to prove herself or himself. I feel that my abilities were at the level necessary to be a contributing and valued member of the counseling staff. We were well prepared by the books. We know our alphabet soup of policies, interventions, and committees. Gysbers, Gladding, Turba, and Stone are like old friends and we can plan out a way to implement the ASCA National Standards with the best of them. The foundation was strong. Theory and planning took a backseat when a child was evicted, a father passed away, college applications were due, and New York State changed the graduation requirements and we were in the midst of it all trying to be a rock of stability and source for answers. This is not a case study and practicum hours don't allow an individual to truly wrestle with these issues.

The theoretical foundation is useful, but learning on the job is going to be an ongoing process for years and years to come. Being a seasoned counselor will be worth more than all the printed knowledge in the end. Theoretically, a feather and a brick fall at the same rate, but we know that isn't what actually occurs in real life. We need to understand a little Newtonian physics to have the big picture make sense and know where to go from there. The books and the internship experience have the same sort of relationship. Theoretically, we know where we need to go and how we may get there, but is takes a bit of pizzazz and chutzpah to get there in an actual school.

It is scary to think that students will be looking to me solely next year, but I am confident that I can handle it. "When in doubt; consult, consult, consult!" That is a lesson from first semester, but probably one of the most valuable in over two years. That needs to be a way of life as a counselor.

*Philip Petrone interned at Westbury High School and Westbury Middle School and graduated from the New York Institute of Technology School Counseling Program.*

## LOOKING BACK: SALIENT POINTS

### Envisioning Your Future

For the past few months you have studied, reflected, and grappled with the traditional and the transformed practices of school counseling and have probably developed a strong belief system in the worth and dignity of each student and formulated in your mind how your beliefs will be demonstrated in your actions. The school counselor who believes that every student can learn and succeed will make this the compass and direction for her or his behavior in day-to-day work. Establish your focus by defining your guiding principles and belief system.

### Preparing for Success as a School Counselor

Learn about your new school beginning with your students' home and **community environment**. Try to determine the climate at your school to determine if there is a sense of camaraderie and cohesiveness among the faculty. Determine if students are engaged, enthusiastic, positive, and motivated. Try to understand the cliques, gangs, and social order of the school environment. Determine the power base for decision making and the formal and informal organizational structure of your school. Try to understand what the administration's and faculty's core belief systems are regarding student learning. Determine if the school uses data to understand student achievement. Observe how teachers interact with students. Walk the hallways, listen, and keenly observe.

Build your support system and your professionalism. You increase your commitment to professional growth when you are an active member of your professional organization. Practice personal wellness as the school counseling job demands both physical and emotional stamina. Try to optimize your physical environment before the first day of school. Set yourself up early in a comfortable arrangement for the year. Get psyched for advocacy by visiting classrooms and reminding yourself why you are there.

### Developing Your School Counseling Program

Write the mission statement for your school counseling program in coordination with the mission statement of the school. Identify an implementation team whose purpose is to institutionalize the preK–12 Comprehensive Counseling Program. Design the program and with the help of the implementation team put the program into operation. Respect the traditions and the established procedures of the school to the greatest extent possible and astutely make your changes so that you can be as effective as possible in the long run. Your comprehensive school counseling program should be in a constant state of growth and change so that it will continue to address the specific needs of all students each year. Make your school counseling program an integral component of the total educational experience of all students.

## KEY TERMS

Steward of equity p. 457

School climate p. 459

Professionalism p. 463

Community environment p. 475

## LEARNING EXTENSIONS/MAKING CONNECTIONS

1. Design a student and parent newsletter to distribute for a school's opening using word processing, graphics, and photos.

2. Create a resource list of websites to distribute to students and a list of websites to use for your own professional development.

3. Visit a school and start to ask questions about how they use relational databases to inform their decision making around school improvement issues. Write up your findings in a two-page summary.

4. Make a list of school report card critical data elements and write up a two-page report of how and why you will discuss these data elements with your principal.

5. Design and deliver a presentation on a school counseling-related issue using presentation software.

6. Put together a mock purchase order describing the equipment you will want for your school counseling office and present a rationale for the purchase of each piece of equipment. Give details such as the components you will want on your computer. Visit equipment retailers via the Internet to learn all you can about the equipment you are ordering.

7. Put together a mock weekly, monthly, and yearly calendar. Do as Karen Kolkedy described and pencil in your activities.

# REFERENCES

Achieve. (2009). *Perspective: News and views from achieve*. Washington DC: Author.

ACLJ Lawsuit Charges Pennsylvania School District Counseled and Facilitated Secret Abortion for Minor Student to Evade State Parental Consent Law. (1999, August 16). *The Free Library*.

Adams, M., Womack, S., Shatzer, R., & Caldarella, P. (2010). Parent involvement in school-wide social skills instruction: Perceptions of a home note program. *Education*, *130*(3), 513–527. doi: 1995179171

Adelman, H. S., & Taylor, L. (2002). Building comprehensive, multifaceted, and integrated approaches to address barriers to student learning. *Childhood Education: Annual Theme*, *78*(5), 261–268.

Adelman, H. S., & Taylor, L. (2002). School counselors and school reform: New directions. *Professional School Counseling*, *5*(4), 235–248.

Adelman, H., & Taylor, L. (2007). *Effective strategies for creating safer schools and communities: Fostering school, family, and community involvement*. Retrieved from http://smhp.psych.ucla.ed/ publications/44 guide 7 fostering school family and community involvement.pdf

Advancement Via Individual Determination. (2010). *Intro to the AVID program*. Retrieved from www.avid.org/intro.html

Aiken, L. R., Jr. (2000). *Psychological testing and assessment* (10th ed.). Boston: Allyn & Bacon.

Akos, P., Lambie, G., Milsom, A., & Gilbert, K. (2007). Early adolescents' aspirations and academic tracking: An exploratory investigation. *Professional School Counseling*, *11*(1), 57–64.

Alexander, K., & Alexander, K. (2010). *Higher education law: Policy and perspectives*. Florence, KY: Routledge.

Algozzine & Ysseldyke, 2006. Teaching students with medical, physical, and multiple disabilities, Corwin Press, 2006.

Allen-Meares, P., Washington, R. O., & Welsh, B. L. (2009). *Social work services in Schools* (6th ed.). Englewood Cliffs, NJ: Prentice Hall.

Alliance for Excellent Education. (2007a). Crisis in American high schools. *Straight A's: Public Education Policy and Progress*, *7*(19). Retrieved from www.all4ed.org/

Alliance for Excellent Education. (2007b). School not preparing students for the global economy. *Straight A's: Public Education Policy and Progress*, *7*(20). Retrieved from www.all4ed.org/

Alliance for Excellent Education. (2007c). The high cost of high school dropouts: New alliance brief pegs cost of class of 2007 dropouts at $329 billion. *Straight A's: Public Education Policy and Progress*, *7*(21). Retrieved from www.all4ed.org/

Amatea, E. S., & Clark, M. A. (2005). Changing schools, changing counselors: A qualitative study of school administrators' conceptions of the school counselor role. *Professional School Counseling*, *9*, 16–27.

Amatea, E. S., & West-Olatunji, C. A. (2007). Joining the conversation about educating our poorest children: Emerging leadership roles for school counselors in high poverty schools. *Professional School Counseling*, *11*, 81–89.

American Association of University Women. (1993). *Hostile hallways*. Washington, DC: Author.

American Association of University Women. (2001). *Hostile hallways: Bullying, teasing and sexual harassment in school*. Washington, DC: Author.

American Counseling Association. (1987). *School counseling: A profession at risk*. Alexandria, VA: American Association for Counseling and Development.

American Counseling Association. (1997). *Sexual harassment in the schools: Background on Title IX of the education amendments of 1972 and guidance issued by the office of civil rights*. Alexandria, VA: Author.

American Counseling Association. (2005a). *Code of ethics and standards of practice*. Retrieved from www.counseling. org

American Counseling Association. (2005b). *Position statement on high stakes testing*. Task Force on High Stakes Testing. Alexandria, VA.

American Counseling Association. (2010). *20/20: A vision for the future of counseling*. Retrieved from www.counseling. org/20-20/index.aspx

American Psychological Association. (2010). *Facing the school dropout dilemma*. Retrieved from www.apa.org/pi/ families/resources/school-dropout-prevention.aspx

American School Counselor Association. (1979). *Standards for guidance and counseling programs*. Falls Church, VA: American Personnel and Guidance Association.

American School Counselor Association. (1994). *The school counselor's role in educational reform*. Alexandria, VA: ASCA Press.

American School Counselor Association. (1997a). *Definition of school counseling*. Alexandria, VA: Author.

American School Counselor Association. (1997b). *Executive summary: The national standards for school counseling programs*. Alexandria, VA: Author.

American School Counselor Association. (1999a). *Position statement: The professional school counselor and comprehensive school counseling*. Alexandria, VA: Author.

American School Counselor Association. (1999b). *Position statement: The role of the professional school counselor*. Alexandria, VA: Author.

American School Counselor Association. (2002). *The professional school counselor and high stakes testing*. Alexandria, VA: Author.

American School Counselor Association. (2003). *American School Counselor Association national model: A framework for school counseling programs.* Alexandria, VA: Author.

American School Counselor Association. (2005). *American School Counselor Association national model: A framework for school counseling programs* (2nd ed.). Alexandria, VA: Author.

American School Counselor Association. (2007). *Position statement: The professional school counselor and high stakes testing.* Alexandria, VA: Author. Retrieved from http://asca2.timberlakepublishing.com//files/PS_High-Stakes%20Testing.pdf

American School Counselor Association. (2008). *The American School Counselor Association national model: A framework for school counseling programs.* Alexandria, VA: Author.

American School Counselor Association. (2009a). *Position statement: The professional school counselor and diversity.* Alexandria, VA: Author.

American School Counselor Association. (2009b) *The American School Counselor Association national model: A framework for school counseling programs.* Alexandria, VA: Author.

American School Counselor Association. (2010a). Ethical standards for school counselors. Retrieved from www.schoolcounselor.org

American School Counseling Association. (2010b). The professional school counselor and students with special needs (Position statement). Retrieved from www.schoolcounselor.org/files/PositionStatements.pdf

American School Counselor Association. (2012). *American School Counselor Association national model: A framework for school counseling programs* (3rd ed.). Alexandria, VA: Author.

Anastasi, A. (1992). What counselors should know about the use of psychological tests. *Journal of Counseling and Development, 70,* 610–615.

Anctil, T., Schenck, P., & Dahir, C. (2009). *School counselors' roles and perceptions of career development.* Poster presentation at the meeting of the National Career Development Association, St. Louis, MO.

Anderson-Butcher, D., & Ashton, D. (2004). Innovative models of collaboration to serve children, youths, families, and communities. *Children and Schools, 26*(1), 39–53.

Annie E. Casey Foundation. (2008). *Kids count data book.* Baltimore, MD: Author

Arman, J. F. (2000). In the wake of the tragedy of Columbine High School. *Professional School Counseling, 3*(3), 218–220.

Arnold v. Board of Education of Escambia County, 880 U.S. F.2d 305 (1989).

Arredondo, P., & Arciniega, G. M. (2001). Strategies and techniques for counselor training based on the multicultural counseling competencies. *Journal of Multicultural Counseling and Development, 29*(4), 263–273.

Arredondo, P., Toporek, R., Brown, S. P., Jones, J., Locke, D., Sanchez, J., et al. (1996). Operationalization of the multicultural counseling competencies. *Journal of Multicultural Counseling and Development, 24,* 42–78.

Arriaza, G. (2004). Making changes that stay made: School reform and community involvement. *The High School Journal, 87*(4), 10–25.

Association for Conflict Resolution, Education Section. (2007). *Recommended Standards for School-Based Peer Mediation Programs 2007.* Washington, DC: Association for Conflict Resolution. Retrieved from www.acrnet.org

Association for Specialists in Group Work. (2007). Group counseling in school: Special issue. *Journal for Specialists in Group Work, 32*(2).

Astramovich, R. L., & Coker, J. K. (2007). Program evaluation: The accountability bridge model for counselors. *Journal of Counseling & Development, 85*(2), 162–172.

Atkins, M., Graczyk, P., Frazier, S., & Abdul-adil, J. (2003). Toward a new model for promoting urban children's mental health: Accessible, effective, and sustainable school-based mental health. *School Psychology Review, 32*(4), 503.

Aud, S., Fox, M., & Kewal-Ramani, A. (2010). *Status and trends in the education of racial and ethnic groups* (NCES 2010-015). U.S. Department of Education, National Center for Education Statistics. Washington, DC: U.S. Government Printing Office.

Aud, S., Hussar, W., Planty, M., Snyder, T., Bianco, K., Fox, M., Frohlich, L., Kemp, J., & Drake, L. (2010). The Condition of Education 2010 (NCES 2010-028). National Center for Education Statistics, Institute of Education Sciences, U.S. Department of Education. Washington, DC.

Auman, M. J. (2007). Bereavement support for children. *The Journal of School Nursing, 23*(1), 34–39.

Axelson, J. (1999). *Counseling and development in a multicultural society.* (3rd ed.). Pacific Grove, CA: Brooks/Cole.

Bailey, S. M. (1993). The current status of gender equity research in American schools. *Educational Psychologist, 28,* 321–339.

Baker, S. B. (2000). *School counseling for the 21st century* (3rd ed.). Upper Saddle River, NJ: Merrill Prentice Hall.

Baker, S. B., & Gerler, E. (2008). *School counseling for the 21st century* (5th ed.). Upper Saddle River, NJ: Merrill Prentice Hall.

Baker, S. B., Robichaud, T. A., Westforth, V. C., Westforth D., Wells, S.C., & Schreck, R. E. (2009). School counselor consultation: A pathway to advocacy, collaboration, and leadership. *Professional School Counseling, 12*(3), 200–206.

Banach, W. (2004). *What students, parents, and staff are saying about schools.* Ray Township, MI: Banach, Banach & Cassidy, Inc.

Bandura, A. (1986). *Social foundations of thought and action: A social cognitive theory.* Upper Saddle River, NJ: Prentice Hall.

Bandura, A. (1993). Perceived self efficacy in cognitive development and functioning. *Educational Psychologist, 28*(2), 117–148.

Bandura, A., & Jeffrey, R. W. (1977). Roles of symbolic coding and rehearsal processes in observational learning. *Journal of Personality and Social Psychology, 26,* 122–130.

Banks, J. A. (2001). *Multicultural education: Issues and perspectives.* (4th ed.). Boston: Allyn & Bacon.

Banks, J. A. (2002). *An introduction to multicultural education* (3rd ed.). Needham, MA: Allyn & Bacon.

Bardwell, R. (2010, March 5). A veteran high school counselor responds to a report critical of the profession. *The New York Times.* Retrieved from http://thechoice.blogs.nytimes.com/2010/03/05/bardwell/?hp

Barth, R. S. (2006). Relationships within the schoolhouse. *Educational Leadership, 63*(6), 8–13.

Bartlett, J. R. (2010). Needs assessments: The key to successful and meaningful school counseling programs. In B. T. Erford (Ed.), *Professional school counseling: A handbook of theories, programs, and practices* (2nd ed., pp. 209–217). Austin, TX: PRO-ED.

Barton, E. A. (2009). *Leadership strategies for safe schools* (2nd ed.). Thousand Oaks, CA: Corwin.

Beale, A. V. (2004, November/December). Questioning whether you have a contemporary school counseling program. *The Clearing House, 78*(2), 73–76.

Beale, A., & Scott, P. (2001). "Bullybusters": Using drama to empower students to take a stand against bullying behavior. *Professional School Counseling, 4*(4), 300–305.

Bellotti v. Baird, 443 U.S. 622, S. Ct. 3035 (1979).

Bemak, F. (2000). Transforming the role of the counselor to provide leadership in educational reform through collaboration. *Professional School Counseling, 3*(5), 323–331.

Bemak, F., & Chung, R. C.-Y. (2005). Advocacy as a critical role for urban school counselor: Working toward equity and social justice. *Professional School Counseling, 8*(3), 196–202.

Bemak, F., & Chung, R. C.-Y. (2008). New professional roles and advocacy strategies for school counselors: A multicultural/social justice perspective to move beyond the nice counselor syndrome. *Journal of Counseling & Development, 86*(3), 372–381.

Benard, B. (2004). *Resiliency: What we have learned*. San Francisco, CA: WestEd

Bernard, M. E. (2006). It's Time We Teach Social-Emotional Competence as Well as We Teach Academic Competence. *Reading and Writing Quarterly*, 22, 103–119.

Benson, P. L., Scales, P. C., Effort, N., & Roehikeepartain, E. C. (1999). *A fragile foundation: The state of developmental assets among American youth*. Minneapolis, MN: The Search Institute.

Bergan, J., & Kratochwill, T. (1990). Behavioral consultation and therapy. New York, NY: Plenum Press.

Bergan, J. R. (1977). *Behavioral consultation*. Columbus, OH: Charles Merrill.

Biles, K., & Eakin, G. (2010, June). *Enhancing intrinsic motivation to change and achieve: Professional development day*. New York: Author.

Bill and Melinda Gates Foundation. (2006). *New report illuminates America's "silent" dropout epidemic*. Retrieved from www.gatesfoundation.orgiUnited States/Education/Transforming High Schools/Announcements/Announce-060302.htm

Bilzing, D. (1996). *Wisconsin Developmental Guidance Model*. Madison, WI: Wisconsin Department of Education.

Blair, J. (2003). New breed of bullies torment their peers on the Internet. *Education Week*, 22(1), 6–7.

Bluestein, J. (2001). *Creating emotionally safe schools*. Deerfield Beach, FL: Health Communications.

Bodine, R., Crawford, D., & Schrumpf, F. (1996). *Creating the peaceable school: A comprehensive program for teaching conflict resolution*. Washington, DC: Office of Juvenile Justice and Delinquency Prevention and Office of Elementary and Secondary Education.

Borders, D. L., & Drury, R. D. (1992). Comprehensive school counseling programs: A review for policy makers and practitioners. *Journal of Counseling and Development*, 70(4), 487–498.

Borum, R., Cornell, D., Modzeleski, W., & Jimerson, S. J. (2010). What can be done about school shootings? A review of the evidence. *Educational Researcher*, 39, 27–35.

Bowers, J., Hatch, T., & Schwallie-Giddis, P. (2001). The brain storm. *ASCA School Counselor*, 42, 17–18.

Boyer, E. L. (1988). Exploring the future: Seeking new challenges. *Journal of College Admissions*, 118, 2–8.

Brand, G. (2005). What a 21st century career and technical education system could look like. In R.Kazis (Ed.), *Remaking career and technical education for the 21st century: What role for high school programs* (pp. 26–28). Aspen, CO: The Aspen Institute.

Brewer, J. M. (1932). *Education as guidance: An examination of the possibilities of curriculum in terms of life activities in elementary and secondary schools and colleges*. New York: Macmillan.

Brigman, G., Campbell, C., & Webb, L. (2007). Building skills for school success: Improving the academic and social competence of students. *Professional School Counseling*, 10(3), 279–288.

Brigman, G., Mullis, F., Webb, L., & White, J. (2005). *School counselor consultation: Skills for working effectively with parents, teachers, and other school personnel*. Hoboken, NJ: John Wiley & Sons.

Brinson, J. A., Kottler, J. A., & Fisher, T. A. (2004). Cross-cultural conflict resolution in the schools: Some practical intervention strategies for counselors. *Journal of Counseling and Development*, 82(3), 294–302.

Brooks, F., & McHenry, B. (2009). *A contemporary approach to substance abuse and addiction counseling*. Alexandria, VA: American Counseling Association.

Brown, C., Dahlbeck, D. T., & Sparkman-Barns, L. (2006). Collaborative relationships: School counselors and non-school mental health professionals working together to improve the mental health needs of students. *Professional School Counseling*, 9(4), 332–335.

Brown, D., & Trusty, J. (2005a). The ASCA national model, accountability, and establishing causal links between school counselors' activities and student outcomes: A reply to Sink. *Professional School Counseling*, 8, 219–228.

Brown, D., & Trusty, J. (2005b). School counselors, comprehensive school counseling programs,and academic achievement: Are school counselors promising more than they can deliver? *Professional School Counseling*, 9, 1–8.

Brown, S., & Lent, W. B. (2005) *Career development and counseling: Putting theory and research to work*. Hoboken, NJ: John Wiley and Sons.

Brownell, M. T., Sindelar, P. T., Kiely, M. T., & Danielson, L. C. (2010). Special education teacher quality and preparation: Exposing foundations, constructing a new model. *Exceptional Children*, 76(3), 357–377.

Bryan, J., & Henry, L. (2008). Strengths-based partnerships: A school-family-community partnership approach to empowering students. *Professional School Counseling*, 12(2), 149–156.

Bryan, J., & Holcomb-McCoy, C. (2004). School counselor's perceptions of their involvement in school-family-community partnerships. *Professional School Counseling*, 7(3), 162–171.

Bryan, J., & Holcomb-McCoy, C. (2007). An examination of school counselor involvement in school-family community partnerships. *Professional School Counseling*, 10(5), 441–454.

Bryan, J., Holcomb-McCoy, C., Moore-Thomas, C., & Day-Vines, N. (2009). Who sees the school counselor for college information? A national study. *Professional School Counseling*, 12(4), 280–291.

Bucher, R. (2008). *Building cultural intelligence (CQ): Nine megaskills*. Upper Saddle River, NJ: Pearson Education.

Buffum, A., Mattos, M., & Weber, C. (2010). The why behind rti. *Educational Leadership*, 68, 10–18.

Bunshaw, W., & Lopez, S. (2010). A time for change: The 42nd annual Phi Delta Kappa/Gallup poll of the public's attitudes toward the public schools. *Kappan*, 92, 8–26.

Burke, K., & Dunn, R. (1998). *Learning style: The clue to you!* Jamaica, NY: St. John's University, Center for the Study of Learning and Teaching Styles.

Burke, K., & Dunn, R. (2003). Learning style–based teaching to raise minority student test scores. *Social Studies*, 94(4), 167–170.

Burnham, J. J., & Jackson, C. M. (2000). School counselor roles: Discrepancies between actual practice and existing models. *Professional School Counseling*, 4, 41–49.

Bursuck, B., & Blanks, B. (2010). Evidence-based early reading practices within a response to intervention system. *Psychology in the Schools*, 47(5), 421–431.

Burtnett, F. (1993, April 28). Move counseling off the back burner of reform. *Education Week*, 32, 22.

Butcher, J. N., Dahlstrom, W. G., Graham, J. R., Tellegen, A., & Kraemmer, B. (1989). *Minnesota Multiphasic Personality Inventory-2 (MMPI-2): Manual for administration and scoring*. Minneapolis, MN: University of Minnesota.

Butler, S. K., & Constantine, M. G. (2005). Collective self-esteem and burnout in professional school counselors. *Professional School Counseling*, 9(1), 55–62.

Campbell, C., & Dahir, C. (1997). *Sharing the vision: The national standards for school counseling programs*. Alexandria, VA: American School Counselor Association.

Campos, D. (2005). *Understanding gay & lesbian youth: Lessons for straight school teachers, counselors, and administrators*. Lanham, MD: Rowman & Littlefield.

Canfield, B. S., Ballard, M. B., Osmon, B. C., & McCune, C. (2004). School and family counselors work together to reduce fighting at school. *Professional School Counseling*, 8, 40–46.

Capuzzi, D., & Gross, D. R. (2000). I don't want to live: The adolescent at risk for suicidal behavior. In D. Capuzzi & D. R. Gross (Eds.), *Youth at risk: A prevention resource for counselors, teachers, and parents* (3rd ed., pp. 319–352). Alexandria, VA: American Counseling Association.

Capuzzi, D., & Gross, D. R. (2003). *Counseling and psychotherapy: Theories and interventions*. (3rd ed.). Upper Saddle River, NJ: Merrill Prentice Hall.

Career Institute for Education and Workforce Development. (2002). *Decisions without direction: Career guidance and decision making among American youth*. Lansing, MI: EPIC-MRA.

Carkhuff, R. (1985). *The art of helping*. (6th ed.). Amherst, MA: Human Resource Development Press.

Carnevale, A., & Desrochers, D. M. (2003a). Preparing students for the knowledge economy: What school counselors need to know. *Professional School Counseling*, 6(4), 228–236.

Carnevale, A., & Desrochers, D. M. (2003b). Standards for what: The economic roots of K–16 reform. Princeton, NJ: Educational Testing Service.

Carney, J. (2008). Perceptions of bullying and associated trauma during adolescence. *Professional School Counseling*, 11, 179–187.

Casey, J. A. (1995). Development Issues for School Counselors Using Technology. *Elementary school guidance & counseling*, 30, 26–34.

Center on Education Policy. (1998). *Public schools: A place where children can learn to get along with others in a diverse society*. Washington, DC: Author.

Center for Mental Health in Schools. (2008). *Community schools: Working towards institutional transformation*. Los Angeles, CA: Author.

Center for Mental Health in Schools at UCLA. (2007). *Violence prevention and safe schools*. Los Angeles, CA: Author.

Centers for Disease Control. (2010). *Understanding school violence fact sheet*. Washington, DC: Author.

Character Education Partnership. (2004). *Eleven principles of character education*. Retrieved from www.goodcharacter.com

Character Education Partnership. (2010). *Eleven principles of character education*. Retrieved from www.goodcharacter.com

Cheek, J., Bradley, L., Reynolds, J., & Coy, D. (2002). An intervention for helping elementary students reduce text anxiety. *Professional School Counseling*, 73, 311–316.

Cheek, J. R., & House, R. M. (2010a). Advocacy in action: The voice of the student. In B. T. Erford (Ed.), *Professional school counseling* (2nd ed., pp. 112–119). Austin, TX: PRO-ED, Inc.

Cheek, J. R., & House, R. M. (2010b). The ASCA national standards: The foundation of the ASCA national model. In B. T. Erford (Ed.), *Professional school counseling: A handbook of theories, programs, and practices* (2nd ed., pp. 112–119). Austin, TX: PRO-ED, Inc.

Chen-Hayes, S. F. (2000). Social justice with lesbian, bisexual, gay, and transgendered persons. In J. Lewis & L. Bradley (Eds.), *Advocacy in counseling: Counselors, clients, and community* (pp. 89–98). Greensboro, NC: CAPS & Eric/CASS.

Chen-Hayes, S. F., Miller, E. M., Bailey, D. F., Getch, Y. Q., & Erford, B. T. (2011).

Leadership and achievement advocacy for every student. In B. T. Erford (Ed.), *Transforming the school counseling profession* (3rd ed.). Upper Saddle River, NJ: Pearson Education, Inc.

Chibbaro, J. (2007). School counselors and the cyber bully: Interventions and implications. *Professional School Counseling*, 11, 65–68.

Children's Defense Fund. (2010). *The State of America's Children 2010: Yearbook 2010*. Washington, DC: Author.

Chisholm, I., & Trumbull, E. (2001). The diverse challenges of multiculturalism. *Education Update*, 43, 1–3.

Clark, M. A., Lee, S. M., Goodman, W., & Yacco, S. (2008). Examining male underachievement in public education action research at a district level. *NASSP Bulletin*, 92, 111–132.

Clark, M. A., & Stone, C. B. (2000a). Evolving our image: School counselors as educational leaders. *Counseling Today*, 42(11), 21–22, 29, 46.

Clark, M., & Stone, C. (2000b). The developmental school counselor as educational leader. In J. Wittmer (Ed.), *Managing your school counseling program: K–12 developmental strategies* (2nd ed., pp. 75–81). Minneapolis, MN: Educational Media.

Clarke, J. H., & Frazer, E. (2003). Making learning personal: Educational practices that work. In J. DiMartino, J. Clarke, & D. Wolk (Eds.), *Personalized learning: Preparing high school students to create their futures* (pp. 174–193). Latham, MD: Scarecrow Press.

Clemens, E. V. (2007). Developmental counseling and therapy as a model for school counselor consultation with teachers. *Professional School Counseling*, 10, 352–359.

Clements, K. D., & Sabella, R. A. (2010). Make it work. *The ASCA Counselor*, 47, 32–35.

Clinchy, E. (1991, November). America 2000: Reform, revolution, or just more smoke and mirrors. *Phi Delta Kappan*, 73(3), 210–218.

Coalition for Community Schools. (2010). *What is a community school?* Retrieved from http://76.227.216.38/aboutschools/what_is_a_community_school.aspx

Cobia, C., & Henderson, D. (2007). *The handbook of school counseling* (2nd ed.). Columbus, OH: Merrill Prentice Hall.

Cohen, M. (2010, June). Achieve applauds final K–12 common core state standards. *Achieve Press Release*. Retrieved from http://achieve.org/achieve-applauds-final-k-12-common-core-state-standards

Cohen, R. (2005). *Students resolving conflict*. Tucson, AZ: Good Year Books.

Comer, J. (1995). Racism and African-American adolescent development. In C. V. Willie et al. (Eds.), *Mental health, racism, and sexism*. (pp. 151–170). Pittsburgh, PA: University of Pittsburgh Press.

Conger, R. D., Conger, K. J., & Elder, G. (1997). Family economic hardship and adolescent academic performance: Mediating and moderating processes. In G. Duncan & J. Brooks-Gunnan (Eds.), *Consequences of growing up poor* (pp. 288–310). New York: Russell Sage Foundation.

Conley, D. (2010). College knowledge: An interview with David Conley. *Kappan*, 92, 28–34.

Conlon, A. L., & Hansen, J. I. (2004). Broadband and narrowband measures of mental and behavioral health. In Wall & Walz (Eds.), *Measuring up: Assessment issues for teachers, counselors, and administrators* (pp. 213–230). Austin, TX: PRO-ED.

Connolly, F., & Protheroe, N. (Eds.). (2009). *Principals and counselors: Partnering for student success*. Washington, DC: Naviance.

Constantine, M. G., & Gainor, K. A. (2001). Emotional intelligence and empathy: Their relation to multicultural counseling knowledge and awareness. *Professional School Counseling*, 5, 131–137.

Constantine, M. G., Hage, S. M., Kindaichi, M. M., & Bryant, R. M. (2007). Social justice and multicultural issues: Implications for the practice and training of counselors and counseling psychologists. *Journal of Counseling and Development*, 85, 24–29.

Cooper, C. R. (1998). *The weaving of maturity: Cultural perspectives on adolescent development*. New York: Oxford University Press.

Corey, G. (2001). *The theory and practice of counseling and psychotherapy* (6th ed.). Pacific Grove, CA: Brooks/Cole.

Corey, G. (2009). *Theory and practice of counseling and psychotherapy*. Belmont, CA: Brooks/Cole.

Corey, G., Corey, M. S., & Callanan, P. (2010). *Issues and ethics in the helping professions*. Pacific Grove, CA: Brooks/Cole.

Corey, G., Corey, M. S., Callanan, P., & O'Phelan, M. L. (1998). *Issues and ethics: In the helping professions*. Pacific Grove, CA: Brooks/Cole.

Corsini, R., & Wedding, D. (1995). *Current psychotherapies* (5th ed.). Itasca, IL: F. E. Peacock.

Cottone, R. R., & Tarvydas, V. M. (2007). *Counseling ethics and decision making*. Upper Saddle River, NJ: Pearson.

Council for Accreditation of Counseling and Related Educational Programs. (2009). *2009 Standards*. Alexandria, VA.

Covey, Stephen. (1990). *The 7 habits of highly effective people*. New York: Simon & Schuster.

Crosson-Tower, C. (2009). *Understanding child abuse and neglect*. Upper Saddle River, NJ: Prentice Hall.

Crothers, L., Hughes, T., & Morine, K. (2008). *Theory and cases in school-based consultation: A resource for school psychologists, school counselors,* special educators, and other mental health professionals. New York, NY: Taylor & Francis.

Crowther, F., Kaagan, S. S., Ferguson, M., & Hann, L. (2002). *Developing teacher leaders: How leadership enhances school success.* Thousand Oaks, CA: Corwin Press.

Cunanan, E., & Maddy-Bernstein, C. (1994, August). *The role of the school counselor.* BRIEF 1, 1, NCRVE: Berkeley.

Cunningham, N. J., & Sandhu, D. S. (2000). A comprehensive approach to school-community violence prevention. *Professional School Counseling, 4,* 126–132.

Curry, J., & Lambie, G. (2007). Enhancing school counselor accountability: The large group guidance portfolio. *Professional School Counseling, 11*(2), 145–148.

Curtis, R., Van Horne, J. W., Robertson, P., Karvonen, M. (2010). Outcomes of a school-wide positive behavioral support program. *Professional School Counseling, 13,* 159–164.

Custred, G. (2002). The primacy of standard language in modem education. *American Behavioral Scientist, 34,* 232–239.

Daggett, W. (2003). School counselors and information literacy from the perspective of Willard Daggett. *Professional School Counseling, 6*(4), 238–242.

D'Agostino, J. V., Murphy, J. A. (2004). A meta-analysis of Reading Recovery in United States schools. *Educational Evaluation and Policy Analysis, 26*(1), 23–38.

Dahir, C. (2000). Principals as partners in school counseling. *ASCA Counselor, 38*(2), 13.

Dahir, C. (2001). The national standards for school counseling programs: Development and implementation. *Professional School Counseling, 4*(5), 320–327.

Dahir, C. (2002, Winter). We have all become important in one day. *NYSSCA Gram-Fall.* Albany, NY: New York State School Counselor Association.

Dahir, C. (2004). Supporting a nation of learners: The development of the national standards for school counseling programs. *Journal of Counseling and Development, 82*(3), 344–353.

Dahir, C. (2009). Where lies the future? Editor, Special Section on School Counseling. *Journal of Counseling and Development, 87,* 3–5.

Dahir, C., Campbell, C., Johnson, L., Scholes, R., & Valiga, M. (1997, March). *Supporting a nation of learners: The development of national standards for school counseling programs.* Paper presented at the annual meeting of the American Educational Research Association, Chicago, IL.

Dahir, C., & Stone, C. (2003). Accountability: A M.E.A.S.U.R.E of the impact school counselors have on student achievement. *Professional School Counseling, 6*(3), 214–221.

Dahir, C., & Stone, C. (2004). No school counselor left behind. *VISTAS: Perspectives on counseling 2004.* Greensboro, NC: CAPSpress.

Dahir, C., & Stone, C. (2007). School counseling at the crossroads of change. *ACA Professional Counseling Digests* (ACAPCD-05). Alexandria, VA: American Counseling Association.

Dahir, C. & Stone, C. (2009). School counselor accountability: The path to social justice and systemic change. *Journal of Counseling and Development, 87,* 12–20.

Dahir, C. A., & Tyson, L. E. (2010). The ASCA national standards: The foundation of the ASCA national model. In B. T. Erford (Ed.), *Professional school counseling: A handbook of theories, programs, and practices* (2nd ed., pp. 166–176). Austin, TX: PRO-ED.

D'Andrea, M. (2004). Comprehensive school-based violence prevention training: A developmental-ecological training method. *Journal of Counseling & Development, 82,* 277–286.

Daniels, J. (2002). Assessing threats of school violence: Implications for counselors. *Journal of Counseling and Development, 80,* 215–218.

Dardig, J. C. (2008). *Involving parents of students with special needs: 25 ready-to-use strategies.* Corwin Press.

Darling-Hammond, L. (1992). *Standards of practice in learner-centered schools.* Albany, NY: New York State Education Department.

Davis v. Monroe County Board of Education et al. 120 F.3d 1390. (Supreme Court, May 24, 1999). Retrieved from http://web.lexis-nexis.com/universe

Davis, K. M., & Lambie, G. W. (2005). Family engagement: A collaborative, systemic approach for middle school counselors. *Professional School Counseling, 9*(2), 144–151.

Davis, T. E., & Osborn, C. J. (2000). *The solution-focused school counselor: Shaping professional practice.* Philadelphia, PA: Accelerated Development.

DeBoer, A. (1995). *Working together: The art of consulting and communicating.* Longmont, CO: Sopris West.

Delaney, E. M., & Kaiser, A. P. (2001). The effects of teaching parents blended communication and behavior support strategies. *Behavioral Disorders, 26*(2), 93–116.

de Shazer, S. (1985). *Keys to solution in brief therapy.* New York: W.W. Norton.

Dettmer, P., Thurston, L. P., & Dyck, N. (2005). *Consultation, collaboration, and teamwork for students with special needs* (5th ed.). Boston: Allyn & Bacon.

Devine, J., & Cohen, J. (2007). *Making your school safe: Strategies to protect children and promote learning.* New York: Teacher's College Press.

Devine, J., & Cohen, J. (2008). *Making your school safe: Strategies to protect children and promote learning.* New York: Teacher's College Press.

DeVoss, J. A. (2010a). Current and future perspectives on school counseling. In B. T. Erford (Ed.), *Professional school counseling: A handbook of theories, programs, and practices* (2nd ed., pp. 23–33). Austin, TX: PRO-ED, Inc.

DeVoss, J. A. (2010b). The professional school counselor and leadership. In B. T. Erford (Ed.), *Professional school counseling: A handbook of theories, programs, and practices* (2nd ed., pp. 94–103). Austin, TX: PRO-ED, Inc.

Dimmitt, C., Carey, J. C., & Hatch, T. (2007). *Evidence-based school counseling: Making a difference with data-driven practices.* Thousand Oaks, CA: Corwin Press.

Dinkes, R., Kemp, J., & Baum, K. (2009). *Indicators of School Crime and Safety: 2008.* NCES 2009-022/NCJ 226343

Dinkmeyer, D., & Caldwell, E. (1970). *Developmental counseling and guidance: A comprehensive school approach.* New York: McGraw-Hill.

Dinkmeyer, D., Jr., & Carlson, J. (2006). *Consultation: Creating school-based interventions* (3rd ed.). New York: Taylor & Francis.

Dinkmeyer, D., Sr., McKay, G., & Dinkmeyer, D., Jr. (1997). *Systematic training for effective parenting.* Circle Pines, MN: American Guidance Services Publishing.

Dollarhide, C. T., Gibson, D. M., & Saginak, K. A. (2008). New counselors' leadership efforts in school counseling: Themes from a year-long qualitative study. *Professional School Counseling, 11*(4), 262–271.

Dollarhide, C., & Lemberger, M. (2006). No Child Left Behind: Implications for school counselors. *Professional School Counseling, 9,* 295–304.

Dorn, M. (2002). Ten common mistakes districts make when developing emergency response plans. *School Superintendent's Insider, 14,* Palm Beach Gardens, FL: LRP Publications.

Dorsey, J. (2000). *Ending school violence: Solutions from America's youth.* Nashville, TN: Archstone Press/Golden Ladder Productions.

Dougherty, A. M. (2009). *Psychological consultation and collaboration in school and community settings* (5th ed.). Belmont, CA: Brooks/Cole, Cengage Learning.

Doyle, L. (2004). Leadership for community building: Changing how we think and act. *The Clearing House, 77*(5), 196.

Dreikurs, R., & Soltz, V. (1990). *Children: The challenge.* New York: Plume.

Drucker, P. (1989). *The new realities.* London: Heinemann Professional Publishing Ltd.

Dryfoos, J. (1994). *Full service schools: A revolution in health and human services for children, youth and families.* San Francisco: Jossey-Bass.

Duffy, M., Giordano, V. A., Farrell, J. B., Paneque, O. M., & Crump, G. B.

(2008). No Child Left Behind: Values and research issues in high-stakes assessments. *Counseling and Values, 53*(1), 53–66.

Duffy, R. D., & Klingaman, E. A. (2009). Ethnic identity and career development among first-year college students. *Journal of Career Assessment, 17,* 286–297.

Duncan, A. (2010, January 20). Duncan carves deep mark on policy in first year. *Education Week, 29.* Retrieved from http://www.edweek.org/ew/articles/2010/01/20/18duncan_ep.h29.html

Dunn, K., & Dunn, R. (1987). Dispelling outmoded beliefs about student learning. *Educational Leadership, 45,* 55–63.

Dunn, K., Dunn, R., & Price, G. E. (2003). *Learning style inventory.* Lawrence, KS: Price Systems.

Dunn, R., & Dunn, K. (1978). *Teaching students through their individual learning styles: A practical approach.* Reston, VA: Reston Publishing Company.

Dwyer, K., Osher, D., & Warger, C. (1998). *Early warning, timely response: A guide to safe schools.* Washington, DC: U.S. Department of Education.

Education Trust. (1997). *Working definition of school counseling.* Washington, DC: Author.

Education Trust. (2001a). *Achievement in America.* Retrieved from http://www2.edtrust.org/edtrust/

Education Trust. (2001b). *National commission on the high school senior year youth at crossroads: Facing high school and beyond.* Washington, DC: Author.

Education Trust. (2003, June 5). The education trust and MetLife Foundation announce the formation of a national center for transforming school counseling. Retrieved from www.edtrust.org/dc/press-room/press-release/the-education-trust-and-metlife-foundation-announce-the-formation-of-a-n

Education Trust. (2009). *Transforming school counseling initiative.* Retrieved from www.2.edtrust.org/EdTrust/Transforming+School+Counseling

Education Trust, National Center for Transforming School Counseling. (2009a). *The new vision for school counseling: Work ready, college ready, same preparation.* Retrieved from www.edtrust.org/dc/tsc/vision

Education Trust, National Center for Transforming School Counseling. (2009b). *The new vision for school counselors: Scope of the work.* Retrieved from www.edtrust.org/sites/edtrust.org/files/Scope%20of%20the%20Work_1.pdf

Education Week. (2010). *Quality counts.* Washington DC: Author. Retrieved from www.edweek.org/ew/toc/2010/01/14/index.html

Education Week. (2010, June 2). *U.S. graduation rate continues to decline.* Washington DC. Author.

Edwards, M. A. (1994). Foreword. In D. G. Burgess & R. M. Dedmond (Eds.),

*Quality leadership and the professional school counselor.* Alexandria, VA: ASCA.

Egan, G. (1994). *The skilled helper* (5th ed.). Monterey, CA: Brooks/Cole.

Eisel v. Board of Education of Montgomery County, 324 Md. 376, 597 A. 2d 447 (Md. Ct. App. 1991).

Eisner, E. W. (1993). Why standards may not improve schools. *Educational Leadership, 51,* 22–24.

Elam, C., Stratton, T., & Gibson, D. (2007). Welcoming a new generation to college: The millennial students. *Journal of College Admission.* Retrieved from Academic Search Premier.

Elias, S. (2008). Fifty years of influence in the workplace: The evolution of the French and Raven power taxonomy. *Journal of Management History, 14*(3), 267–283.

Epstein, J., & Sheldon, S. (2002). Present and accounted for: Improving student attendance through family and community involvement. *The Journal of Educational Research, 95*(5), 308.

Epstein, J. L. (2001). *School, family, and community partnerships: Preparing educators and improving schools.* Boulder, CO: Westview Press.

Epstein, J. L., Sanders, M. G., Sheldon, S. B., Simon, B. S., Salinas, K. C., Jansorn, N. R., Van Voorhis, F. L., Martin, C. S., Thomas, B. G., Greenfield, M. D., Hutchins, D. J., & Williams, K. J. (2009). *School, family, and community partnerships: Your handbook for action.* Thousand Oaks, CA: Corwin Press.

Erchul, W. P., & Sheridan, S. M. (Eds.). (2008). *Handbook of research in school consultation.* New York: Taylor & Francis.

Erford, B. (2010). *Professional school counseling: A handbook of theories, programs, and practices* (2nd ed.). Austin, TX: Pro-Ed.

Erford, B. T. (2011a). Accountability: Evaluating programs, assessing needs, and determining outcomes. In B. T. Erford (Ed.), *Transforming the school counseling profession* (3rd ed., pp. 245–287). Upper Saddle River, NJ: Pearson Education.

Erford, B. T. (2011b). Consultation, collaboration, and parent involvement. In B. T. Erford (Ed.), *Transforming the school counseling profession* (3rd ed., pp. 222–244). Upper Saddle River, NJ: Pearson Education.

Erford, B. T. (2011c). *Transforming the school counseling profession.* Upper Saddle River, NJ: Pearson.

Erford, B. T., & McCaskill, K. (2010). Professional school counseling: Integrating theory and practice into a data-driven, outcomes-based approach. In B. T. Erford (Ed.), *Professional school counseling: A handbook of theories, programs, and practices* (2nd ed., pp. 2–8). Austin, TX: PRO-ED.

Erickson, E. H. (1963). *Childhood and society.* New York: W.W. Norton.

Erickson, E. H. (1968). *Identity, youth and crisis.* New York: W.W. Norton.

Family Education Rights and Privacy Act of 1974 (FERPA), 20 U.S.C. § 1232g (1974).

Farmer, T., Farmer, E., Estell, D., Hutchins, B. (2007).The developmental dynamics of aggression and the prevention of school violence. *Journal of Emotional and Behavioral Disorders, 15,* 197–208.

Feller, R. W. (2003) Aligning school counseling: The changing workplace, and career development assumptions. *Professional School Counseling.* Retrieved from www.findarticles.com/cftrvgnt/

Feller, R. W. (2009, September/October). STEM: Career launch pad. *ASCA School Counselor, 47*(1). 37–41.

Feller, R. W. (2010, Spring). Comprehensive school counseling programs and STEM careers. *Career Developments, 26*(2), 16–17.

Fields, T. H., & Hines, P. L. (2010). The professional school counselor's role in raising student achievement. In B. T. Erford (Ed.), *Professional school counseling* (2nd ed., pp. 120–127). Austin, TX: PRO-ED, Inc.

Fink, E., & Resnick, L. B. (2001). Developing principals as instructional leaders. *Phi Delta Kappan, 82,* 598–606.

Finkelstein, D. (2009). *A closer look at the principal-counselor relationship: A survey of principals and counselors.* Retrieved from http://professionals.collegeboard.com/profdownload/a-closer-look.pdf

Fischer, G. P., & Sorenson, L. (1996). *School law for counselors, psychologists and social workers* (3rd ed.). White Plains, NY: Longman.

Fischer, K., & Kettl, P. (2001). Trends in school violence: Are our schools safe? In M.Shafii & S. L.Shafii (Eds.), *School violence: Assessment, management, prevention.* Washington, DC: American Psychiatric Publishing, Inc.

Fischer, L., Schimmel, D., & Stellman, L. R. (2010). *Teachers and the law.* Upper Saddle River, NJ: Prentice Hall.

Fitch, T. J., & Marshall, J. L. (2004). What counselors do in high-achieving schools: A study on the role of the school counselor. *Professional School Counseling, 7,* 172–178.

FL§ 1006.42. Title 48.K-20 Education Code (Chs. 1000-1013); Chapter 1006. Support for Learning; Part I. Public K–12 Education Support for Learning and Student Services, (2010).

Frankl, V. L. (1963). *Man's search for meaning.* Boston: Beacon.

Franklin, J. (2001). The diverse challenges of multicultural education. *Education Update, 43,* 2.

Fredrickson, B. L. (2001). The role of positive emotions in positive psychology. *American Psychologist, 56,* 218–226.

French, J. R. P., Jr., & Raven, B. H. (1959). *The bases of social power.* In D.Cartwright et al., *Studies in social power* (pp. 1150–1167) Ann Arbor, MI: Institute for Social Research.

Friend, M., & Cook, L. (2009). *Interactions: Collaboration skills for school professionals* (6th ed.). Upper Saddle River, NJ: Prentice Hall.

Frisén, A., Jonsson, A., & Persson, C. (2007). Adolescents' perception of bullying: Who is the victim? Who is the bully? What can be done to stop bullying? *Adolescence, 42*, 749–761.

Fuchs, D., Fuchs, L. S. (2006). Introduction to Response to Intervention: What, why, and how valid is it? Reading Research Quarterly, 41, doi: 10.1598/RRQ.41.1.4

Fullan, M. (1993). Innovation, reform and restructuring strategies. Challenges and Achievements of American Education, the 1993 ASCD Yearbook. *Association of Supervision in Curriculum and Development, 4*, 14.

Fullan, M. (2002). Leadership and sustainability. *Principal Leadership, 3*(4), 14–17.

Fullan, M. (2004). *Leadership and sustainability.* Thousand Oaks, CA: Corwin Press.

Fusco, J. (2009). *State records shed light on weapons incidents in Mohawk Valley schools.* Retrieved from www.uticaod.com/news/x1331538639/State-records-shed-light-on-weapons-incidents-in-Mohawk-Valley-schools

Galassi, J., & Akos, P. (2004a). Déjà vu and moving the conversation: Reactions to an underutilized partnership. *The Counseling Psychologist, 32*, 215–244.

Galassi, J., & Akos, P. (2004b). Developmental advocacy: Twenty-first century school counseling. *Journal of Counseling and Development, 82*, 146–157.

Galassi, J. P., & Akos, P. (2007). *Strengths-based school counseling: Promoting student development and achievement.* New York: Lawrence Erlbaum Associates.

Galassi, J. P., Griffin, D., & Akos, P. (2008). Strength-based school counseling and the ASCA National Model. *Professional School Counseling, 12*(2), 176–181.

Gappa, J. M., Austin, A. E., & Trice, A. G. (2007). *Rethinking faculty work: Higher education's strategic imperative.* San Francisco, CA: Jossey-Boss.

Garbarino, J. (1999). *Lost boys: Why our sons turn violent and how we can save them.* Chicago: Simon & Schuster.

Garbarino, J., & Stott, F. M. (1989). *What children can tell us.* San Francisco: Jossey-Bass.

Gardner, H. (1999). *Intelligence reframed: Multiple intelligences for the 21st century.* New York: Simon & Schuster.

Geltner, J. A., & Leibforth, T. N. (2008). Advocacy in the IEP process: Strength-based school counseling in action. *Professional School Counseling, 12*(2), 162–165.

Gerler, E. R. (1992). What we know about school counseling: A reaction to Borders and Drury. *Journal of Counseling and Development, 70*, 499–500.

George, R., & Cristiani, T. (1995). *Counseling: Theory and practice* (4th ed.) Needham Heights, MA: Simon and Schuster.

Geroski, A. M., & Knauss, L. (2000). Addressing the needs of foster children in a school counseling program. *Professional School Counseling, 3*, 152–161.

Gestwiki, C. (2010). *Home, school, and community* (7th ed.). Belmont, CA: Wadsworth.

Gibson, D. M. (2010). Consulting in the schools: The role of the professional school counselor. In B. T. Erford (Ed.), *Professional school counseling: A handbook of theories, programs, and practices* (2nd ed., pp. 303–311). Austin, TX: PRO-ED, Inc.

Gilligan, C. (1993). *In a different voice: Psychological theory and women's development.* Cambridge, MA: Harvard University Press.

Gladding, S. T. (2004). *Counseling: A comprehensive profession* (5th ed.). Upper Saddle River, NJ: Pearson Education, Inc.

Gladding, S. T. (2009). *Counseling: A comprehensive profession* (5th ed.). Upper Saddle River, NJ: Pearson Education, Inc.

Glasser, W. (1986). *Control theory in the classroom.* New York: Harper & Row.

Glasser, W. (1998). *Choice theory.* New York: Harper Collins.

Glasser, W. (2000a). *Every student can succeed.* Chula Vista, CA: Black Forest Press.

Glasser, W. (2000b). School violence from the perspective of William Glasser. *Professional School Counseling, 4*, 77–80.

GLSENTalk. (1998, October). *GLSEN Hudson Valley co-sponsors youth conference.* Available by email from Glsentalk@glsen.org

Goldman, D. (1995). *Emotional intelligence.* New York: Bantam.

Goldstein, A., & Kodluboy, D. (1998). *Gangs in schools: Signs, symbols and solutions.* Champaign, IL: Research Press.

Goodnough, G., & Lee, V. (2004). Group counseling in schools. In B. T.Erford (Ed.), *Professional school counseling: A handbook of theories, programs, and practices.* (pp. 173–182). Austin, TX: PRO-ED.

Gordon, E. E. (2005). *Peer tutoring: A teacher's resource guide.* Lanham, MD: Scarecrow Education.

Gordon, E. W. (2006). Establishing a system of public education in which all children achieve at high levels and reach their full potential. In T. Smiley (Ed.), *The covenant with Black America* (pp. 23–45). Chicago: Third World Press.

Gordon, I. J. (1977). Parent education and parent involvement: Retrospect and prospect. *Childhood education, 54*, 71–77.

Gore, P. A., & Leuwerke, W. C. (2000). Information technology for career assessment on the Internet. *Journal of Career Assessment, 8*(1), 3–19.

Gottfredson, D. (2001). *School-based crime prevention of problem behavior: What works … under what conditions?* Paper presented at the 2001 Office of Safe and Drug Free Schools Technical Assistance Meeting, Washington, DC.

Graham, S., & Taylor, A. Z. (2002). Ethnicity, gender and the development of achievement values. In A. Wigfield & J. S. Eccles (Eds.), *Development of achievement motivation: A volume in the educational psychology series* (pp. 121–146). San Diego, CA: Academic Press.

Green, A., & Keys, S. (2001). Expanding the developmental school counseling paradigm: Meeting the needs of the 21st century student. *Professional School Counseling, 5*(2), 84–95.

Green, A. G., Conley, J. A. & Barnett, K. (2005). Urban school counseling: Implications for practice and training. *Professional School Counselor Journal, 8*, 189–195.

Greenberg, K. (2003). *Group counseling in schools.* Upper Saddle River, NJ: Pearson Education.

Green, A., & Keys, S. (2001). Expanding the developmental school counseling paradigm: Meeting the needs of the 21st century student. *Professional School Counseling, 5*(2), 84–95.

Greene, J. P., & Winters, M. A. (2005). Public high school graduation rates and college readiness rates: 1991–2002. *Education Working Paper, 8*, 1–27.

Griffin, D., & Farris, A. (2010). School counselors and collaboration: Finding resources through community asset mapping. *Professional School Counseling, 13*(5), 248–256.

Griffin, D., & Steen, S. (2010). School-family-community partnerships: Applying Epstein's theory of the six types of involvement to school counselor practice. *Professional School Counseling, 13*(4), 218–226. doi: 2018215341

Grossman v. S. Shore Pub. Sch. Dist., 507 F.3d 1097 (7th Cir. 2007).

Grotberg, E. (1998). I am, I have, I can: What families worldwide taught us about resilience. *Reaching Today's Youth: The Community Circle of Caring, 1*(3), 36–39.

Guindon, M. H. (2003). Assessment. In B. T. Erford, *Transforming the school counseling profession.* Upper Saddle River, NJ: Merrill Prentice Hall.

Gurian, M. (2001). *Boys and girls learn differently: A guide for teachers and parents.* San Francisco, CA: Jossey-Bass

Gysbers, N. C. (2001). School guidance and counseling in the 21st century: Remember the past into the future. *Professional School Counseling, 5*(2), 96–105.

Gysbers, N. C. (2004). Comprehensive guidance and counseling programs: The evolution of accountability. *Professional School Counseling*, 8(1), 1–14.

Gysbers, N. C., & Henderson P. (1994). *Developing and managing your school guidance program* (2nd ed.). Alexandria, VA: American Counseling Association.

Gysbers, N. C., & Henderson, P. (2000). *Developing and managing your school guidance program* (3rd ed.). Alexandria, VA: American Counseling Association.

Gysbers, N. C., & Henderson, P. (2001). Comprehensive guidance and counseling programs: A rich history and a bright future. *Professional School Counseling*, 4(4), 246–256.

Gysbers, N. C., & Henderson, P. (2002). *Leading and managing comprehensive school guidance programs.* (ERIC Document Reproduction Service No. ED462670) Greensboro, NC: ERIC/CASS Digest.

Gysbers, N. C., & Henderson, P. (2006). *Developing and managing your school guidance program* (4th ed.). Alexandria, VA: American Counseling Association.

Gysbers, N. C., & Henderson, P. (2012). *Developing and managing your school guidance program* (5th ed.). Alexandria, VA: American Counseling Association.

Gysbers, N. C., & Moore, E. J. (1981). *Improving guidance programs.* Englewood Cliffs, NJ: Prentice-Hall.

H. L. v. Matheson, 450 U.S. 398 (1981).

Hackman, R. (2002). *Leading teams: Setting the stage for great performances.* Boston, MA: Harvard Business School Press.

Halford, J. M. (1999). A different mirror: A conversation with Richard Takaki. *Educational Leadership*, 56(7), 8–13.

Hallahan, D. P. (1992). Some thoughts on why the prevalence of learning disabilities has increased. *Journal of Learning Disabilities*, 25(8), 523–528.

Hallahan, D. P., Kauffman, J. M., & Pullen, P. C. (2009). *Exceptional learners: An introduction to special education.* Boston, MA: Pearson.

Hammond, B. (2010). *Schools can't be social workers and fix problems rooted in the home: Or should they?* Retrieved from www.oregonlive.com/education/index.ssf/2010/02/schools_cant_be_social_workers.html

Handy, C. (2002). *The elephant and the flea.* London: Hutchinson.

Harris, H. L., Wierzalis, E. A., & Coy, D. R. (2010). Parental involvement in schools. In B. T.Erford (Ed.), *Professional school counseling: A handbook of theories, programs, and practices* (2nd ed., pp. 973–981). Austin, TX: Pro-Ed.

Harris, M. B., & Bliss, K. G. (1997). Coming out in a school setting: Former students' experiences and opinions about disclosure. In M. B. Harris (Ed.), *School experiences of gay and lesbian youth* (pp. 85–100). New York: Harrington Park Press.

Hart, P., & Jacobi, M. (1992). *Gatekeeper to advocate.* New York: College Board Press.

Hawkins, D. L., Pepler, D. J., & Craig, W. M. (2001). Naturalistic observations of peer interventions in bullying. *Social Development*, 10(4), 512–527.

Hawkins, J. D., Farrington, D. P., & Catalano, R. F. (1998). Reducing violence through the schools. In D. S.Elliott, B. A. Hamburg, & K. R.Williams (Eds.), *Violence in American schools: A new perspective* (pp. 188–216). Cambridge, England: Cambridge University Press.

Hawkins, J. D., Herrenkohl, T., Farrington, D. B., Catalano, R., Harachl, T., & Cothern, L. (2000, April). Predictors of youth violence. *Juvenile Justice Bulletin.* Retrieved from http://ncjrs.org/html/jojdp/jjbul2000_04_5/contents.html

Haycock, K. (2001). Closing the achievement gap. *Educational Leadership*, 58(6), 6–11.

Haycock, K., & Hines, P. (2006, January). School counsel's role in college admission. In R. Way (Chair), *ASCA Board Meeting.* Symposium conducted at the meeting of the American School Counseling Association, Washington, DC.

Hayden, L., Poynton, T. A., & Sabella, R. A. (2008). School counselors' use of technology within the ASCA National Model's delivery system. *Journal of Technology in Counseling*, 5(1). Retrieved from http://jtc.colstate.edu/Vol5_1/Hayden.htm

Hazler, R. J. (2000). When victims turn aggressors: Factors in the development of deadly school violence. *Professional School Counseling*, 4, 105–112.

Heinzmann, G. S. (2002). Parental violence in youth sports: Facts, myths and videotape. *Parks & Recreation*, 37, 66–73.

Heller, K. A., Holtzman, W. H., & Messick, S. (1982). *Placing children in special education: A strategy for equity.* Washington, DC: National Academy Press.

Helms, J. (2004). Fair and valid use of educational testing in grades K–12. In Wall J. & Walz, G. (Eds.), *Measuring up: Assessment issues for teachers, counselors, and administrators* (pp. 81–88). Austin, TX: PRO-ED.

Henderson, A. T., Mapp, K. L., Johnson, V. R., & Davies, D. (2007). *Beyond the bake sake: The essential guide to family-school partnerships.* New York: New Press.

Henderson, D., & Thompson, C. (2011). *Counseling children* (8th ed.). Belmont, CA: Brooks/Cole.

Henderson, N., & Milstein, M. (1996). *Resiliency in schools: Making it happen for students and educators.* Thousand Oaks, CA: Corwin Press.

Hernández, T. J., & Seem, S. R. (April 2004). A safe school climate: A systemic approach and the school counselor. *Professional School Counseling.* 7(4), 256–262.

Herr, E. L. (1979). *Guidance and counseling in the schools. Perspectives on the past, present, and future.* Falls Church, VA: American Personnel and Guidance Association.

Herr, E. L. (1997). *Career development and work-bound youth.* University of North Carolina at Greensboro, NC: ERIC/CASS. (ERIC Document Reproduction Service Document No. ED051199)

Herr, E. L. (2001). The impact of national policies, economics, and school reform on comprehensive guidance programs. *Professional School Counseling*, 4(4), 236–245.

Hilliard, A. (1991). Do we have the will to educate all children? *Educational Leadership*, 48, 31–36.

Hipolito-Delgado, C. P., & Lee, C. C. (2007). Empowerment theory for the professional school counselor: A manifesto for what really matters. *Professional School Counseling*, 10(4), 327–332.

Holcomb, E. (2009). *Asking the right questions: Tools for collaboration and school change* (3rd ed.). Thousand Oaks, CA: Corwin Press.

Holcomb-McCoy, C. (2004). Assessing the multicultural competence of school counselors: A checklist. *Professional School Counseling*, 7, 178–186.

Holcomb-McCoy, C. (2005). Investigating school counselors' perceived multicultural competence. *Professional School Counseling*, 8, 414–423.

Holcomb-McCoy, C. (2007). *School counseling to close the achievement gap: A social justice framework for success.* Thousand Oaks, CA: Corwin Press.

Holland, J. L. (1994). *Self-directed search.* Odessa, FL: Psychological Assessment Resources.

Holland, J. L. (1997). *Making vocational choices. A theory of vocational personalities and work environments* (3rd ed.). Odessa, FL: Psychological Assessment Resources.

Holland, J. L., Fritzsche, B. A., & Powell, A. B. (1994a). *The self-directed search technical manual.* Odesssa, FL: Psychological Assessment Resources.

Holland, J. L., Magoon, T. M., & Spokane, A. R. (1981). Counseling psychology: Career interventions, research, and theory. *Annual Review of Psychology*, 32, 279–305.

Honigsfeld, A., & Dunn, R. (2009). Learning-style responsive approaches for teaching typically performing and at-risk adolescents. *The Clearing House*, 82(5), 220–224. Retrieved from Research Library. (Document ID: 1719481381)

Hookway, C. (2005). Pragmatism. In R. B. Goodman (Ed.), *Pragmatism: Critical concepts in philosophy* (pp. 285–311). New York: Routledge.

Hord, S. M., & Sommers, W. A. (2008). *Leading professional learning communities: Voices from research and practice*. Thousand Oaks, CA: Corwin Press.

Horner, R., & Sugai, G. (2000). School-wide behavior support: An emerging initiative. *Journal of Positive Behavior Interventions*, 2(4), 231–232.

Horner, R. H., Sugai, G., Smolkowski, K., Eber, L., Nakasato, J., Todd, A., & Esperanza, J. (2009). A randomized, waitlist-controlled effectiveness trial assessing school-wide positive behavior support in elementary schools. *Journal of Positive Behavior Interventions*, 11, 133–144.

House, R., & Martin, P. (1998). Advocating for better futures for all students: A new vision for school counselors. *Education*, 119, 284–286.

House, R. M., & Hayes, R. L. (2002). School counselors: Becoming key players in school reform. *Professional School Counseling*, 5, 249–256.

Howard, G. R. (1999). We can't teach what we don't know. New York: Columbia University, Teachers College.

Howe, N., & Strauss, W. (2000). *Millenials rising: The next great generation*. New York: Vintage Books.

Hoyt, K. B. (2001). Helping high school students broaden their knowledge of postsecondary options. *Professional School Counseling*, 5, 6–12.

Hoyt, K. B. (2002). The right tools. *ASCA School Counselor*, 39, 19–23.

Hoyt, K. B., & Wickwire, P. N. (2001). Knowledge-information-service era changes in work and education and the changing role of the school counselor in career education. *Career Development Quarterly*, 49(3), 238–249.

Huey, W. C., & Remley, T. P., Jr. (1988). Confidentiality and the school counselor: A challenge for the 1990s. *The School Counselor*, 41, 23–30.

Huerta, N. E. (2008). The promise and practice of the Individuals with Disabilities Education Act. In T. Jiménez & V. Graf (Eds.), *Education for all* (pp. 1–33). San Francisco, CA: Jossey-Bass.

Hull, N. E. H., & Hoffer, P. C. (2001). *Roe v. Wade: The abortion rights controversy in American history*. Lawrence, KS: University Press of Kansas.

Huss, S., Bryant, A., & Mulet, S. (2008). Managing the quagmire of counseling in a school: Bringing the parents onboard. *Professional School Counseling*, 11(6), 362–367.

Isaacs, M. L. (2003). Data-driven decision making: The engine of accountability. *Professional School Counseling*, 6, 288–295.

Isaacs, M. L., & Stone, C. (1999). School counselors and confidentiality: Factors affecting professional choices. *The Professional School Counselor*, 2, 258–266.

Ivey, A. E., & Ivey, M. B. (2010). *Intentional interviewing and counseling in a multicultural society* (7th ed.). Pacific Grove, CA: Brooks/Cole.

Ivey, A. E., Ivey, M. B., & Simek-Morgan, L. (1993). *Counseling and psychotherapy: A multicultural perspective*. Boston: Allyn & Bacon.

Jacobsen, K. E., & Bauman, S. (2007). Bullying in schools: School counselors' responses to three types of bullying incidents. *Professional School Counseling*, 11, 1–9.

Janosz, M., Archambault, I., Morizot, J., & Pagani, L. (2008). School engagement trajectories and their differential predictive relations to dropout. *Journal of Social Issues*, 64(1), 21–40. doi: 10.1111/j.1540-4560.2008.00546.x

Janson, C. (2008). *High school counselors' perceptions of their leadership behaviors: A Q methodology study*. Unpublished doctoral dissertation, Kent State University, Kent, OH.

Janson, C., & Militello, M. (2009). Where do we go from here? Eight elements of effective school counselor-principal relationships. In F.Connolly & N. Protheroe (Eds.), *The school principal field manual for working with counselors* (pp. 159–164). Washington, DC: Educational Research Service and Naviance, Inc.

Janson, C., Militello, M., & Kosine, N. (2008). Four views of the professional school counselor-principal relationship: A Q-methodology study. *Professional School Counseling*, 11, 353–361.

Janson, C., Stone, C., & Clark, M. A. (2009). Stretching leadership: A distributed perspective for school counselor leaders. *Professional School Counseling*, 13(2), 98–106.

Jennings, K. (2010). OSDFS national conference highlights *The Challenge*, 16, 3. p. 1.

Jiménez, T. C., & Graf, V. L. (2008). *Education for all: Critical issues in the education of children and youth with disabilities*. San Francisco, CA: Jossey-Bass.

Johnson, C. D., & Johnson, S. K. (1991). The new guidance: A system approach to pupil personnel programs. *CACD Journal*, 11, 5–14.

Johnson, C. D., & Johnson, S. K. (2001). *Results-based student support programs: Leadership academy workbook*. San Juan Capistrano, CA: Professional Update.

Johnson, C. D., & Johnson, S. K. (2002). *Building stronger school counseling programs: Bringing futuristic approaches into the present*. Greensboro, NC: Caps Publishers.

Johnson, J., Duffet, A. (2005). *Life after high school: Young people talk about their hopes and prospects*. New York: Public Agenda.

Johnson, J., Rochkind, J., Ott, A., & DuPont, S. (2010). *Can I get a little advice here?* San Francisco, CA: Public Agenda. Retrieved from www.publicagenda.org/theirwholelivesaheadofthem?qt_active=1

Johnson, L. S. (1995). Enhancing multicultural reactions: Intervention strategies for the school counselor. *The School Counselor*, 43(2), 103–113.

Johnson, L. S. (2000). Promoting professional identity in an era of educational reform. *Professional School Counseling*, 4, 31–40.

Johnson, S. K., & Johnson, C. D. (2003). Results-based guidance: A systems approach to student support programs. *Professional School Counseling*, 6(3), 180–184.

Johnson, S. K., Johnson, C. D., & Downs, L. (2006). *Building a results-based student support program*. Boston, MA: Houghton Mifflin.

Kachgal, M., Romano, J. L., & Peterson, J. (2001). *Changes in counseling preparation programs: Early findings*. Minneapolis, MN: University of Minnesota, Center for Applied Research and Educational Improvement.

Kaiser, A., & Hancock, T. (2003). Teaching parents new skills to support their young children's development. *Infants and Young Children*, 16, 9–21.

Kampwirth, T. J. (2006). *Collaborative consultation in the schools: Effective practices for students with learning and behavior problems* (3rd ed.). Upper Saddle River, NJ: Prentice Hall.

Kaplan, L. S. (1996). Outrageous or legitimate concerns: What some parents are saying about school counseling. *The School Counselor*, 43, 165–170.

Karcher, M. (2009). Increases in academic connectedness and self-esteem among high school students who serve as cross-age peer mentors. *Professional School Counseling*, 12(4), 292–299.

Kazie, R. (2005, April). *Remaking career and technical education for the 21st century: What role for high school programs?* Aspen, CO: The Aspen Institute.

Kennedy, S. S. (2009). What can schools do about cyber bullying? *The Challenge*, 16, 4. Office of Safe and Drug Free Schools: Boulder, CO: Montana Safe Schools Center.

Kerr, M., & Dahir, C. (2007). Fundamentals of professional school counseling. In J. Gregorie & C. Jungers (Eds.), *The counselor's companion: What every beginning counselor needs to know* (pp. 360–375). Mahwah, NJ: Lawrence Erlbaum Associates.

Keys, S. G. (2000). Living the collaborative role: Voices from the field. *Professional School Counseling*, (3)5, 332.

Killen v. Independent School District no. 706, CX-95-2505 113 (Mn Ct. App.1996).

Kimmel, M. (2003). I am not insane; I am angry. In M. Sadowski (Ed.), *Adolescents at school: Perspectives on youth, identity, and education*. Cambridge, MA: Harvard University Press.

Kipnis, D., Schmidt, S. M., & Wilkinson, I. (1980). Intraorganizational influence tactics: Explorations in getting one's way. *Journal of Applied Psychology*, 65(4), 440–452.

Kiselica, M. S., & Robinson, M. (2001). Bringing advocacy counseling to life: The history, issues, and human dramas of social justice work in counseling. *Journal of Counseling & Development*, 79, 387–397.

Kitchener, K. S. (1986). Teaching applied ethics in counselor education: An integration of psychological processes and philosophical analysis. *Journal of Counseling and Development*, 64, 306–310.

Klotz, M. B., & Canter, A. (2006). Culturally competent assessment and consultation. *Principal Leadership*, April, 2006, p. 11–15.

Klotz, M. B., & Canter, A. (2007). Response to intervention (RtI): A primer for parents. Retrieved from www.nasponline.org/resources/handouts/revisedPDFs/rtiprimer.pdf

Kohlberg, L. (1984). *The psychology of moral development: The nature and validity of moral stages.* San Francisco: Harper & Row.

Kohm, B., & Nance, B. (2009). Creating collaborative culture. *Educational Leadership*, 67(2), 67–72.

Kosciw, J. G., Diaz, E. M., & Greytak, E. A. (2008). 2007 *National School Climate Survey: The experiences of lesbian, gay, bisexual and transgender youth in our nation's schools.* New York: GLSEN.

Kottler, J. A. (2000). *Doing good: Passion and commitment for helping others.* Philadelphia, PA: Taylor & Francis Group.

Kottler, J. A., & Kottler, E. (2007). Counseling skills for teachers. (2nd ed.) Thousand Oaks, CA: Corwin Press.

Krumboltz, J. D. (1998). Counsellor actions needed for the new career perspective. *British Journal of Guidance and Counselling*, 26, 559–564.

Krumboltz, J. D., & Levin. A. (2004). *Luck is no accident: Making the most of happenstance in your life and career.* Atascadero, CA: Impact Publishers.

Krumboltz, J. D., Mitchell, A. M. & Jones, G. B. (1976). A Social Learning Theory of Career Selection. *The Counselling Psychologist*, 6(1), pp. 71–81.

Kutash, K. & Duchnowski, A. (2006). *Creating environments that work for all youth: Increasing the use of evidence-based strategies by special education Teachers.* Improving Secondary Education and Transition Services Through Research. v.5.: National Center on Education and Transition.

Laird, J. (1998). Theorizing culture: Narrative ideas and practice principles. In M. McGoldrick (Ed.), *Re-visioning family therapy* (pp. 20–36). New York: Guilford.

Lane, K. L., Mahdavi, J. N., & Borthwick-Duffy, S. (2003). Teacher perceptions of the pre-referral intervention process: A call for assistance with school-based interventions. *Preventing School Failure*, (47)4, 148.

Langhout, R. D., Rappaport, J., & Simmons, D. (2002). Integrating community into the classroom: Community gardening, community involvement, and project-based learning. *Urban Education*, 37(3), 323.

Lapan, R., Aoyagi, M., & Kayson, M. (2007). Helping rural adolescents make successful postsecondary transitions: A longitudinal study. *Professional School Counseling*, 10, 266–272.

Lapan, R. T. (2001). Results-based comprehensive guidance and counseling program: A framework for planning and evaluation. *Professional School Counseling*, 4, 289–299.

LaRocque, M. (2007, January 1). Closing the achievement gap: The experience of a middle school. *Clearing House: A Journal of Educational Strategies, Issues and Ideas*, 80(4), 157.

Lassonde, C. A., & Israel, S. E. (2010). *Teacher collaboration for professional learning: Facilitating study, research, and inquiry communities.* San Francisco, CA: Jossey-Bass.

Lawhorn, W. (2004, Spring). The 2002–12 job outlook in brief. *Occupational Outlook Quarterly*, 48(1) 2-5. Washington, DC: U.S. Department of Labor.

Lawson, H. A., & Barkdull, C. (2000). Gaining the collaborative advantage and promoting systems and cross-systems change. In A. Sallee, K. Briar-Lawson, & H. A. Lawson (Eds.), *New century practice with child welfare families* (pp. 245–270). Las Cruces, NM: Eddie Bowers Education.

Lee, C. (1998). *Counseling for diversity: A guide for school counselors and related professionals.* Alexandria, VA: American Counseling Association.

Lee, C. (2001). Culturally responsive school counselors and programs: Addressing the needs of all students. *Professional School Counseling*, 4(4), 257–261.

Lee, C. C. (Ed.). (2007a). *Counseling for social justice* (2nd ed.). Alexandria, VA: American Counseling Association.

Lee, C. C. (2007b). Multicultural issues in counseling: New approaches to diversity. Alexandria, VA: American Counseling Association.

Lee, C. C., & Rodgers, R. A. (2009). Counselor advocacy: Affecting systemic change in the public arena. *Professional School Counseling*, 87, 284–287.

Lee, C. C., & Walz, G. R. (Eds.). (1998). *Social action: A mandate for counselors.* Alexandria, VA: American Counseling Association.

Lee, Courtland C. (2007, April 1). Empowerment theory for the professional school counselor: A manifesto for what really matters. *The Free Library*. (2007). Retrieved from http://www.thefreelibrary.com/Empowerment theory for the professional school counselor: a manifesto...-a0165235177

Lee, S. M., Daniels, M. H., Puig, A., Newgent, R., & Nam, S. K. (2008). A data-based model to predict postsecondary educational attainment of low-socio-economic-status students. *Professional School Counselor*, 11, 306–316.

Leffert, N., & Scales, P. (1999). *Developmental assets.* Minneapolis, MN: Search Institute.

Legum, H. (2005). Finding Solutions. Retrieved from www.schoolcounselor.org/article.asp?article=776&paper=91&cat=137

Lehrer, W., & Sloan, J. (2003). *Crossing the blvd: Strangers, neighbors, aliens in a new America.* New York: W.W. Norton & Company.

Leibforth, T. N. (2008). School counselors and individualized education plan (IEP) meetings: Opportunity for meaningful involvement. *New York State School Counseling Journal*, 5(1), 34–42.

Leinbaugh, T. C. (2010). Understanding special education policies and procedures. In B. T. Erford (Ed.), *Professional school counseling: A handbook of theories, programs, and practices* (2nd ed., pp. 741–748). Austin, TX: Pro-Ed.

Leinhardt, A. M., & Willert, H. J. (2002). Involving stakeholders in resolving school violence. *NASSP Bulletin*, 86, 32–43.

Leithwood, K., Begley, P., & Cousins, J. B. (1992). *Developing expert leadership for future schools.* Washington, DC: The Falmer Press.

Leithwood, K., Steinbach, R., & Jantizi, D. (2002). School leadership and teachers' motivation to implement accountability policies. *Educational Administration Quarterly*, 38(1), 94–119.

Lenhardt, A. M., Farrell, M., & Graham, L. (2010, April–June). Providing anchors reclaiming our troubled youth: Lessons for leaders from a student, *The Educational Forum*, 74, 104–116. doi: 10.1080/00131721003604405

Lerner, R. M., & Benson, P. L. (2002). Developmnetal assets and assets building communities. NY: Kluwer Academic/Plenum Publishers.

Lesko, N. (2001). *Act your age! A cultural construction of adolescence.* New York: Routledge Falmer.

Lewis, J., & Bradley, L. (Eds.). (2000). *Advocacy in counseling: Counselors, clients, & community.* Greensboro, NC: Caps Publications and ERIC/CASS.

Lewis, J. A., Lewis, M. D., Daniels, J. A., & D'Andrea, M. J. (1998). *Community counseling: Empowerment strategies for a diverse society* (2nd ed.). Pacific Grove, CA: Brooks/Cole.

Lieberman, A. (2004). Confusion regarding school counselor functions: School leadership impacts role clarity. *Education*, 124, 552.

Likona, T. (2004). *Character matters.* Carmichael, CA: Touchstone Press.

Likona, T., Schaps, E., & Lewis, C. (2000). *Eleven principles of effective character education.* Retrieved from www.character.org

Limar, S. (2009). Bullying in the digital age. *The Challenge*, 16, 2. Boulder, CO: Office of Safe and Drug Free Schools.

Lindahl, R. (2008). Shared leadership: Can it work in schools? *The Educational Forum, 72,* 289–307.

Linde, L., & Stone, C. (2010). Code of ethics and ethical and legal considerations for students, parents, and professional school counselors. In B. T. Erford (Ed.), *Professional school counseling: A handbook of theories, programs, and practices* (2nd ed., pp. 45–60). Austin, TX: Pro-Ed.

Lister, D. (2005). Effects of traditional versus tactual and kinesthetic learning-style responsive instructional strategies on Bermudian learning-support sixth-grade students' social studies achievement and attitude-test scores. *Research for Educational Reform, 10*(2), 24–40.

Lockwood, A. L. (2008). *The case for character education: A developmental approach.* New York: Teachers College Press.

Loewen, J. W. (1995). *Lies my teacher told me: Everything your American history textbook got wrong.* New York: The New Press.

Loveless, T. (1999). *The tracking and ability group debate.* Washington, DC: Thomas B. Fordham Foundation.

Lowry, R., Powell, K. E., Kann, L., Collins, J. L., & Kolbe, L. J. (1998). Weapon carrying, physical fighting and fight related injuries among U.S. adolescents. *American Journal of Preventive Medicine, 14,* 122–129.

Luck, L., & Webb, L. (2009). School counselor action research: A case example. *Professional School Counseling, 12*(6), 408–412.

Lunenburg, F. C., & Ornstein, A. C. (2008). *Educational administration: Concepts and practices* (5th ed.). Belmont, CA: Thomson Learning, Inc.

Luongo, P. F. (2000). Partnering child welfare, juvenile justice and behavioral health with children. *Professional School Counseling, 3,* 308–314.

L. W. vs. Toms River Regional Schools Board of Education. A-111-05 (2007).

MacGregor, J. (2004). Unpublished video, September 15, 2003.

Maddy-Bernstein, C. (2000). Career development issues affecting secondary schools. *The Highlight Zone Research @ Work.* Retrieved from www.nccte.org/publications/infosynthesis/highlightzone/highlight01/highlight01-careerdevelopment.pdf

Maine Commission on Secondary Education. (1998). *Promising futures: A call to improve learning for Maine's secondary students.* Augusta: Maine Department of Education

Marnik, G. (1997). *A glimpse at today's high schools.* Presented at Successful Transitions conference by the College of Education and Human Development, University of Maine, Orono.

Marsten, D., Muyskens, P., Lau, M., & Canter, A. (2003). Problem solving model for decisions making with high incidence disabilities: The Minneapolis experience. *Learning Disabilities Research & Practice, 18*(3), 187–200.

Martin, P. (1998). *Transforming school counseling.* Unpublished manuscript. Washington, DC: The Education Trust.

Martin, P. J. (2002). Transforming school counseling: A national perspective. *Theory Into Practice, 41,* 148–154.

Martin, P. J. (2004). *The school counselor's role in closing the achievement gap.* Presentation delivered at the Teaching and Learning Academy. March 16, 2004. Memphis, TN.

Martin, P. J., & Robinson, S. G. (2011). Transforming the school counseling profession. In B. T. Erford (Ed.), *Transforming the school counseling profession* (3rd ed., pp. 1–18). Upper Saddle River, NJ: Pearson Education, Inc.

Marzano, R. J. (2000). Implementing standards in schools. *National Association of Secondary School Principals Bulletin, 82,* 2–4.

Mason, E. C. M., & McMahon, H. G. (2009). Leadership practice of school counselors. *Professional School Counseling, 13*(2), 107–115.

Mason, M. J. (2009). Rogers redux: Relevance and outcomes of motivational interviewing across behavioral problems. *Journal of Counseling and Development, 87,* 357–362.

Mathewson, R. H. (1962). *Guidance policy and practice.* New York: Harper & Bros.

Matsunaga, M. (2009). Parents don't (always) know their children have been bullied: Child parent discrepancy on bullying and family-level profile of communication. *Human Communication Research, 35,* 221–247.

May, R. (1950). *Love and will.* New York: W.W. Norton.

May, R., & Yalom, I. (1995). Existential psychotherapy. In R. Corsini & D. Wedding (Eds.), *Current psychotherapies* (5th ed., pp. 262–292). Itasca, IL: Peacock.

McAuliffe, G., Grothaus, T., Pare, D., & Wininger, A. (2008). The practice of culturally alert counseling. In G. McAuliffe, *Culturally alert counseling: A comprehensive introduction* (pp. 570–631). Thousand Oaks, CA: Sage.

McDevitt, T. M., & Ormond, J. E. (2007). *Child development and education* (3rd ed.) Upper Saddle River, NJ: Merrill Prentice Hall.

McDivitt, P. J. (2010). The standards-based educational reform movement. In B. T. Erford (Ed.), *Professional school counseling: A handbook of theories, programs, and practices* (2nd ed., pp. 158–165). Austin, TX: PRO-ED, Inc.

McEachern, A. (2003). School counselor preparation to meet the guidance needs of exceptional students: A national study. *Counselor Education and Supervision, 42*(4), 314.

McFarland, W. P., & Dupuis, M. (2001). The legal duty to protect gay and lesbian students from violence in schools. *Professional School Counseling, 4,* 171–179.

McLoyd, V. C. (1998). Socio-economic disadvantage and child development. *American Psychologist, 53*(2), 185–204.

McNeely, C. A., & Blum, R. W. (2002). Promoting student connectedness to school: Evidence from the national longitudinal study of adolescent health. *Journal of School Health, 72,* 4.

McWhirter, E. H. (1997). Empowerment, social activism, and counseling. *Counseling and Human Development, 29,* 1–14.

Menzies, H., & Falvey, M. A. (2008). Inclusion of students with disabilities in general education. In T. Jimenez & V. Graf (Eds.), *Education for all* (pp. 71–99). San Francisco, CA: Jossey-Bass.

Meyer, M. J., & Furlong, M. J. (2010). How safe are our schools? *Educational Researcher, 39,* 14–24.

Militello, M., & Janson, C. (2007). Socially focused, situationally driven practice: A study of distributed leadership among school principals and counselors. *Journal of School Leadership, 17*(4), 409–442.

Miller, D. G. (2006). How collaboration and research can affect school counseling practices: The Minnesota store. *Professional School Counseling, 9*(3), 238–244.

Miller, W. R., & Rollnick, S. (2002). *Motivational interviewing: Preparing people for change* (2nd ed) New York: Guilford Press.

Milsom, A., & Bryant, J. (2006). School counseling departmental web sites: What message do we send? *Professional School Counseling, 10,* 210–217.

Milsom, A., Goodnough, G., & Akos, P. (2007). School counselor contributions to the individualized education program (IEP) process. *Preventing School Failure, 52*(1), 19–24.

Minke, K. M., & Anderson, K. J. (2005). Family-school collaboration and positive behavior support. *Journal of Positive Behavior Interventions, 7,* 181–185.

Mitchell, L. K., & Krumboltz, J. D. (1996). Krumboltz's learning theory of career choice and counseling. In D. Brown, L. Brooks, & Associates (Eds.), *Career choice and development* (3rd ed., pp. 233–276). San Francisco: Jossey-Bass.

Modzeleski, W., Feucht, T., Rand, M., Hall, J. T., Simon, T. A., & Butler, L. (2008). School associated student homicides 1992–2006. *Morbidity and Mortality Weekly Report, 57,* 33–36.

Moe, J. (2001, June). *Helping students build their strength.* Paper presented at the American School Counselor Association Annual Conference, Portland, OR.

Moore, D. (2003). Community Partners. *Leadership for Student Activities, 32*(3), 27.

Moore-Thomas, C. (2010). Comprehensive developmental school counseling programs. In B. T. Erford (Ed.), *Professional school counseling: A handbook of theories, programs, and practices* (pp. 201–208). Austin, TX: PRO-ED.

Mubenga, P. (2006, January 16). Closing the achievement gap between African American children and their Caucasian counterparts using collaboration learning setting. *Online Submission* (ERIC Document Reproduction Service No. ED 490762)

Muller-Ackerman, B., & Shelton, C. (2006). Practitioners' perspective on school counseling and emotional intelligence. In J. Pellitteri, R. Stern, C. Shelton, & B. Muller-Acherman (Eds.), *Emotionally intelligent school counseling* (pp. 17–28). Mahwah, NJ: Lawrence Erlbaum Associates.

Murrow-Taylor, C., Foltz, B. M., McDonald, A. B., Ellis, M. R., & Culbertson, K. (1999). A multicultural career fair for elementary school students. *Professional School Counseling, 2,* 241–243.

Myers, H. N. F. (2005). How elementary school counselors can meet the needs of students with disabilities. *Professional School Counseling, 8*(2), 442–450.

Myrick, R. D. (1997). *Developmental guidance and counseling: A practical approach* (3rd ed.). Minneapolis, MN: Educational Media Corporation.

Myrick, R. D. (2000). *Developmental guidance and counseling: A practical approach* (4th ed.). Minneapolis, MN: Educational Media Corporation.

Myrick, R. D. (2003a). Accountability: Counselors count. *Professional School Counseling, 6*(3), 174–179.

Myrick, R. D. (2003b). *Developmental guidance and counseling: A practical handbook.* (5th ed.) Minneapolis, MN: Educational Media Corporation.

NAEP. (2009). Grade 8 national results. Retrieved from http://nationsreportcard.gov/reading_2009/nat_g8.asp?tab_id=tab2&subtab_id=Tab_1

National Association of Secondary School Principals. (1996). *Breaking ranks: Changing an American institution.* Reston, VA: Author.

National Association of Secondary School Principals. (2004). *Breaking ranks II: Strategies for leading high school reform.* Reston, VA: Author.

National Association of State Directors of Special Education [NASDSE]. (2006). *Response to intervention: Policy considerations and implementation.* Alexandria, VA: Author.

National Career Development Guidelines. (1989). Retrieved from www. acrnetwork.org

National Career Development Guidelines. (2004). Retrieved from www.ncda.org.

National Center for Education Statistics. (2008). *Condition of education.* Washington, DC: Author.

National Center for Education Statistics. (2010). *Condition of education.* Washington, DC: Author.

National Center for Injury Prevention and Control. (2002). *National youth violence resource center.* Atlanta, GA: Author.

National Center of Educational Statistics. (2010). *Table A-6-1. Number and percentage distribution of 3- to 21-year olds served under the Individuals with Disabilities Education Act (IDEA). Selected school years, 1976–77 through 2007–08.* Washington, DC: Author.

National Center on Response to Intervention. (March, 2010). *Essential components of RtI—A closer look at response to intervention.* Washington, DC: U.S. Department of Education, Office of Special Education Programs, National Center on Response to Intervention: Author.

National Commission on Excellence in Education. (1983). *A nation at risk: The imperative for educational reform.* Washington, DC: Author.

National Council on Education Standards and Testing. (1991). Retrieved from www.eric.ed.gov/PDFS/ED335403.pdf

National Dissemination Center for Children with Disabilities. (2010b). Categories of disability under IDEA law. Retrieved from www.nichcy.org/Disabilities/Categories/

National Dropout Prevention Center/ Network. (2009). *School-community collaboration.* Retrieved from www. dropoutprevention.org/effstrat/school_community_collab/overview.htm

National Education Goals Panel. (1992). *Promises to keep.* Washington, DC: U.S. Department of Education.

National Occupational Information Coordinating Committee. (1989). *National career development guidelines: Local handbook.* Washington, DC: Author. (ERIC Document Reproduction Service No.: Elementary School Level— ED317879; Middle School/Junior High School Level—ED317878; High School Level—ED317877; Postsecondary Level —ED317876; Community and Business Organizations—ED317875)

National Occupational Information Coordinating Committee. (2004). *National career development guidelines.* Washington, DC: Author.

National Office for School Counselor Advocacy. (2010). *Eight components for college and career readiness* (p. 6). New York: College Board.

National Women's Law Center. (2007). *How to protect students from sexual harassment: A primer for schools.* Retrieved from www.sde.ct.gov/sde/lib/sde/pdf/equity/title_ix/studentsfromsexual harassment.pdf

N.C. v. Bedford Central School District, 04 CIV. 2627 (SCR) 32 (United States District Court for The Southern District of New York. 2004).

Nelson, J., Bustamante, R., Wilson, E., & Onwuegbuzie, A. (2008). The school-wide cultural competence observation

checklist for school counselors: An exploratory factor analysis. *Professional School Counseling, 11*(4), 207–217.

Newsome, D. W., & Harper, E. S. (2010). Counseling individuals and groups in schools. In B. T. Erford (Ed.), *Transforming the school counseling profession* (2nd ed., pp. 178–201). Columbus, OH: Merrill Prentice Hall.

New York State Center for School Safety. (2010, September 8). *Dignity for all act.* Retrieved from www.ny.gov/governor/press/090810-DignityStudentsAct.html

New York State Office of Mental Health. (2008). *Engaging in the next step: Children's mental health plan.* Albany, NY: Author.

Nichols, M. P., & Schwartz, R. C. (2006). *Family therapy concepts and methods.* (7th ed.). Boston: Pearson.

Niles, S. G., & Goodnough, G. (1996). Life long salience and values: A review of recent research. *Career Development Quarterly, 45,* 65–86.

Niles, S. G., & Harris-Bowlsbey, J. (2002). *Career development intervention in the 21st century.* Upper Saddle River, NJ: Prentice-Hall.

No Child Left Behind Act of 2001, 20 U.S.C. § 6319 (2008).

Nugent, F. A. (1994). *An introduction to professional counseling.* New York: Merrill.

O'Connor, C. (1997). Dispositions towards struggle and educational resilience in the inner city: A case analysis of six African-American high school students. *American Educational Research Journal, 34,* 593–629.

Office for Civil Rights. (2001). *Revised sexual harassment policy guidance: Harassment of students by school employees, other students or third parties.* Retrieved from www.ed.gov/offices/OCR/shguide/index.html

Office of Safe and Drug Free Schools. (2009). Preventing school violence: Plans make it possible. *The Challenge, 15,* 1.

Office of Safe and Drug Free Schools. (2010). The school bully in cyberspace. *The Challenge, 16,* 1.

O'Hanlon, B. (1999). *Do one thing different.* New York: HarperCollins.

Olweus, D. (1993). Victimization by peers: Antecedents and long-term outcomes. In K. H. Rubin & J. B. Asendorf (Eds.), *Social withdrawal, inhibition, and shyness* (pp. 315–334). Hillsdale, NJ: Erlbaum.

Orfield, G., & Paul, F. G. (1994). *High hopes: A major report on hoosier teens and the American dream* (ED378463). Retrieved from www.eric.ed.gov/PDFS/ED378463.pdf

Ormsbee, C. (2001). Effective pre-assessment team procedures: Making the process work for teachers and students. *Intervention in School and Clinic, 36*(3), 146.

Orton, G. L. (1997). *Strategies for counseling children and families.* Pacific Grove, CA: Brooks/Cole.

Osborn, D. S., & Baggerly, J. M. (2004). School counselor's perceptions of career counseling and career testing: Preferences, priorities, and predictors. *Journal of Career Development 31*, 45–59. doi: 10.1177/089484530403100104

Osborne, J. L., Collison, B. B., House, R. M., Gray, L. A., Firth, J., & Lou, M. (1998). Developing a social advocacy model for counselor education. *Counselor Education and Supervision, 37*(3), 190–202.

Osborne, A., & Russo, C. (2006). *Special education and the law: A guide for practitioners*. Thousand Oaks, CA: Corwin Press.

Osgood, R. L. (2008). *The history of special education: A struggle for equality in American public schools*. Westport, CT: Praeger.

Oswald, D. P., Coutinho, M. J., Best, A. M., & Singh, N. N. (1999). Ethnic representation in special education: The influence of schoolrelated economic and demographic variables. *The Journal of Special Education, 32*(1), 194–206.

Owings, W., & Kaplan, L. (2000). Learning of standards. *Virginia ASCD, 3*, 1–6.

Page v. Rotterdam-Mohonasen Central School District, et. al., 109 Misc. 2d 1049, 441 N.Y.S.2d 323 (1981).

Parker, J. (2001). Language: A pernicious and powerful tool. *The English Journal, 91*, 74–78.

Parsons, F. (1909). *Choosing a vocation* (rep. 1989). Garret Park, MD: Garrett Park Press.

Parsons, R. D., & Kahn, W. J. (2005). *The school counselor as consultant: An integrated model for school-based consultation*. Belmont, CA: Thomson Brooks/Cole.

Parrott, J. (2002). Are advisors risking lawsuits for misadvising students? *The mentor: An academic advising journal*. Retrieved from www.psu.edu/dus/mentor

Partnership for Twenty-First Century Skills. (2006). *Results that matter: Twenty-first century skills and high school reform*. Tuscon, AZ: Author.

Patterson, J. (2009). Beyond an elementary approach. Retrieved from www.counseling.org/Publications/CounselingTodayArticles.aspx?AGuid=2634a8dd-7e07-4a74-a47b-b79d8075cd25

Paulson, A. (2010, March 23). No Child Left Behind embraces college and career readiness. *The Christian Science Monitor*. Retrieved from www.csmonitor.com/layout/set/print/content/view/print/288883

Payne, K. J., & Biddle, B. J. (1999). Poor school funding, child poverty, and mathematic achievement. *Educational Researcher, 28*(6), 4–12.

Payne, R. (2008, April). Whose problem is poverty? *Educational Leadership, 65*, 48–52.

Pedersen, P. B. (1991). Multiculturalism as a generic approach to counseling. *Journal of Counseling & Development, 70*, 6–12.

Peebles-Wilkins, W. (2003). Collaborative interventions. *Children and Schools, 25*(4), 195.

Perls, F. (1969). *Gestalt therapy verbatim*. Lafayette, CA: Real Person.

Perry, N. (1991). The school counselor's role in education reform. *NASSP Bulletin, 79*, 24–29.

Perry, N., & Schwallie-Giddis, P. (1993). The counselor and reform in tomorrow's schools. *The Journal of Counseling and Human Development, 25*, 1–8.

Phelps, P. H. (2008). Helping teachers become leaders. *The Clearing House, 81*(3), 119–122.

Piaget, J. (1952). *The origins of intelligence in children*. New York: International Universities Press.

Pierangelo, R., & Guiliani, G. (2007). *100 frequently asked questions about the special education process*. Thousand Oaks, CA: Corwin Press.

Plamp v. Mitchell School District no. 17-2, No. 08-2700 450 (United States Court of Appeals for the Eighth Circuit, 2009).

Plank, S. (2001). *Career and technology education in the balance: An analysis of high school persistence, academic achievement, and postsecondary destinations*. Columbus, OH: The Ohio State and Technical Education, and St. Paul, MN: University of Minnesota, National Research Center for Career and Technical Education.

Pollack, W. (1998). *Real boys: Rescuing our sons from the myths of boyhood*. New York: Henry Holt.

Ponec, D. L., & Brock, B. L. (2000). Relationships among elementary school counselors and principals: A unique bond. *Professional School Counseling, 3*, 208–217.

Ponterotto, J. Utsey, S., & Pedersen, P. (2006). *Preventing prejudice* (2nd ed.). Thousand Oaks, CA: Sage Publications.

Pope, M. (2004). Sexual minority youth in the schools: Issues and desirable counselor responses. In G.Walz & R.Yep (Eds), *Vistas: Perspectives on counseling 2004*. Alexandria, VA: American Counseling Association.

Portner, J. (2002). Suicide: Many schools fall short on prevention. *Education Week*. Retrieved from www.edweek.org/ew/eprintstory.cfm?slug=32solution.h19

Postsecondary Education Opportunity. (2010). *Education and training pay*. Oskaloosa, IO: Author; Retrieved from www.postsecondary.org/default.asp

Potts, P. (2003). *Inclusion in the city: Selection, schooling and community*. London: RoutledgeFalmer.

Quigney, T. A., & Studer, J. R. (1998). Touching strands of the educational web: The professional school counselor's role in inclusion. *Professional School Counseling, 2*(1), 77–81.

Quiroz, H. C., Arnette, J. L., & Stephens, R. D. (2006). *Bullying in schools: Fighting the bully battle*. Retrieved from www.schoolsafety.us

Rai, A., & Amatea, E. (2009). Engaging in collaborative problem solving with families. In E.Amatea (Ed.), *Building culturally responsive family-school partnerships: From theory to practice*. Boston, MA: Merrill.

Ramirez, Z., & Smith, K. A. (2007). Case vignette's of school psychologists consultations invoving Hispanic youth. *Journal of Education and Psychological Consultation, 17*, 79–93.

Ratts, M. J. (2008). A pragmatic view of social justice advocacy: Infusing micro-level social justice advocacy strategies into counseling practices. *Counseling and Human Development, 41*(1), 1–8.

Ratts, M. J., DeKruyf, L., & Chen-Hayes, S. F. (2007). The ACA advocacy competencies: A social justice advocacy framework for professional school counselors. *Professional School Counseling, 11*(2), 90–97.

Raven, B. (1965). Social influence and power. In I. D. Steiner & M. Fishbein (Eds.), *Current studies in social psychology* (pp. 371–382). New York: Holt Rinehart & Winston.

Reid, K. (2001, May 2). Iowa's high court holds counselors liable. *Education Week*. Retrieved from www.edweek.org/ew/ewstory.cfm?slug=33guide.h20

Remley, T. P., & Herlihy, B. (2009). Ethical, legal, and professional issues in counseling. Upper Saddle River, NJ: Prentice Hall.

Ripley, V., Erford, B. T., Dahir, C., & Eschbach, L. (2003). Planning and implementing a 21st century comprehensive developmental school counseling program. In B. T.Erford (Ed.), *Transforming the school counseling profession*, (pp. 63–120). Columbus, OH: Merrill Prentice Hall.

Roberts, M. E. P. (1997, October 31). Who's looking out for Tiffany? *Washington City Paper*, p. 23.

Roberts, S. (2010, April 29). Listening to (and saving) the world's languages. *New York Times*, New York edition, p. A1.

Roberts, S. M., & Pruitt, E. Z. (2009). *Schools as professional learning communities: Collaborative activities and strategies for professional development* (2nd ed.). Thousand Oaks, CA: Corwin Press.

Rogers, C. (1961). *On becoming a person*. Boston: Houghton Mifflin.

Rogers, C. (1980). *A way of being*. Boston: Houghton Mifflin.

Rollins, J. (2008). *Emerging client issues*. Retrieved from www.counseling.org/Publications/CounselingTodayArticles.aspx?AGuid=f7127725-484b-4d16-b2cd-d6e3080bc473

Rollins, J. (2010). *Making definitive progress*. Retrieved from www.counseling.

org/Publications/CounselingToday Articles.aspx?AGuid=dd8a7048-4433-45e8-85ce-7b42d0b777a4

Rollnick, S., & Miller, W. R. (1995). *What is motivational interviewing?* Retrieved from http://motivationalinterview.org/clinical/whatismi.html

Rollnick, S., Miller, W. R., & Butler, C. (2008). *Motivational interviewing in health care: Helping patients change behavior.* New York: Guilford Press.

Rosenbaum, J. E. (1976). *Making inequality: The hidden current of high school tracking.* New York: Wiley.

Rosengran, D. (2009). *Building motivational interviewing skills: A practitioner workbook.* New York: Guilford Press.

Rothstein, R. (2004). *Class and schools: Using social, economic, and educational reform to close the black-white achievement gap.* New York: Economic Policy Institute and Teachers College.

Rothstein, R. (2008, April). Whose problem is poverty? *Educational Leadership, 65,* 8–13.

Rothstein, R., Jacobsen, R., & Wilder, T. (2008). *Grading education: Getting accountability right.* Washington, DC: Teachers College Press.

Rubie-Davies, C. M. (2010). Teacher expectations and perceptions of student attributes: Is there a relationship? *The British Journal of Educational Psychology, 80,* 121–135.

Rubin, H. (2009). *Collaborative leadership: Developing effective partnerships in communities and schools* (2nd ed.). Thousand Oaks, CA: Corwin Press.

Ruble, D., & Martin, C. (1998). Gender development. In W. Damon (Editor-in-Chief) & N. Eisenberg (*Vol. Ed.*), *Handbook of child psychology: Social, emotional, and personality development* (Vol. 3, 5th ed., pp. 993–1016). New York: Wiley.

Rueda, R., Klingner, J., Sager, N., & Velasco, A. (2008). Reducing disproportionate representation in special education. In T. Jiménez & V. Graf (Eds.), *Education for all* (pp. 131–166). San Francisco, CA: Jossey-Bass.

Ryan, T., & Zeran, F. (1972). *Organization and administration of guidance services.* Danville, IL: Interstate.

Sabella, R. A. (2003). *SchoolCounselor.com: A friendly and practical guide to the World Wide Web* (2nd ed.). Minneapolis, MN: Educational Media Corporation.

Sabella, R. A., Poynton, T. A, & Isaacs, M. L. (2010). School counselors perceived importance of counseling technology competencies. *Computers in Human Behavior, 26*(4), 609–617. Retrieved from www.elsevier.com/locate/comphumbeh

Sadker, D., & Zittleman, K. (2006). *Teachers schools and society: A brief introduction to education.* New York: McGraw Hill.

Sadker, M., & Sadker, D. (2005). *Teachers, schools, and society* (7th ed.). New York: McGraw Hill.

Sain v. Cedar Rapids Community School District, 626 N.W.2d 115 (Iowa 2001).

Samuels, C. (2010). Guidance says bullying may violate civil rights. Retrieved from www.Edweek.org

Sanders, M. G. (2000). Schools, families, and communities: Partnerships for school success. Reston, VA: National Association of Secondary School Principals. Retrieved from www.principals.org/pdf/schls_fmles_Cmntes.pdf

Sanders, M. G. (2006). *Building school-community partnerships: Collaboration for student success.* Thousand Oaks, CA: Corwin Press.

Sandhu, D. S. (2000). Alienated students: Counseling strategies to curb school violence. *Professional School Counseling, 4,* 81–85.

Sandomierski, T., Kincaid, D., Algozzine, B. (2007). Response to intervention and positive behavior support: Brothers from different mothers or sisters with different misters? *PBIS Newsletter, 4*(2), 1

Sanford, S. (2001, January). General Colin Powell: Keeping America's promise. Retrieved from www.centerdigitaled.com/converge/?pg=magstory&id=3284

Sapon-Shevin, M. (2001). Schools fit for all. *Educational Leadership, 58,* 34–39.

Scales, P., & Taccogna, J. (2000). Caring to try: How building students' developmental assets can promote school engagement and success. *NASSP Bulletin, 84,* 69–78.

Scarborough, J. L. (2005). The school counselor activity rating scale: An instrument for gathering process data. *Professional School Counseling, 8*(3), 274–283.

Scarborough, J. L., & Luke, M. (2008). School counselors walking the walk and talking the talk: A grounded theory of effective program implementation. *Professional School Counseling, 11*(6), 404–416.

Schanfield, M. (2010). Advisory advice. *ASCA School Counselor, 47,* 18–22.

Schellenberg, R. (2008). *The new school counselor: Strategies for universal academic achievement.* Lanham, MD: Rowan & Littlefield.

Schellenberg, R., Parks-Savage, A., & Rehfuss, M. (2007). Reducing levels of elementary school violence with peer mediation. *Professional School Counseling, 10,* 475–481.

Schmidt, J. J. (2007). *Counseling in schools: Essential services and comprehensive programs* (5th ed.). Needham Heights, MA: Allyn & Bacon.

Schwallie-Giddis, P., & Kobylarz, L. (2000). Career development: The counselor's role in preparing K–12 students for the 21st century. In J. Wittmer (Ed.), *Managing your school counseling program: K–12 developmental strategies* (2nd ed., pp. 211–218). Minneapolis, MN: Educational Media Corporation.

Schwallie-Giddis, P., ter Maat, M., & Park, M. (2003). Initiating leadership by introducing and implementing the ASCA national model. *Professional School Counseling, 6*(3), 170–173.

Sciarra, D. T. (2004). *School counseling: Foundations and contemporary issues.* Belmont, CA: Brooks/Cole.

Search Institute. (1997, 2007). *The forty developmental assets.* Minneapolis, MN: Author. Retrieved from http://www.search-institute.org/assets/40Assets.pdf

Search Institute. (2010). *Developmental assets: An overview.* Retrieved from www.search-institute.org/assets

Seligman, L. (2001). *Systems, strategies, and skills of counseling and psychotherapy.* Columbus, OH: Merrill Prentice Hall.

Sewall, G. (1991, November). America 2000: An appraisal. *Phi Delta Kappan, 72,* 204–209.

Shafii, M., & Shafii, S. L. (1992). Clinical manifestations and developmental psychopathology of depression. In M. Shafii & S. L.Shafii (Eds.), *Clinical guide to depression in children and adolescents* (pp. 3–42). Washington DC: American Psychiatric Press.

Shafii, M., & Shafii, S. L. (2001). *School violence: Assessment, management, prevention.* Washington, DC: American Psychiatric Press.

Shapiro, J. P., & Stefkovich, J. A. (2005). *Ethical leadership and decision making in education: Applying theoretical perspectives to complex dilemmas.* Mahwah, NJ: Lawrence Erlbaum Associates, Inc.

Sheridan, S. M., Clarke, B. L., & Burt, J. D. (2008). Conjoint behavioral consultation: What do we know and what do we need to know? In W. Erchul, & S. Sheridan (Eds.), *Handbook of research in school consultation* (pp. 177–202). New York: Taylor & Francis.

Sherwin, G., & Jennings, T. (2006). Feared, forgotten, or forbidden: Sexual orientation topics in secondary teacher preparation programs in the USA. *Teaching Education (17)* 3, 207–223.

Shipman, N. J., Queen, J. A., & Peel, H. A. (2007). *Transforming school leadership with ISLLC and ELCC.* Larchmont, NY: Eye on Education.

Simcox, A. G., Nuijens, L., & Lee, C. C. (2006). School counselors and school psychologists: Collaborative partners in promoting culturally competent schools. *Professional School Counseling, 9*(4), 272–277.

Simmons, D. (2010). D. C. mulls anti-bullying law. Retrieved from www.Washington Times.com.

Simpson, M. (1999a). Student suicide: Who's liable? *National Education Association, 5*(17), 1–25.

Simpson, M. (1999). *The suicide of a child is an unthinkable tragedy. But can parents hold school employees legally liable?* National Education Association.

Singh, A. A., Urbano, A., Haston, M., & McMahon, E. (2010). School counselors' strategies for social justice change: A grounded theory of what works in the real world. *Professional School Counseling, 13*(3), 135–145.

Singh, N., Lancioni, G., Singhjoy, S., Winton, A., Sabaawi, M., Wahler, R., & Singh, J. (2007). Adolescents with conduct disorder can be mindful of their aggressive behavior. *Journal of Emotional and Behavioral Disorders, 15*, 56–63.

Sink, C. (2009). School counselors as accountability leaders: Another call for action. *Professional School Counseling, 13*(2), 68–74.

Sink, C. A., & Mc Donald, G. (1998). The status of comprehensive guidance and counseling in the United States. *Professional School Counseling, 2*, 88–94.

Sistek-Chandler, C. (2001, May). The incredible expanding classroom of Marco Torres. *Converge, 4*, 44.

Skiba, R. J., & Peterson, R. L. (1999). The dark side of zero tolerance: Can punishment lead to safe schools? *Phi Delta Kappan, 80*, 372–382.

Smith, D. C., & Sandhu, D. S. (2004). Toward a positive perspective on violence prevention in schools: Building connections. *Journal of Counseling & Development, 82*, 287–293.

Smith, D. E. (2000). Schooling for inequity. *Journal of Women in Culture and Society, 25*, 1147–1151.

Smith, S. C., & Piele, P. K. (2006). *School leadership: Handbook for excellence in student learning* (4th ed.). Thousand Oaks, CA: Corwin Press.

Smith, S. D., Reynolds, C. A., & Rovnak, A. (2009). A critical analysis of the social advocacy movement in counseling. *Journal of Counseling & Development, 87*(4), 483–491.

Snell, L. (2005). *School violence and No Child Left Behind: Best practices to keep kids safe.* Los Angeles: Reason Foundation.

Sornson, R., Frost, F. & Burns, M. (2005). Instructional support teams. *Communique, 33* (5), 28–29.

Southern Poverty Law Center. (2010). *Teaching tolerance.* Retrieved from www.tolerance.org

Spies, R. A., Carlson, J., & Geisinger, K. K. (Eds.). (2010). *The Eighteenth Mental Measurements Buros Center for Testing.* Lincoln, NE: Buros Institute for Mental Measurement.

Spradlin, L. K., & Parsons, R. D. (2008). *Diversity matters: Understanding diversity in schools.* Belmont, CA: Wadsworth.

Staley, W. L., & Carey, A. L. (1997, May). The role of school counselors in facilitating a quality twenty-first century workforce. *The School Counselor, 44*, 377–381.

Stanciak, L. (1995). Reforming the high school counselor's role: A look at developmental guidance. *NASSP Bulletin, 79*, 60–68.

Stein, R., Richin, R., Banyon, R., Banyon, F., & Stein, M. (2001). *Connecting character to conduct: Helping students do the right things.* Alexandria, VA: Association of Supervision and Curriculum Development.

Sternberg, R. J. (1985). *Beyond IQ: A triarchic theory of human intelligence.* New York: Cambridge University Press.

Stone, C. (1996). Unpublished successful grant application for the Transforming School Counseling DeWitt-Wallace Grant.

Stone, C. (1998). Leveling the playing field: An urban school system examines access to mathematics curriculum. *Urban Review, 30*, 295–307.

Stone, C. (2001). *Legal and ethical issues in working with minors in schools* [Film]. Alexandria, VA: American Counseling Association.

Stone, C. (2002). Negligence in academic advising and abortion counseling: Courts rulings and implications. *Professional School Counselor: Special Issue on Legal and Ethical Issues, School Counselor, 6*(1).

Stone, C. (2003). Ethical and legal considerations for students, parents, and school counselors. In B.Erford (Ed.), *The school counselor handbook.* Michigan: ERIC/CASS.

Stone, C. (2003, April). The new school counselor: Agent of change. *The College Board Review, 199*, 45–48.

Stone, C. (2003, September). School counselors: Educators first with mental health expertise. *Counseling Today, 46*(3), 14–15.

Stone, C. (2010a). *School counseling principles: Ethics and law* (2nd ed.). Alexandria, VA: American School Counselor Association.

Stone, C. (2010b). [Writing letters for problem students]. Unpublished raw data. (Document ID: 969285161)

Stone, C., & Dahir, C. (2004). *School counselor accountability: A measure of student success.* Upper Saddle River, NJ: Pearson Education.

Stone, C. B., & Dahir, C. A. (2006). *The transformed school counselor.* Boston, MA: Houghton Mifflin Company.

Stone, C., & Dahir, C. (2007). *School counselor accountability: A measure of student success* (2nd ed.). Upper Saddle River, NJ: Pearson Education, Inc.

Stone, C., & Dahir, C. (2011). *School counselor accountability: A measure of student success* (3rd ed.). Upper Saddle River, NJ: Prentice Hall.

Stone, C., & Hanson, C. (2002). Selection of school counselor candidates: Future directions at two universities. *Counselor Education and Supervision, 41*(3), 175–192.

Stone, C., & Turba, R. (1999). School counselors using technology for advocacy. *Journal of Technology in Counseling, 1*(1). Retrieved from http://jtc.colstate.edu/vol1_1/advocacy.htm

Stone, C. B., & Clark, M. (2001). School counselors and principals: Partners in support of academic achievement. *National Association of Secondary School Principals Bulletin, 85*(624), 46–53.

Strom, P. S., & Strom, R. D. (2005). Cyberbullying by adolescents: A preliminary assessment. *The Educational Forum, 70*(1), 21–36.

Studer, Q. (2006). Self-test: Are you an engaged leader? *Healthcare Financial Management, 60*(1), 97–98. Retrieved from www.ncbi.nlm.nih.gov/pubmed/16433390

Sue, D. W., Arredondo, P., & Mc Davis, R. J. (1992). Multicultural counseling competencies and standards: A call to the profession. *Journal of Counseling and Development, 70*, 447–483.

Sullivan, A. L., A'Vant, E., Baker, J., Chandler, D., Graves, S., McKinney, E., & Sayles, T. (2009). Understanding the problem of disproportionality. *National Association of School Psychologists, 8*(1), 1–3.

Sullivan, D. R. (2005). *Learning to lead.* New Jersey: Pearson Education.

Super, D. E. (1980). A life-span approach to career development. *Journal of Vocational Behavior, 16*, 282–298.

Super, D. E., Savickas, M. L., & Super, C. M. (1996). The life span, life-space approach to careers. In D.Brown & L.Brooks (Eds.), *Career choice and development: Applying contemporary theories to practice* (3rd ed., pp. 121–178). San Francisco: Jossey-Bass.

Swearer, S., Espelage, D., Vaillancourt, T., & Hymel, S. (2010) What can be done about school bullying? Research to educational practice. *Educational Researcher, 39*, 38–43.

Swick, K. (2004). Empowering parents, families, schools, and communities during the early childhood years. Champaign, IL: Stipes

Swick, K.J. (2008). Empowering the parent–child relationship in homeless and other high-risk parents and families. *Early Childhood Education Journal, 36*, 149–153. DOI: 10.1007/s10643-007-0228-x.

Tang, M., & Erford, B. T. (2010). The history of school counseling. In B. T. Erford (Ed.), *Professional school counseling: A handbook of theories, programs, and practices* (2nd ed., pp. 9–22). Austin, TX: PRO-ED, Inc.

Tarver-Behring, S., & Spagna, M. E. (2005). Counseling with exceptional children. *Counseling and Human Development, 37*(9), 1–12.

Teaching Tolerance. (2003). *Responding to hate at school.* Southern Poverty Law Center. Montgomery, AL: Author.

Thompson, C., & Henderson, P. (2007). *Counseling children* (7th ed.). Pacific Grove, CA: Brooks/Cole.

Thompson, C. L., & Rudolph, L. B. (2000). *Counseling children* (5th ed.). Pacific Grove, CA: Brooks/Cole.

Trolley, B. (2008). Editor's message. *New York State School Counseling Journal, 5*(1), 9.

Truscott, S. D., Cohen, C. D., Sams, D. P., Sanborn, K. J., & Frank, A. J. (2005). The current state(s) of preferably intervention teams: A report from two national surveys. *Remedial and Special Education, 26*(3), 130–140.

Turner, S., Conkel, J., Starkey, M., Landgraf, R., Lapan, R., Stewart, J., & Huang, J. (2008). Gender differences in Holland vocational personality types: Implications for school counselors. *Professional School Counseling, 11*(5), 317–326.

Turner S., & Lapan, R. T. (2002) Career self-efficacy and perceptions of parent support in adolescent career. *Career Development Quarterly, 51*, 44–55.

Tyler, J. M., & Sabella, R. A. (2004). *Using technology to improve counseling practice: A primer for the 21st century.* Alexandria, VA: American Counseling Association.

U.S. Census Bureau. (2008). Current population survey, 2010. U.S. Census Bureau, American Community Survey. Retrieved from http://factfinder.census.gov

U.S. Census Bureau. (2009). U.S. Census Bureau, Population Projections. Retrieved from http://factfinder.census.gov

U.S. Census Bureau. (2010). U.S. Census Bureau, American Community Survey. Retrieved from http://factfinder.census.gov

U.S. Council on Competitiveness. (2007). *Competitiveness index: Where America stands.* Retrieved from www.compete.org/publications/detail/357/competitiveness-index-where-america-stands/

U.S. Department of Education. (1987). *What works: Research about teaching and learning.* Washington, DC: Author.

U.S. Department of Education. (1990). *America 2000: An education strategy.* Washington, DC: Author.

U.S. Department of Education. (1994). *Goals 2000: The Educate America Act.* Washington, DC: Author.

U.S. Department of Education. (1994b). *School to Work Opportunities Act.* Washington, DC: Author.

U.S. Department of Education. (1998a). *Gaining early awareness and readiness for undergraduate programs.* Washington, DC: Author.

U.S. Department of Education. (1998b). *Early warning, timely response: A guide to safe schools.* Washington, DC: Author.

U.S. Department of Education. (2001). *No Child Left Behind* (ERIC Document No. ED 447 608). Washington, DC: Author.

U.S. Department of Education. (2002a). *Exemplary and promising safe, disciplined, and drug free schools.* Washington, DC: Author.

U.S. Department of Education. (2002b). *No Child Left Behind: A desktop reference.* Washington, DC: Author.

U.S. Department of Education. (2002c). *Preventing bullying: A manual for schools and communities.* Washington, DC: Author.

U.S. Department of Education. (2004). *Individuals with Disabilities Education Improvement Act of 2004.* Retrieved from www2.ed.gov/about/offices/list/osers/osep/index.html?src=mr

U.S. Department of Education. (2005). *The guidance counselor's role in ensuring equal educational opportunity.* Retrieved from www.ed.gov/about/offices/list/ocr/docs/hq43ef.html

U.S. Department of Education, National Center for Education Statistics. (2007). *Digest of Education Statistics.* Washington, DC: U.S. Government Printing Office.

U.S. Department of Education, National Center for Education Statistics (2009). *Digest of Education Statistics.* Washington, DC: U.S. Government Printing Office.

U.S. Department of Education, National Center for Education Statistics (2010). *Digest of Education Statistics.* Washington, DC: U.S. Government Printing Office.

U.S. Department of Education, Office of Civil Rights. (2008). *Sexual harassment it's not academic.* Retrieved from www2.ed.gov/about/offices/list/ocr/docs/ocrshpam.pdf

U.S. Department of Education, Office of Planning, Evaluation and Policy Development. (2010). *ESEA Blueprint for Reform,* Washington, DC: Author.

U.S. Department of Education & U.S. Department of Justice. (2003). *Annual report on school safety.* Washington, DC: Author.

U.S. Department of Education, U.S. Department of Justice, & American Institute of Research. (2002). *Safeguarding our children: An action plan.* Washington, DC: Author.

U.S. Department of Education & U.S. Secret Service. (2002a). *The final report and findings of the safe school initiative: Implications for the prevention of school attacks in the United States.* Washington, DC: Author.

U.S. Department of Education & U.S. Secret Service. (2002b). *Threat assessment in schools: A guide to managing threatening situations and creating safe school climates.* Washington, DC: Author.

U.S. Department of Labor. (2004). *Occupational Outlook Quarterly.* Spring 2004. Washington, DC: Author.

U.S. Department of Labor. (2010). *Occupational Outlook Handbook, 2010.* Bureau of Labor Statistics. Washington, DC: Author.

U.S. Preventive Services Task Force. (2004). Screening for suicide risk: Recommendations and rationale. *American Family Physician, 70*, 2187–2190.

Uwah, C. J., McMahon, G. H., & Furlow, C. F. (2008). School belonging, educational aspirations, and academic self-efficacy among African American male high school students: Implications for school counselors. *Professional School Counseling, 11*(5), 296–305.

Vanderbilt Mental Health Center & Tennessee Department of Education. (2007). *Tennessee schools: Prepare.* Nashville, TN: Author.

Van Horn, S. M., & Myrick, R. D. (2001). Computer technology and the 21st century school counselor. *Professional School Counseling, 5*(2), 124–130.

Van Velsor, E. (2009). Introduction: Leadership and corporate social responsibility. *Corporate Governance, 9*(1), 3–6. DOI 1636445221)

Vaughn, S., & Fuchs, L. S. (2003). Redefining learning disabilities as inadequate response to instruction: The promise and potential problems. *Learning Disabilities Research & Practice, 18,* 137–146.

Velsor, P. V. (2009). School counselors as social-emotional learning consultants: Where do we begin? *Professional School Counseling, 13,* 50–58.

Vernon, A. (2004). *Counseling children and adolescents.* Denver, CO: Love Publishing.

Vigoda, E. (2002). From responsiveness to collaboration: Governance, citizens, and the next generation of public administration. *Public Administration Review, 62*(5), 527.

Wadsworth, D., & Remaley, M. (2007) What families want. *Educational Leadership, 64* (6) 23–27.

Walker, J. (2006). Principals and counselors working for social justice: A complementary leadership team. *Guidance and Counseling, 21*(2), 114–124.

Wall, J. E., & Walz, G. R. (2004). *Measuring up: Assessment issues for teachers, counselors, and administrators.* Austin, TX: PRO-ED.

Wallis, C., & Steptoe, S. (2006, December 10). How to bring our schools out of the 20th century. Retrieved from www.time.com.time/magazine/article/0,91711568480,000.html

Walser, N. (2007). Response to intervention: A new approach to reading instruction aims to catch struggling readers early. *Harvard Education Letter, 23,* 1.

Walsh, M. E., Barrett, J. G., & DePaul, J. (2007). Day to day activities of school counselors: Alignment with new directions in the field and the ASCA national model. *Professional School Counseling, 10*(4), 370–378.

Wang, J., Iannotti, R., & Nansel, T. R. (2009a). Bullying: We need to increase our efforts and broaden our focus. *Journal of Adolescent Health, 45,* 323–325.

Wang, J., Iannotti, R. J., & Nansel, T. R. (2009b). School bullying among adolescents in the United States: Physical, verbal, relational, and cyber. *Journal of Adolescent Health, 45,* 368–375.

Ward, J. (2002). School rules. In *The Jossey-Bass reader on gender in education* (pp. 510–542). San Francisco: Jossey-Bass.

Watson, T. S., Watson, T. S., & Weaver, A. D. (2010). Direct behavioral consultation: An effective method for promoting school collaboration. In B. T. Erford (Ed.), *Professional school counseling: A handbook of theories, programs, and practices* (2nd ed., pp. 295–302). Austin, TX: Pro-Ed.

Weaver, R. L., Martin, E. C., Klein, A. R., Zwier II, P. J., Eades, R. W., & Bauman, J. H. (2009). *Mastering Tort Law.* Durham, NC: Carolina Academic Press.

Wesley, D. C. (2001, February). The administrator-counselor team: The relationship between counselor and administrator can enhance or exhaust a school's ability to meet the needs of its students. *Principal Leadership,* 60–63.

West, J. F., & Idol, L. (1987). School consultation: An interdisciplinary perspective on theory, models, and research. *Journal of Learning Disabilities, 20*(7), 385–408.

Wheeler, A. M., & Bertram, B. (2008). *The counselor and the law: A guide to legal and ethical practice* (5th ed.). Alexandria, VA: American Counseling Association.

Whiston, S. C. (2002). Response to the past, present, and future of school counseling: Raising some issues. *Professional School Counseling, 5,* 148–155.

Whiston, S. C., & Sexton, T. L. (1998). A review of school counseling outcome research: Implications for practice. *Journal of Counseling and Development, 4,* 412–426.

Whitbread, K. M., Bruder, M. B., Fleming, G., & Park, H. J. (2007). Collaboration in special education: Parent-professional training. *Teaching Exceptional Children, 39* (4), 6–14.

White, S. W., & Kelly, F .D. (2010). The school counselor's role in school dropout prevention. *Journal of Counseling and Development, 88,* 227–235.

White House. (n.d.). Education: Reform and invest in K–12 education. Retrieved from http://www.whitehouse.gov/isues/education

Wiggins, G. (1991). Standards, not standardization: Evoking quality student work. *Educational Leadership,* 18–25.

Wilczenski, F. L., & Coomey, S. M. (2006). Cyber-communication: Finding its place in school counseling practice, education, and professional development. *Professional School Counseling, 9,* -327–331.

Wilkerson, K. (2009). An examination of burnout among school counselors guide by Stress-Strain-Coping Theory. *Journal of Counseling and Development, 87*(4), 428–437.

Willard, N. (2006). *Cyberbullying and cyberthreats: Responding to the challenge of online social cruelty, threats, and distress.* Eugene, OR: Center for Safe and Responsible Internet Use.

William T. Grant Commission on Work, Family and Citizenship. (1988). *The forgotten half: Pathways to success for America's youth and young families.* Washington, DC: Author.

Williams, J., & Noguera, P. (2010). Poor schools or poor kids?: To some, fixing education means taking on poverty and health care. *Education Next, 10*(1). Retrieved from http://educationnext.org/poor-schools-or-poor-kids/

Wiseman, R. (2002). The hidden world of bullying. *Principal Leadership, 3* (4) 18–23.

Wittmer, J. (Ed.). (2000). *Managing your school counseling program: K–12 developmental strategies* (2nd ed.). Minneapolis, MN: Educational Media.

Wittmer, J. & Clark, M. A. (Eds.). (2007). *Managing your school counseling program: Developmental strategies* (3rd ed.). Minneapolis, MN: Educational Media Corporation.

Wolchick, S. A., Ma, Y., Tein, J., Sandler, I. N., & Ayers, T. S. (2008). Parentally bereaved children's grief: Self-system beliefs as mediators of the relations between grief and stressors and caregiver-child relationship quality. *Death Studies, 32*(7), 597–620.

Wolfe, D., Crooks, C., Chiodo, D., & Jaffe, P. (2009). Child maltreatment, bullying, gender-based harassment, and adolescent dating violence: Making the connections. *Psychology of Women Quarterly, 33,* 21–24.

Wolfensberger, W. (1972). *The principle of normalization in human services.* Toronto: National Institute on Mental Retardation.

Woodcock, R. W., McGrew, K. S., & Mather, N. (2001). *Woodcock-Johnson III.* Itasca, IL: Riverside Publishing.

Woolfolk, A. (2001). *Educational psychology* (8th ed.). Boston: Allyn & Bacon.

Woolfolk, A. (2009). *Educational psychology* (11th ed.). Boston: Allyn & Bacon.

Worthington, R. L., & Juntunen, C. L. (1997). The vocational development of non–college bound youth: Counseling psychology and the school to work transition movement. *Counseling Psychologist, 25,* 323–363.

Wrenn, G. (1962). *The counselor in a changing world.* Washington, DC: American Personnel and Guidance Association.

Wubbolding, R. E. (2000). *Reality therapy for the 21st century.* Bristol, PA: Accelerated Development.

Wyke v. The Polk County School Board, 129 F.3d 560 (11th cir. 1997).

Yalom, I. (1980). *Existential psychotherapy.* New York: Basic Books.

Young, A., Hardy, V., Hamilton, C., Biernesser, K., Sun, L. L., & Niebergall, S. (2009). Empowering students: Using data to transform a bullying prevention and intervention program. *Professional School Counseling, 12,* 413–419.

Ysseldyke, J., & Algozzine, B. (2006). *Public policy, school reform, and special education: A practical guide for every teacher.* Thousand Oaks, CA: Corwin Press.

Yukl, G., & Tracey, J. B. (1992). Consequences of influence tactics used with subordinate, peers, and the boss. *Journal of Applied Psychology, 77,* 522–535.

Zehr, M. (2004, January 14). Report updates portrait of LEP students 2004. *Education Week, 23*(18), 3.

Zirkel, P. (1991, April). End of story. *Phi Delta Kappan, 72*(8), 640–642.

Zirkel, P. (2001a, March). A pregnant pause? *Phi Delta Kappan, 82*(7), 557–558.

Zirkel, P. (2001b, September). Ill advised. *Phi Delta Kappan, 83*(1), 98–99.

# NAME INDEX

# SUBJECT INDEX